DIABETES PUBLIC HEALTH

DIABETES PUBLIC HEALTH

FROM DATA TO POLICY

EDITED BY

K. M. Venkat Narayan, MD
Guest Researcher, Division of Diabetes Translation, National Center for Chronic Disease
Prevention and Health Promotion, Centers for Disease Control and Prevention *and*
Ruth and O.C. Hubert Professor, Emory University, Atlanta, GA

Desmond Williams, MD, PhD
Associate Branch Chief, Team Lead for the CDC Chronic Kidney Disease Initiative,
Epidemiology and Statistics Branch (ESB), Division of Diabetes Translation, National Center
for Chronic Disease Prevention and Health Promotion, Centers for Disease Control and
Prevention, Atlanta, GA

Edward W. Gregg, PhD
Branch Chief, Epidemiology and Statistics Branch, Division of Diabetes Translation, National
Center for Chronic Disease Prevention and Health Promotion, Centers for
Disease Control and Prevention, Atlanta, GA

Catherine C. Cowie, PhD, MPH
Director, Diabetes Epidemiology Program, National Institute of Diabetes and Digestive and
Kidney Diseases, National Institutes of Health, Bethesda, MD

TECHNICAL WRITER-EDITORS:

Peter L. Taylor, MBA
Senior Editor, Palladian Partners, Silver Spring, MD

Juanita Mondesire
Senior Editorial Coordinator, Division of Diabetes Translation, National Center for Chronic
Disease Prevention and Health Promotion, Centers for Disease Control and Prevention,
Atlanta, GA

Susana Moran
Editorial Assistant, Division of Diabetes Translation, National Center for Chronic Disease
Prevention and Health Promotion, Centers for Disease Control and Prevention, Atlanta, GA

OXFORD
UNIVERSITY PRESS
2011

OXFORD
UNIVERSITY PRESS

Oxford University Press, Inc., publishes works that further
Oxford University's objective of excellence
in research, scholarship, and education.

Oxford   New York
Auckland   Cape Town   Dar es Salaam   Hong Kong   Karachi
Kuala Lumpur   Madrid   Melbourne   Mexico City   Nairobi
New Delhi   Shanghai   Taipei   Toronto

With offices in
Argentina   Austria   Brazil   Chile   Czech Republic   France   Greece
Guatemala   Hungary   Italy   Japan   Poland   Portugal   Singapore
South Korea   Switzerland   Thailand   Turkey   Ukraine   Vietnam

Published by Oxford University Press, Inc.
198 Madison Avenue, New York, New York 10016
www.oup.com

Oxford is a registered trademark of Oxford University Press

Library of Congress Cataloging-in-Publication Data

Diabetes public health : from data to policy / edited by K.M. Venkat
Narayan ... [et al.]; technical writer-editors, Peter L. Taylor,
Juanita Mondesire; Susana Moran, editorial assistant.
p. ; cm.
Includes bibliographical references.
ISBN 978-0-19-531706-0
1. Diabetes—Prevention.   2. Diabetes—Epidemiology.   I. Narayan, K. M. Venkat.
[DNLM: 1. Diabetes Mellitus.   2. Health Policy.   3. Public Health Practice.   WK 810]
RA645.D5D546 2010
362.196'462—dc22
2010032158

9 8 7 6 5 4 3 2 1
Printed in the United States of America
on acid-free paper

FOREWORD

A world free of the devastation of diabetes is not only an admirable vision, but is a vital necessity. In the United States lifetime risk estimates of diabetes indicate that one in three children born in the year 2000 will develop diabetes sometime in their lifetime, and this statistic is closer to one in two for high-risk ethnic populations. Globally, an estimated 285 million adults have diabetes, and this is expected to rise to 439 million by 2030. Although diabetes is most common among older adults, prevalence rates are increasing substantially among younger populations. Diabetes remains the leading cause of adult blindness, kidney failure, and nontraumatic lower-limb amputation, a significant contributor to heart disease and stroke, is responsible for pregnancy complications, and is now associated with dementia and some forms of cancer. Thus, diabetes has far reaching human and economic implications as the prevalence continues to rise.

Numerous research programs have developed over the last decade to improve the understanding of causes, prevention, and treatment of diabetes and its complications. These programs have emerged from diverse sources, including national and state-based surveillance systems, community surveys, cohort studies, randomized controlled trials, and health service and managed care systems. These research programs have also benefited from the development of novel methods in areas such as health services research, systematic reviews, statistical and economical modeling, as well as progress in the areas of genomics, diagnostics, and therapeutic technologies. An efficient synthesis of the data and information from these diverse sources is crucial to effectively prioritize interventions and assemble resources for the implementation of public health programs that will reduce the burden of diabetes. *Diabetes Public Health: From Data to Policy* is a comprehensive state-of-the art book on diabetes and public health that provides this much-needed synthesis. This book shares both the successes and future challenges in diabetes. It exposes the scope, magnitude, and threat of the problem and highlights effective interventions that have been developed.

What is it going to take to achieve a world that is free of the devastation of diabetes? The effort will certainly require new discoveries in treating, preventing, and curing diabetes and its complications. But it also requires implementing and sustaining the discoveries that have already been made to a scale that reaches the vast majority of the affected population—discoveries must be translated. Importantly, research, interventions, and policies must target not only individuals with or at risk for diabetes, but also their families and the communities and societies where they live, work, and play. Please take the information provided in *Diabetes Public Health: From Data to Policy* and use it to support your contributions to achieving a world free of the devastation of diabetes.

—Ann Albright, PhD, RD
Director, Division of Diabetes Translation
National Center for Chronic Disease Prevention and Health Promotion
Centers for Disease Control and Prevention
Atlanta, GA

CONTENTS

CONTRIBUTORS

Ronald T. Ackermann, MD, MPH
Associate Professor of Medicine
Affiliated Scientist of the Regenstrief
    Institute for Healthcare
Indiana University School of Medicine
Indianapolis, IN

Amanda I. Adler, MD, PhD, FRCP
Consultant Physician
Addenbrooke's Hospital
Institute of Metabolic Sciences
Cambridge, UK

Roger T. Anderson, PhD
Professor and Chief, Division of Health
    Services Research
Department of Public Health Sciences
Penn State University College of
    Medicine
Hershey, PA

Pablo Arias, MD, PhD
Assistant Professor
Department of Physiology and
    Biophysics
University of Buenos Aires Medical School
Buenos Aires, Argentina

David C. Aron, MD, MS
Associate Chief of Staff/Education
Louis Stokes Cleveland Department of
    Veterans Affairs Medical Center
and
Co-Director, VA, HSRD Center for
    Implementation Practice and
    Research Support
Professor of Medicine and
    Epidemiology and Biostatistics
School of Medicine
and
Professor of Organizational Behavior
Weatherhead School of Management
Case Western Reserve University
Cleveland, OH

Rajesh Balkrishnan, PhD
Director, Center for Medication Use,
    Policy, and Economics
Associate Professor, Department of
    Clinical, Social and Administrative
    Sciences
Associate Professor, Department of
    Health Management and Policy
The University of Michigan
Ann Arbor, MI

Evan M. Benjamin, MD
Associate Professor of Medicine
Tufts University School of Medicine
Senior Vice President, Healthcare
    Quality
Baystate Medical Center
Springfield, MA

Peter H. Bennett, MB, ChB, FRCP
Scientist Emeritus
National Institute of Diabetes and
    Digestive and Kidney Diseases
National Institutes of Health
Phoenix, AZ

Alain G. Bertoni, MD, MPH
Associate Professor
Department of Epidemiology and
    Prevention, Division of Public Health
    Sciences
Department of Internal Medicine
Wake Forest University Baptist Medical
    Center
Winston-Salem, NC

**Andrew J. M. Boulton, MD, DSc
    (Hon), FRCP**
Professor of Medicine, University of
    Manchester
Consultant Physician, Manchester
    Royal Infirmary
Vice-President and Director of
    Postgraduate Education for the
    European Association for the Study
    of Diabetes
Manchester, UK
and
Division of Endocrinology, Metabolism,
    and Diabetes
University of Miami School of Medicine
Miami, FL

Frank L. Bowling, BSc, DPodM, PhD
Honorary Research Fellow
University of Manchester
Manchester Royal Infirmary
Manchester, UK

Arleen F. Brown, MD, PhD
Associate Professor
UCLA Division of General Internal
    Medicine and Health Services
    Research
Los Angeles, CA

Wändi Bruine de Bruin, PhD
Assistant Professor
Carnegie Mellon University
Department of Social and Decision
    Sciences
Department of Engineering and Public
    Policy
Pittsburgh, PA

Nilka R. Burrows, MT, MPH
Epidemiologist
Division of Diabetes Translation
National Center for Chronic Disease
    Prevention and Health Promotion
Centers for Disease Control and
    Prevention
Atlanta, GA

Fabian Camacho, MS
Senior Instructor
Department of Public Health Sciences
Penn State University College of
    Medicine
Hershey, PA

Hae Mi Choe, PharmD, CDE
Assistant Professor of Pharmacology
Department of Clinical Sciences,
    College of Pharmacy
University of Michigan
Ann Arbor, MI

Charles M. Clark Jr., MD
Associate Dean, Continuing Medical
    Education Professor of Medicine
Indiana University School of Medicine
Director, WHO/PAHO Diabetes
    Collaborating Center for Continuing
    Health
Professional Education Division of
    Continuing Medical Education
Indianapolis, IN

Jeanne M. Clark, MD, MPH
Associate Professor of Medicine and
    Epidemiology
The Johns Hopkins University School of
    Medicine and Bloomberg School of
    Public Health
Baltimore, MD

**Adolfo Correa-Villaseñor, MD, MPH,
    PhD**
Medical Officer
Division of Birth Defects and
    Developmental Disabilities
Centers for Disease Control and
    Prevention
Atlanta, GA

Catherine C. Cowie, PhD, MPH
Director, Diabetes Epidemiology
    Program
National Institute of Diabetes and
    Digestive and Kidney Diseases
National Institutes of Health
Bethesda, MD

Jeffrey M. Curtis, MD, MPH
Staff Clinician
Diabetes Epidemiology and Clinical
    Research Section
National Institute of Diabetes and
    Digestive and Kidney Diseases
National Institutes of Health
Phoenix, AZ

Dana Dabelea, MD, PhD
Associate Professor
Department of Epidemiology
Colorado School of Public Health
University of Colorado Denver
Aurora, CO

Julie S. Downs, PhD
Assistant Research Professor
Carnegie Mellon University
Department of Social and Decision
    Sciences
Pittsburgh, PA

Mark S. Eberhardt, PhD
Science Officer
Centers for Disease Control and
    Prevention
National Center for Health Statistics
Division of Health and Nutrition
    Examination Survey
Hyattsville, MD

Leonard E. Egede, MD, MS
Professor of Medicine
Director, Center for Health Disparities
    Research
Medical University of South Carolina
Charleston, SC

Kristina L. Ernst, BSN, RN, CDE
Program Consultant
Division of Diabetes Translation,
    Program Development Branch
National Center for Chronic Disease
    Prevention and Health Promotion
Centers for Disease Control and
    Prevention
Atlanta, GA

Baruch Fischhoff, PhD
Howard Heinz University Professor
Carnegie Mellon University
Department of Social and Decision
  Sciences
Department of Engineering and Public
  Policy
Pittsburgh, PA

Terrence Forrester MB, BS, DM, PhD
Director, Tropical Medicine Research
  Institute
The University of The West Indies
Mona, Jamaica

Joanne M. Gallivan, MS, RD
Director, National Diabetes Education
  Program
National Institutes of Health
Office of Communications and Public
  Liaison, National Institute of
  Diabetes and Digestive and Kidney
  Diseases
National Institutes of Health
Bethesda, MD

Linda S. Geiss, MA
Diabetes Surveillance Team Lead
Division of Diabetes Translation
National Center for Chronic Disease
  Prevention and Health Promotion
Centers for Disease Control and
  Prevention
Atlanta, GA

Christopher H. Gibbons, MD, MMSc
Assistant Professor of Neurology,
  Harvard Medical School
Beth Israel Deaconess Medical Center
Boston, MA

David C. Goff Jr., MD, PhD
Professor and Chair, Department
  of Epidemiology and Prevention,
  Division of Public Health Sciences
Professor, Department of Internal
  Medicine
Wake Forest University School of
  Medicine
Winston-Salem, NC

Edward W. Gregg, PhD
Branch Chief, Epidemiology and
  Statistics Branch
Division of Diabetes Translation
National Center for Chronic Disease
  Prevention and Health Promotion
Centers for Disease Control and
  Prevention
Atlanta, GA

Robert L. Hanson, MD, MPH
Staff Scientist
Diabetes Epidemiology and Clinical
  Research Section
National Institute of Diabetes and
  Digestive and Kidney Diseases
National Institutes of Health
Phoenix, AZ

Mary Hoskin, MS, RD
Program Coordinator, Diabetes
  Prevention Program Outcomes Study
Diabetes Epidemiology and Clinical
  Research Section
National Institute of Diabetes and
  Digestive and Kidney Diseases
National Institutes of Health
Phoenix, AZ

Giuseppina Imperatore, MD, PhD
Medical Epidemiologist
Team Lead, Epidemiology Section
Division of Diabetes Translation
National Center for Chronic
    Disease Prevention and Health
    Promotion
Centers for Disease Control and
    Prevention
Atlanta, GA

Shailaja Kale, MD
Associate Professor
King Edward Memorial Hospital
Pune, India

Andrew J. Karter, PhD
Senior Investigator
Division of Research
Kaiser Permanente Northern
    California
Oakland, CA

Jane Kelly, MD
Former Director
National Diabetes Education Program
Division of Diabetes Translation
National Center for Chronic Disease
    Prevention and Health Promotion
Centers for Disease Control and
    Prevention
Atlanta, GA

Catherine Kim, MD MPH
Assistant Professor of Medicine and
    Obstetrics & Gynecology
Division of General Internal Medicine
Departments of Medicine and
    Obstetrics & Gynecology
University of Michigan
Ann Arbor, MI

Barbara E. K. Klein, MD, MPH
Professor, Department of
    Ophthalmology and Visual Sciences
University of Wisconsin School of
    Medicine and Public Health
Madison, WI

Ronald Klein, MD, MPH
Professor, Department of
    Ophthalmology and Visual Sciences
University of Wisconsin School of
    Medicine and Public Health
Madison, WI

David C. Klonoff, MD, FACP
Medical Director, Diabetes Research
    Institute
Mills-Peninsula Health Services
San Mateo, CA
and
Clinical Professor of Medicine, U.C.
    San Francisco
San Francisco, CA

William C. Knowler, MD, DrPH
Chief
Diabetes Epidemiology and Clinical
    Research Section
National Institute of Diabetes and
    Digestive and Kidney Diseases
National Institutes of Health
Phoenix, AZ

Yeong Kwok, MD
Assistant Professor of Medicine
Division of General Internal Medicine
Department of Medicine
University of Michigan
Ann Arbor, MI

Ronald E. LaPorte, PhD
Professor
Department of Epidemiology
Graduate School of Public Health
University of Pittsburgh
Pittsburgh, PA

Jean M. Lawrence, ScD, MPH, MSSA
Research Scientist and Epidemiologist
Department of Research and Evaluation
Kaiser Permanente Southern California
Research Associate Professor
Department of Preventive Medicine
Keck School of Medicine
University of Southern California
Los Angeles, CA

Rui Li, MD, PhD
Health Economist
Division of Diabetes Translation
National Center for Chronic Disease
    Prevention and Health Promotion
Centers for Disease Control and
    Prevention
Atlanta, GA

Astrid M. Libman, MD, MPH
Assistant Lecturer
Department of Semiology
University of Rosario Medical School
Rosario, Argentina

Ingrid M. Libman, MD, PhD
Assistant Professor
Division of Pediatric Endocrinology
    and Diabetes
Children's Hospital of Pittsburgh of
    UPMC
Pittsburgh, PA

Barbara Linder, MD, PhD
Senior Advisor
Childhood Diabetes Research
Division of Diabetes
Endocrinology and Metabolic Diseases
National Institute of Diabetes and
    Digestive and Kidney Diseases
Bethesda, MD

Cinzia Maraldi, MD
Consultant Physician
Section of Internal Medicine,
    Gerontology, and Geriatrics
Department of Clinical and
    Experimental Medicine
University of Ferrara
Ferrara, Italy

Jessica A. Marcinkevage, MSPH
Oak Ridge Institute for Science and
    Education Fellow
Oak Ridge Institute for Science and
    Education
Oak Ridge, TN
Division of Nutrition Sciences
Emory University
Atlanta, GA

David G. Marrero, PhD
J. O. Ritchey Professor of Medicine
Division of Endocrinology &
    Metabolism
Indiana University School of Medicine
Indianapolis, IN

Elizabeth J. Mayer-Davis, PhD
Professor, Departments of Nutrition
    and Medicine
University of North Carolina at Chapel
    Hill
Chapel Hill, NC

James B. Meigs, MD, MPH
Associate Professor of Medicine
Harvard Medical School
General Medicine Division
Massachusetts General Hospital
Boston, MA

Viswanathan Mohan, MD, FRCP
  (Lond, Edin, Glasg & Ire), PhD,
  DSc, FNASc
Director & Chief of Diabetes Research
Madras Diabetes Research Foundation
  and Dr. Mohan's Diabetes
  Specialities Centre
Chennai, India

Juanita Mondesire
Senior Editorial Coordinator
Division of Diabetes Translation
National Center for Chronic Disease
  Prevention and Health Promotion
Centers for Disease Control and
  Prevention
Atlanta, GA

Susana Moran
Editorial Assistant
Division of Diabetes Translation
National Center for Chronic Disease
  Prevention and Health Promotion
Centers for Disease Control and
  Prevention
Atlanta, GA

Indra Mustapha, DDS, MS
Assistant Professor and Faculty
Department of Periodontology
Howard University
Washington, DC

K. M. Venkat Narayan, MD
Guest Researcher
Division of Diabetes Translation
National Center for Chronic Disease
  Prevention and Health Promotion
Centers for Disease Control and
  Prevention
and
Ruth and O.C. Hubert Professor
Emory University
Atlanta, GA

Robert G. Nelson, MD, PhD
Investigator, Diabetes Epidemiology
  and Clinical Research Section
National Institute of Diabetes and
  Digestive and Kidney Diseases
National Institutes of Health
Phoenix, AZ

Meda E. Pavkov, MD, PhD
Medical Epidemiologist
Division of Diabetes Translation
National Center for Chronic
  Disease Prevention and Health
  Promotion
Centers for Disease Control and
  Prevention
Atlanta, GA

Manjiri D. Pawaskar, PhD
Research Associate
Ohio State University
Columbus, OH
and
Research Scientist
US Outcomes Research
Endocrine/Obesity/MetS
Eli Lilly and Company
Lilly Technology Center
Indianapolis, IN

Matt Petersen
Director, Information Resources and
  Professional Engagement
American Diabetes Association
Alexandria, VA

David J. Pettitt, MD
Senior Scientist
Sansum Diabetes Research Institute
Santa Barbara, CA

Leonard M. Pogach, MD, MBA
Director, Health Services Research
    Center for Healthcare Knowledge
    Management
Department of Veterans Affairs New
    Jersey Healthcare System
East Orange, NJ
and
Clinical Coordinator, VHA Diabetes
    Quality Enhancement Research
    Initiative (QUERI)
Professor, Departments of Medicine
    and Preventive Medicine
University of Medicine and Dentistry
    of New Jersey—New Jersey Medical
    School
Newark, NJ

Rajendra Pradeepa, MSc, PhD
Head, Research Grants Division
Madras Diabetes Research Foundation
    and Dr. Mohan's Diabetes
    Specialities Centre
Chennai, India

**Ambady Ramachandran, MD, PhD,
    DSc, FRCP (Lond), FRCP (Edin)**
Professor/Doctor
President—India Diabetes Research
    Foundation and Chairman—
    Dr. A. Ramachandran's Diabetes
    Hospitals
India Diabetes Research Foundation
and
Dr. A. Ramachandran's Diabetes
    Hospitals
Chennai, India

**Kaushik Ramaiya, MBBS, MMed
    (Int Med)**
Consultant Physician & Asst. Medical
    Administrator
Shree Hindu Mandal Hospital and
Hon. Lecturer
Department of Internal Medicine
Muhimbili University of Health &
    Allied Sciences
Dar es Salaam, Tanzania

Jinan B. Saaddine, MD, MPH
Medical Epidemiologist
Vision Health Initiative Team Leader
Division of Diabetes Translation
National Center for Chronic Disease
    Prevention and Health Promotion
Centers for Disease Control and
    Prevention
Atlanta, GA

Sharon H. Saydah, PhD
Senior Scientist
Division of Diabetes Translation
National Center for Chronic Disease
    Prevention and Health Promotion
Centers for Disease Control and
    Prevention
Atlanta, GA

Dean Schillinger, MD
UCSF Professor of Medicine in
    Residence
Director, UCSF Center for Vulnerable
    Populations
San Francisco General Hospital
San Francisco, CA

Chamukuttan Snehalatha, MSc, DPhil, DSc
Doctor
Director—Research
India Diabetes Research Foundation/
  Head—Biochemistry
Dr. A. Ramachandran's Diabetes
  Hospitals
Chennai, India

Jeremy B. Soule, MD
Associate Professor
Ralph H. Johnson VA Medical Center
and
Division of Endocrinology, Metabolism,
  and Medical Genetics
Medical University of South Carolina
Charleston, SC

Nikhil Tandon, MD, PhD (Cantab)
Professor
Department of Endocrinology and
  Metabolism
All India Institute of Medical Sciences
New Delhi, India

Peter L. Taylor, MBA
Senior Editor
Palladian Partners
Silver Spring, MD

Karen Teff, PhD
Member
Monell Chemical Senses Center
Director
Translational Research
Institute for Diabetes, Obesity and
  Metabolism
University of Pennsylvania
Philadelphia, PA

Patricia Thompson-Reid, MAT, MPH
Community-Based Systems Specialist
Division of Diabetes Translation
National Center for Chronic Disease
  Prevention and Health Promotion
Centers for Disease Prevention and
  Control
Atlanta, GA

Marshall Tulloch-Reid, MBBS, MPhil, DSc, FACE
Lecturer in Epidemiology
Epidemiology Research Unit, TMRI
The University of the West Indies
Consultant Endocrinologist
Oxford Medical Centre & The Heart
  Institute of the Caribbean
Mona, Jamaica

Frank Vinicor, MD, MPH
Associate Director for Public Health
  Practice
National Center for Chronic Disease
  Prevention and Health Promotion
Centers for Disease Control and
  Prevention
Atlanta, GA

Stefano Volpato, MD, MPH
Assistant Professor
Section of Internal Medicine,
  Gerontology, and Geriatrics
Department of Clinical and
  Experimental Medicine
University of Ferrara
Ferrara, Italy

Elizabeth A. Walker, PhD, RN, CDE
Professor, Department of Medicine and
  Epidemiology and Population Health
Director, Prevention and Control Care
Einstein Diabetes Research and
  Training Center
Albert Einstein College of Medicine
Bronx, NY

Desmond Williams, MD, PhD
Associate Branch Chief
Team Lead for the CDC Chronic
    Kidney Disease Initiative
Epidemiology and Statistics Branch
    (ESB)
Division of Diabetes Translation
National Center for Chronic Disease
    Prevention and Health Promotion
Centers for Disease Control and
    Prevention
Atlanta, GA

Jennifer Wyckoff, MD
Assistant Professor of Medicine
Division of Metabolism, Endocrinology,
    and Diabetes, Department of
    Medicine
University of Michigan
Ann Arbor, MI

Chittaranjan S. Yajnik, MD, FRCP
Director, Diabetes Unit
King Edward Memorial Hospital
Pune, India
and
Visiting Professor
Peninsula Medical School
Plymouth, UK

Ping Zhang, PhD
Senior Health Economist
Division of Diabetes Translation
National Center for Chronic Disease
    Prevention and Health Promotion
Centers for Disease Control and
    Prevention
Atlanta, GA

INTRODUCTION

Edward W. Gregg, K. M. Venkat Narayan, Desmond Williams,
and Catherine C. Cowie

Diabetes is a prototypical chronic public health problem. The disease sequalae and economic burden of diabetes are extensive owing to its degenerative nature despite the best available treatments. Effective delivery of preventive strategies to delay progression of the disease and its complications are challenging at best, with the persistent need for interventions integrating individual, clinical, system, and society-level approaches that span the full course of life. Prevalence has now surpassed 10% in U.S. adults, and at least 25 countries around the world have reported even higher estimates (Cowie et al. 2009; Diabetes Atlas). The absolute numbers of individuals affected by diabetes are daunting, with current reports of 24 million in the United States and 285 million adults worldwide and projections of 48 million Americans by 2050 and 439 million worldwide by 2030. This causes or contributes to at least 230,000 deaths per year in the United States and has a devastating impact on multiple body systems including the heart and vasculature, nerves, kidneys, eyes, limbs, and the brain. Diabetes more than doubles the costs of care for the average individual in western countries; in developing countries it threatens to undermine the family and national economic progress, as it substantially impacts the working-age population.

Fortunately, clinical trials have armed clinicians with numerous effective approaches, leading to some improvement in rates of diabetes complications (Gregg et al. 2009). However diabetes' extensive demands on the individual and on the healthcare system, its multiple etiologies and complications, and its intricate basis in culture and society make it beyond what clinical approaches alone can control. The breadth of the diabetes problem has fostered the attention and interest of multiple disciplines of population health research, ranging from epidemiologic surveillance and monitoring to effectiveness trials, and translation research to health economic studies. Thus the evidence base for diabetes clinical and public health now includes the broad spectrum of community and population surveys, cohort studies, randomized controlled trials, health services research, systematic reviews, and statistical and economic modeling. Considerable progress has also been made in the areas of genomics, diagnostic and therapeutic technologies, and bioinformatics. Accordingly, interventions now span direct population-based clinical and health service-based approaches as well as health promotion and policy approaches. Although the progress is encouraging, the scope, speed, and diversity of new information and changes in knowledge present ongoing challenges for clinicians, researchers, public health professionals, and policy makers.

Efficient synthesis of these data and knowledge is crucial to prioritize interventions effectively and to make the information accessible and friendly to the end-user. We have designed this book and organized the sections to follow the natural continuum: (1) surveillance, as the basic science of public health in order to prioritize the subconditions and populations in need of interventions; (2) effectiveness and cost-effectiveness research in order to prioritize interventions; and (3) the processes and resources that can guide public health decision making. Section 1 highlights the continued growth of the epidemic of diabetes (type 1, type 2, and gestational diabetes) and emphasizes the need to view the epidemic from an ecologic and life-course perspective. This section summarizes both the contemporary and emerging risk factors and current understanding of the mechanistic links between risk factors and the disease. Section 2 summarizes the current epidemiology and etiology of traditional acute glycemic complications as well as the microvascular, macrovascular, and neurologic damage wrought by the disease. This section highlights the persistent burden of both coronary and noncoronary cardiovascular disease and the alarming growth of diabetes kidney disease. Stubborn disparities remain among many of the diabetes complications, despite knowledge about modifiable risk factors at individual, clinical, and community levels. This section also brings to light the diverse impact of diabetes, ranging from digestive and liver diseases to disability, cognitive decline and geriatric syndromes, and to sexual dysfunction.

Section 3 reviews the evidence for prevention of diabetes and its complications and for diverse modes of translation of this evidence to outside of the clinical setting, ranging from proof-of-concept clinical trials to the evolution of national movements to improve quality of care and to organize and integrate care. This section describes the gradual improvements in quality of care but stresses the importance of new-generation measures to improve the yet-inadequate levels of diabetes care in the United States. This section brings attention to the potential promise of models of clinical-community partnerships but also depicts the ambiguity of current evidence for environmental approaches. Finally, this section summarizes the economic burden of diabetes and reviews the cost-effectiveness of primary and secondary prevention interventions and the impact of interventions on quality of life, underscoring the wide range of high-value interventions that are now available but that require efficient implementation.

Section 4 describes two of the major mechanisms for implementation of public health programs in the United States, the congressionally funded *Diabetes*

Prevention and Control Programs and the *National Diabetes Education Program.* Section 5 describes the current application and variation of prevention and control programs in developing countries. These chapters serve as a reminder that the entire world can benefit from the expansion and dissemination of clinical and public health science, but the application of this science will always have to be context-specific to be effective.

Section 6 reviews many of the newly emerging issues concerning the diabetes public health burden along with some of the frontiers of future public health action. The last decade has seen the impact of diabetes in youth expand beyond that of type 1 diabetes, for which the evidence base for interventions remains unclear in many areas. This period has also witnessed the identification of dozens of genes and potential gene-environment interactions as well as many promising technological advances with applications ranging from clinical therapeutics to self-management to population-disease management. The evidence for effectiveness of these approaches is young as well, but it demands the same rigor of evaluation as traditional clinical approaches. Finally, this section provides a unique summary of public health information resources to assist clinicians, researchers, and public health specialists in their attempt to advance public health efforts against diabetes.

We hope that this integration of the surveillance, clinical and population-based epidemiology, health services research and economics, along with emerging sciences will provide for a more seamless transition from science to effective public health action. While we are confronted with an increasingly widespread global diabetes epidemic, effective interventions exist, which if systematically and aggressively implemented across populations can more than halve the incidence of diabetes and of its complications. The motivation behind this book is to provide clinicians, public health practitioners, and policy makers with a synthesis of science-based information to help them deliver the public health challenge of diabetes prevention and control.

SECTION 1

BURDEN OF DIABETES IN THE U.S. POPULATION

1. EVOLUTION OF CLASSIFICATION AND DIAGNOSTIC CRITERIA FOR DIABETES AND OTHER FORMS OF HYPERGLYCEMIA

Peter H. Bennett

■ Introduction

Diabetes mellitus has become a major public health problem. The prevalence and incidence of diabetes mellitus have increased considerably over the past 50 years, and increases have been seen in both developed and developing nations. Globally it is estimated that there will be some 330 million cases by 2025 (International Diabetes Federation 2007; Wild et al. 2004). The disease is associated with metabolic and vascular complications, which affect primarily the eye, kidneys, peripheral nerves, and heart. These complications are responsible for most of the excess morbidity and mortality associated with the disease, and there are an estimated 2.9 million excess deaths per year attributable to the disease (Roglic et al. 2005). Increased morbidity from blindness, heart disease, and renal failure vastly increase the direct and indirect medical costs associated with the disease. In the United States alone it is estimated that the health care expenditures for diabetes exceed 200 billion dollars per year (International Diabetes Federation 2007). Diabetes mellitus is a heterogeneous disease, and in the past 40 years considerable advances have been made in understanding the etiology and pathogenesis of its various forms, in large part as the result of standardization of the classification and acceptance of uniform criteria for its diagnosis.

Entities currently defined as diabetes have been recognized for some 3500 years (Ahmed 2002). Early descriptions date back to 1550 B.C., where it was described in the Ebers papyrus as a condition with the passing of too much urine (Loriaux 2009). In the first century A.D. Aretaeus used the term to describe a disease characterized by "melting down of flesh and limbs into urine." By the 5th and 6th centuries A.D. the sweet honey-like taste of the urine in polyuric patients that attracted ants and other insects was reported by Indian physicians, and at this time two forms, one in older more obese people and the other in thin people who did not survive for long, were described. In the 17th century the sweetness of diabetic urine was rediscovered in Europe. At this time the term "mellitus" was introduced to distinguish it from diabetes insipidus, also recognized as a cause of polyuria but not associated with sweetness in the urine. Thomas Willis (1621–1675) noted that "although the disease was rare in ancient times its frequency is increasing." These developments led to urine tasting as the predominant means of diagnosis. In the 19th and early 20th centuries more objective methods of identifying sugar in the urine, and later in the blood, were devised. In this same era it was also recognized that reducing substances in the urine were not specific to diabetes mellitus and that sugars other than glucose, such as lactose and galactose, could result in a false diagnosis. Although elevation of blood glucose was documented in the early part of the 19th century, measurement of glucose levels was cumbersome and expensive, thereby limiting its usefulness in clinical practice. Until the middle of the 20th century, identification of reducing substances in the urine remained the mainstay for clinical diagnosis.

In the early part of the 20th century the idea emerged that oral glucose tolerance tests (OGTTs) would be useful in the diagnosis of diabetes mellitus. Administration of a large oral glucose load resulted in high blood levels among individuals with glycosuria. Attempts to standardize such tests eventually led to the British Diabetic Association in 1964 recommending glucose criteria for diagnosis based on the administration of a 50-g oral glucose load (FitzGerald and Keen 1964) and, in 1969, to the American Diabetes Association (ADA) recommending criteria based on blood glucose levels after a 100-g oral glucose load (American Diabetes Association 1969). Criteria for the diagnosis of diabetes using this test had been formulated by Fajans and Conn, who administered OGTTs to normal healthy individuals and considered glucose levels that fell beyond the mean plus two standard deviations to be abnormal (Fajans and Conn 1959). This led to values that became the most widely used criteria for diagnosis of diabetes mellitus in the United States (American Diabetes Association 1969).

The use of OGTTs also identified individuals with abnormal glucose tolerance who did not have the classic diabetes mellitus symptoms of polydipsia, polyuria, polyphagia, and overt glycosuria—symptoms that historically had been considered characteristic of the disease. Furthermore, glucose tolerance testing in populations indicated that in most there was not a discreet subset of individuals characterized by hyperglycemia. This led to the question as to whether or not diabetes mellitus should be considered a discreet entity or simply represented the upper end of a continuous distribution. Yet it was well recognized that persons who had unequivocally elevated glucose levels were at high risk of developing specific types of complications, such as retinopathy and kidney disease, that were important causes of morbidity and mortality. Population studies also suggested that post-load glucose values in apparently healthy subjects appeared to change with age, suggesting perhaps that criteria for diagnosis should vary according to age (Andres 1967).

In 1965 a World Health Organization (WHO) Study Group on diabetes mellitus made recommendations that, it was hoped, would result in standardization and international acceptance of criteria for diagnosis (WHO Expert Committee 1965). However, these recommendations were not widely adopted, and debate as to what constituted diabetes mellitus and whether there were better tests for its diagnosis continued throughout the late 1960s and the 1970s without standardized definitions and with much variation in the criteria used for diagnosis (West 1975). At the same time it was generally believed that there were two major common forms of the disease, then most commonly described as adult-onset and juvenile-onset diabetes, as well as other forms of the disease associated with chronic pancreatitis, hemochromatosis, and endocrinopathies, such as Cushing's syndrome and acromegaly, often grouped together as "secondary diabetes."

Uniform classifications and diagnostic criteria were needed to plan and conduct clinical research, to serve as a framework for the collection of epidemiologic data on etiology, natural history, and the impact and costs of diabetes, and to aid the clinician in categorizing patients so that appropriate treatment could be given. To meet these needs the National Diabetes Data Group (NDDG) in the United States in 1979 (National Diabetes Data Group 1979) and WHO in 1980 (WHO Expert Committee 1980) made new recommendations for classification and diagnosis.

1979 NDDG and 1980 WHO Recommendations

During the 1970s definitive evidence of differences in the two major types of diabetes had emerged. It was recognized that those who often had an early age of onset and who were most likely to develop diabetic ketoacidosis if not treated with insulin were characterized by certain HLA types and circulating islet cell antibodies as well as very low fasting and stimulated plasma insulin and C-peptide concentrations. In contrast, those with an older age of onset, many of whom were obese, did not show any association with particular HLA types, did not have islet cell antibodies, were less likely to develop ketoacidosis, and could often obtain control of hyperglycemia with either dietary treatment or oral hypoglycemic agents. At the same time some populations with a high prevalence of diabetes were shown to have bimodality in the frequency distributions of their fasting and post-load plasma glucose levels, and those who fell into the upper component of the glucose distributions were more likely to have specific complications such as diabetic retinopathy and diabetic renal disease (Rushforth et al. 1971; Rushforth, Miller, and Bennett 1979). Data from the Bedford, U.K. study indicated a substantial increase in the frequency of retinopathy at and above the glucose levels that corresponded to optimal cut-point for bimodality in glucose distributions among the Pima Indians (Jarrett and Keen 1976; WHO Study Group 1985). These observations influenced the choice of definition of diabetes as a disease characterized by chronic hyperglycemia and with a high risk of specific complications, and thereby the choice of the recommended diagnostic criteria. The NDDG and WHO made similar recommendations for a clinical classification of diabetes that included two major clinical classes, insulin-dependent diabetes mellitus (IDDM) and non-insulin-dependent diabetes mellitus (NIDDM)

TABLE 1.1   *NDDG (1979) and WHO (1980) Classification of Diabetes and Other Categories of Glucose Intolerance*

Clinical classes:

Insulin-dependent type—type 1

Non-insulin-dependent—type 2

Other types—include diabetes mellitus associated with certain conditions and syndromes: pancreatic disease, diseases of hormonal etiology, drug- or chemical-induced conditions, insulin receptor abnormalities, and certain genetic syndromes

Impaired glucose tolerance

Gestational diabetes

and at the same time recognized that there were many other less common types (see Table 1.1).

The proposed diagnostic cut-points for diabetes were well above glucose levels considered normal for healthy individuals. Uncertainty remained about glucose levels above those seen in normal healthy individuals but lower than those associated with the increased risk of the specific diabetic complications. This uncertainty, together with information suggesting that such individuals had a high likelihood of future worsening of glucose tolerance and progression to diabetes, led to designation of the class of impaired glucose tolerance (IGT), a category introduced primarily to stimulate further research into the significance of this abnormality.

During the late 1960s and 1970s evidence had emerged that women who developed abnormal glucose tolerance in pregnancy, but who often reverted to normal glucose tolerance postpartum, had an increased risk of having babies who were large for gestational age and who were prone to hyperbilirubinemia and respiratory distress syndrome (O'Sullivan and Mahan 1964). This led to such women being classified as having gestational diabetes mellitus (GDM).

Although both the 50-g and the 100-g oral glucose loads had been widely used in different parts of the world, it was recommended that the load used for OGTTs should be standardized. Consensus emerged that a 75-g oral glucose load should be used in the future. In support of this were studies using this load that indicated glucose levels that were associated with the development of complications (Rushforth, Miller, and Bennett 1979) and that, in pregnant women, were associated with excess levels of macrosomia in the newborn (Pettitt et al. 1980).

The 1979 NDDG and 1980 WHO reports both recommended measurement of glucose concentrations in venous plasma rather than whole blood. This was because variation in red cell volume results in differences in glucose levels when measured in whole blood, but not in plasma, as well as the belief that the plasma value represented a more physiological exposure.

The NDDG diagnostic criteria were that diabetes should be diagnosed on the basis of fasting venous plasma glucose levels of 140 mg/dL or over or 2-hour post 75-g oral glucose load venous plasma levels of 200 mg/dL or over. Criteria for IGT were defined as fasting plasma glucose levels of less than 140 mg/dL and 2-hour post-load plasma glucose levels of 140 to 199 mg/dL. The WHO group made similar recommendations but with cut-off values stated in SI units.

An unresolved issue between NDDG and WHO recommendations concerned criteria for the diagnosis of GDM. The WHO group recommended that glucose levels based on a 75-g OGTT conducted at the end of the second or beginning of the third trimester of pregnancy should be used for diagnosis of GDM and that the glucose concentrations recommended for diabetes diagnosis in nonpregnant adults should also be used in pregnancy. On the other hand, NDDG recommended a continuation of the "O'Sullivan criteria" that had been used increasingly in the United States during the 1970s (O'Sullivan and Mahan 1964). These criteria were based on two-stage testing, first a screening test with glucose measurement 1-hour after a 50-g oral glucose load, followed by a 3-hour glucose tolerance test using a 100-g oral glucose load for those who have a positive screening test (National Diabetes Data Group 1979).

1985 WHO Revised Classification

In 1985 the WHO Expert Committee added a further clinical class—malnutrition-related diabetes mellitus (MRDM) (WHO Study Group 1985). This was added because of evidence, particularly from developing countries, that diabetes mellitus associated with malnutrition did not fall clearly into the classes of IDDM or NIDDM. MRDM was believed to have two forms, one due to pancreatic calculi giving rise to fibrocalculus pancreatitis and the other thought to be the result of nutritional protein deficiency, so-called protein deficient malnutrition-related diabetes. There were also slight modifications made to the WHO diagnostic cut-off values to more correctly align the glucose concentrations (mmol/L and mg/dL) previously recommended in 1980.

1997 ADA and 1998–1999 WHO Reports

The 1997 ADA (Gavin et al. 1997) and 1998-99 WHO (WHO Consultation Group 1999) recommendations represented a major change from those of 1979 and 1980. A two-dimensional classification was proposed involving clinical stages, which could be recognized regardless of the underlying cause of the abnormalities, and an etiological classification (see Fig. 1.1). The etiological classification was driven in large part by the increased knowledge that some types of diabetes by now had identifiable etiologies, albeit that the most common forms of diabetes, which were relabeled as type 1 and type 2 diabetes, were still of uncertain etiology (see Table 1.2).

Since the quality and standardization of plasma glucose measurement had improved since the 1980s, a fasting plasma glucose value for diabetes diagnosis that

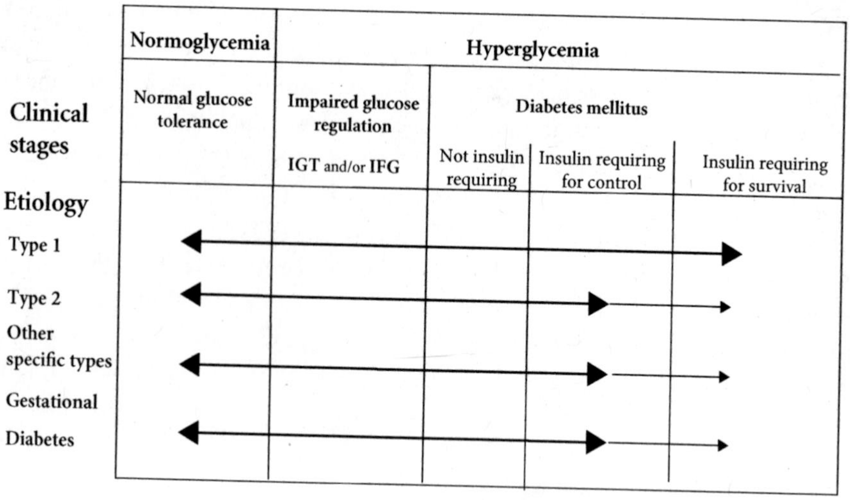

Normoglycemia	Hyperglycemia			
Normal glucose tolerance	Impaired glucose regulation IGT and/or IFG	Diabetes mellitus		
		Not insulin requiring	Insulin requiring for control	Insulin requiring for survival

Clinical stages

Etiology

Type 1 ◄──►

Type 2 ◄────────────────────────────►─────────►

Other specific types ◄────────────────────►──────►

Gestational Diabetes ◄────────────────────►──────►

FIGURE 1.1. Classification of clinical stages and etiological types

TABLE 1.2   *ADA (1997) and WHO (1999) Etiological Classification of Disorders of Glycemia*

Type 1

    Autoimmune

    Idiopathic

Type 2

Other specific types

    Genetic defects of β-cell function

    Genetic defects in insulin action

    Diseases of the exocrine pancreas

    Drug- or chemical-induced

    Infections

    Uncommon forms of immune-mediated diabetes

    Other genetic syndromes sometimes associated with diabetes

Gestational diabetes*

*WHO gestational diabetes now also includes the former category of gestational impaired glucose intolerance, whereas the 1997 ADA classification does not.

was close to "equivalent" to the 2-hour post-75-g venous plasma glucose level of ≥11.1 mol/L (200 mg/dL) was now deemed appropriate for diagnosis. Thus, a fasting glucose level of ≥7.0 mmol/L (126 mg/dL) was recommended to replace the previous value of ≥7.8 mmol/L (140 mg/dL). The clinical stages that replaced the previous clinical classes were normal glucose tolerance, IGT, impaired fasting glycemia (IFG), and diabetes mellitus (DM). The category of IFG was introduced as a possible analog of IGT, which had been shown to be clinically useful as it was highly predictive of future diabetes (Edelstein et al. 1997). Because IFG was also likely to be predictive of future diabetes, it would have clinical utility, especially as fasting glucose determinations were widely used in clinical practice. Thus, it seemed likely that the designation of IFG would result in identification of many more people who might benefit from preventative measures to reduce risk of progression to diabetes.

The 1997 ADA/1998–99 WHO recommendations were the first for an international etiological classification of diabetes mellitus. It was now recognized that the previous classes of IDDM and NIDDM were not etiologically homogeneous and that the etiology for some types of diabetes that previously fell into these classes had become more distinctive. The categories of IDDM and NIDDM were abandoned, and in their place the terms type 1 and type 2 diabetes were adopted. For type 1 diabetes there appeared to be at least two underlying pathophysiological processes, one associated with autoimmune destruction of pancreatic β cells and another whose etiology was obscure but that was not associated with the presence of islet cell or other autoantibodies. Consequently the subtypes of autoimmune and idiopathic type 1 diabetes were chosen. The etiology of type 2 diabetes remained uncertain. Although the syndrome was characterized by abnormalities of both insulin resistance and insulin secretion, the underlying etiologic basis was still unclear. However, more information on other types of diabetes had emerged. Thus, the category of "other specific types" now was extended to include specific genetic defects that defined forms of maturity-onset diabetes of the young, specific genetic defects of insulin action, diseases of the exocrine pancreas, other endocrinopathies, drug or chemically induced diabetes, diabetes due to specific agents such as congenital rubella, and distinctive genetic syndromes often associated with hyperglycemia even though the specific underlying etiology might still be obscure, for example, Turner syndrome, Klinefelter syndrome, and others.

The fasting plasma venous glucose level recommended for the diagnosis of diabetes was reduced to 7.0 mmol/L (126 mg/dL) from 7.8 mmol/L (140 mg/dL). This change, together with acknowledgment that fasting plasma glucose levels of 6.1 mmol (110 mg/dL) and over were abnormal, led to the criteria for IFG as plasma glucose levels between 6.1 and less than 7 mmol/L (110–125 mg/dL) as well as modifications to the criteria for IGT that were consequent upon the change in diagnostic fasting glucose values.

Some differences in recommendations remained as the American Diabetes Association recommended use of fasting glucose levels for both screening and diagnosis and discouraged use of the OGTT. On the other hand, the WHO recommendation was that the fasting glucose level was useful for screening and diagnosis but with the important caveat that "if resources allow, it is recommended that all those with IFG have an OGTT to exclude the diagnosis of diabetes."

Introduction of the category of IFG immediately led to investigations to determine if this category were indeed equivalent to IGT, whose utility as a predictive factor for the development of diabetes was now widely accepted. However, it was soon shown that individuals with IGT and IFG were largely different segments of the population. Only half of individuals who manifested IFG had IGT; the majority of individuals with IGT did not have IFG; and the prevalence of IGT was greater than that of IFG. Yet several studies showed that IFG and IGT alone and in combination were associated with a substantial risk for diabetes. The risks were greater when both IFG and IGT were present, but isolated IFG and isolated IGT each had strong predictive value for development of diabetes. Furthermore, the underlying pathophysiology of IGT and IFG differed, with IFG representing hepatic abnormalities due to defects in insulin secretion, whereas isolated IGT reflected insulin resistance in the presence of only a relative deficiency of insulin secretion.

2003 ADA Recommendations

Differences in IFG and IGT led the American Diabetes Association to reconsider its recommendations concerning cut-off values for fasting plasma glucose levels in 2003 (Genuth et al. 2003). In an effort to make the cut-off values for IFG and IGT more equivalent, especially in view of the clinical trials that indicated both lifestyle and drug interventions in persons with IGT were effective in preventing progression to diabetes (Diabetes Prevention Program Research Group 2002; Pan et al. 1997), it was felt that if a larger proportion of the at-risk population were identified by using fasting plasma glucose there would be more effective prevention. Based on five studies that investigated the predictive value of both IFG and IGT, the recommended cut-off value for IFG was lowered to ≥5.6 mmol/L (100 mg/dL) (Genuth et al. 2003).

2006 WHO Report

WHO did not react immediately to the 2003 ADA recommendations, but in 2005 a joint WHO/International Diabetes Federation (IDF) technical group considered the following issues: (1) Should the current diagnostic criteria for diabetes be changed? (2) How should normal plasma glucose levels be defined? (3) How should IGT be defined? (4) How should IFG be defined? and (5) Which diagnostic tests should be used to define glycemic status (WHO/IDF Consultation Group 2006)?

The group felt that there was inadequate justification to recommend changes in diagnostic criteria for diabetes that had been in place for a decade. Whereas the specific diagnostic cut-off points had been determined originally based on identifying individuals who had an increased risk of the specific microvascular complications, in particular retinopathy, and the occurrence of bimodality in glucose distributions in some populations, the group emphasized that it is cardiovascular disease that is the primary cause of excess morbidity and mortality in diabetes; yet this has not played a role in determining the criteria for the disease. However there were no data to suggest a clear cut-point for diagnostic criteria based on increased cardiovascular morbidity or mortality.

The group also recommended that the definition of IGT, as defined in 1980, should be maintained but recognized that this category of glycemia may not be optimal in identifying those at risk of diabetes and that in future consideration should be given to replacing this category by an overall risk assessment for diabetes and cardiovascular disease that would likely include glucose measurement as a continuous variable.

Whether or not the fasting plasma glucose cut-point for IFG should be changed was considered, but the final recommendation was that the 1997–99 WHO recommendation of fasting venous plasma glucose levels of 6.1–7.0 mmol/L (110–125 mg/dL) should remain. Reasons for not adopting the 2003 American Diabetes Association IFG recommendation were based on concerns about the large increase in IFG prevalence that would occur if the lower cut-point were adopted, the related impact on health systems, and the lack of evidence of benefit in reducing adverse outcomes or progression to diabetes among those with fasting plasma glucose levels of 5.6 to 6.0 mmol/L (100 to 109 mg/dL). Also, persons with these levels of fasting plasma glucose have a more favorable cardiovascular risk profile and only half the risk of developing diabetes as those who are between the cut-points for IFG of 6.1–7.0 mmol/L (110–125 mg/dL).

Because both IFG and IGT represent states of glycemia that are neither unequivocally normal nor diagnostic of diabetes, it was recommended that the term "intermediate hyperglycemia" be adopted to describe such levels, and the term "prediabetes," as suggested by the ADA, was discouraged to avoid the stigma associated with the word diabetes and the fact that many people in this category do not progress to diabetes as the term implies.

The currently recommended WHO/IDF criteria for diabetes and other categories of hyperglycemia are shown in Figure 1.2.

Whether or not alternative diagnostic tests should be used to define glycemic status was considered. The recommendations were to continue to use venous plasma glucose level as the standard measurement together with steps to prevent glycolysis and the consequent reduction in glucose concentrations. Blood should be separated and plasma glucose measured immediately after collection or collected into a tube containing glycolytic inhibitors and placed in ice water until plasma is separated. The group also recommended that the 75-g OGTT should be retained as the "gold standard" for diagnostic testing because fasting plasma glucose levels alone fail to identify approximately 30% of those with undiagnosed diabetes, is frequently needed to confirm or exclude an abnormality of glucose tolerance in asymptomatic people, and because the OGTT is the only means of identifying people with IGT.

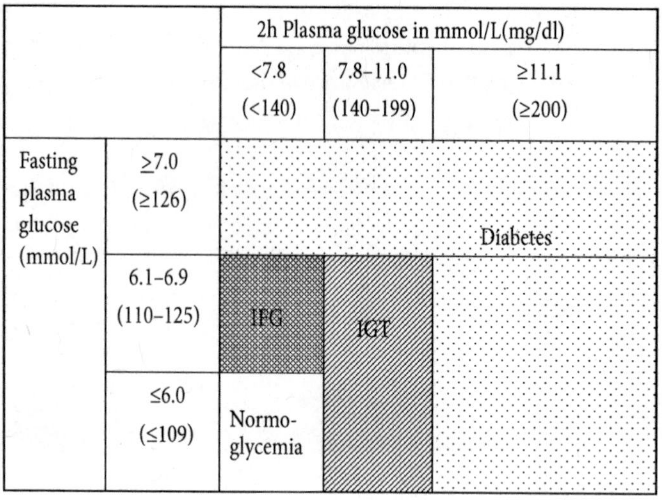

		2h Plasma glucose in mmol/L(mg/dl)		
		<7.8 (<140)	7.8–11.0 (140–199)	≥11.1 (≥200)
Fasting plasma glucose (mmol/L)	≥7.0 (≥126)	Diabetes		
	6.1–6.9 (110–125)	IFG	IGT	
	≤6.0 (≤109)	Normo-glycemia		

FIGURE 1.2. The 2006 WHO criteria for diabetes and other categories of glycemia. (From WHO/IDF Consultation Group 2006.)

The 1999 recommendation that an OGTT should be used in individuals with IFG to determine whether or not they might also have diabetes was reaffirmed.

Whether or not hemoglobin A1C (HbAlC) levels should be considered as a suitable diagnostic test for diabetes or intermediate hyperglycemia was considered. However, because the lack of availability of HbAlC determinations in many developing regions, it was felt that the use of HbAlC for diagnosis was premature, although it seemed likely that this may eventually become appropriate.

■ Conclusions

Whether current criteria for the definition of diabetes and other forms of hyperglycemia are optimal remains an open question. Although the current diagnostic criteria for diabetes define levels of glycemia that are associated with a high risk of microvascular complications, whether or not this is the most appropriate means of defining criteria for diabetes is debatable. Whether cardiovascular disease risk should be considered in formulating the diagnostic criteria needs further investigation. Similarly, whether the currently defined intermediate states of hyperglycemia are the most useful means to identify those at risk for developing diabetes is questionable, and a risk score based on other factors, perhaps not even including glucose levels, may be a better way to identify those in whom preventative measures are appropriate. It is likely that the diagnostic criteria for diabetes and other forms of hyperglycemia will be modified in the future, and HbA1C determinations may eventually supplant glucose as the analyte of choice for diagnostic purposes. Indeed, in

2010 the American Diabetes Association recommended that diabetes could also be diagnosed in the presence of a confirmed HbA1C concentration of 6.5% or greater, and that at-risk individuals could be identified if HbA1C is between 5.7% and 6.4% provided that the HbA1C assay is appropriately standardized (American Diabetes Association 2010). As understanding of the etiology of different forms of diabetes progresses, additional specific types of diabetes will be recognized, and quite different methods for diagnosis may be recommended. On the other hand, the current diagnostic criteria that have been accepted internationally have endured with only modest changes for 30 years.

■ References

Ahmed AM (2002). History of diabetes mellitus. *Saudi Medical Journal* **23** (4), 373–8.

American Diabetes Association (1969). Standardization of the oral glucose tolerance test. *Diabetes* **18**, 299–310.

American Diabetes Association (2010). Standards of Medical Care in Diabetes-2010. *Diabetes Care*, **33** (Supplement 1), S11-S61.

Diabetes Prevention Program Research Group (2002). Reduction in the incidence of type 2 diabetes with lifestyle intervention or metformin. *New England Journal of Medicine* **346** (6), 393–403.

Fajans SS, Conn JW (1959). The early recognition of diabetes mellitus. *Annals of the New York Academy of Sciences* **82**, 208–18.

FitzGerald M, Keen H (1964). Diagnostic classification of diabetes. *British Medical Journal* **1**, 1568.

Genuth S et al. (2003). Follow-up report on the diagnosis of diabetes mellitus. *Diabetes Care* **26**(11), 3160–7.

International Diabetes Federation (2007). *Diabetes Atlas*. 3rd ed. Brussels: International Diabetes Federation.

Jarrett RJ, Keen H (1976). Hyperglycaemia and diabetes mellitus. *Lancet* **2** (7993), 1009–12.

National Diabetes Data Group (1979). Classification and diagnosis of diabetes mellitus and other categories of glucose intolerance. *Diabetes* **28** (12), 1039–57.

O'Sullivan JB (1970). Gestational diabetes and its significance. *Advances in Metabolic Disorders* **1** (Suppl.).

O'Sullivan JB, Mahan CM (1964). Criteria for the oral glucose tolerance test in pregnancy. *Diabetes* **13**, 278–85.

Pettitt DJ et al. (1980). Gestational diabetes: infant and maternal complications of pregnancy in relation to third-trimester glucose tolerance in the Pima Indians. *Diabetes Care* **3** (3), 458–64.

Roglic G et al. (2005). The burden of mortality attributable to diabetes: realistic estimates for the year 2000. *Diabetes Care* **28** (9), 2130–5.

Rushforth NB et al. (1971). Diabetes in the Pima Indians. Evidence of bimodality in glucose tolerance distributions. *Diabetes* **20** (11), 756–65.

Rushforth NB, Miller M, Bennett PH (1979). Fasting and two-hour post-load glucose levels for the diagnosis of diabetes. The relationship between glucose levels and complications of diabetes in the Pima Indians. *Diabetologia* **16** (6), 373–9.

West KM (1965). Substantial differences in the diagnostic criteria used by diabetes experts. *Diabetes* **24**(7), 641–4.

WHO Consultation Group (1999). Definition, diagnosis and classification of diabetes mellitus and its complications. Part 1: diagnosis and classification of diabetes mellitus: report of a WHO consultation. WHO/NCD/NCS/99.2. Geneva: World Health Organization.

WHO Expert Committee on Diabetes Mellitus (1965). Report of a WHO Expert Committee. *WHO Technical Report Series* **310**, 1–44. Geneva: World Health Organization.

WHO Expert Committee on Diabetes Mellitus (1980). *WHO Technical Report Series.* **646**, 1–80. Geneva: World Health Organization.

WHO Study Group (1985). Diabetes Mellitus. Report of a WHO Study Group. *WHO Technical Report Series* **727**, 1–113. Geneva: World Health Organization.

WHO/IDF Consultation Group (2006). Definition and diagnosis of diabetes mellitus and intermediate hyperglycaemia: report of a WHO/IDF consultation. Geneva: World Health Organization.

Wild S et al. (2004). Global prevalence of diabetes: estimates for the year 2000 and projections for 2030. *Diabetes Care* **27** (5), 1047–53.

2. Type 2 Diabetes and Persons at High Risk of Diabetes

Linda S. Geiss and Catherine C. Cowie

■ Main Public Health Messages

- Diabetes is a growing, worldwide public health problem.
- In the United States, the tremendous increase in the number of people with diabetes is likely the result of population growth, changing population demographics, and societal and environmental changes that promote sedentary lifestyles, unhealthy diets, overconsumption of food, and subsequent obesity.
- Since 1990 both the prevalence and incidence of diabetes have continued to increase sharply in the United States; this growth, which has been concomitant with the rise in obesity, shows no signs of slowing.
- Predictions of the future burden of diabetes are disheartening, and the aged and disadvantaged populations will be disproportionately affected.
- Diabetes will continue to be a major public health problem in the United States until effective interventions and policies are implemented to prevent the continued and concomitant growth of diabetes and obesity.

■ Introduction

This chapter documents the past growth of diabetes in the United States, and it warns readers about a possible future in which effective public health policies to prevent or reduce the public health burden of diabetes have not been implemented. The chapter documents trends in the prevalence and incidence of diabetes, identifies population groups that are particularly vulnerable to the disease, briefly discusses leading risk factors (for a more detailed discussion see chapter 3), examines trends in prediabetes and gestational diabetes, and analyzes projections of the future burden of diabetes. Because epidemiologic sources of disease data are unable to distinguish between types of diabetes, and because the vast majority of people with diabetes have type 2, the data presented within this report reflect type 2 diabetes.

■ Historical Perspective and Sources of Data

Because studies that involve serial screening and follow-up of nationally representative samples of Americans do not exist, monitoring the growth of diabetes within the United States is challenging and requires a diversity of data sources. Sources for monitoring diabetes, prediabetes, and gestational diabetes in the United States include national health surveys, health care administrative data, birth certificates, and community-based research. These sources provide different but valuable insights into diabetes and those persons at high risk of developing the disease.

National Health Survey Data

Three surveys of the Centers for Disease Control and Prevention (CDC) are the most frequently used surveys to monitor trends in diabetes. The National Health Interview Survey (NHIS), conducted continuously since 1958 (http://www.cdc.gov/nchs/nhis.htm), is the oldest household interview survey in North America and provides data on long-term trends in diagnosed diabetes. The state-based Behavioral Risk Factor Surveillance System (BRFSS), an ongoing telephone health survey system conducted continuously since 1984 (http://www.cdc.gov/brfss), provides state-specific estimates of the prevalence of diagnosed diabetes and thus information on the geographic distribution of the disease across the United States. The third survey is the National Health and Nutrition Examination Survey (NHANES) (http://www.cdc.gov/nchs/nhanes.htm), which has been conducted periodically over the last four decades but is now conducted on a continuous basis. This survey has an examination component that includes blood and biochemical measurements that, when combined with interview data, allow estimation of both diagnosed and undiagnosed diabetes and thus of all persons with the disease, as well as estimation of prediabetes. In the analyses of NHANES data reported in this chapter, American Diabetes Association (ADA) diagnostic criteria based on fasting plasma glucose (FPG) were used to determine whether people without diagnosed diabetes had undiagnosed diabetes (FPG ≥7.0 mmol/L) or impaired fasting glucose (IFG) (FPG 5.6 to <7.0 mmol/L) (Expert Committee on the Diagnosis and Classification of Diabetes Mellitus 2003).

Health Care Administrative Data

In many countries with universal health care, health care administrative data provide a primary means to monitor diabetes. However in the United States such health care administrative data typically exist only for special populations whose health care is provided for or paid by a governmental agency, such as the Medicare, Medicaid, Veterans Affairs, and the Indian Health Service. In health care administrative data, hospitalization and physician claims or encounter data are characteristically used to identify cases of diabetes. Hospital discharge data have been used to identify cases of gestational diabetes.

Birth Certificate Data

In 2003 the U.S. standard certificate of birth was changed to collect information on preexisting and gestational diabetes among mothers. As of 2007 about 24 states have adopted the new standard. Many states collected such data before the new standard and have examined trends in gestational diabetes using these data.

Community-Based Research

Cross-sectional and longitudinal community-based studies conducted in selected locations or populations have contributed to our understanding of diabetes and persons at high risk for the disease. Cohort studies, which follow people over time, are particularly useful for studying the natural history of a disease, including investigating the incidence of diabetes and its risk factors.

■ Data Limitations

Studies based solely on interview surveys and administrative databases can not identify undiagnosed diabetes or prediabetes. Additionally, due to short-term intraindividual variation in both fasting glucose and 2-hour glucose values, survey estimates of undiagnosed diabetes that use single laboratory measurements of blood glucose are higher than estimates that would be obtained if a confirmatory second measurement were required (Selvin et al. 2007). Although both interview survey data and administrative data are moderately sensitive and highly specific in identifying people with diagnosed diabetes (Hux et al. 2002; Saydah et al. 2004), neither survey nor administrative data are sensitive or specific in identifying persons with prediabetes. The use of telephones to conduct health surveys, such as the BRFSS, may introduce bias because households without landline telephones are not included. However, bias from noncoverage is currently not a large problem for telephone surveys (Blumberg, Luke, and Cynamon 2006). Another shortcoming of national surveys is that because they collect data for a variety of purposes they generally do not allow collection of in-depth information on any one topic. Also, samples for subpopulations (e.g., race and ethnicity) might be small, limiting the ability to examine or detect differences when they do exist.

Questions on gestational diabetes have not been consistently included on national surveys, thus ruling out the examination of trends in gestational diabetes from self-reports, and it is generally believed that gestational diabetes is underreported in birth certificate and hospital discharge data (Lydon-Rochelle et al. 2005). Further, both administrative data and birth certificate data have limited information on socioeconomic status, health behaviors, and risk factors.

Although community-based studies may overcome several of the limitations of survey and administrative data, data from community-based studies reflect small geographic areas or special population subgroups that will probably not represent the experience of the general U.S. population. Further, such studies tend to differ in methodology, time period, definitions used, and length of follow-up, making summary statements difficult.

■ Prevalence of Diabetes, Prediabetes, and Gestational Diabetes

Prevalence and Trends

Diagnosed Diabetes in the United States

In 1958, based on self-reports, an estimated 1.6 million Americans had been diagnosed with diabetes (Kenny, Aubert, and Geiss 1995) (Fig. 2.1). That number grew to 23.6 million in 2007 (CDC 2008) and is expected to increase to 48.3 million by 2050 (Narayan et al. 2006). The prevalence of diagnosed diabetes among Americans of all ages increased from 0.9% in 1958 (Kenny et al. 1995) to 5.9% in 2005 (CDC 2007) (see Fig. 2.1) and is expected to increase to 12.0% in 2050 (Narayan et al. 2006). Further, it is predicted that 33% of American children born in the year 2000 will be diagnosed with diabetes during their lifetime (Narayan et al. 2003).

In general, the prevalence of diagnosed diabetes rises with age (CDC 2007; Cowie et al. 2006). In 1999–2002, prevalence ranged from 1.7% among persons aged 20–39 to 15.8% among persons aged ≥65 years (Cowie et al. 2006). In this same time period age-adjusted prevalence was similar in men (7.0%) and women (6.1%), and prevalence adjusted for both age and gender was about twice as high in

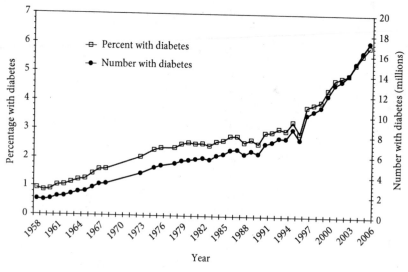

FIGURE 2.1. Number of people with diagnosed diabetes and prevalence of diagnosed diabetes in the United States 1958–2006

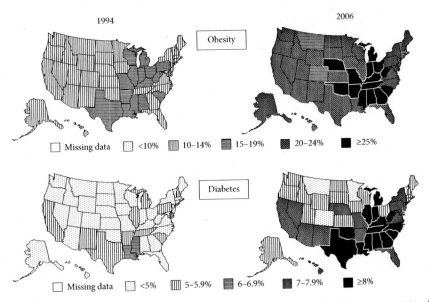

FIGURE 2.2. Age-adjusted prevalence of self-reported obesity and diabetes per 100 adult population, United States, 1994 and 2006 (Source: CDC's Behavioral Risk Factor Surveillance System Age-adjusted to 2000 US standard population.)

non-Hispanic blacks (11.0%) and Mexican Americans (10.4%) as in non-Hispanic whites (5.2%).

Since 1990 the prevalence of diagnosed diabetes has risen sharply, and this trend shows no signs of slowing (Fig. 2.1) (CDC 2007; Geiss, Wang, and Gregg 2007). This growth of diagnosed diabetes is apparent in all age groups, in both genders, and in all racial/ethnic groups for which data are available (CDC 2007). Among adults, the growth in prevalence is found in all of the states, as shown in Figure 2.2. This growth has been concomitant with the growth of obesity.

Undiagnosed Diabetes and the Ratio of Undiagnosed to Total Diabetes

About a quarter of persons with diabetes are unaware that they have the disease (CDC 2008). In 2007 this group represented about 5.7 million persons (CDC 2008). Like diagnosed diabetes, the prevalence of undiagnosed diabetes in U.S. adults rises with age (Cowie et al. 2006; Harris et al. 1998). Unlike diagnosed diabetes, the prevalence of undiagnosed diabetes adjusted for both age and gender in 1999–2002 was similar by race (2.7% for non-Hispanic whites, 3.6% for non-Hispanic blacks, 3.0% for Mexican Americans) (Cowie et al. 2006). However the percentage of diabetes that was undiagnosed (number of undiagnosed divided by the number of diagnosed *plus* the number of undiagnosed) was higher in non-Hispanic whites (34%) than in Mexican Americans (21.8%). The age-adjusted prevalence of undiagnosed diabetes was higher in men (3.6%) than in women (2.1%), as was the percentage of total diabetes that was undiagnosed (34.3% in men vs. 25.5% in women).

The age- and gender-adjusted prevalence of undiagnosed diabetes among persons aged ≥20 years in 1999–2002 (2.8%) was not different from the prevalence of undiagnosed diabetes in 1988–1994 (2.8%) (Cowie et al. 2006). Further, an analysis of three consecutive NHANES from 1976 to 2000 suggests that there has been no decrease in the prevalence of undiagnosed diabetes over the last three decades (Gregg et al. 2004). However this trend varied by body mass index (BMI), defined as weight in kilograms divided by height in meters squared. Those most obese (individuals with a BMI ≥35) had the highest increase in diagnosed diabetes (from 8.6% in 1976–1980 to 15.1% in 1999–2000) but experienced a decline in the prevalence of undiagnosed diabetes (from 12.5% to 3.2%), suggesting increased detection in people who are most obese.

Total Diabetes (Diagnosed and Undiagnosed)

In 2007 an estimated 7.8% of the total U.S. population (23.6 million people) had diabetes (either diagnosed or undiagnosed) (CDC 2008). In adults aged ≥20 years, the prevalence was 10.7%. Estimated prevalence in 2007 ranged from 0.2% in the population aged <20 years to 23.1% among persons aged 60 years or older. In 1999–2002, age- and gender-adjusted diabetes prevalence in non-Hispanic blacks (14.6%) and Mexican Americans (13.5%) was almost twice that of non-Hispanic whites (7.8%), and this differential did not decline in the last decade (Cowie et al. 2006). Age-adjusted prevalence of diabetes in non-Hispanic whites was higher in men than women, but prevalence was similar by gender among non-Hispanic blacks and Mexican Americans.

The age-adjusted prevalence of total diabetes among adults aged 20–74 years increased from 5.3% in 1976–1980 to 8.2% in 1999–2000 (Gregg et al. 2004). During that same time period, the age-adjusted prevalence of diagnosed diabetes increased from 3.3% to 5.8%, while the prevalence of undiagnosed diabetes showed little change (2.0% to 2.4%). Because the prevalence of total diabetes was relatively stable within BMI levels, these data suggest that obesity may be the predominant force behind the growth of diabetes (Gregg et al. 2004).

Vulnerable Groups

The aged, minority groups, and those with low socioeconomic status are among the groups disproportionately burdened by diabetes.

Aged. The prevalence of diabetes rises sharply with age in all gender and racial groups (CDC 2007; Cowie et al. 2006). The only exception to this rule is a decline in the oldest age group that is sometimes observed, probably due to selective mortality. In 1999–2002 the prevalence of diagnosed and undiagnosed diabetes among Americans aged 65 years or older (21.6%) was about 10 times as high as among those aged 20–39 years (2.3%) (Cowie et al. 2006). The prevalence of diabetes among elderly in minority groups was particularly high, exceeding 30%.

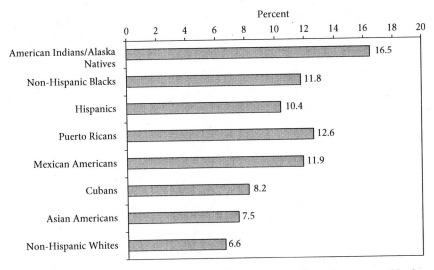

FIGURE 2.3. Age-adjusted prevalence of diagnosed diabetes in people aged 20 years or older, by race/ ethnicity, United States, 2004–2006 (Source: With the exception of American Indian/Alaska Native prevalence, estimated diagnosed diabetes prevalence was calculated using the 2004–2006 National Health Interview Survey data. The prevalence of diagnosed diabetes among American Indians/ Alaska Natives were derived from the 2005 outpatient database of the Indian Health Service.)

Minority groups. Race/ethnicity is a risk factor for diabetes incidence (Brancati et al. 2000; Burke et al. 1999; CDC 2007; Geiss et al. 2006; Kenny et al. 1995; McBean et al. 2004; Resnick et al. 1998). Generally the prevalence of diabetes is higher in racial and ethnic minority populations (Burrows et al. 2000; CDC 2008; Cowie et al. 2006; Kenny et al. 1995) (see Fig. 2.3). Furthermore, in minority populations diabetes develops at younger ages, leaving individuals in those populations even more vulnerable to developing complications of the disease at younger ages. Although there is significant variability across populations and tribes, American Indians and Alaska Natives in the United States are disproportionately affected by diabetes, with rates two to five times as great as among whites (Burrows et al. 2000). Most other minority populations within the United States, including Hispanic/Latino Americans and non-Hispanic blacks, also have a higher prevalence of diabetes than do their white counterparts (CDC 2007; Cowie et al. 2006). In 2004–2006, among the racial and ethnic groups examined, the age-adjusted prevalence of diagnosed diabetes was lowest for non-Hispanic white adults and highest among American Indians and Alaska Natives (Fig. 2.3) (CDC 2008). Higher rates of diabetes among minority populations may reflect differing environmental exposures, greater genetic susceptibility, higher levels of risk factors for diabetes, or a combination of these and other factors.

Low socioeconomic status. Low socioeconomic status—whether measured by income or educational level—is associated with an elevated risk of diabetes (Geiss et al. 2006; Maty et al. 2005; Robbins et al. 2001, 2005). The mechanisms by which socioeconomic status affects the development of diabetes are not well understood. Those with lower socioeconomic status may have higher levels of risk factors for diabetes and other chronic diseases (Brancati et al. 2000; Maty et al. 2005; Robbins et al. 2005), less access to care, higher levels of stress, unhealthy environmental exposures, and/or low levels of health literacy that may affect both self-care and medical care (Berkman et al. 2004).

Prevalence and Trends in Prediabetes

People with prediabetes have blood glucose levels higher than normal but not high enough to be classified as diabetes. Prediabetes is defined as having IFG (defined as fasting glucose of 100–125 mg/dl), IGT (defined as glucose of 140–199 mg/dl after a 2-hour oral glucose tolerance test), or both IFG and IGT (Expert Committee on the Diagnosis and Classification of Diabetes Mellitus 2003). In a cross-sectional sample of U.S. adults aged 40–74 years who were tested during the period 1988–1994, 33.8% had IFG, 15.4% had IGT, and 40.1% had prediabetes (IGT or IFG or both) (CDC 2008). When these percentages were applied to the U.S. population in 2000, an estimated 35 million adults aged 40–74 had IFG, 16 million had IGT, and 41 million had prediabetes. More recent nationally representative data are not available on IGT, but the 2003–2006 prevalence of IFG in the U.S. population was 25.9% (CDC 2008). Applying this percentage to the 2007 U.S. population yields an estimated 57 million adults with IFG.

In 1999–2002 the prevalence of IFG rose with age, ranging from 15.9% among persons aged 20–39 years to 39.1% among persons aged 65 years or older (Cowie et al. 2006). Age-adjusted IFG prevalence was higher in men (32.8%) than in women (19.5%). Age- and gender-adjusted rates were lower in non-Hispanic whites (26.1%) than in Mexican Americans (31.6%), and they were lowest in non-Hispanic blacks (17.7%). The age- and gender-adjusted prevalence of IFG in 1999–2002 (26.0%) was similar to the 1988–1994 prevalence of 25.5%, indicating no increase between the time periods. However, data from earlier time periods using a more restrictive definition of IFG (110 to <126 mg/dl) in samples of the U.S. population aged 40–74 years found an increase in IFG between 1976–1980 (6.5%) and 1988–1994 (9.7%) but no increase in IGT (15.6% in both time periods) (Harris et al. 1998).

Prevalence and Trends for Gestational Diabetes

Gestational diabetes (GDM) is defined as glucose intolerance that is first recognized during pregnancy. Diagnosis of GDM is currently based on a 3-hour 100-g oral glucose tolerance test with two or more plasma glucose concentrations meeting or exceeding defined levels (American Diabetes Association 2004). The definition does not exclude the possibility that unrecognized glucose intolerance may have begun before or concomitantly with the pregnancy. Glucose intolerance, usually type 2 diabetes, persists immediately after pregnancy in about 5%–10% of women (Kim, Newton, and Knopp 2002). Women in whom glucose intolerance subsides are at increased risk of future GDM and have a 20%–60% chance of developing diabetes (usually type 2) in the next 5–10 years. Compared with offspring of mothers without diabetes, offspring of women with GDM have higher birth weight, and they face higher perinatal morbidity and mortality and notably higher risks of obesity, glucose intolerance, and diabetes in late adolescence and young adulthood.

Data from small clinic populations prior to the early 1990s suggested that GDM may occur in 1%–14% of all pregnancies, with variation due to the diagnostic criteria used and populations studied (Coustan 1995). More recently, in 2001 the prevalence of GDM based on birth certificate data in New York City was reported to be 3.8% (95% confidence interval [CI] 3.7–3.9) (Thorpe et al. 2005), but data from birth certificates are likely to underestimate prevalence. Among screened pregnancies in members of the Northern California Kaiser Permanente Medical Care Program in 2000, the age- and race-adjusted prevalence of GDM defined by hyperglycemia was 6.2%, and defined by either hyperglycemia or a hospital discharge diagnosis, it was 6.9% (Ferrara et al. 2004). The age-adjusted prevalence in Kaiser Permanente of Colorado in 2002, using a standard protocol to universally screen for GDM, was lower at 4.1%; the lower prevalence may be explained by the use of older diagnostic criteria with a higher glucose threshold (Dabelea et al. 2005). An assumption that approximately 7% of pregnancies are complicated by GDM translates to some 200,000 cases each year. Regardless of the study, the prevalence of GDM is substantially higher in minority groups, and in the Northern California study it was highest among Asians and Hispanics, intermediate among African Americans, and lowest among non-Hispanic whites; the Colorado study found GDM to be highest in Asian women. Other risk factors include increasing maternal age, obesity, a history of GDM, a family history of diabetes, and increasing calendar year of diagnosis.

As noted above, the prevalence of GDM is increasing over time, a finding that is consistent across studies. In the Colorado study, the significance of increasing calendar year of diagnosis was independent of a history of GDM and not related to parity or gravidity. The age-adjusted prevalence of GDM in Colorado rose from 2.1% in 1994 to 4.1% in 2002, a 95% increase. The age- and race-adjusted prevalence of GDM in the Northern California study rose from 3.7% in 1991 to 6.2% in 2000 based on hyperglycemia alone (a 68% increase) and from 5.1% to 6.9% during the same time period based on either hyperglycemia or a diagnosis (a 35% increase). Based on birth certificate data in the New York City study, prevalence increased by 46% from 1990 to 2001. Coordinated efforts are needed to alter these trends in GDM in order to prevent diabetes in GDM patients and their offspring.

■ Incidence of Diabetes

Magnitude and Trend

In 2005, the incidence of diagnosed diabetes among U.S. adults aged 18–79 years was 7.4 per 1000, representing 1.4 million new cases (CDC 2007) (see Fig. 2.4). Incidence

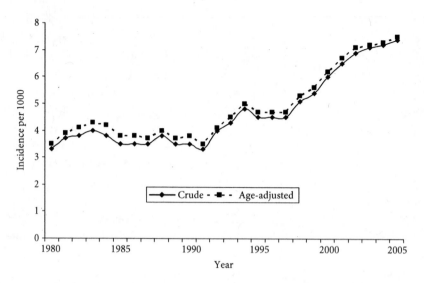

FIGURE 2.4. Crude and age-adjusted incidence of diagnosed diabetes per 1000 population aged 18–79 years, United States, 1980–2005

rose with age from 3.4 per 1000 among persons aged 18–44 years to 13.1 per 1000 among persons aged 65–79 years. Age-adjusted incidence was similar for men and women (7.4 and 7.5 per 1000, respectively) but varied by race and ethnicity. Age-adjusted incidence was 6.9 per 1000 among whites, 10.4 per 1000 among blacks, and 10.2 per 1000 among Hispanics.

Overall, the incidence of diagnosed diabetes among U.S. adults aged 18–79 years showed little change from 1980 to 1990 but began to increase sharply in 1990 (CDC 2007; Geiss, Wang, and Gregg 2007) (Fig. 2.4). Between 1990 and 2005, the incidence of diagnosed diabetes more than doubled, increasing from 3.5 per 1000 in 1990 to 7.4 per 1000 in 2005 (CDC 2007). During this period, incidence increased in all ages, both genders, and in all racial/ethnic groups examined. Medicare administrative data confirm increasing incidence among the aged (McBean et al. 2004), with a 37% increase in this high-risk population between 1994 and 2001.

Most community-based studies in the United States conducted in earlier periods and using differing methodologies also indicate that incidence is increasing (Burke et al. 1999, 2002; Fox et al. 2006; Leibson et al. 1997). Between 1970–1974 and 1990–1994 among residents of Rochester, Minnesota who were aged 30 or older, age-adjusted incidence rose 67% for men and 42% for women (Burke et al. 2002). Among Mexican Americans and non-Hispanic whites aged 25 to 64 years who participated in the San Antonio Heart Study, incidence almost tripled from 1987 to 1996 (Burke et al. 1999). Also, in the Framingham Offspring Study cohort of individuals aged 40–55 years, the incidence of diabetes doubled in the 20 years from 1971 to 1991 (Fox et al. 2006).

Modifiable Risk Factors

Various measures of adiposity are associated with the incidence of diabetes (Vazquez et al. 2007). The incidence of diabetes increases sharply with BMI, and obesity is a major factor in the development of the disease (Edelstein et al. 1997; Fox et al. 2006; Gurwitz et al. 1994; Hara, Egusa, and Yamakido 1996; Hu et al. 2001; Lee et al. 2002; Lipton et al. 1993; Stevens et al. 2001; Weinstein et al. 2004; Williams, Stern, and Gonzalez-Villalpando 2004). Increasing diabetes prevalence and incidence coincide with increasing obesity in the United States (Fig. 2.2). Incidence is also higher among people who are overweight (Fox et al. 2006; Geiss et al. 2006; Hu et al. 2001), and weight gain is associated with incidence, regardless of BMI (Colditz et al. 1995; Ford, Williamson, and Liu 1997; Koh-Banerjee et al. 2004; Oguma et al. 2005). Abdominal fat and waist circumference are also associated with incidence (Cassano et al. 1992; Koh-Banerjee et al. 2004; Wei et al. 1997).

Physical inactivity, independent of the effects of obesity, further elevates the risk of diabetes (Hu et al. 2001; Jeon et al. 2007; Kriska et al. 2003; Weinstein et al. 2004). Other lifestyle factors associated with incidence include smoking (Foy et al. 2005; Hu et al. 2001; Manson et al. 2000; Rimm et al. 1995), no or excessive alcohol consumption (Koppes et al. 2005; Rimm et al. 1995; Wei et al. 2000), and certain dietary components (Hodge et al. 2007; Hu et al. 2001; Hu, van Dam, and Liu 2001; Lindström 2006; Liu et al. 2000; Salmeron et al. 1997; Schulze et al. 2004). These and other lifestyle risk factors often precede or contribute to the development of obesity. Risk factors for diabetes are discussed in more detail in chapter 3.

■ Future Burden of Diabetes

In the United States it is projected that 48.3 million people will have diagnosed diabetes in 2050 (Narayan et al. 2006). This will represent about 12% of the U.S. population in that year, essentially twice the prevalence in 2005. Age-specific increases in the projected number of persons with diagnosed diabetes are expected to be the largest for the two oldest age groups: a 220% increase among those aged 65–74 years and a 449% increase among those aged ≥75 years. Increases in the absolute number of people with diabetes will be especially large for minority groups, with the number of persons with diagnosed diabetes projected to increase 481% among Hispanics, 208% among blacks, and 113% among whites.

For persons born in the United States in the year 2000, the lifetime risk of diagnosed diabetes is high, approximately 32.8% for males and 38.5% for females (Narayan et al. 2003). Estimated lifetime risk for individuals born in 2000 is higher for non-Hispanic blacks and Hispanics than for non-Hispanic whites. For men born in 2000, the risk is 26.7% for non-Hispanic whites, 40.2% for non-Hispanic blacks, and 45.4% for Hispanics. For women born in the same year, the lifetime risk is 31.2% for non-Hispanic whites, 49.0% for non-Hispanic blacks, and 52.5% for Hispanics.

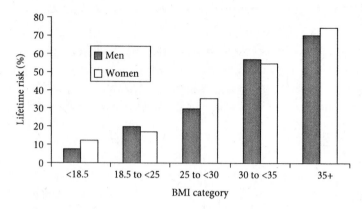

FIGURE 2.5. Lifetime risk of being diagnosed with diabetes among persons 18 years of age, by baseline BMI and gender

Lifetime risks for diagnosed diabetes are similar to or higher than the lifetime risks of many other common diseases and conditions, including breast cancer, hip fracture, and coronary heart disease.

Overweight and obesity substantially increase the lifetime risk of diagnosed diabetes among adults (Narayan et al. 2007) (see Fig. 2.5). Among 18-year-old men the remaining lifetime risk of diagnosed diabetes ranges from 7.6% for those with BMI <18.5 to 70.3% for those with BMI ≥35. For 18-year-old women the remaining lifetime risk of diagnosed diabetes ranges from 12.2% for those with BMI <18.5 to 74.4% for those with BMI ≥35. These risks are generally higher among minority groups within both genders and within all baseline BMI strata.

Underlying these projections and lifetime risks are a number of assumptions that could lead to either underestimation or overestimation. These include an assumption that the incidence of diabetes and life expectancy among people with diabetes will not change, that changes in diagnostic criteria will not occur, and that there will be no advances in diabetes prevention. If the incidence of diabetes continues to rise, the impact on the future numbers with diagnosed diabetes will be much more overwhelming.

■ Areas of Uncertainty or Controversy

Numerous factors could be causing the growth in diabetes in the United States. These include changes in diagnostic criteria for diabetes, increased detection, demographic changes in the population (e.g., the growth of minority populations and aging), improved life expectancy, and a true increase in incidence due to increases in important risk factors for diabetes (e.g., obesity). The relative contribution of each of these factors and others to the growth in diabetes is unknown.

Although it is widely believed that the increasing adiposity of the U.S. population is the primary force behind the increase in diabetes, without nationwide studies involving serial screening for diabetes, the magnitude of the effect of increasing adiposity cannot be determined with absolute certainty. However, two community-based studies (Fox et al. 2006; Williams et al. 2004) that included serial testing for diabetes found that increasing adiposity was a large factor—although not the sole factor—in increasing the incidence of diabetes. Using different methods, the San Antonio Heart Study estimated that 28% of the increase in incidence could be attributed to an increase in obesity (Williams et al. 2004), and the study of middle-aged adults in Framingham, Massachusetts, documented about a 30% reduction in incident diabetes after adjustment for BMI (Fox et al. 2006). However, neither study incorporated other measures of adiposity such as waist circumference, weight gain, and distribution of body fat, which would further characterize the impact of changes in adiposity on the incidence of diabetes. In contrast to these community-based studies that used incidence data to calculate the attribution of adiposity, a study using nationally representative prevalence data suggested that about 85% of type 2 diabetes in North America and Cuba is attributable to a BMI >21.0 (James et al. 2003).

Regardless of the magnitude of the effect of increasing adiposity on the incidence of diabetes, lifestyle changes that include weight loss, increased physical activity, and diet modification have been shown to reduce the risk of progression to diabetes among individuals with IGT (Diabetes Prevention Program Research Group 2002; Pan et al. 1997; Tuomilehto et al. 2001). The weight loss that is key to reducing risk is best achieved through reduced caloric intake or increased physical activity or both.

■ Future Developments

Over the past 15 years both the prevalence and incidence of diagnosed diabetes have increased sharply, and these trends show no signs of slowing. This growth is apparent across most population subgroups and has followed the growth of overweight and obesity within the United States Too many people are prematurely dying from diabetes-related complications and will continue to do so unless further gains are made in preventing the onset of complications and premature mortality.

Predictions of the future burden of diabetes are disheartening, with the aged and disadvantaged populations expected to be disproportionately affected. As the U.S. population continues to increase and to age, and as its minority populations increase, both the incidence and prevalence of diabetes are likely to increase. Further, the annual number of newly diagnosed cases of diabetes each year exceeds the number of deaths among adults with diabetes, adding to the increasing prevalence of diabetes. This imbalance is likely to continue to grow if premature mortality among persons with diabetes continues to decrease and incidence continues to increase. Incidence is likely to increase in the U.S. population if the prevalence of lifestyle risk factors for obesity and diabetes continues to increase. Because current diabetes projection models are based only on projected population demographic changes and do not account for the possibility of a continued increase in the incidence of diabetes, the disease's future burden will likely be even greater than currently predicted. Vulnerable populations, including the elderly, minorities, and the economically disadvantaged, will more than likely be disproportionately affected. Prevention efforts to slow the rate of increase of diabetes are needed to alter the devastating forecasts of the future burden of diabetes.

■ References

American Diabetes Association (2004). Gestational diabetes mellitus. *Diabetes Care* **27**, S88–90.

Berkman ND et al. (2004). *Literacy and health outcomes.* Agency for Healthcare Research and Quality, Rockville, MD. Evidence Report/Technology Assessment 87.

Blumberg SJ, Luke JV, Cynamon ML (2006). Telephone coverage and health survey estimates: evaluating the need for concern about wireless substitution. *American Journal of Public Health* **96**, 926–31.

Brancati FL et al. (2000). Incident type 2 diabetes mellitus in African American and white adults: the Atherosclerosis Risk in Communities Study. *JAMA* **283**, 2253–9.

Burke JP et al. (1999). Rapid rise in the incidence of type 2 diabetes from 1987 to 1996: results from the San Antonio Heart Study. *Archives of Internal Medicine* **159**, 1450–6.

Burke JP et al. (2002). Impact of case ascertainment on recent trends in diabetes incidence in Rochester, Minnesota. *American Journal of Epidemiology.* **155**, 859–65.

Burrows NR et al. (2000). Prevalence of diabetes among Native Americans and Alaska Natives, 1990–1997: an increasing burden. *Diabetes Care* **23**, 1786–90.

Cassano PA et al. (1992). Obesity and body fat distribution in relation to the incidence of non-insulin-dependent diabetes mellitus. A prospective cohort study of men in the normative aging study. *American Journal of Epidemiology.* **136**, 1474–86.

Centers for Disease Control and Prevention. National Diabetes Surveillance System (2007). Available from: http://apps.nccd.cdc.gov/ddtstrs/default.aspx. Accessed November 27, 2007.

Centers for Disease Control and Prevention (2008). *National Diabetes Fact Sheet: General Information and National Estimates on Diabetes in the United States, 2007.* Atlanta, GA: U.S. Department of Health and Human Services, Centers for Disease Control and Prevention.

Colditz GA et al. (1995). Weight gain as a risk factor for clinical diabetes mellitus in women. *Annals of Internal Medicine* **122**, 481–6.

Coustan DR (1995). Gestational diabetes. In: Harris M et al., eds. *Diabetes in America,* 2nd ed., pp 703–17. Bethesda: National Institutes of Health.

Cowie CC et al. (2006). Prevalence of diabetes and impaired fasting glucose in adults in the U.S. population, National Health and Nutrition Examination Survey 1999-2002. *Diabetes Care* **29**, 1263–8.

Dabelea D et al. (2005). Increasing prevalence of gestational diabetes mellitus (GDM) over time and by birth cohort: Kaiser Permanente of Colorado GDM Screening Program. *Diabetes Care* **28**, 579–84.

Diabetes Prevention Program Research Group (2002). Reduction in the incidence of type 2 diabetes with lifestyle intervention or metformin. *New England Journal of Medicine* **346**, 393–403

Edelstein SL et al. (1997). Predictors of progression from impaired glucose tolerance to NIDDM: an analysis of six prospective studies. *Diabetes* **46**, 701–10.

Expert Committee on the Diagnosis and Classification of Diabetes Mellitus (2003). Report of the expert committee on the diagnosis and classification of diabetes mellitus. *Diabetes Care* **26**, S5–20.

Ferrara A et al. (2004). An increase in the incidence of gestational diabetes mellitus: Northern California, 1991–2000. *Obstetrics and Gynecology* **103**, 526–33.

Ford ES, Williamson DF, Liu S (1997). Weight change and diabetes incidence: findings from a national cohort of US adults. *American Journal of Epidemiology* **146**, 214–22.

Fox CS et al. (2006). Trends in the incidence of type 2 diabetes mellitus from the 1970s to the 1990s: the Framingham Heart Study. Circulation **113**, 2914–8.

Foy CG et al. (2005). Smoking and incidence of diabetes among U.S. adults: findings from the Insulin Resistance Atherosclerosis Study. *Diabetes Care* **28**, 2501–7.

Geiss LS et al. (2006). Changes in incidence of diabetes in U.S. Adults, 1997-2003. *American Journal of Preventive Medicine* **30**, 371–7.

Geiss LS, Wang J, Gregg EW (2007). Long term trends in the prevalence and incidence of diagnosed diabetes (0125-R). *Diabetes* **56**, A33.

Gregg EW et al. (2004). Trends in the prevalence and ratio of diagnosed to undiagnosed diabetes according to obesity levels in the U.S. *Diabetes Care* **27**, 2806–12.

Gurwitz JH et al. (1994). Risk factors for non-insulin-dependent diabetes mellitus requiring treatment in the elderly. *Journal of the American Geriatric Society.* **42**, 1235–40.

Hara H, Egusa G, Yamakido M (1996). Incidence of non-insulin-dependent diabetes mellitus and its risk factors in Japanese-Americans living in Hawaii and Los Angeles. *Diabetic Medicine* **13**, S133–42.

Harris MI et al. (1998). Prevalence of diabetes, impaired fasting glucose, and impaired glucose tolerance in U.S. adults. The Third National Health and Nutrition Examination Survey, 1988–1994. *Diabetes Care* **21**, 518–24.

Hodge AM et al. (2007). Plasma phospholipid and dietary fatty acids as predictors of type 2 diabetes: interpreting the role of linoleic acid. *American Journal of Clinical Nutrition* **86**, 189–97.

Hu FB et al. (2001). Diet, lifestyle, and the risk of type 2 diabetes mellitus in women. *New England Journal of Medicine* **345**, 790–7.

Hu FB, van Dam RM, Liu S (2001). Diet and risk of Type II diabetes: the role of types of fat and carbohydrate. *Diabetologia* **44**, 805–17.

Hux JE et al. (2002). Diabetes in Ontario: determination of prevalence and incidence using a validated administrative data algorithm. *Diabetes Care* **25**, 512–6.

James WPT et al. (2003). Overweight and obesity (high body mass index). In: Ezzati M et al., eds. *Comparative Quantification of Health Risks. Global and Regional Burden of Disease Attributable to Selected Major Risk Factors*, pp 496–596. Volume 1. Geneva: World Health Organization.

Jeon CY et al. (2007). Physical activity of moderate intensity and risk of type 2 diabetes: a systematic review. *Diabetes Care* **30**, 744–52.

Kenny SJ, Aubert RE, Geiss L (1995). Prevalence and incidence of non-insulin-dependent diabetes. In: Harris M et al., eds. *Diabetes in America*, 2nd ed., pp. 47–67. Bethesda: National Institutes of Health.

Kim C, Newton KM, Knopp RH (2002). Gestational diabetes and the incidence of type 2 diabetes: a systematic review. *Diabetes Care* 25:1862–8.

Koh-Banerjee P et al. (2004). Changes in body weight and body fat distribution as risk factors for clinical diabetes in US men. *American Journal of Epidemiology* **159**, 1150–9.

Koppes LL et al. (2005). Moderate alcohol consumption lowers the risk of type 2 diabetes: a meta-analysis of prospective observational studies. *Diabetes Care* **28**: 719–25.

Kriska AM et al. (2003). Physical activity, obesity, and the incidence of type 2 diabetes in a high-risk population. *American Journal of Epidemiology*. **158**, 669–75.

Lee ET et al. (2002). Incidence of diabetes in American Indians of three geographic areas: the Strong Heart Study. *Diabetes Care* **25**, 49–54.

Leibson CL et al. (1997). Relative contributions of incidence and survival to increasing prevalence of adult-onset diabetes mellitus: a population-based study. *American Journal of Epidemiology* **146**, 12–22.

Lindstrom J et al. (2006). High-fibre, low-fat diet predicts long-term weight loss and decreased type 2 diabetes risk: the Finnish Diabetes Prevention Study. *Diabetologia* **49**, 912–20.

Lipton RB et al. (1993). Determinants of incident non-insulin-dependent diabetes mellitus among blacks and whites in a national sample. The NHANES I Epidemiologic Follow-up Study. *American Journal of Epidemiology* **138**, 826–39.

Liu S et al. (2000). A prospective study of whole-grain intake and risk of type 2 diabetes mellitus in US women. *American Journal of Public Health* **90**, 1409–15.

Lydon-Rochelle MT et al. (2005). The reporting of pre-existing maternal medical conditions and complications of pregnancy on birth certificates and in hospital discharge data. *American Journal Obstetrics and Gynecology* **193**,125–34

Manson JE et al. (2000). A prospective study of cigarette smoking and the incidence of diabetes mellitus among US male physicians. *American Journal of Medicine* **109**, 538–42.

Maty SC et al. (2005). Education, income, occupation, and the 34-year incidence (1965–99) of Type 2 diabetes in the Alameda County Study. *International Journal of Epidemiology* **34**, 1274–81.

McBean AM et al. (2004). Differences in diabetes prevalence, incidence, and mortality among the elderly of four racial/ethnic groups: whites, blacks, Hispanics, and Asians. *Diabetes Care* **27**, 2317–24.

Narayan KM et al. (2003). Lifetime risk for diabetes mellitus in the United States. *JAMA* **290**, 1884–90.

Narayan KM et al. (2006). Impact of recent increase in incidence on future diabetes burden: U.S., 2005–2050. *Diabetes Care* **29**, 2114–6.

Narayan KM et al. (2007). Effect of BMI on lifetime risk for diabetes in the U.S. *Diabetes Care* **30**, 1562–6.

Oguma Y et al. (2005). Weight change and risk of developing type 2 diabetes. *Obesity Research* **13**, 945–51.

Pan XR et al. (1997). Effects of diet and exercise in preventing NIDDM in people with impaired glucose tolerance. The Da Qing IGT and Diabetes Study. *Diabetes Care* **20**, 537–44.

Resnick HE et al. (1998). Differential effects of BMI on diabetes risk among black and white Americans. *Diabetes Care* **21**, 1828–35.

Rimm EB et al. (1995). Prospective study of cigarette smoking, alcohol use, and the risk of diabetes in men. *British Medical Journal* **310**, 555–9.

Robbins JM et al. (2001). Socioeconomic status and type 2 diabetes in African American and non-Hispanic white women and men: evidence from the Third National Health and Nutrition Examination Survey. *American Journal of .Public Health* **91**, 76–83.

Robbins JM et al. (2005). Socioeconomic status and diagnosed diabetes incidence. *Diabetes Research and Clinica Practice* **68**, 230–6.

Salmeron J et al. (1997). Dietary fiber, glycemic load, and risk of NIDDM in men. *Diabetes Care* **20**, 545–50.

Saydah SH et al. (2004). Review of the performance of methods to identify diabetes cases among vital statistics, administrative, and survey data. *Annals of .Epidemiology* **14**, 507–16.

Schulze MB et al. (2004). Glycemic index, glycemic load, and dietary fiber intake and incidence of type 2 diabetes in younger and middle-aged women. *American Journal of Clinical Nutrition* **80**, 348–56.

Selvin E et al. (2007). Short-term variability in measures of glycemia and implications for the classification of diabetes. *Archive of Internal Medicine* 167:1545–51

Stevens J et al. (2001). Sensitivity and specificity of anthropometrics for the prediction of diabetes in a biracial cohort. *Obesity Research.* **99**, 696–705

Thorpe LE et al. (2005). Trends and racial/ethnic disparities in gestational diabetes among pregnant women in New York City, 1990–2001. *American Journal of .Public Health* **95**, 1536–9.

Tuomilehto J et al. (2001). Prevention of type 2 diabetes mellitus by changes in lifestyle among subjects with impaired glucose tolerance. *New England Journal of Medicine* **344**, 1343–50.

Vazquez G et al. (2007). Comparison of body mass index, waist circumference, and waist/hip ratio in predicting incident diabetes: a meta-analysis. *Epidemiologic Reviews* **29**, 115–28.

Wei M et al. (1997). Waist circumference as the best predictor of noninsulin dependent diabetes mellitus (NIDDM) compared to body mass index, waist/hip ratio and other anthropometric measurements in Mexican Americans—a 7-year prospective study. *Obesity Research* **55**, 16–23.

Wei M et al. (2000). Alcohol intake and incidence of type 2 diabetes in men. *Diabetes Care* **23**, 18–22.

Weinstein AR et al. (2004). Relationship of physical activity vs. body mass index with type 2 diabetes in women. *JAMA* **292**, 1188–94.

Williams K, Stern MP, Gonzalez-Villalpando C (2004). Secular trends in obesity in Mexico City and in San Antonio. *Nutrition Reviews* **62**, S158–62.

3. Risk Factors for Type 2 and Gestational Diabetes

Elizabeth J. Mayer-Davis, Dana Dabelea, Jean M. Lawrence, James B. Meigs, and Karen Teff

■ Main Public Health Messages

- Multiple risk factors for the development of type 2 diabetes have been identified, offering opportunities for primary prevention.
- An ecologic perspective is needed to consider numerous variables that affect risk for type 2 diabetes and overall health: genetic and pathophysiologic pathways, individual behavior, social relationships, living conditions, neighborhoods and communities, institutions, and social policies.
- Risk factors for type 2 diabetes may emerge over the life course from its very beginning—the intrauterine environment and growth trajectories and behaviors during early life may contribute to overall risk of diabetes.
- Obesity, the leading modifiable risk factor for development of type 2 diabetes, operates through a variety of critical metabolic mechanisms. Data from clinical trials provide compelling evidence for the efficacy of moderate weight loss through lifestyle intervention to reduce the risk of type 2 diabetes.
- Race and ethnicity are critical to understanding patterns of risk for type 2 diabetes and thus opportunities for primary prevention, but interactions of race/ethnicity with obesity and socioeconomic position must be considered.
- Several dietary variables, such as intake of fiber, as well as factors such as dysfunctional sleep, depression, smoking, maternal diabetes, and infant feeding, may be risk factors for type 2 diabetes.
- Risk factors for gestational diabetes are generally the same as those for type 2 diabetes, and women with a history of gestational diabetes are at markedly increased risk for type 2 diabetes.

■ Introduction

A global epidemic of type 2 diabetes has emerged unchecked into the 21st century (Engelgau et al. 2004). Concurrent global phenomena that are facilitating this epidemic include increases in migration and associated patterns of acculturation, affluence, urbanization, and obesity (Misra and Ganda 2007). In this setting an *ecologic perspective* is needed to consider genetic and pathophysiologic pathways, individual behavior, social relationships, living conditions, neighborhoods and communities, institutions, and social and economic policies as major forces that affect risk for type 2 diabetes and overall health. Such a perspective was described by Susser and Susser in 1996 (Susser and Susser 1996) in the context of epidemiologic studies and was further developed and promoted by the Institute of Medicine in 2003 (Gebbie 2003; Smedley and Syme 2001).

One can further consider that complex interactions among multiple determinants of health unfold over the *life course* of individuals, families, and communities to shape health status, as depicted in Figure 3.1. For type 2 diabetes this perspective is critical because risk factors for the disease emerge over the life course, and indeed, the intrauterine environment and early-life growth trajectories and behaviors all contribute to overall diabetes risk, as will be described later in this chapter.

The ecologic paradigm as it plays out over the life course may differ by population subgroup. The constructs of *race* and *ethnicity* in biomedical research have been hotly debated in recent years (Burchard et al. 2003; Cooper 2003; Rotimi 2003), with concerns raised regarding the validity of using race in a biological or genetic sense rather than for its social and cultural aspects or for ethnic self-identification. Some researchers have promoted a "race-neutral approach" in the absence of clear

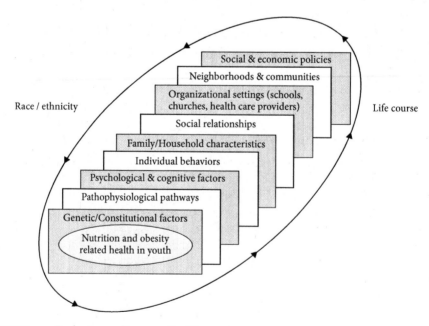

FIGURE 3.1. Ecologic paradigm over the life course

evidence for biological or genetic significance of the term "race" (Cooper, Kaufman, and Ward 2003; Fullilove 1998). However, particularly in the areas of obesity and type 2 diabetes, marked differences in health outcomes and risk factors for health outcomes have been identified between subgroups of individuals defined according to U.S. Census-based self-identification of race and ethnicity. Accordingly many researchers promote use of self-identified race and ethnicity as the most valid measure for most types of epidemiologic studies (Karter 2003), and many studies cited in this chapter will highlight race and ethnicity as key risk factors themselves for development of type 2 diabetes.

■ The Development of Type 2 Diabetes

Consistent with the ecologic framework, an understanding of the key *pathophysiologic* pathways through which type 2 diabetes develops is critical to identification of risk factors for this disease. It is well accepted that both insulin resistance and relative deficiency in the secretion of insulin are involved in the etiology of type 2 disease (Kahn, Hull, and Utzschneider 2006). *Genetic* and *environmental factors* interact to increase risk for obesity, insulin resistance, and β-cell dysfunction. Accordingly risk factors for type 2 diabetes include those that are modifiable, and thus present opportunities for prevention, and those that cannot be modified. Family history of diabetes and aging are two important, non-modifiable risk factors. The most obvious non-modifiable risk factor is the presence of susceptibility genes, but the presence of a susceptibility gene does not make the development of type 2 diabetes inevitable. Recent data from large genetic association studies point to genetic susceptibility in β-cells as key to the pathogenesis of type 2 (Sladek et al. 2007; Zeggini et al. 2007; Grant et al. 2006). A plausible global hypothesis of the pathogenesis of type 2 diabetes posits obesity and novel risk factors as exacerbating insulin resistance and conferring an environmental stress that leads to type 2 disease in the setting of genetic predisposition to β-cell failure (Elbein, Wegner, and Kahn 2000).

The following sections will provide an overview of key risk factors for type 2 diabetes, beginning with metabolic risk factors, including those that are related directly to obesity, followed by discussions of overweight itself with consideration of the obesity epidemic; behavioral risk factors; early-life risk factors; demographic, social, and community factors; and a discussion of risk factors for gestational diabetes mellitus (GDM). Engelgau and colleagues (Engelgau et al. 2004) note the importance of broad approaches to primary prevention of diabetes, approaches that would include considerations of policy and health care systems as well as individual-level social and economic circumstances in order to effectively support the behavioral changes that are important to sustainable reduction of diabetes risk.

■ Metabolic Risk Factors

Overview of the Pathophysiology of Type 2 Diabetes

An excellent review published by Kahn and co-workers in 2006 (Kahn et al. 2006) focused on the various mechanisms that link obesity to insulin resistance and to β-cell dysfunction. Briefly, in obese individuals, excess body fat, particularly in the viscera, results in increased release of nonesterified fatty acids (NEFAs), which leads to the development of hepatic and whole-body *insulin resistance*. Also related to obesity, increases in pro-inflammatory cytokines (e.g., c-reactive protein [CRP] and tumor necrosis factor [TNF]-α) contribute to insulin resistance, as do declines in other hormones such as adiponectin. Even in lean individuals, excess visceral fat can contribute to development of insulin resistance because of the increased metabolic activity of visceral fat.

In healthy individuals the magnitude of *insulin secretion* depends on exogenously derived stimulants (e.g., ingested macronutrients) and insulin resistance. For example individuals with greater insulin sensitivity require less insulin secretion to achieve normal glucose levels. In the presence of insulin resistance, the production of insulin by the pancreatic β-cells is increased, and hepatic clearance of insulin is reduced to maintain normoglycemia. This increase in insulin secretion is a function of both the responsiveness and mass of the β-cells. However when the β-cells become dysfunctional, impaired glucose tolerance and type 2 diabetes ensue because relative insulin insufficiency leads to reduced uptake of glucose by target tissues and to increased hepatic production of glucose. Both elevated glucose concentrations (termed "glucotoxicity") and increased release of NEFAs (termed "lipotoxicity") contribute to evolving β-cell dysfunction. Insulin resistance may be long-standing and does not always lead to diabetes, but once β-cell failure is apparent, frank diabetes appears to develop within a few years (Ferrannini et al. 2004). Type 2 diabetes is itself a progressive disease, owing substantially to increasing β-cell dysfunction over time.

Obesity-Related Metabolic Processes

In humans the accumulation of adipose tissue initiates a cascade of changes in metabolic pathways, many of which have the potential to initiate or exacerbate insulin resistance, thereby leading to an increased risk of type 2 diabetes. Many of these changes are localized to fat tissue, specifically adipocytes, which over the past decade have been increasingly viewed as an active endocrine tissue. Adipocytes secrete hormones such as adiponectin, which protects against insulin resistance, as well as a multitude of inflammatory cytokines that contribute to insulin resistance.

Adiponectin, the most abundant protein in the adipocyte, increases the oxidation of muscle fat and also has been shown to exhibit anti-inflammatory properties. The protein is less abundant in obese and type 2 diabetes patients than in healthy volunteers and is inversely correlated with insulin resistance (Arita et al. 1999). Furthermore one locus for genetic susceptibility to type 2 diabetes has been associated with the adiponectin gene, and mutations in this locus are higher in patients with type 2 disease (Comuzzie et al. 2001).

In contrast to adiponectin, which is inversely related to adiposity, the inflammatory cytokines are positively associated with obesity. Central-body adiposity (Panagiotakos et al. 2005) and, specifically, insulin resistance (McLaughlin et al. 2002; Guldiken et al. 2007) are associated with increased systemic levels of inflammatory markers such as TNF-α, interleukin 6 (IL-6), and CRP as well as pro-inflammatory markers such as monocyte chemoattractant protein (MCP-1) (Dahlman et al. 2005). Increases in cytokines, such as TNF-α and IL-1β, may induce insulin resistance in adipocytes, thereby increasing lipolysis and elevating levels of free fatty acids, which are key regulators of insulin sensitivity.

Based on an analysis of the Women's Health Initiative Observational Study, TNF-α receptor 2, IL-6, and high-sensitivity CRP are all associated with increased risk of diabetes (Liu et al. 2007). However from the Nurses' Health Study, variants of IL-6R were not found to be associated with risk of diabetes (Qi, Rifai, and Hu 2007), and the authors argued that it remains to be determined whether IL-6 is causal for diabetes.

Of the myriad of circulating hormones and neuropeptides proposed as regulators of body weight and/or adiposity, the present discussion will highlight leptin, insulin, ghrelin, and retinol-binding protein. Leptin and insulin are the only two hormones that have been consistently shown to be involved in regulation of body weight. Both hormones are secreted peripherally, transported across the blood-brain barrier, and act on specific areas in the central nervous system to regulate behavior and body weight. Although both hormones are thought to act as satiety factors in the brain, in human obesity, both hormones have elevated concentrations because of tissue resistance to circulating levels. Therefore, it is often difficult to determine the risk associated with elevated leptin levels that is independent of either obesity and/or insulin resistance (Schmidt et al. 2006; Wannamethee et al. 2007).

Ghrelin, which is synthesized in the gastrointestinal tract, is an orexigenic hormone shown to promote food intake in animals (Tschop, Smiley, and Heiman 2000) and humans (Wren et al. 2001). Two studies have shown an association between low ghrelin levels and indexes of insulin sensitivity based on fasting levels of insulin and glucose (Ukkola, Poykko, and Antero 2006; Poykko et al. 2003) Furthermore, mutations in the ghrelin gene have been associated with the metabolic syndrome (Steinle et al. 2005).

Serum retinol-binding protein (RBP4) is another relatively novel factor also expressed in adipose tissue. Serum RBP4 has been found to be elevated in individuals with impaired glucose tolerance, obese insulin-resistant participants in a prospective study (Cho et al. 2006), and lean, normoglycemic individuals with a strong family history of diabetes (Yang et al. 2005). In general, serum RBP4 correlates inversely with insulin sensitivity. Two studies have found genetic polymorphisms in the RBP4 gene that were associated with insulin resistance and/or type 2 diabetes (Craig, Chu, and Elbein 2007; Munkhtulga et al. 2007).

Metabolic Predictors of Type 2 Diabetes

Proxy measures validated against detailed physiologic study consistently show both insulin resistance (usually measured using a homeostasis model of insulin resistance or as fasting insulin concentration) and β-cell function (assessed with a variety of surrogate measures most commonly derived from oral or intravenous glucose tolerance tests) to be strong independent risk factors for type 2 diabetes (Lillioja et al. 1993; Hanson et al. 2000; Haffner et al. 1996).

Insulin resistance is a potent and complex risk factor for diabetes. Whereas insulin resistance alone triples the risk of diabetes, when it occurs in the setting of a cluster of risk factors for cardiovascular disease (CVD) called metabolic syndrome (typically including hyperglycemia, hypertension, dyslipidemia, and central adiposity), it is an especially common and powerful risk factor for type 2 diabetes (Ford 2005; Hanson et al. 2002; Meigs et al. 2007b). Insulin resistance and the clustering of CVD risk factors appear to confer much of the risk for diabetes commonly associated with excess adiposity (Meigs et al. 2006). Metabolic syndrome increases risk of diabetes by about a factor of 7 and accounts for about 50% of diabetes cases on a population basis (Wilson et al. 2005). Indeed, metabolic syndrome appears synonymous with prediabetes and can be used as an efficient tool for predicting diabetes (Wilson et al. 2007; Stern MP et al. 2004).

Beyond risk factors included in the metabolic syndrome, diverse novel metabolic factors are associated with insulin resistance and diabetes risk. Novel risk factors include the inflammatory cytokines, hormones, and neuropeptides discussed in the previous section, increased free fatty acid flux (Groop et al. 1991; Pankow et al. 2004), hepatic steatosis (Kotronen et al. 2007; Andre et al. 2007; Lee et al. 2004), generalized subclinical inflammation (Schmidt et al. 1999; Pradhan et al. 2001; Festa et al. 2000), hemolytic and arterial endothelial dysfunction (Weyer et al. 2002; Vita et al. 2004; Sakkinen et al. 2000; Meigs et al. 2006), and heightened oxidative stress (Houstis, Rosen, and Lander 2006; Meigs et al. 2007a). In epidemiologic studies the markers most consistently associated with risk of diabetes have included elevated plasma levels of γ-glutamyltransferase, IL-6, and CRP. The relative risks associated with some of these novel risk factors are quite large, suggesting important roles in the pathogenesis of diabetes. For instance in one study subjects in the top fifth of the CRP distribution had a relative risk of approximately 4 for incident diabetes when the lowest fifth of the CRP distribution was used as the referent (Hu et al. 2004). However the large relative risks notwithstanding, few novel risk factors improve the ability to predict diabetes when added to traditional risk factors (e.g., obesity) in prediction models (Wilson et al. 2007).

Obesity as a Risk Factor for Diabetes: Observational
Epidemiology and Clinical Trials

By far the most important risk factor for development of type 2 diabetes is excess body fat. Evidence for a causal link between obesity and type 2 diabetes is well documented relative to key pathophysiologic mechanisms (Kahn et al. 2006) and has been observed clearly in prospective observational studies (Hu et al. 2001; Moore et al. 2000). Hu and colleagues (Hu et al. 2001) estimated that 91% of type 2 cases among women could be attributed to lifestyle factors, with factors related to obesity being by far the most important. Most convincing is the fact that randomized clinical trials have shown undeniable efficacy for substantially reducing risk for developing type 2 diabetes through modest weight loss, whether achieved via lifestyle interventions (Chiasson et al. 2002; Tuomilehto et al. 2001), pharmacologic intervention (Heymsfield et al. 2000), or surgical intervention (Sjostrom et al. 2004). These studies have documented risk reduction as high as 58% over periods of 2 to 10 years. Results from key clinical trials of lifestyle interventions for primary prevention of type 2 diabetes have been reviewed recently (Burnet et al. 2006; Pi-Sunyer 2007) and are summarized in Table 3.1.

■ The Obesity Epidemic

From scientists and health care providers to policy makers, politicians, and journalists, a great variety of people have focused attention on the obesity epidemic. Such attention is well placed. Increases in obesity-associated mortality and in several chronic diseases, including diabetes, that are associated with obesity have been recently reviewed (Bray and Ballenger 2006). Self-reported data from the U.S. Behavioral Risk Factor Surveillance System documented a 24% increase in the prevalence of overweight and obesity in adults for the period 1995–2004 (Pearson 2007), and data from the Framingham study show that the incidence of overweight and obesity has increased progressively over the last 50 years in the population under study (Parikh et al. 2007).

Data from the nationally representative U.S. National Health and Nutrition Examination Survey (NHANES) demonstrated striking increases in the prevalence of objectively measured obesity through the 1980s and 1990s (Flegal et al. 2002). Most recently, Ogden and co-workers (Ogden et al. 2006) reported the prevalence of overweight (defined as a body mass index [BMI] of 25–29 when calculated as weight in kilograms divided by height in meters squared) and obesity (BMI ≥ 30) in the United States for the years 1999–2004; key findings are given in Figure 3.2. For the period 2003–2004 the prevalence of overweight or obesity among men was 70.8%, ranging from 60.7% among non-Hispanic blacks to 74.7% among Mexican Americans. There was a statistically significant increase in the prevalence of obesity in men between 1999–2000 (27.5%) and 2003–2004 (31.1%). Among women

TABLE 3.1 *Lifestyle Trials to Prevent or Delay Diabetes*

	Diabetes Prevention Program (DPP)[a,b]	Diabetes Prevention Study (DPS)[c,d]	Da-Qing IGT and Diabetes Study[e]	Malmö Feasibility Study[f]
Population				
Country	United States	Finland	China	Sweden
Years	1996 to 2001	1993 to 2000	1986 to 1992	1974 to 1985
N	3234	522	577	415
Inclusion criteria	IGT and ↑FPG	IGT	IGT	Mild DM (no symptoms), IGT, normal controls
Age (y, mean ± SD)	50.6 ± 10.7	55 ± 7	45.0 ± 9.1	Range = 47 to 49
BMI (mean ± SD)	34.0 ± 6.7	31.3 ± 4.6 (intervention group)	25.8 ± 3.8	27.7 ± 3.7 (group 1; DM, lifestyle)
		31.0 ± 4.5 (control group)		26.6 ± 3.1 (group 2; IGT, lifestyle)
				26.7 ± 4.0 (group 3; IGT controls)
				24.3 ± 2.8 (group 4; normal controls)
Follow-up (mean y)	2.8	3.2	6	5
Race	55% white	100% white	100% Asian	100% white
	20% African American			

16% Hispanic			
5% American Indian			
4% Asian American			

Study design

	Study 1	Study 2	Study 3	Study 4
Type	RCT; individuals randomized	RCT; individuals randomized	RCT; clinics randomized	Nonrandomized feasibility study. Baseline differences in groups.
Number of sites	27	5	33	1
Arms	4 arms:	2 arms:	4 arms:	Lifestyle intervention:
	Lifestyle intervention, $n = 1079$	Lifestyle intervention, $n = 265$	Diet alone, $n = 130$	Group 1 (DM), $n = 41$
	Metformin, $n = 1073$	Control group, $n = 257$	Exercise alone, $n = 141$	Group 2 (IGT), $n = 181$
	Troglitazone (discontinued 1998)		Diet ± exercise, $n = 126$	No intervention:
	Control, $n = 1082$		Control, $n = 133$	Group 3 (IGT), $n = 79$
				Group 4 (normals), $n = 114$

Goals

Weight loss	7% weight loss	≥5% weight loss	For BMI <25: none	Not mentioned
			For BMI ≥25: 0.5 to 1.0 kg loss/ mo until BMI = 23	

(continued)

TABLE 3.1 *(continued)*

	Diabetes Prevention Program (DPP)[a,b]	Diabetes Prevention Study (DPS)[c,d]	Da-Qing IGT and Diabetes Study[e]	Malmö Feasibility Study[f]
Diet	<25% kcal from fat	<30% kcal from fat <10% saturated fat ≥15 g fiber/1000 kcal	BMI <25: 25 to 30 kcal/kg intake 55% to 65% carbohydrates 10% to 15% protein 25% to 30% fat BMI ≥25: ↓kcal intake	↓Simple carbohydrates ↑Complex carbohydrates ↓Saturated fats Substitute polyunsaturated fats ↓Kilocalories for obese subjects
Physical activity	150 min physical activity per week	30 min moderate intensity physical activity per day	↑Leisure physical activity by 1 to 2 study-specific units per day*	Not mentioned

Intermediate outcomes

Weight change

	Diabetes Prevention Program (DPP)[a,b]	Diabetes Prevention Study (DPS)[c,d]	Da-Qing IGT and Diabetes Study[e]		Malmö Feasibility Study[f]
			Did not develop DM	Did develop DM	
kg (mean)	Lifestyle ↓5.6 Metformin ↓2.1 Placebo ↓0.1	Lifestyle ↓4.2 at 1 y ↓3.5 at 2 y Control ↓0.8 at 1 y ↓0.8 at 2 y	Control: ↑0.27 DM diet: ↑0.93 Exercise: ↑0.71 Diet + exercise: ↓1.77	↓1.55 ↓2.43 ↓1.93 ↓3.33	Lifestyle (groups 1 and 2) ↓6 at 1 y ↓2.0 to 3.3 at 5 y Control (groups 3 and 4) ↓0.2 to 2.0 at 5 y

% subjects meeting weight loss goal	50% in lifestyle arm	By year 1: 43% lifestyle group 13% control group	
% subjects maintaining weight loss goal	38% in lifestyle arm		82% group 1 & 71% group 2 maintained overall weight reduction over 5 y
Physical activity			
% subjects meeting activity goal	74% in lifestyle arm	By year 1: 86% lifestyle group 71% control group	
% subjects maintaining activity goal	58% in lifestyle arm		
Diabetes outcomes			
Incidence	Cumulative 3-y DM incidence: Control 28.9% Lifestyle 14.4% Metformin 21.7%	Cumulative 2-y DM incidence: Control 14% Lifestyle 6% Cumulative 4-y DM incidence: Control 23% Lifestyle 11%	Cumulative 6-y DM incidence: Control 67.7% Diet 43.8% Exercise 41.1% Diet ± exercise 46.0%
			Cumulative 6-y DM incidence: Lifestyle (group 2) 10.6% Control (group 3) 28.6% Control (group 4) 0%

(continued)

TABLE 3.1 *(continued)*

	Diabetes Prevention Program (DPP)[a,b]	Diabetes Prevention Study (DPS)[c,d]	Da-Qing IGT and Diabetes Study[e]	Malmö Feasibility Study[f]
Risk reduction in intervention vs control group	DM risk reduction over 3 y:	DM risk reduction over 6 y:	DM risk reduction over 6 y:	DM risk reduction over 6 y:
	Lifestyle 58%	Lifestyle 58%	Diet 31%	Lifestyle 63%
	Metformin 31%		Exercise 46%	
			Diet ± exercise 42%	(group 2 vs group 3)

One study-specific physical activity unit=30 minutes of mild intensity (e.g., slow walking) or 20 minutes of moderate intensity (e.g., brisk walking) or 10 minutes of strenuous intensity (e.g., slow running) or 5 minutes of very strenuous intensity (e.g., jumping rope) exercise.

IGT, impaired glucose tolerance; FPG, fasting plasma glucose; DM, type 2 diabetes mellitus; BMI, body mass index [weight in kilograms/(height in meters)²]; RCT, randomized controlled trial; kcal, kilocalories.

[a]Eriksson KF, Lindgarde F (1991). Prevention of type 2 (non-insulin-dependent) diabetes mellitus by diet and physical exercise: the 6-year Malmö feasibility study. *Diabetologia* **34**, 891–8.

[b]American Diabetes Association (2004). Screening for type 2 diabetes. *Diabetes Care* **27**, S11–3.

[c]Tuomilehto J et al. (2001). Prevention of type 2 diabetes mellitus by changes in lifestyle among subjects with impaired glucose tolerance. *New England Journal of Medicine* **344**, 1343–50.

[d]Hillier TA, Pedula KL (2003). Complications in young adults with early-onset type 2 diabetes. *Diabetes Care*, **26**, 2999–3005.

[e]U.S. Department of Agriculture (2005). *Dietary guidelines for Americans 2005.* Available at: http://www.health.gov/dietaryguidelines/dga2005/document/. Accessed April 1, 2005.

[f]United States Department of Health and Human Services (2001). *The Surgeon General's call to action to prevent and decrease overweight and obesity.* U.S. Department of Health and Human Services, Public Health Service, Office of the Surgeon General, Rockville, MD.

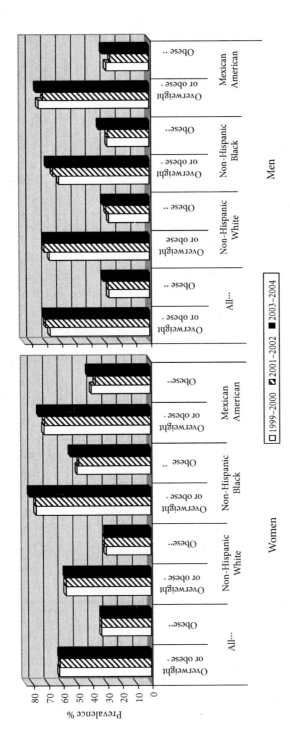

FIGURE 3.2. Prevalence of overweight and obesity in men and women by racial/ethnic group. Body mass index (BMI), calculated as weight in kilograms divided by the square of height in meters, was rounded to the nearest tenth. Pregnant women were excluded. *Overweight or obese defined as BMI of 25 or higher. **Obese defined as BMI of 30 or higher. ***Includes racial/ethnic groups not shown separately. (Taken from Ogden et al. 2006.)

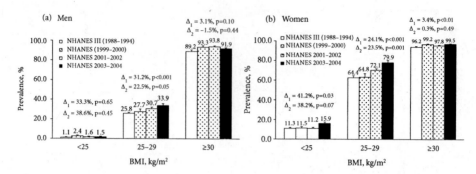

FIGURE 3.3. Age-adjusted prevalence of abdominal obesity (NCEP ATP III: WC >102 cm for men and >88 cm for women) among U.S. adults ≥20 years of age according to BMI, NHANES III (1988–1994) to NHANES 2003–2004. Δ_1 = difference between NHANES 2003–2004 and NHANES III (1988–1994). Δ_2 = difference between NHANES 2003–2004 and NHANES 1999–2000.

the prevalence of overweight or obesity was 61.8%, ranging from 58.0% among non-Hispanic whites to 81.6% among non-Hispanic black women. Interestingly, there was no statistically significant increase in the prevalence of obesity among women between 1999–2000 and 2003–2004. This seemingly positive finding is off-set by the simple fact that one-third of all women, for each of those time periods, were obese.

Increasing trends in waist circumference and abdominal obesity among U.S. men and women (Li et al. 2007) also constitute a cause for concern because of the elevated risk for metabolic disturbances associated with visceral adiposity. Figure 3.3 (Li et al. 2007) shows the interplay of BMI and abdominal obesity based on the NHANES data. Of note is the increase in prevalence of abdominal obesity over time within the subgroup of individuals with BMI of 25–29, for both men and women.

Behavioral Risk Factors

Weight Management

The most critical behavioral risk factors to consider for diabetes prevention relate to weight management (Hamman et al. 2006); Klein and colleagues have recently reviewed issues pertinent to weight management (Klein et al. 2004). Approaches include lifestyle intervention and augmentation of lifestyle change with weight-loss medication or bariatric surgery; each of these approaches has been shown in clinical trials to reduce risk for diabetes (Franz et al. 2002; Torgerson et al. 2004). Despite recently renewed interest in high-protein, low-carbohydrate diets to facilitate weight loss, neither of the two published clinical trials that followed patients for 12 months demonstrated greater weight loss for such a diet than for conventional low-fat (25–30% energy) diets (Foster et al. 2003; Stern L et al. 2004). One clinical trial showed that a Mediterranean diet moderate in fat (35% energy) may enhance long-term (18- to 30-month) adherence and success in weight loss

(McManus, Antinoro, and Sacks 2001). The current consensus is that weight-loss strategies need to incorporate increased energy expenditure and reduced intake of total energy with an emphasis on reduced consumption of foods with added sugars, fats, and alcohol that provide calories but few essential nutrients (U.S. Department of Health and Human Services and U.S. Department of Agriculture 2005). Other chapters in this book will deal with approaches to effective delivery of lifestyle interventions designed for weight management and prevention of type 2 diabetes.

Dietary Intake of Fat

Reduced intake of total fat, particularly saturated fat, may reduce risk for diabetes independent of weight status (Franz et al. 2002; van Dam et al. 2002b). It appears that all types of dietary fat (except n-3 fatty acids) may have an adverse effect on insulin sensitivity (Mayer-Davis et al. 1997), particularly among obese individuals. Saturated fats may have the greatest adverse effect on insulin sensitivity, especially as compared with monounsaturated fats (Vessby et al. 2001). Increased intake of polyunsaturated fat, in the context of appropriate total energy intake for weight management, may reduce the risk of type 2 diabetes (Meyer et al. 2001).

Dietary Intake of Carbohydrate

Studies have provided consistent evidence for reduced risk of diabetes with increased intake of whole grains and dietary fiber (Franz et al. 2002; Meyer et al. 2000; Schulze et al. 2004a; Stevens et al. 2002). Intake of foods containing whole grains has been associated with higher insulin sensitivity, independent of obesity (Liese et al. 2003), and the amount of dietary fiber has been associated with higher insulin sensitivity as well as a higher disposition index that reflects the ability of the pancreas to secrete insulin adequately relative to insulin resistance (Liese et al. 2005).

There is considerable debate as to the potential role of the glycemic index and glycemic load (both surrogates of expected glucose excursion following ingestion of food containing carbohydrates) in preventing type 2 diabetes (Sheard et al. 2004). Associations of glycemic index and glycemic load with diabetes incidence have been reported inconsistently (Hodge et al. 2004; Meyer et al. 2000; Salmeron et al. 1997; Schulze et al. 2004a; Stevens et al. 2002). These inconsistencies may relate to the methodological difficulties inherent in applying the concept of the glycemic index (derived from data on glucose excursions from test foods consumed in the fasting state) to the concept of usual dietary intake (incorporating foods consumed in the fasting and postprandial states, prepared variously over time) (Mayer-Davis et al. 2006).

Whether as a function of glucose excursions or simply excess caloric intake, consumption of sweetened beverages (e.g., soda, fruit punch) has been associated with increased risk for weight gain and the development of type 2 diabetes (Schulze et al. 2004b), although the literature regarding associated risk for type 2 diabetes is inconsistent (Paynter et al. 2006).

Other Dietary Factors

Selected micronutrients may affect glucose and insulin metabolism (Franz et al. 2002), but to date, data to document their role in the development of diabetes remain relatively scant. Evidence is mounting for a protective effect of higher levels of plasma vitamin E, but this effect appears to occur only in the range of vitamin E intake readily available from food, with no protective advantage of high-dose supplementation (Mayer-Davis et al. 2002). Increased intake of low-fat dairy products may reduce risk for type 2 diabetes, independent of BMI (Choi et al. 2005), which may be due to beneficial effects of calcium (Ma et al. 2006; Sanchez et al. 1997; Schrager 2005) or magnesium (Lopez-Ridaura et al. 2004; Ma et al. 2006; Rosolova, Mayer, and Reaven 2000; Song et al. 2004). Recent studies suggest that consumption of nuts (including peanut butter) may reduce risk for diabetes (Jiang et al. 2002), and, contrary to what would be predicted, increased intake of nuts may not result in increased weight (Alper and Mattes 2002) perhaps because of the high satiety value of nuts. Moderate alcohol intake (versus either low or high intake) has been related to improved insulin sensitivity (Bell et al. 2000) and, based on a meta-analysis of 15 observational cohort studies, with reduced risk for diabetes (Koppes et al. 2005). If alcohol is consumed, recommendations from the U.S. Department of Agriculture (USDA) *Dietary Guidelines for Americans 2005* of up to one drink per day for women and two drinks per day for men should be followed (U.S. Department of Health and Human Services and U.S. Department of Agriculture 2005).

"Western" dietary patterns, characterized by relatively high intake of red and processed meats, sweets, fried foods, and refined grains, have been associated with higher risk for type 2 diabetes than dietary patterns characterized by higher intake of vegetables, fruits, fish, poultry, and whole grains (Fung et al. 2004; Hodge et al. 2007; van Dam et al. 2002a).

Physical Activity

Physical activity is a key contributor to prevention or delay of type 2 diabetes via sustained weight loss (Hamman et al. 2006). In addition both moderate and vigorous physical activity have been associated with higher insulin sensitivity (Mayer-Davis et al. 1998), a relationship mediated partly by BMI. A meta-analysis of prospective studies of moderate-intensity physical activity and development of type 2 diabetes found a significant protective effect (relative risk 0.83) even after adjustment for BMI (Jeon et al. 2007). Of note for implementation of primary prevention programs, even regular walking (typically ≥2.5 hours/week) compared with almost no walking was significantly associated with lower risk for type 2 diabetes.

Dysfunctional Sleep

Long (more than 8 hours) and short (less than 7 hours) duration of sleep and disordered breathing during sleep (e.g., obstructive sleep apnea, snoring) have been associated with increased risk for insulin resistance and type 2 diabetes, although some differences by gender may exist (Chaput et al. 2007; Knutson et al. 2007; Spiegel et al. 2005; Tuomilehto et al. 2007, 2008). Adverse effects of abnormal sleep patterns may occur regardless of whether sleep deprivation or excess sleep is by personal choice or due to a medical condition such as obstructive sleep apnea. Knutson and colleagues (Knutson et al. 2007) reviewed three potential mechanisms, including alterations in glucose metabolism, upregulation of appetite via neuroendocrine control, and decreased energy expenditure, and found that all three contributed. In addition, increased release of pro-inflammatory cytokines due to stress hypoxia in obstructive sleep apnea may contribute to insulin resistance and type 2 diabetes (Alam et al. 2007). Although dysfunctional sleep patterns are potentially promising as an approach to prevention of type 2 diabetes, to date there have been no clinical trials in which alterations in sleep patterns have been used for this purpose.

Smoking

Smoking has been identified as a risk factor for type 2 diabetes in several prospective cohorts (van Dam 2003). Increased number of cigarettes and consumption of nicotine and tar were recently associated with increased risk for type 2 diabetes (Meisinger et al. 2006), although potential mechanisms are not clear. Smoking has also been associated with insulin resistance, although studies have been inconsistent (Reaven and Tsao 2003). Caution may be in order when one reviews these observational studies, however, because insufficient control for potential confounding by negative health behaviors that may co-occur with smoking may have led to some degree of overestimation of the adverse impact of smoking on risk of type 2 diabetes (van Dam 2003). Further, a large clinical trial of the effect of changes in lifestyle habits on parameters of the metabolic syndrome showed some negative effects for smoking cessation, including increases in insulin concentration, waist circumference, and BMI in men as well as increases in waist circumference and BMI among women (Balkau et al. 2006).

Depression

Depression has been associated with type 2 diabetes, but it is not clear whether this represents a true etiologic risk factor or primarily a response to obesity or the challenges of living with diabetes (Iafusco et al. 2002; Talbot and Nouwen 2000). Rubin and Peyrot have reviewed this topic (Rubin and Peyrot 2002) and call for new research to clarify this issue. In their opinion, although depression may confer some degree of excess diabetes risk based on biological pathways, this is most likely to occur among individuals otherwise at high risk by virtue of other well-documented risk factors such as obesity, family history, or inactivity.

■ Risk Factors from Early in Life

Several risk factors for type 2 diabetes that operate during fetal life or soon after birth have been described. Although the amount of diabetes in adulthood that can be attributed uniquely to such exposures is probably small, they all appear to act through increasing the risk of obesity at early ages.

Birth Weight

Being either small or large for gestational age is associated with the development of type 2 diabetes later in life (Hales et al. 1991; Valdez et al. 1994; McCance et al. 1994; Dabelea et al. 1999). The association between low birth weight and type 2 diabetes has been explained as representing long-term effects of nutritional deprivation in utero, through biological programming, on future risk of diabetes (the "thrifty phenotype" hypothesis) (Hales and Barker 1992). The highest risk is typically among adults who were small at birth and became overweight during childhood and early adulthood (Ong et al. 2000).

The alternative hypothesis is that the association between low birth weight and type 2 diabetes follows from pleiotropic effects of genes that influence both fetal growth and susceptibility to diabetes (McCarthy 1998). Fetuses that carry the heterozygous mutation in the glucokinase gene responsible for the development of one form of maturity-onset diabetes of the young (MODY 2) are also approximately half a kilogram lighter at birth than their unaffected siblings (Hattersley et al. 1998). Compared with the normal population, these individuals are of low birth weight only when they inherit the mutation from their father. A similar association among paternal, but not maternal, type 2 diabetes, low birth weight, and type 2 diabetes in offspring was reported in Pima Indians (Lindsay et al. 2000).

In Utero Exposure to Diabetes

Offspring whose mothers had diabetes during pregnancy, either preexisting or gestational diabetes, are seven times as likely to develop impaired glucose tolerance (Silverman et al. 1991) and 32 times as likely to develop type 2 diabetes (Pettitt et al. 1988) later in life as are the offspring of mothers without diabetes. By the age of 20–24 years type 2 diabetes is present in 45.5% of the Pima Indian offspring of mothers with diabetes, compared with 8.6% and 1.4% in the respective offspring of prediabetic mothers and mothers without diabetes (Pettitt 1985). The higher rate of diabetes in these offspring is only partially mediated by the earlier development of obesity (Pettitt 1985). Although these offspring have increased genetic susceptibility for the disease, within the same family, siblings born after a mother's diagnosis of diabetes have over three times the risk of developing diabetes at an early age as those born before the diagnosis of diabetes in the mother (Dabelea et al. 2000). These data suggest that exposure to the diabetic intrauterine environment, with alterations of fetal fuels, predisposes the child to the development of diabetes later in life, an effect that is in addition to any inherited susceptibility genes.

Exposure to intrauterine maternal hyperglycemia was the strongest (odds ratio 10.4; 95% confidence interval 4.4–25.1, $p < 0.0001$) single risk factor for type 2 diabetes in Pima Indian youth (Dabelea et al. 1998). As of 1996 the diabetic pregnancy accounted for almost 40% of diabetes in the offspring (Dabelea et al. 1998). It has been suggested that a vicious cycle results, explaining at least in part the increase in type 2 diabetes seen over the past several decades (Dabelea et al. 1998). That the vicious cycle of the diabetic pregnancy may be operating in racial/ethnic groups other than American Indians is possible, but this question has not yet been adequately investigated. Initial data from the SEARCH for Diabetes in Youth Case-Control Study suggest that exposure to maternal diabetes in utero is strongly associated with type 2 diabetes in various subpopulations of youth, including African Americans, Hispanics, and non-Hispanic whites, with a magnitude of effect similar to that seen among Pima Indians (Dabelea et al. 2008).

Diet in Early Infancy

Recent meta-analyses primarily drawing from white populations concluded that having been breast-fed is associated with 13%–22% reduced odds for overweight or obesity later in life (Owen et al. 2005; Arenz et al. 2004) in a dose-dependent fashion (Harder et al. 2005). Both behavioral and metabolic explanations for the apparent benefit of breast-feeding on later development of obesity have been proposed (Hall 1975; Lucas et al. 1980).

Among adults, breast-feeding in infancy has been associated with reduced risk of type 2 diabetes (Owen et al. 2006). Studies in young Native American populations have shown that individuals with type 2 diabetes were less likely to have been breast-fed as infants than were those without type 2 diabetes (Pettitt et al. 1997; Young et al. 2002). Recently, the SEARCH Case-Control Study reported similar results in a group of youth of non-Hispanic white, Hispanic, and African American origin (Mayer-Davis et al. 2008), a result that was attenuated after inclusion of attained childhood weight status. These data suggest that breast-feeding may protect against the development of type 2 diabetes regardless of race/ethnicity, a degree of protection that is mediated in part by attained weight status later in life.

■ Demographic, Social, and Community Factors

The prevalence of diabetes in the United States is higher among African American, Hispanic, Asian and Pacific Islander, and American Indian populations than among non-Hispanic white populations (Dagogo-Jack 2003; Egede and Dagogo-Jack 2005; Kurian and Cardarelli 2007; Mokdad et al. 2003). In addition, lower socioeconomic position has been associated with increased prevalence of type 2 disease (Mokdad et al. 2003) (Agardh et al. 2007) and of the metabolic syndrome, particularly among women (Loucks et al. 2007). Food insecurity, defined as inadequate access to food due to inadequate household income, also has been associated with increased prevalence of type 2 diabetes, even after adjustment for a variety of sociodemographic factors, for physical activity, and for BMI (Seligman et al. 2007).

Of critical importance to diabetes prevention is a realization that both minority and lower-socioeconomic-position groups have been disproportionately affected by the obesity epidemic. Associations of overweight and obesity with socioeconomic position are quite complex and vary according to race/ethnicity, gender, whether the setting is in a developed country or a developing country, and over time, as recently reviewed (Ball and Crawford 2005; McLaren 2007; Parikh et al. 2007). Both individual- and community-level markers of socioeconomic position are important (Robert and Reither 2004; Wang et al. 2007). In developing countries it is first important to note that despite the presence of hunger and inadequate nutrition, obesity is emerging as a real public health threat, particularly in more urbanized regions (Prentice 2006). Within low-development countries indicators of higher socioeconomic position are associated with higher obesity, whereas the reverse is true in more developed countries (McLaren 2007). Interestingly this contrast is observed to a lesser extent in more recent studies than in older studies, and this difference has been attributed to the influence of globalization.

In the United States studies consistently show a marked racial/ethnic difference in obesity among women and much smaller racial/ethnic differences among men (Wang et al. 2007). These differences by race or ethnicity are explained in part by socioeconomic position, with lower socioeconomic position associated with a higher prevalence of obesity. However among African American women, those with less than a high school education had a lower prevalence of obesity than those with higher educational attainment. The literature regarding the impact of socioeconomic position on weight change among men and women of different races/ethnicities is inconsistent but provides some support for increased rates of weight gain in the setting of lower socioeconomic position (Ball and Crawford 2005; Baltrus et al. 2005; Bennett, Wolin, and James 2007).

Geographic variation in the prevalence of both obesity and diabetes in the United States has been documented (Ford et al. 2005; Mokdad et al. 2003), and it is not clear what specific characteristics of regions of the country, or communities, contribute to variation in risk. In terms of preventing diabetes, coherent analysis and development of prevention strategies will benefit from an ecologic perspective (see Fig. 3.1) for the most effective intervention.

■ Gestational Diabetes: Are the Risk Factors the Same
   as Those for Type 2 Diabetes?

GDM, which is defined as glucose intolerance with onset or first recognition during pregnancy, includes women whose glucose intolerance may have been present but was unrecognized prior to pregnancy (American Diabetes Association 2007). Risk factors for GDM are similar to those for type 2 diabetes. Among the numerous risk factors for GDM are older maternal age; maternal low birth weight (< 2500 gm); being Hispanic, African, Native American, Asian, or Pacific Islander (when compared with non-Hispanic white women); high pre-gravid BMI (overweight or obese); having characteristics of the metabolic syndrome; having polycystic ovary syndrome; smoking; having a first-degree relative with diabetes; being exposed to diabetes in utero; having a previous macrosomic baby; and carrying a large-for-gestational-age fetus in the current pregnancy (Bottalico 2007; Egeland, Skjaerven, and Irgenns 2000; Solomon et al. 1997). There may also be genetic determinants of GDM, but at this time it is uncertain whether they are different from and independent of those associated with type 2 diabetes (Watanabe et al. 2007).

Women with a history of GDM are at increased risk for future occurrence of GDM, prediabetes (impaired glucose tolerance and impaired fasting glucose), and developing type 2 diabetes. β-Cell defects in GDM result from autoimmune disease, monogenic causes, and insulin resistance, the same cadre of conditions that cause other forms of hyperglycemia (Buchanan et al. 2007). Recurrence of GDM in a subsequent pregnancy is quite common, particularly for women from minority populations. The rate of recurrence has been estimated to be 30% to 84%, depending upon the study population (Kim, Berger, and Chamany 2007). Women who have GDM are at high risk of developing type 2 diabetes in the future, with estimates from a recent review ranging from 3% to 70% after follow-up from 6 weeks to 28 years (Kim, Newton, and Knopp 2002). The development of type 2 diabetes occurred fairly rapidly in the first years after a GDM-affected pregnancy and then leveled off. Among women with GDM who participated in the Diabetes Prevention Program, both the lifestyle intervention and metformin reduced risk for development of type 2 diabetes.

The debate continues about whether GDM is a unique disease state or whether pregnancy with its associated metabolic challenges is a litmus test that identifies women who are susceptible to hyperglycemia and subsequent development of diabetes. Ultimately, the strong association between GDM and diabetes provides women, their health care providers, and the public health community with a significant incentive to take action to improve the health of women with a history of GDM.

■ Summary and Conclusions

The context and key risk factors for type 2 diabetes, and the opportunities for primary prevention, are given in summary form at the beginning of this chapter under "Key Public Health Messages." Type 2 diabetes is a complex disease, driven by a multitude of genetic, environmental, and behavioral factors, which is rapidly emerging as one of the most critical public health threats of our time. There is, however, reason for optimism with a dose of realism. Opportunities for primary prevention derive from the clear and compelling evidence that sustained, moderate weight loss can markedly reduce risk for development of type 2 diabetes. To reverse the direction of the type 2 epidemic, it appears necessary to reverse the direction of the epidemic of obesity worldwide and to do so effectively across all ages. Consistent with a philosophy of an ecologic approach to disease prevention and health promotion, this will require multiple strategies at the individual, family, and community levels. Success will likely demand sustained efforts across the scientific, medical, educational, industrial, and political arenas.

■ References

Agardh EE et al. (2007). Socio-economic position at three points in life in association with type 2 diabetes and impaired glucose tolerance in middle-aged Swedish men and women. *International Journal of Epidemiology* **36**, 84–92.

Alam I et al. (2007). Obesity, metabolic syndrome and sleep apnoea: all pro-inflammatory states. *Obesity Reviews* **8**, 119–27.

Alper CM, Mattes RD. (2002). Effects of chronic peanut consumption on energy balance and hedonics. *International Journal of Obesity and Related Metabolic Disorders* **26**, 1129–37.

American Diabetes Association (2007). Diagnosis and classification of diabetes mellitus. *Diabetes Care* **30** (Suppl. 1), S42–7.

Andre P et al. (2007). Gamma-glutamyltransferase activity and development of the metabolic syndrome (International Diabetes Federation Definition) in middle-aged men and women: data from the Epidemiological Study on the Insulin Resistance Syndrome (DESIR) cohort. *Diabetes Care* **30**, 2355–61.

Arenz S et al. (2004). Breast-feeding and childhood obesity—a systematic review. *International Journal of Obesity and Related Metabolic Disorders.* **28**, 1247–56.

Arita Y et al. (1999). Paradoxical decrease of an adipose-specific protein, adiponectin, in obesity. *Biochemical and Biophysical Research Communications* **257**, 79–83.

Balkau B et al. (2006). The impact of 3-year changes in lifestyle habits on metabolic syndrome parameters: the DESIR study. *European Journal of Cardiovascular Prevention and Rehabilitation* **13**, 334–40.

Ball K, Crawford D (2005). Socioeconomic status and weight change in adults: a review. *Social Science & Medicine* **60**, 1987–2010.

Baltrus PT et al. (2005). Race/ethnicity, life-course socioeconomic position, and body weight trajectories over 34 years: the Alameda County Study. *American Journal of Public Health* **95**, 1595–601.

Bell RA et al. (2000). Associations between alcohol consumption and insulin sensitivity and cardiovascular disease risk factors: the Insulin Resistance and Atherosclerosis Study. *Diabetes Care* **23**, 1630–6.

Bennett GG, Wolin KY, James SA. (2007). Lifecourse socioeconomic position and weight change among blacks: the Pitt County study. *Obesity (Silver Spring)* **15**, 172–81.

Bottalico JN (2007). Recurrent gestational diabetes: risk factors, diagnosis, management, and implications. *Seminars in Perinatology.* **31**, 176–84.

Bray GA, Bellanger T (2006). Epidemiology, trends, and morbidities of obesity and the metabolic syndrome. *Endocrine* **29**, 109–17.

Buchanan TA et al. (2007). What is gestational diabetes? *Diabetes Care* **30** (Suppl. 2), S105–11.

Burchard EG et al. (2003). The importance of race and ethnic background in biomedical research and clinical practice. *New England Journal of Medicine* **348**, 1170–5.

Burnet DL et al. (2006). Preventing diabetes in the clinical setting. *Journal of General Internal Medicine* **21**, 84–93.

Chaput JP et al. (2007). Association of sleep duration with type 2 diabetes and impaired glucose tolerance. *Diabetologia* **50**, 2298–304.

Chiasson JL et al. (2002). Acarbose for prevention of type 2 diabetes mellitus: the STOP-NIDDM randomised trial. *Lancet* **359**, 2072–7.

Cho YM et al. (2006). Plasma retinol-binding protein-4 concentrations are elevated in human subjects with impaired glucose tolerance and type 2 diabetes. *Diabetes Care* **29**, 2457–61.

Choi HK et al. (2005). Dairy consumption and risk of type 2 diabetes mellitus in men: a prospective study. *Archives of Internal Medicine* **165**, 997–1003.

Comuzzie AG et al. (2001). The genetic basis of plasma variation in adiponectin, a global endophenotype for obesity and the metabolic syndrome. *Journal of Clinical Endocrinology and Metabolism* **86**, 4321–5.

Cooper RS (2003). Race, genes, and health—new wine in old bottles? *International Journal of Epidemiology* **32**, 23–5.

Cooper RS, Kaufman JS, Ward R. (2003). Race and genomics. *New England Journal of Medicine.* **348**, 1166–70.

Craig RL, Chu WS, Elbein SC (2007). Retinol binding protein 4 as a candidate gene for type 2 diabetes and prediabetic intermediate traits. *Molecular Genetics and Metabolism* **90**, 338–44.

Dabelea D et al. (1998). Increasing prevalence of Type II diabetes in American Indian children. *Diabetologia* **41**, 904–10.

Dabelea D et al. (1999). Birth weight, type 2 diabetes, and insulin resistance in Pima Indian children and young adults. *Diabetes Care* **22**, 944–50.

Dabelea D et al. (2000). Intrauterine exposure to diabetes conveys risks for type 2 diabetes and obesity: a study of discordant sibships. *Diabetes* **49**, 2208–11.

Dagogo-Jack S (2003). Ethnic disparities in type 2 diabetes: pathophysiology and implications for prevention and management. *Journal of the National Medical Association* **95**, 774, 779–89.

Dabelea D et al. (2008). Association of intrauterine exposure to maternal diabetes and obesity with type 2 diabetes in youth: SEARCH Case-Control Study. *Diabetes Care* **31**, 1422–6.

Dahlman I et al. (2005). A unique role of monocyte chemoattractant protein 1 among chemokines in adipose tissue of obese subjects. *Journal of Clinical Endocrinology and Metabolism* **90**, 5834–40.

Edelstein SL et al. (1997). Predictors of progression from impaired glucose tolerance to NIDDM: an analysis of six prospective studies. *Diabetes* **46**, 701–10.

Egede LE, Dagogo-Jack S (2005). Epidemiology of type 2 diabetes: focus on ethnic minorities. *Medical Clinics of North America* **89**, 949–75, viii.

Egeland GM, Skjaerven R, Irgens LM (2000). Birth characteristics of women who develop gestational diabetes: population based study. *British Medical Journal* **321**, 546–7.

Elbein SC, Wegner K, Kahn SE (2000). Reduced B-cell compensation to the insulin resistance associated with obesity in members of Caucasian familial type 2 diabetic kindred. *Diabetes Care* **23**, 221–7.

Engelgau MM et al. (2004). Prevention of type 2 diabetes: issues and strategies for identifying persons for interventions. *Diabetes Technology & Therapeutics* **6**, 874–82.

Ferrannini E et al. (2004). Mode of onset of type 2 diabetes from normal or impaired glucose tolerance. *Diabetes* **53**, 160–5.

Festa A et al. (2000). Chronic subclinical inflammation as part of the insulin resistance syndrome: the Insulin Resistance Atherosclerosis Study (IRAS). *Circulation* **102**, 42–7.

Flegal KM et al. (2002). Prevalence and trends in obesity among US adults, 1999–2000. *JAMA* **288**, 1723–7.

Ford ES (2005). Risks for all-cause mortality, cardiovascular disease, and diabetes associated with the metabolic syndrome: a summary of the evidence. *Diabetes Care* **28**, 1769–78.

Ford ES et al. (2005). Geographic variation in the prevalence of obesity, diabetes, and obesity-related behaviors. *Obesity Research* **13**, 118–22.

Foster GD et al. (2003). A randomized trial of a low-carbohydrate diet for obesity. *New England Journal of Medicine* **348**, 2082–90.

Franz MJ et al. (2002). Evidence-based nutrition principles and recommendations for the treatment and prevention of diabetes and related complications. *Diabetes Care* **25**, 148–98.

Fullilove MT (1998). Comment: abandoning "race" as a variable in public health research—an idea whose time has come. *American Journal of Public Health* **88**, 1297–8.

Fung TT et al. (2004). Dietary patterns, meat intake, and the risk of type 2 diabetes in women. *Archives of Internal Medicine* **164**, 2235–40.

Gebbie K (2003). *Who Will Keep the Public Healthy? Educating Public Health Professionals for the 21st Century*. Washington, DC: National Academy Press.

Grant SF et al. (2006). Variant of transcription factor 7-like 2 (TCF7L2) gene confers risk of type 2 diabetes. *Nature Genetics* **38**, 320–3.

Groop LC et al. (1991). The role of free fatty acid metabolism in the pathogenesis of insulin resistance in obesity and noninsulin-dependent diabetes mellitus. *Journal of Clinical Endocrinology and Metabolism* **72**, 96–107.

Guldiken S et al. (2007). The levels of circulating markers of atherosclerosis and inflammation in subjects with different degrees of body mass index: soluble CD40 ligand and high-sensitivity C-reactive protein. *Thrombosis Research* **119**, 79–84.

Haffner SM et al. (1996). A prospective analysis of the HOMA model. The Mexico City Diabetes Study. *Diabetes Care* **19**, 1138–41.

Hales CN, Barker DJ (1992). Type 2 (non-insulin-dependent) diabetes mellitus: the thrifty phenotype hypothesis. *Diabetologia* **35**, 595–601.

Hales CN et al. (1991). Fetal and infant growth and impaired glucose tolerance at age 64. *British Medical Journal* **303**, 1019–22.

Hall B (1975). Changing composition of human milk and early development of an appetite control. *Lancet* **1**, 779–81.

Hamman RF et al. (2006). Effect of weight loss with lifestyle intervention on risk of diabetes. *Diabetes Care* **29**, 2102–7.

Hanson R et al. (2000). Evaluation of simple indices of insulin sensitivity and insulin secretion for use in epidemiologic studies. *American Journal of Epidemiology* **151**, 190–8.

Hanson RL et al. (2002). Components of the "metabolic syndrome" and incidence of type 2 diabetes. *Diabetes* **51**, 3120–7.

Harder T et al. (2005). Duration of breastfeeding and risk of overweight: a meta-analysis. *American Journal of Epidemiology* **162**, 397–403.

Hattersley AT et al. (1998). Mutations in the glucokinase gene of the fetus result in reduced birth weight. *Nature Genetics* **19**, 268–70.

Heymsfield SB et al. (2000). Effects of weight loss with orlistat on glucose tolerance and progression to type 2 diabetes in obese adults. *Archives of Internal Medicine* **160**, 1321–6.

Hodge AM et al. (2004). Glycemic index and dietary fiber and the risk of type 2 diabetes. *Diabetes Care* **27**, 2701–6.

Hodge AM et al. (2007). Dietary patterns and diabetes incidence in the Melbourne Collaborative Cohort Study. *American Journal of Epidemiology* **165**, 603–10.

Houstis N, Rosen ED, Lander ES (2006). Reactive oxygen species have a causal role in multiple forms of insulin resistance. *Nature* **440**, 944–8.

Hu FB et al. (2001). Diet, lifestyle, and the risk of type 2 diabetes mellitus in women. *New England Journal of Medicine* **345**, 790–7.

Hu FB et al. (2004). Inflammatory markers and risk of developing type 2 diabetes in women. *Diabetes* **53**, 693–700.

Iafusco D et al. (2002). Permanent diabetes mellitus in the first year of life. *Diabetologia* **45**, 798–804.

Jeon CY et al. (2007). Physical activity of moderate intensity and risk of type 2 diabetes: a systematic review. *Diabetes Care* **30**, 744–52.

Jiang R et al. (2002). Nut and peanut butter consumption and risk of type 2 diabetes in women. *JAMA* **288**, 2554–60.

Kahn SE, Hull RL, Utzschneider KM (2006). Mechanisms linking obesity to insulin resistance and type 2 diabetes. *Nature* **444**, 840–6.

Karter AJ. (2003). Commentary: race, genetics, and disease—in search of a middle ground. *International Journal of Epidemiology* **32**, 26–8.

Kim C, Berger DK, Chamany S (2007). Recurrence of gestational diabetes mellitus: a systematic review. *Diabetes Care* **30**, 1314–9.

Kim C, Newton KM, Knopp RH (2002). Gestational diabetes and the incidence of type 2 diabetes: a systematic review. *Diabetes Care* **25**, 1862–8.

Klein S et al. (2004). Weight management through lifestyle modification for the prevention and management of type 2 diabetes: rationale and strategies: a statement of the American Diabetes Association, the North American Association for the Study of Obesity, and the American Society for Clinical Nutrition. *Diabetes Care* **27**, 2067–73.

Knutson KL et al. (2007). The metabolic consequences of sleep deprivation. *Sleep Medicine Reviews* **11**, 163–78.

Koppes LL et al. (2005). Moderate alcohol consumption lowers the risk of type 2 diabetes: a meta-analysis of prospective observational studies. *Diabetes Care* **28**, 719–25.

Kotronen A et al. (2007). Liver fat in the metabolic syndrome. *Journal of Clinical Endocrinology and Metabolism* **92**, 3490–7.

Kurian AK, Cardarelli KM (2007). Racial and ethnic differences in cardiovascular disease risk factors: a systematic review. *Ethnicity and Disease* **17**, 143–52.

Lee DH et al. (2004). gamma-Glutamyltransferase, obesity, and the risk of type 2 diabetes: observational cohort study among 20,158 middle-aged men and women. *Journal of Clinical Endocrinology and Metabolism* **89**, 5410–4.

Li C et al. (2007). Increasing trends in waist circumference and abdominal obesity among US adults. *Obesity (Silver Spring)* **15**, 216–24.

Liese AD et al. (2003). Whole-grain intake and insulin sensitivity: the Insulin Resistance Atherosclerosis Study. *American Journal of Clinical Nutrition* **78**, 965–71.

Liese AD et al. (2005). Dietary glycemic index and glycemic load, carbohydrate and fiber intake, and measures of insulin sensitivity, secretion, and adiposity in the Insulin Resistance Atherosclerosis Study. *Diabetes Care* **28**, 2832–8.

Lillioja S et al. (1993). Insulin resistance and insulin secretory dysfunction as precursors of non-insulin-dependent diabetes mellitus. Prospective studies of Pima Indians. *New England Journal of Medicine* **329**, 1988–92.

Lindsay RS et al. (2000). Type 2 diabetes and low birth weight: the role of paternal inheritance in the association of low birth weight and diabetes. *Diabetes* **49**, 445–9.

Liu S et al. (2007). A prospective study of inflammatory cytokines and diabetes mellitus in a multiethnic cohort of postmenopausal women. *Archives of Internal Medicine* **167**, 1676–85.

Lopez-Ridaura R et al. (2004). Magnesium intake and risk of type 2 diabetes in men and women. *Diabetes Care* **27**, 134–40.

Loucks EB et al. (2007). Socioeconomic disparities in metabolic syndrome differ by gender: evidence from NHANES III. *Annals of Epidemiology* **17**, 19–26.

Lucas A et al. (1980). Breast vs bottle: endocrine responses are different with formula feeding. *Lancet* 1, 1267–9.

Ma B et al. (2006). Dairy, magnesium, and calcium intake in relation to insulin sensitivity: approaches to modeling a dose-dependent association. *American Journal of Epidemiology* 164, 449–58.

Mayer-Davis EJ et al. (1997). Dietary fat and insulin sensitivity in a triethnic population: the role of obesity. The Insulin Resistance Atherosclerosis Study (IRAS). *American Journal of Clinical Nutrition* 65, 79–87.

Mayer-Davis EJ et al. (1998). Intensity and amount of physical activity in relation to insulin sensitivity: the Insulin Resistance Atherosclerosis Study. *JAMA* 279, 669–74.

Mayer-Davis EJ et al. (2002). Plasma and dietary vitamin E in relation to incidence of type 2 diabetes: the Insulin Resistance and Atherosclerosis Study (IRAS). *Diabetes Care* 25, 2172–7.

Mayer-Davis EJ et al. (2006). Towards understanding of glycaemic index and glycaemic load in habitual diet: associations with measures of glycaemia in the Insulin Resistance Atherosclerosis Study. *British Journal of Nutrition* 95, 397–405.

Mayer-Davis EJ et al. (2008). Breast-feeding and type 2 diabetes in the youth of three ethnic groups: the SEARCH for diabetes in youth case-control study. *Diabetes Care* 31, 470–5.

McCance DR et al. (1994). Birth weight and non-insulin dependent diabetes: thrifty genotype, thrifty phenotype, or surviving small baby genotype? *British Medical Journal* 308, 942–5.

McCarthy M (1998). Weighing in on diabetes risk. *Nature Genetics* 19, 209–10.

McLaren L (2007). Socioeconomic status and obesity. *Epidemiologic Reviews* 29, 29–48.

McLaughlin T et al. (2002). Differentiation between obesity and insulin resistance in the association with C-reactive protein. *Circulation* 106, 2908–12.

McManus K, Antinoro L, Sacks F (2001). A randomized controlled trial of a moderate-fat, low-energy diet compared with a low fat, low-energy diet for weight loss in overweight adults. *International Journal of Obesity and Related Metabolic Disorders* 25, 1503–11.

Meigs JB et al. (2006). Hemostatic markers of endothelial dysfunction and risk of incident type 2 diabetes: the Framingham Offspring Study. *Diabetes* 55, 530–7.

Meigs JB et al. (2007a). Association of oxidative stress, insulin resistance, and diabetes risk phenotypes: the Framingham Offspring Study. *Diabetes Care* 30, 2529–35.

Meigs JB et al. (2007b). Impact of insulin resistance on risk of type 2 diabetes and cardiovascular disease in people with metabolic syndrome. *Diabetes Care* 30, 1219–25.

Meisinger C et al. (2006). Association of cigarette smoking and tar and nicotine intake with development of type 2 diabetes mellitus in men and women from the general population: the MONICA/KORA Augsburg Cohort Study. *Diabetologia* 49, 1770–6.

Meyer KA et al. (2000). Carbohydrates, dietary fiber, and incident type 2 diabetes in older women. *American Journal of Clinical Nutrition* 71, 921–30.

Meyer KA et al. (2001). Dietary fat and incidence of type 2 diabetes in older Iowa women. *Diabetes Care* **24**, 1528–35.

Misra A, Ganda OP (2007). Migration and its impact on adiposity and type 2 diabetes. *Nutrition* **23**, 696–708.

Mokdad AH et al. (2003). Prevalence of obesity, diabetes, and obesity-related health risk factors, 2001. *JAMA* **289**, 76–9.

Moore LL et al. (2000). Can sustained weight loss in overweight individuals reduce the risk of diabetes mellitus? *Epidemiology* **11**, 269–73.

Munkhtulga L et al. (2007). Identification of a regulatory SNP in the retinol binding protein 4 gene associated with type 2 diabetes in Mongolia. *Human Genetics.* **120**, 879–88.

Ogden CL et al. (2006). Prevalence of overweight and obesity in the United States, 1999–2004. *JAMA* **295**, 1549–55.

Ong KK et al. (2000). Association between postnatal catch-up growth and obesity in childhood: prospective cohort study. *British Medical Journal* **320**, 967–71.

Owen CG et al. (2005). Effect of infant feeding on the risk of obesity across the life course: a quantitative review of published evidence. *Pediatrics* **115**, 1367–77.

Owen CG et al. (2006). Does breastfeeding influence risk of type 2 diabetes in later life? A quantitative analysis of published evidence. *American Journal of Clinical Nutrition* **84**, 1043–54.

Panagiotakos DB et al. (2005). The implication of obesity and central fat on markers of chronic inflammation: the ATTICA study. *Atherosclerosis* **183**, 308–15.

Pankow JS et al. (2004). Fasting plasma free fatty acids and risk of type 2 diabetes: the atherosclerosis risk in communities study. *Diabetes Care* **27**, 77–82.

Parikh NI et al. (2007). Increasing trends in incidence of overweight and obesity over 5 decades. *American Journal of Medicine* **120**, 242–50.

Paynter NP et al. (2006). Coffee and sweetened beverage consumption and the risk of type 2 diabetes mellitus: the atherosclerosis risk in communities study. *American Journal of Epidemiology* **164**, 1075–84.

Pearson WS (2007). Ten-year comparison of estimates of overweight and obesity, diagnosed diabetes and use of office-based physician services for treatment of diabetes in the United States. *Preventive Medicine* **45**, 353–7.

Pettitt DJ et al. (1985). High plasma glucose concentrations in normal weight offspring of diabetic women (Abstract). *Diabetes Research and Clinical Practice* S445.

Pettitt DJ et al. (1988). Congenital susceptibility to NIDDM. Role of intrauterine environment. *Diabetes* **37**, 622–8.

Pettitt DJ et al. (1997). Breastfeeding and incidence of non-insulin-dependent diabetes mellitus in Pima Indians. *Lancet* **350**, 166–8.

Pi-Sunyer FX (2007). How effective are lifestyle changes in the prevention of type 2 diabetes mellitus? *Nutrition Reviews* **65**, 101–10.

Poykko SM et al. (2003). Low plasma ghrelin is associated with insulin resistance, hypertension, and the prevalence of type 2 diabetes. *Diabetes* **52**, 2546–53.

Pradhan AD et al. (2001). C-reactive protein, interleukin 6, and risk of developing type 2 diabetes mellitus. *JAMA* **286**, 327–34.

Prentice AM (2006). The emerging epidemic of obesity in developing countries. *International Journal of Epidemiology* **35**, 93–9.

Qi L, Rifai N, Hu FB (2007). Interleukin-6 receptor gene variations, plasma interleukin-6 levels, and type 2 diabetes in US women. *Diabetes* **56**, 3075–81.

Reaven G, Tsao PS (2003). Insulin resistance and compensatory hyperinsulinemia: the key player between cigarette smoking and cardiovascular disease? *Journal of the American College of Cardiology* **41**, 1044–7.

Robert SA, Reither EN (2004). A multilevel analysis of race, community disadvantage, and body mass index among adults in the US. *Social Science & Medicine* **59**, 2421–34.

Rosolova H, Mayer O Jr, Reaven GM (2000). Insulin-mediated glucose disposal is decreased in normal subjects with relatively low plasma magnesium concentrations. *Metabolism* **49**, 418–20.

Rotimi CN (2003). Genetic ancestry tracing and the African identity: a double-edged sword? *Developing World Bioethics* **3**, 151–8.

Rubin RR, Peyrot M. (2002). Was Willis right? Thoughts on the interaction of depression and diabetes. *Diabetes/Metabolism Research and Reviews* **18**, 173–5.

Sakkinen PA et al. (2000). Clustering of procoagulation, inflammation, and fibrinolysis variables with metabolic factors in insulin resistance syndrome. *American Journal of Epidemiology* **152**, 897–907.

Salmeron J et al. (1997). Dietary fiber, glycemic load, and risk of non-insulin dependent diabetes in women. *JAMA* **277**, 472–7.

Sanchez M et al. (1997). Oral calcium supplementation reduces intraplatelet free calcium concentration and insulin resistance in essential hypertensive patients. *Hypertension* **29**, 531–6.

Schmidt MI et al. (1999). Markers of inflammation and prediction of diabetes mellitus in adults (Atherosclerosis Risk in Communities study): a cohort study. *Lancet* **353**, 1649–52.

Schmidt MI et al. (2006). Leptin and incident type 2 diabetes: risk or protection? *Diabetologia* **49**, 2086-96.

Schrager S. (2005). Dietary calcium intake and obesity. *Journal of the American Board of Family Practice.* **18**, 205–10.

Schulze MB et al. (2004a). Glycemic index, glycemic load, and dietary fiber intake and incidence of type 2 diabetes in younger and middle-aged women. *American Journal of Clinical Nutrition* **80**, 348–56.

Schulze MB et al. (2004b). Sugar-sweetened beverages, weight gain, and incidence of type 2 diabetes in young and middle-aged women. *JAMA* **292**, 927–34.

Seligman HK et al. (2007). Food insecurity is associated with diabetes mellitus: results from the National Health Examination and Nutrition Examination Survey (NHANES) 1999–2002. *Journal of General Internal Medicine* **22**, 1018–23.

Sheard NF et al. (2004). Dietary carbohydrate (amount and type) in the prevention and management of diabetes: a statement by the American Diabetes Association. *Diabetes Care* **27**, 2266–71.

Silverman BL et al. (1991). Long-term prospective evaluation of offspring of diabetic mothers. *Diabetes* **40**(Suppl. 2), 121–5.

Sjostrom L et al. (2004). Lifestyle, diabetes, and cardiovascular risk factors 10 years after bariatric surgery. *New England Journal of Medicine*. **351**, 2683–93.

Sladek R et al. (2007). A genome-wide association study identifies novel risk loci for type 2 diabetes. *Nature* **445**, 881–5.

Smedley BD, Syme SL. (2001). Promoting health: intervention strategies from social and behavioral research. *American Journal of Health Promotion* **15**, 149–66.

Solomon CG et al. (1997). A prospective study of pregravid determinants of gestational diabetes mellitus. *JAMA* **278**, 1078–83.

Song Y et al. (2004). Dietary magnesium intake in relation to plasma insulin levels and risk of type 2 diabetes in women. *Diabetes Care* **27**, 59–65.

Spiegel K et al. (2005). Sleep loss: a novel risk factor for insulin resistance and type 2 diabetes. *Journal of Applied Physiology* **99**, 2008–19.

Steinle NI et al. (2005). Variants in the ghrelin gene are associated with metabolic syndrome in the Old Order Amish. *Journal of Clinical Endocrinology and Metabolism* **90**, 6672–7.

Stern L et al. (2004). The effects of low-carbohydrate versus conventional weight loss diets in severely obese adults: one-year follow-up of a randomized trial. *Annals of Internal Medicine* **140**, 778–85.

Stern MP et al. (2004). Does the metabolic syndrome improve identification of individuals at risk of type 2 diabetes and/or cardiovascular disease? *Diabetes Care* **27**, 2676–81.

Stevens J et al. (2002). Dietary fiber intake and glycemic index and incidence of diabetes in African-American and white adults: the ARIC study. *Diabetes Care* **25**, 1715–21.

Susser M, Susser E. (1996). Choosing a future for epidemiology: II. From black box to Chinese boxes and eco-epidemiology. *American Journal of Public Health* **86**, 674–7.

Talbot F, Nouwen A. (2000). A review of the relationship between depression and diabetes in adults: is there a link? *Diabetes Care* **23**, 1556–62.

Torgerson JS et al. (2004). Xenical in the prevention of diabetes in obese subjects (XENDOS) study: a randomized study of orlistat as an adjunct to lifestyle changes for the prevention of type 2 diabetes in obese patients. *Diabetes Care* **27**, 155–61.

Tschop M, Smiley DL, Heiman ML (2000). Ghrelin induces adiposity in rodents. *Nature* **407**, 908–13.

Tuomilehto H et al. (2007). Sleep duration is associated with an increased risk for the prevalence of type 2 diabetes in middle-aged women — the FIN-D2D survey. *Sleep Medicine* **9**, 221–7.

Tuomilehto H et al. (2008). Sleep-disordered breathing is related to an increased risk for type 2 diabetes in middle-aged men, but not in women — the FIN-D2D survey. *Diabetes, Obesity & Metabolism* **10**, 468–75.

Tuomilehto J et al. (2001). Prevention of type 2 diabetes mellitus by changes in lifestyle among subjects with impaired glucose tolerance. *New England Journal of Medicine* **344**, 1343–50.

U.S. Department of Health and Human Services, U.S. Department of Agriculture (2005). *Dietary guidelines for Americans.* U.S. Government Printing Office, Washington, DC.

Ukkola O, Poykko SM, Antero KY (2006). Low plasma ghrelin concentration is an indicator of the metabolic syndrome. *Annals of Medicine* **38**, 274–9.

Valdez R et al. (1994). Birthweight and adult health outcomes in a biethnic population in the USA. *Diabetologia* **37**, 624–31.

van Dam RM (2003). The epidemiology of lifestyle and risk for type 2 diabetes. *European Journal of Epidemiology* **18**, 1115–25.

van Dam RM et al. (2002a). Dietary patterns and risk for type 2 diabetes mellitus in U.S. men. *Annals of Internal Medicine* **136**, 201–9.

van Dam RM et al. (2002b). Dietary fat and meat intake in relation to risk of type 2 diabetes in men. *Diabetes Care* **25**, 417–24.

Vessby B et al. (2001). Substituting dietary saturated for monounsaturated fat impairs insulin sensitivity in healthy men and women: The KANWU Study. *Diabetologia* **44**, 312–9.

Vita JA et al. (2004). Brachial artery vasodilator function and systemic inflammation in the Framingham Offspring Study. *Circulation* **110**, 3604–9.

Wang MC et al. (2007). Socioeconomic and food-related physical characteristics of the neighbourhood environment are associated with body mass index. *Journal of Epidemiology and Community Health* **61**, 491–8.

Wannamethee SG et al. (2007). Adipokines and risk of type 2 diabetes in older men. *Diabetes Care* **30**, 1200–5.

Watanabe RM et al. (2007). Genetics of gestational diabetes mellitus and type 2 diabetes. *Diabetes Care* **30** (Suppl. 2), S134–40.

Weyer C et al. (2002). Humoral markers of inflammation and endothelial dysfunction in relation to adiposity and in vivo insulin action in Pima Indians. *Atherosclerosis* **161**, 233–42.

Wilson PW et al. (2005). Metabolic syndrome as a precursor of cardiovascular disease and type 2 diabetes mellitus. *Circulation* **112**, 3066–72.

Wilson PW et al. (2007). Prediction of incident diabetes mellitus in middle-aged adults: the Framingham Offspring Study. *Archives of Internal Medicine* **167**, 1068–74.

Wren AM et al. (2001). Ghrelin enhances appetite and increases food intake in humans. *Journal of Clinical Endocrinology and Metabolism* **86**, 5992.

Yang Q et al. (2005). Serum retinol binding protein 4 contributes to insulin resistance in obesity and type 2 diabetes. *Nature* **436**, 356–62.

Young TK et al. (2002). Type 2 diabetes mellitus in children: prenatal and early infancy risk factors among native Canadians. *Archives of Pediatrics and Adolescent Medicine* **156**, 651–55.

Zeggini E et al. (2007). Replication of genome-wide association signals in UK samples reveals risk loci for type 2 diabetes. *Science* **316**, 1336–41.

4. NON-TYPE 2 DIABETES

Prevalence, Incidence, and Risk Factors

Ingrid M. Libman, Ronald E. LaPorte, Astrid M. Libman,
and Pablo Arias

■ Main Public Health Messages

- Non-type 2 diabetes, which in addition to type 1 disease includes maturity-onset diabetes of youth, neonatal diabetes, diabetes associated with exocrine pancreatic disease, drug- and toxin-induced diabetes mellitus, and diabetes associated with other genetic syndromes, may account for less than 10% of all cases of diabetes in the United States, but its profound impact should not be underestimated.
- Among U.S. children type 1 continues to be the major type of diabetes; its appearance early in life imposes considerable demands on children, their families, and society, and for patients, it marks the beginning of a protracted, costly experience in obtaining the services and supplies they will require during the duration of their lives.
- The incidence of type 1 diabetes is increasing worldwide, with the greatest rise seen in the group under age 5 years. This rise cannot be explained solely by genetics; environmental factors clearly play a role.
- Greater recognition has been given to inherited forms of the disease such as maturity-onset diabetes of youth (MODY), which can currently be confirmed by genetic testing. Although infrequent (but not rare, because it might affect up to 2% of all Americans with diabetes—approximately 400,000 people), a diagnosis of monogenic diabetes definitely makes a difference in terms of treatment, prognosis, and genetic counseling.
- Non-type 2 diabetes is also seen in individuals with cystic fibrosis. Early screening for diabetes related to cystic fibrosis might improve both quality of life and survival in that disease.
- Continuous surveillance is imperative for understanding the epidemiologic patterns of non-type 2 disease, identifying risk factors, assessing the efficacy of prevention strategies, and facilitating the appropriate allocation of health care funds.

■ Introduction

Although type 2 is the most frequent type of diabetes around the world, type 1 remains the main form of diabetes in childhood (SEARCH for Diabetes in Youth Study Group 2007). Inherited diabetes syndromes, such as MODY, have also received attention in recent years as more information has become available on their pathophysiology and optimal management. This chapter summarizes available information on the prevalence and incidence of non-type 2 diabetes and its risk factors. The chapter includes discussion of type 1 diabetes and diabetes that is (1) related to genetic defects of β-cell function such as MODY and neonatal diabetes, (2) associated with pancreatic disease such as cystic fibrosis-related diabetes (CFRD), (3) caused by drugs and toxins, and (4) related to certain common genetic syndromes such as Down syndrome.

■ Background and Historical Perspective

Diabetes mellitus has been known to medicine for well over 2000 years. First descriptions of the frequency of the disease were by Galen, who in the second century A.D. referred to diabetes as being a "rare condition," and by Arataeus the Cappadocian, who described it as "not being very frequent among men." Around the 12th century Maimonides wrote that diabetes was "seldom seen in cold Europe and frequently encountered in warm Africa" (Libman and LaPorte 2005). About a century ago the heterogeneous characteristics of this disease were being described by numerous clinicians and scientists in Europe and the United States, including Elliott Joslin from the United States (Gale 2001). By the 1970s the two main types of diabetes were loosely divided into "juvenile onset" and "maturity onset." The first comprehensive report on the frequency of the disease and trends worldwide was not compiled until that decade, when West (West 1978) summarized the available clinical and population-based studies and highlighted the many gaps in diabetes epidemiology.

It was not until well into the 1970s that formal classifications were put in place. The first one was introduced in 1976 by the U.S. National Diabetes Data Group (National Diabetes Data Group 1979) and then endorsed by the World Health Organization Expert Committee on Diabetes Mellitus. This classification was based on the absolute need of insulin for therapy: thus, the juvenile-onset type was renamed insulin-dependent diabetes mellitus (IDDM, or type I diabetes), while the maturity-onset type was called non-insulin-dependent diabetes mellitus (NIDDM, or type II diabetes). An additional distinct category included malnutrition-related diabetes. A revision took place in 1997, based on pathophysiology and not therapy: absolute insulin deficiency states were to be known as type 1 diabetes mellitus, and the combination of insulin resistance and relative insulin deficiency would be known as type 2 diabetes (see Fig. 4.1) (The Expert Committee on the Diagnosis and Classification of Diabetes Mellitus 1997). In addition, the fasting glucose concentration was chosen as the diagnostic method of choice because of its simplicity and

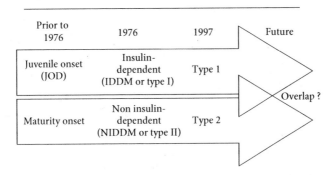

FIGURE 4.1. Epidemiology of name changes for the main two types of diabetes: time line

availability, and a cutoff value was selected to define the disease. The form of disease termed malnutrition-related diabetes was eliminated and reclassified as fibrocalculous pancreatopathy, a disease of the exocrine pancreas.

Over the last 25–30 years the standardization of definitions and methodology, combined with international collaboration, has fueled our knowledge about the frequency of diabetes and its trends. However it was recognized early on that the new classification scheme created challenges for routine care and epidemiologic studies, a point raised by the European Diabetes Epidemiology Group. These concerns included, among others, the recommendation to use a fasting glucose value for routine clinical use as well as for estimates of diabetes prevalence and incidence. This approach will not identify subjects with a high 2-hour value after a glucose challenge, and changing the diagnostic criteria would make it difficult or virtually impossible to compare temporal trends in the prevalence and incidence of type 2 diabetes in epidemiologic studies (European Diabetes Epidemiology Group 1998).

■ Burden of Disease

Type 1 Diabetes

Type 1 diabetes is characterized by β-cell destruction usually leading to absolute insulin deficiency. In most cases, this destruction is of autoimmune origin (called type 1a diabetes). In others, there is no known etiology.

Type 1a Diabetes

Type 1a diabetes is an organ-specific autoimmune disease characterized by T-cell-mediated destruction of pancreatic β-cells that results in absolute dependence on exogenous insulin for survival and maintenance of health. Although first-degree relatives of patients with type 1 disease are at increased risk, most cases of type 1, approximately 90%, occur in individuals with no family history of the disease. The presence of autoantibodies to one of several islet cell autoantigens, such as glutamic acid decarboxylase

65 protein (GAD65 Ab) or insulin, is taken as evidence of autoimmune diabetes. However, in many settings there is no attempt to assess the presence of these autoantibodies, and many studies do not differentiate type 1a from type 1 diabetes generally.

Type 1b Diabetes, or Idiopathic Diabetes

Although most cases of type 1 diabetes have an autoimmune etiology, some forms have no known cause. These patients have permanent insulinopenia and are prone to ketoacidosis, but there is no evidence of autoimmunity. Although only a small percentage of patients fall into this category, most who do are of African or Asian ancestry. This form of diabetes is strongly inherited, lacks immunologic evidence, and is not HLA (human leukocyte antigen) associated. Individuals with this form of diabetes suffer from episodic ketoacidosis and exhibit varying degrees of insulin deficiency between episodes, but they need insulin for survival (American Diabetes Association 2007). Very limited data are available on the frequency of this condition; in Japan, it seems to account for about 10% of patients with type 1 diabetes (Abiru, Kawasaki, and Eguch 2002).

Incidence Data for Type 1 Diabetes

More than half of individuals with type 1 disease are diagnosed before the age of 15 years (Daneman 2006). In western countries type 1 still accounts for more than 90% of diabetes seen in childhood and adolescence. In the 1980s the need was recognized for rigorous epidemiologic methods that could assess the burden of type 1, and this led to the creation of the World Health Organization-sponsored DIAbetes MONDiale (DIAMOND) Project and the EURODIAB study. One of the main goals of the two projects was the creation of population-based registries to monitor trends in children below age 15; DIAMOND and EURODIAB used standardized definitions and data collection forms and a standardized method to validate completeness of the registries. The DIAMOND Project included more than 110 registries in 57 countries, representing 84,000,000 children around the world, with a data set of 43,000 children diagnosed between 1990 and 1999. The EURODIAB study included 44 European centers, covering about 30,000,000 youth and including 47,000 children in its registries (DIAMOND Project Group 2006; Soltesz et al. 2007). More recently efforts like those of the SEARCH for Diabetes in Youth Study Group in the United States, a population-based observational study of physician-diagnosed diabetes among youth aged < 20 years, have further contributed to our knowledge of the disease in childhood (SEARCH for Diabetes in Youth Study Group 2006; The Writing Group for the SEARCH for Diabetes in Youth Study Group 2007).

A key finding from these efforts was the extremely wide variation in the incidence of the disease worldwide, more than a 350-fold difference. The overall standardized annual incidence (per 100,000) varied from 0.1 in China (DIAMOND Project Group 2006) to more than 38 in Sardinia (Casu et al. 2004) and 45 in Finland (Podar et al.

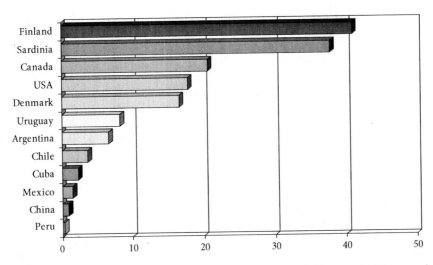

FIGURE 4.2. Age-standardized incidence of type 1 diabetes in children under 15 years of age (per 100,000/year)

2001). Overall, the incidence was higher in populations of European or Caucasian origin, including countries in Europe, the United States, and Canada. Countries elsewhere in which a high percentage of the population was of Caucasian origin had a higher relative incidence within their respective regions, such as Argentina and Uruguay in South America and Australia and New Zealand in the Western Pacific area. On the other hand, the incidence was quite low in countries with a high percentage of other ethnic groups, countries such as Mexico, Peru, and China (see Fig. 4.2) (DIAMOND Project Group 2006).

In general, the incidence increases with age, with a peak at puberty. The DIAMOND data have shown that, using children aged 0–4 years as the referent, children aged 5–9 years have a risk ratio of 1.62 (95% confidence interval [CI] 1.57–1.66), and those aged 10–14 years have a risk ratio of 1.94 (95% CI 1.89–1.98) (DIAMOND Project Group 2006).

Among children, boys and girls are at similar risk. A minor excess for males has been reported in populations of European origin and a slight excess for females in populations of African/Asian origin. In contrast, in type 1 populations of exclusively European origin aged 15–40 years, male excess is a constant finding (Gale and Gillespie 2001).

Seasonality of onset has been reported in many northern hemisphere studies and in some southern hemisphere studies, with a peak occurring in winter, a feature usually observed in both sexes and in all age groups. This phenomenon is more pronounced in countries with a marked difference between summer and winter temperatures (Levy-Marchal et al. 1995).

Children who subsequently develop type 1 diabetes seem to have a different seasonality of birth than is seen in the background population, but the literature is controversial. Analysis of data from 19 EURODIAB regions provided no consistent evidence that environmental factors, which vary from season to season, have any influence in fetal and neonatal life that would determine the onset of type 1 disease. Significant seasonality was confirmed in only two of five regions of Great Britain (McKinney et al. 2001). More recently, a seasonality pattern was observed in ethnically homogeneous populations (such as Ashkenazi Jews; Israeli Arabs; residents of Sardinia and Canterbury, New Zealand; and African Americans) but not in heterogeneous populations (such as in Sydney, Australia; Allegheny County, Pennsylvania [U.S.A.]; and Denver, Colorado [U.S.A.]) (Laron et al. 2005).

Various temporal trends have been identified that were unlikely to be the result of changes in methodology (Gale 2000). A systematic review considering worldwide incidence trends for the period 1960–1996 noted a significant increase in incidence in 24 of 37 studies (65%) from 27 countries, with an upward tendency in another 12 (32%), and only 1 reporting a small (and nonsignificant) decline. The global average annual increase was 3.0% (95% CI 2.6%–3.3%), with a more pronounced relative increase in the populations with a lower incidence (Onkamo et al. 1999). Data from the DIAMOND study found a mean annual increase in incidence of 2.8% (95% CI 2.4%–3.2%) from 103 centers. From 1990 to 1994, the average annual increase was 2.4% (95% CI 1.3%–3.4%); from 1995 to 1999, the annual increase was higher at 3.4% (95% CI 2.7%–4.3%) (DIAMOND Project Group 2006).

A large European survey for 1989–1998 showed a 3.2% (95% CI 2.7%–3.7%) annual increase, most marked in some Central and Eastern European countries. In absolute terms, the increase was similar in the 0–4, 5–9, and 10–14 age groups, but the most rapid increase relative to baseline was in the youngest group (Green et al. 2001). Several studies in Europe have found that the highest rate of increase is occurring in children below the age of 5 years (Karvonen et al. 1999; Schoenle et al. 2001). This may be related to earlier clinical manifestation or to a true increase in the causative factors of the disease. More recently, data from Sardinia for 1989–1999 showed a significant increase in incidence, with a yearly increase of 2.8% (95% CI 1.0%–4.7%) (Casu et al. 2004). Data from Victoria, Australia, for 1999–2002 showed an average increase of 9.3% per year, with a greater relative increase in children aged 0 to 4 years (Chong et al. 2007).

In the United Sstates data from the Allegheny County Registry showed a rapid increase during 1985–1989, with an overall increase of 83% for 1966–1989. The most rapid increase was in nonwhite males and in the 0–4 age group (Dokheel et al. 1993). In the last update a higher incidence of diabetes (per 100,000 population) for African Americans (17.6) than for whites (16.5) was described. This higher incidence among African Americans was explained by their much higher incidence of diabetes in the 15–19 age group, which at 30.7 was almost three times that of whites (11.2). The 1990–1994 incidence for African Americans was two and three times as high, respectively, as that reported in 1985–1989 and 1980–1984 (Libman et al. 1998). Part of this increase could have been due to the inclusion of some children with other types of diabetes, but this would be unlikely to have accounted for an increase of this magnitude.

More recently, the SEARCH for Diabetes in Youth Study identified new diabetes cases in geographically defined populations in Ohio, Washington state, South Carolina, and Colorado and among health plan enrollees in Hawaii and California for 2002–2003 and found an annual incidence (per 100,000 population) of 24.3 (95% CI 23.3–25.3). Regardless of race/ethnicity, most children under age 10 with diabetes had type 1 disease. The highest rates of type 1 were observed in non-Hispanic white youth (18.6, 28.1, and 32.9 for age groups 0–4, 5–9, and 10–14 years, respectively) (The Writing Group for the SEARCH for Diabetes in Youth Study Group 2007).

Only a few studies have examined the incidence of type 1 diabetes in adults, mainly because of (1) the lack of a standard definition of diabetes that has been practically and consistently applied in the adult diabetes population and (2) the difficulty in distinguishing between different types of diabetes. The incidence of type 1 seems to decrease in the third decade of life, only to increase in the fifth to seventh decades (Molbak et al. 1994). Recent data suggest that about 40%–50% of those with type 1 are older than age 16–18 at initial presentation (Daneman 2006). Autoimmune diabetes in adults may comprise a spectrum, with some individuals presenting with evidence of diabetes-associated autoantibodies but not requiring insulin initially, a condition described as latent autoimmune diabetes in adults. Patients with this disorder seem to comprise 5%–10% of newly diagnosed diabetes patients who do not require insulin (David et al. 2006). This varies, however, by mode of ascertainment, definition of the disease, sourced population, and the age of the patients (the condition is more frequent in younger age groups).

Prevalence Data for Type 1 Diabetes

Only a few studies have estimated the prevalence of type 1 diabetes, and their findings should be treated cautiously, as they covered different time periods, assessed limited geographic areas, and used different definitions and methods to collect the information. An early study, conducted in the 1970s via a mail survey, found a prevalence of 1.6 per 1000 among Michigan schoolchildren (Gorwitz, Howen, and Thompson 1976). Rates were higher for females than males and for whites than nonwhites and increased with advancing age. In this study, 15.5% of those with diabetes reportedly did not receive insulin. A study among schoolchildren living in Minnesota published during the same decade found a prevalence of 1.89 per 1000, with 95% receiving insulin (Kyllo and Nuttall 1978).

A Finnish study that used 1979 data found a somewhat higher prevalence, 262/100,000 for children aged 0–19 years (Reunanen and Tuomilehto 1982). In contrast, data for the same age group from Benghazi, Lybia, yielded a prevalence of 37.3/100,000 (95% CI 30.5–45.4) in 1990. This prevalence reflected a rise from 1981 with 23.5/100,000 (95% CI 17.1–37.5) (Kadiki and Moawad 1993). Other studies from the 1990s include one from Avellaneda, Argentina, among schoolchildren aged 3–20 years that obtained a prevalence of 0.45/1000 in those aged 3–12 years and 1.25/1000 in the 13–20 group (Marti et al. 1994), and another from

Leicestershire, United Kingdom, among white and South Asian children aged 0–14 years (Gujral et al. 1994). That study estimated a prevalence of 0.75/1000 (95% CI 0.61–0.89) among the white children and 0.77/1000 (95% CI 0.41–1.13) among the South Asians (Gujral et al. 1994). More recent data, this from the early 2000s and obtained in Kuwait, showed a prevalence of 269.9/100,000 for the group aged 6–18 years (Moussa et al. 2005).

Early data from Funen County in Denmark that included the whole population (all ages) and were based on insulin prescriptions from pharmacies found prevalence rates of 3.6/1000 for males and 3.3/1000 for females (Green et al. 1981). Later, 1988 data from Estonia indicated a prevalence of 1.72/1000 for all age groups combined, with the highest in the 40–49 group (3.04 in males and 2.77 in females) (Kalits and Podar 1990).

In the United States data from the SEARCH for Diabetes in Youth Study, using standardized methodology, found a prevalence in 2001 of 1.82 diabetes cases per 1000 youth aged <20, with rates of 0.70 for those aged 0–9 years and 2.8 for those 10–19 years. Among younger children type 1 accounted for over 80% of diabetes (83% in American Indians, 93% in Asians/Pacific Islanders, and over 95% in non-Hispanic whites); among older youth, the proportion of diabetes that was type 2 ranged from 6% (0.19 cases per 1000 among non-Hispanic whites) to 76% (1.74 cases per 1000 among American Indians) (SEARCH for Diabetes in Youth Study Group 2006).

Risk Factors for Type 1 Diabetes

These diabetes registries have given rise to numerous studies evaluating the risk factors for childhood-onset type 1 diabetes, but what is missed is that the most important factor for determining risk is the country of residence. For example, a child in Finland is 400 times more likely to develop diabetes than a child in Beijing, China (DIAMOND Project Group 2006). This, to our knowledge, is the greatest geographic variation for any non-communicable disease.

Temporal trends in diabetes have provided important clues for understanding the disease, most likely reflecting environmental changes more than differences in genetic susceptibility and leading to the generation of hypotheses trying to explain these increases. What is striking is that across the world and the diversity of the world's children, almost all countries have shown a rise in incidence, indicating that the drivers of the increase are global. Although unproven, it can be postulated that the almost universal reduction of infectious diseases might play a role. In this scenario, termed the "hygiene hypothesis," the lack of early exposure to a range of infectious agents gives rise to a failure of the immune system to regulate potential harmful consequences of inflammatory responses and leads to the development of different diseases such as type 1 diabetes and asthma (Gale 2002). The so-called polio hypothesis expands the hygiene hypothesis by arguing that diabetes is increasing rapidly in countries like Finland and Sweden where the frequency of enterovirus infections has tended to decrease over the last decades (Hyoty 2004).

On the other hand data from animal studies, the seasonality of incidence, as well as clustering in time and space suggest that infectious diseases are involved (Jun and Yoon 2003). Conflicting results have been obtained in retrospective studies. For example unspecified infections before the onset of diabetes may be associated with an increased risk (Yoon 1995), but attendance at preschool day care, a proxy for early infection load, has been indicated to be protective (Kaila and Taback 2001). And yet population-based collection of maternal sera during pregnancy or at the time of delivery has clearly indicated an association with enteroviruses, and a large Finnish prospective cohort on high-risk individuals indicated an association between enteroviral exposure and onset of diabetes.

A number of population-based studies have identified associations with maternal age, preeclampsia, delivery by cesarean section, increased birth weight, gestational age, birth order, and incompatibility of the blood group (between mother and fetus). Many of these associations were confirmed in the EURODIAB Study, where blood group incompatibility was the strongest risk factor (Dahlquist et al. 1999; Soltesz et al. 2007). It has also been suggested that vaccinations could increase the risk of type 1 diabetes, but none of the routine childhood immunizations have been shown to increase the risk of this disease (DeStefano et al. 2001; EURODIAB Substudy 2 Study Group 2000).

Early exposure to diabetes through feeding patterns was suspected to be a risk factor based on the epidemiologic observation that children with diabetes had been breastfed for a shorter time than children without diabetes. This has been reviewed in a number of studies, including a meta-analysis (Gerstein 1994; Norris and Scott 1996). Following from this observation about duration of breastfeeding, numerous epidemiologic and experimental studies started to analyze whether early introduction of cow's milk protein or cereal products could be the explanation for an increase in diabetes rather than the loss of a protective effect from breast milk. A prospective intervention study, Trial to Reduce IDDM in the Genetically at Risk (TRIGR), is designed to answer the question of what effect the early introduction of formula feeding may have on development of type 1 diabetes (Akerblom et al. 2005). The Diabetes Autoimmunity Study in the Young (DAISY) study, which followed newborns from birth, has to date found no evidence that ingestion of bovine milk contributes to the risk of diabetes. Recent reports, including one from the DAISY study and another from the German BABYDIAB, however, have suggested that early ingestion of cereal or gluten increases risk of type 1 disease (Norris et al. 2003; Ziegler et al. 2003). Other interesting hypotheses, which are based on the reported north-south gradient and the seasonality of incidence, are that sunshine and vitamin D are protective factors. In agreement with a series of experimental animal studies, a large European population-based case control study clearly indicated that vitamin D protects against diabetes in children (Diabetes Epidemiology Research International Group 1988; The EURODIAB Substudy 2 Study Group 1999).

Another possibility is that the increased weight of the world's children is playing a role, with obesity pushing the incidence rates upward. Not only higher birth weight but also greater growth in early childhood have been associated with increasing risk for type 1 diabetes in a number of population-based studies based on prospectively recorded growth data (Johansson, Samuelsson, and Ludvigsson 1994; Hypponen, Kenward, and Virtanen 1999). The largest study, which was based on five EURODIAB centers, involved almost 500 diabetic children and 1350 control subjects. Height and weight standard deviation scores were significantly increased among patients from 1 month after birth, and the maximum risk difference occurred between ages 1 and 2 years (EURODIAB Substudy 2 Study Group 2002).

Moreover, an increasing prevalence of overweight has been found in children with type 1 diabetes, with 25% having a body mass index ≥85th percentile at onset of the disease in 1990–1998 (Libman et al. 2003). According to the accelerator hypothesis, excessive weight gain causes insulin resistance that accelerates the apoptosis of β-cells and leads to early presentation of type 1 disease (Wilkin 2001). Accelerated growth and excess weight gain because of improved nutrition or even overconsumption during infancy and childhood may be risk factors that help to explain the raising incidence of type 1 diabetes.

The identification of exogenous factors that trigger and potentiate the destruction of β-cells suggests there may be ways to prevent type 1 disease. With this possibility in mind, the TEDDY consortium (The Environmental Determinants in Diabetes of the Young) was formed; six clinical centers in the United States or Europe are involved. The primary objective is to identify infectious agents, dietary factors, or other environmental exposures that are associated with increased risk of autoimmunity and type 1 diabetes. The observational cohort studies included in TEDDY enroll newborns from the general population who are younger than 4 months and have high-risk HLA alleles or who are first-degree relatives of patients affected with type 1 diabetes (Hagopian 2006).

Diabetes Related to Genetic Defects of β-Cell Function

Maturity-Onset Diabetes of Youth

Introduction. MODY represents a clinically heterogeneous group of disorders characterized by non-ketotic diabetes mellitus, an autosomal-dominant mode of inheritance, usual onset before age 25 years, and a primary defect in the function of the β-cells of the pancreas. In most cases, patients with MODY do not exhibit the characteristics of the metabolic syndrome, have normal insulin sensitivity, and are of Caucasian origin (American Diabetes Association 2007; Owen et al. 2002).

Data on incidence and prevalence. Early observations of what became known as MODY were made in Europe as well as the United States. Joslin's 1924 textbook mentioned four patients with a strong family history of diabetes who were diagnosed before age 20 and survived for 9–21 years on diet alone. In 1928 dominant inheritance of a mild form of diabetes was proposed (Njolstad, Molven, and Sovik 2005). In the decade following the introduction of sulfonylureas, Fajans and Conn studied and described a group of lean children and youngsters with mild, tolbutamide-treated diabetes who showed good metabolic control, even after years of observation (Fajans and Conn 1960), and in the mid-1970s Tattersall and Fajans (1975) published their descriptions of the mode of inheritance and other characteristic and unique clinical findings. These two authors coined the term "maturity onset-type diabetes of childhood or of young people," still in common usage as the acronym MODY. The nosological definition (and the resulting acronym) was based on the outdated classification of diabetes into juvenile-onset and maturity-onset diabetes. MODY is now defined as a genetic defect in β-cell function with subclassifications according to the gene involved: the expanding MODY gene family comprises at present six well-characterized members (Table 4.1). All these genes are expressed in β-cells, and mutation of any of them leads to β-cell dysfunction and diabetes mellitus.

MODY is most commonly seen as MODY2 or MODY3. MODY2 (associated with mutations in the glucokinase gene) is characterized by mild hyperglycemia. Less than 50% of affected subjects present with overt diabetes, and many patients are diagnosed only by oral glucose tolerance testing during pregnancy or in familial studies. MODY3, which results from mutations in the hepatic nuclear factor (HNF-1α) gene, represents a more severe form of diabetes and is often mistaken for type 1 disease or evolves to an insulin requirement (up to 30%–40% of these patients need insulin to attain adequate metabolic control) (Fajans, Bell, and Polonsky 2001).

In most white populations the estimated prevalence of MODY is less than 5% of diabetes patients (Velho and Froguel 1998). However, these are probably underestimates, as mild hyperglycemia can remain undiagnosed, or patients may be misdiagnosed as suffering from type 2 diabetes or even type 1 (Lambert et al. 2003). The prevalence of MODY in the white U.K. population is estimated at 1%–2% of all persons with diabetes (Shepherd et al. 2001). In the UK Prospective Diabetes Study (UKPDS), systematic screening for HNF-1α mutations in newly diagnosed patients has shown that MODY3 accounts for approximately 3% of cases of adult type 2 diabetes (Cox et al. 1999). More recently, the crude minimum population prevalence of pediatric MODY in the United Kingdom was estimated as 0.17/100,000 in a cross-sectional survey that collected data on all children with non-type 1 diabetes (Ehtisham et al. 2004). The prevalence of the known MODY genes has been considerably lower in Japanese and Chinese series than has been reported in European white populations. Porter et al. have shown that MODY due to mutations in the HNF-1α and in the glucokinase genes is present in U.K. Asian children; the clinical phenotype is similar to that observed in white U.K.

TABLE 4.1 *Subtypes of Maturity-Onset Diabetes of the Young and the Genes Involved*

MODY Type	Gene Locus	Gene Name	Frequency	Onset of Diabetes	Clinical Features of Heterozygous State
MODY 1	20q	Hepatocyte nuclear factor 4 α	Rare	Adolescence/early adulthood	Diabetes, microvascular complications, decrease in serum triglycerides, apolipoproteins AII and CIII and Lp(a) lipoprotein
MODY 2	7p	Glucokinase	10–65%	Early childhood	IFG, IGT, diabetes
MODY 3	12q	Hepatocyte nuclear factor 1 α	20–75%	Adolescence/Early adulthood	Diabetes, microvascular complications, renal glycosuria, increased sensitivity to sulfonylurea drugs
MODY 4	13q	Insulin promoter factor 1	Rare	Early adulthood	Diabetes
MODY 5	17q	Hepatocyte nuclear factor 1 β	Rare		Diabetes, renal cysts, and other abnormalities of renal development, internal genital abnormalities (in female carriers)
MODY 6	2q32	Neurogenic differentiation 1	Rare	Early adulthood	Diabetes

Source: Adapted from Fajans et al. 2001 and Vaxillaire et al. 2006.

patients, and the number of families referred for testing for MODY is lower than expected assuming equal prevalence between ethnic groups (Porter et al. 2006).

Monogenic forms of diabetes associated with MODY genotypes are seldom described as a cause of hyperglycemia in African American children and young adults (Nakamura, House, and Winter 1997). However, these results may arise from racial disparities in access to health care and in diagnosis, resulting in a lower number of minority families referred for genetic testing.

Risk factors. Monogenic forms of diabetes usually present in the second to fourth decade of life, and hence the pediatrician/clinician may be faced with a wide differential diagnosis of hyperglycemic syndromes that may be attributable to insulin resistance, autoimmune disorders, or genetic etiologies. As most cases are likely to be type 2, strategies should be developed to identify those in whom genetic testing will be beneficial so that resources can be directed appropriately.

At present, the traditional criteria used to diagnose MODY syndromes (age of onset <25 years and parental history of diabetes) are insufficient to differentiate MODY from type 2 diabetes, as many type 2 patients are diagnosed well before the age of 25, and approximately equal numbers of MODY and type 2 patients report a parent with diabetes (Owen et al. 2002). Moreover, with the prevalence of obesity increasing, it may be difficult to use obesity as a criterion to distinguish between different types of diabetes.

Neonatal Diabetes

Hyperglycemia that requires insulin in the first 3–6 months of life is known as neonatal diabetes mellitus and presents in two variants: transient and permanent. This rare condition (1 in 500,000 births) may be associated with intrauterine growth retardation, especially the transient type (Sperling 2006a). It is not associated with high-risk type 1 diabetes, HLA DQ alleles, and islet-specific autoantibodies. Approximately half of the cases are transient and have been associated with paternal isodisomy (the inheritance of two chromosome homologs from the father only) and other imprinting defects of chromosome 6. Patients with transient neonatal diabetes, however, may develop permanent diabetes later in life. Permanent cases have been associated with pancreatic aplasia, activating mutations of KCNJ11, which is the gene encoding the adenosine-triphosphate-sensitive potassium channel subunit Kir6.2 (7p15-p13), as well as ABCC8 (sulfonylurea receptor 1 (SUR1), also in the same chromosome region, and with mutations of the insulin promoter factor-1 (IPF-1) (chromosome 7). In this last instance there is pancreatic aplasia, complete glucokinase deficiency (chromosome 7), and mutations of the FOXP3 gene (T-cell regulatory gene) as part of the IPEX syndrome (Metz el al. 2002; Sperling 2006a,b).

Diabetes Related to Disorders of the Exocrine Pancreas

Cystic-Fibrosis-Related Diabetes

Introduction. In the white population, cystic fibrosis is the most commonly inherited life-threatening disease. In the United States the incidence is 1 in 3000 live births in whites, 1 in 14,000 African Americans, and 1 in 25,000 Asians (Greening 2000; FitzSimmons 1993). Pulmonary disease and pancreatic insufficiency are the most common manifestations. Since it was first described in 1936, survival rates for cystic fibrosis have increased substantially. In the 1940s around 80% of those with the disease died within the first few years of life, but median survival was over 30 years in the 1990s (Riggs, Seaquist, and Moran 1999). With improved survival, impaired glucose tolerance and CFRD are becoming more frequent secondary complications. Insulin deficiency is believed to be the primary cause of CFRD, but insulin resistance is also present during acute illness that is secondary to infections or from the use of medications such as glucocorticoids (Hardin and Moran 1999).

Incidence. A 5-year prospective study among cystic fibrosis patients that relied on annual oral glucose tolerance tests from the age of 2 years reported an average annual incidence rate of CFRD of 3.8%, increasing with age. Patients over age 10 and over age 20 had a 5.0% and 9.3% incidence, respectively (Greening 2000).

Prevalence. The estimated prevalence of CFRD among patients with cystic fibrosis varies from 5% to 50%, with an additional 15%–40% of patients having impaired glucose tolerance. The 2003 Cystic Fibrosis Foundation Patient Registry Annual Report, which reflected data from 21,742 patients at 117 accredited care centers, stated that 16.9% of cystic fibrosis patients in the United States aged >13 years had CFRD requiring chronic insulin therapy. In contrast, a survey of 1348 cystic fibrosis patients at six European centers reported an overall prevalence of CFRD of 4.9%. When annual systematic screening with oral glucose tolerance tests is performed, the prevalence has been reported to increase regularly with age, with less than 10% of CFRD cases occurring before the age of 10 to more than 40% of these cases appearing over the age of 30 (Marshall et al. 2005).

Risk factors. The prevalence of CFRD increases with age; the median age at onset is close to 20 years. Risk factors include female sex, pancreatic insufficiency, and δ F508 homozygous genotype. A recent study from the Epidemiology Study of Cystic Fibrosis, a longitudinal, encounter-based patient registry in the United States, reported that patients with CFRD have more severe pulmonary disease, more frequent pulmonary exacerbations, and poorer nutritional status than affected patients without diabetes. However, this study was not longitudinal and can not be used as proof of causality (Marshall et al. 2005). Screening recommendations vary from obtaining a random blood glucose level annually in all children with cystic fibrosis aged ≥14 years to performing an annual oral glucose tolerance test in all those aged 10 or more.

Diabetes Associated with Pancreatic Disease

Depending on the extent of the lesion, acquired pancreatic processes resulting in tissue destruction may cause permanent diabetes. This "pancreatogenic" diabetes was recognized in earlier classifications of diabetes mellitus (Cudworth 1976; National Diabetes Data Group 1979), and these forms of diabetes may account for 0.5% of all cases of diabetes mellitus (Del Prato, Coppelli, and Tiengo 2004). The prevalence is heightened in populations with heavy drinking habits (which increase the rate of alcohol-related pancreatitis) and in tropical countries where chronic fibrocalculous pancreatitis is endemic.

Pancreatitis. Acute pancreatitis can be accompanied by transient (3–6 weeks) hyperglycemia in up to 50% of cases, but permanent diabetes is uncommon unless further attacks or chronic pancreatitis develops. Remnant impaired glucose tolerance is found in about 10% of patients (Del Prato et al. 2004; Banks, Marks, and Vinik 1975).

In contrast secondary diabetes is frequent in chronic pancreatitis: a prospective cohort study of 500 patients with chronic pancreatitis found that after 25 years of follow-up the cumulative rate of diabetes mellitus was 83%, with 54% of these patients on insulin treatment (Malka et al. 2000; Banks et al. 1975).

Fibrocalculous pancreatic diabetes, a later stage of tropical chronic pancreatitis, is seen almost exclusively in developing countries in the tropics. Younger age of onset, absence of exposure to alcohol, the presence of large intraductal calculi, and a high susceptibility to pancreatic cancer are some of the distinctive features of this form of chronic pancreatitis. Diabetes mellitus affects more than 90% of these patients, commonly occurring 10–20 years after onset. The prevalence of tropical chronic pancreatitis in Southern India has been estimated at 125/100,000, and in western countries it is reported to be 10–15/100,000 (Balaji et al. 1993; Copenhagen Pancreatic Study Group 1990).

Pancreatic cancer. Pancreatic adenocarcinoma is a neoplasm with a high incidence and very poor prognosis (it is the fourth-most common cause of cancer death in the U.S. male population). In patients with this cancer, diabetes is frequently of recent onset and is only partially caused by growth of the tumor. Recognition that atypical diabetes (such as a case involving a middle-aged lean adult without a family history who rapidly progresses to insulin dependence) may be the first sign that a patient has pancreatic cancer might improve survival. At diagnosis, 40–50% of all pancreatic cancer patients are hyperglycemic, and approximately 80% show impaired glucose tolerance. Glycemic control can be difficult, in spite of insulin treatment, and the coexistence of diabetes is associated with a worse prognosis (Ghadirian, Lynch, and Krewski 2003; Pfeffer et al. 1999; Saruc and Pour 2003; Del Prato et al. 2004).

Hemochromatosis. The hereditary form of hemochromatosis is fairly common in whites of northern European ancestry. In the United States it affects 1 in 200–500 individuals, with the prevalence somewhat higher in whites than in other races/ethnicities (Steinberg et al. 2001; O'Reilly et al. 1997). Diabetes mellitus affects over 75% of all hereditary hemochromatosis patients and develops early in the disease process, often preceding the diagnosis of iron accumulation disease (Milman et al. 2001). Insulin secretion, as well as muscle and hepatic insulin sensitivity, is reduced due to iron deposition in Langerhans' islets, muscle, and liver (Ferrannini 2000).

Secondary iron deposition due to frequent blood transfusions leads to insulin resistance and diabetes. Patients with thalassemia major and secondary hemochromatosis show a 5% prevalence of diabetes mellitus, and glucose tolerance is impaired in up to 50% of these patients. The use of iron chelation therapy with deferoxamine and/or deferiprone has been shown to reduce or reverse glucose intolerance in patients with thalassemia major (Merket et al. 1988; Cario et al. 2003; Platis et al. 2004).

Drug- and Toxin-Induced Diabetes Mellitus

Drugs, chemical agents, and toxins that cause diabetes mellitus directly or by precipitating this condition in already predisposed individuals were included in classification systems of diabetes as early as 1979 (National Diabetes Data Group 1979). These agents may influence glucose metabolism by decreasing pancreatic insulin secretion, increasing peripheral insulin resistance, altering liver metabolism, or by a combination of these mechanisms. Some antihypertensives (thiazide diuretics, chlorthalidone or β-adrenergic receptor antagonists), steroid hormones (such as glucocorticoids), anticonvulsants (phenytoin), and drugs acting on the immune system (α-interferon) have well-known effects on glucose and lipid metabolism. Newer substances and drug combinations used increasingly in recent years should be added to this list, including drugs used for treating transplant rejection, schizophrenia, and infection with the human immunodeficiency virus (HIV). Increased attention has also been paid to the association between environmental contaminants (including persistent organic pollutants such as biphenyls and dioxins, as well as arsenic) and an increased risk of developing diabetes.

Unfortunately, accurate data on the incidence or prevalence of diabetes secondary to drugs or chemicals are not available. Regardless, they should not be neglected as possible causative agents, since according to the indirect estimations, diabetes secondary to these agents may account for 1%–5% of all diagnosed cases of diabetes in the United States (American Diabetes Association 2007; Ganda 1995).

Antihypertensives

Various prospective studies have shown an increased risk of developing diabetes in patients treated with thiazide diuretics, chlorthalidone, or β-adrenergic receptor antagonists. In a case-control study performed in the setting of the New Jersey Medicaid program, the estimated relative risk for initiation of antihyperglycemic therapy (oral drugs or insulin) was 1.40 (95% CI 1.26–1.58) for patients receiving thiazide diuretics and 1.93 (95% CI 1.75–2.13) when a thiazide was used in concert with another antihypertensive drug, most commonly a β-blocker. The metabolic effects of thiazides are dose dependent and can be reduced by lowering the dose; fortunately, the newer adrenergic antagonists combining α- and β-adrenergic antagonistic properties, such as carvedilol, do not seem to exert these metabolically untoward effects (Gurwitz et al. 1993; Zillich et al. 2006; Bell 2004).

Glucocorticoids

Glucocorticoids have profound effects on the metabolism of carbohydrates, lipids, and proteins, as they generate insulin resistance and thus decrease use of glucose; stimulate lipolysis and proteolysis; and enhance the production of hepatic glucose. Long-term treatment with corticosteroids results in a significant, dose-dependent increase in the risk of developing hyperglycemia. In a community-based case-control study, the estimated relative risk for developing hyperglycemia that required treatment was 2.23 (95% CI 1.92–2.59) in all patients using oral glucocorticoids, and the adjusted odds ratio for initiation of antidiabetic medication (oral drugs or insulin) was 1.77 for an average daily steroid dose of 1–39 mg but 10.34 for a daily steroid dose of 120 mg or more (expressed in hydrocortisone-equivalent mg) (Gurwitz et al. 1994). It should be stressed that oral (adjusted rate ratio 2.31, 95% CI 2.11–2.54) but not inhaled corticosteroid was related to the development of diabetes in a population-based study using administrative databases that was performed in elderly patients (Blackburn et al. 2002).

Posttransplant Diabetes Mellitus

A major adverse effect of immunosuppressive drugs that affects a widely variable proportion of recipients (2%–50% during the first year, according to different series), posttransplant diabetes mellitus has a significant impact on short-term patient and graft survival, and it affects long-term morbidity and mortality as well. Because in the modern era, organ recipients live longer, the vascular complications of drug-induced diabetes and dyslipidemia assume greater relevance, resulting in poorer cardiovascular outcomes (Kasiske et al. 2003; Montori et al. 2002). Most reports deal with solid-organ transplantation, but survivors of hematopoietic cell transplants who receive immunosuppressive drugs may also be affected (Hoffmeister, Storer, and Sanders 2004). Beyond the mere phenomenic description (i.e., development of diabetes after transplantation) there is no consensus, and there are no established criteria regarding the definition of posttransplant diabetes. Lack of a uniform definition of this condition surely hampers intercenter comparisons and poses a great difficulty in obtaining and analyzing the published results.

The use of newer drugs or treatment modalities has resulted in a decline in the cumulative incidence of posttransplant diabetes. Among 11,659 Medicare beneficiaries receiving their first kidney transplant between 1996 and 2000 who were registered in the United States Renal Data System, the cumulative incidence of posttransplant diabetes was 9.1% at 3 months, 16.0% at 12 months, and 24.0% at 36 months (Kasiske et al. 2003). Although calcineurin inhibitors such as cyclosporine A and tacrolimus may affect insulin release and sensitivity, their immunosuppresive potency has led to improved graft survival and avoided the use of high-dose corticosteroid therapy, considered the main causative factor for posttransplant diabetes in the early era of transplantation. It is hoped that the introduction of newer immunosuppressants, such as sirolimus, will contribute to reducing the incidence of metabolic complications such as diabetes (Penfornis and Kury-Paulin 2006).

Additive risk is conferred by the recipient's age and ethnicity (nonwhite transplant patients are more frequently affected), the presence of obesity and a family history of diabetes, and various transplant-related factors (deceased donor, number of HLA mismatches, rejection, repeat transplant, delayed graft function). Hepatitis C virus infection has also been associated with the development of posttransplant diabetes (Kiberd, Panek, and Kiberd 2006; Araki et al. 2006).

Choosing an adequate immunosuppressive combination and tackling modifiable risk factors (e.g., lowering pretransplant weight in overweight/obese patients) will contribute to reducing the incidence of this complication. There is a need for randomized trials to assess the feasibility and convenience of tight glycemic control and other issues related to posttransplant diabetes (e.g., use of oral antidiabetic drugs versus insulin, effect of treatment on long-term outcomes). Absolutely requisite is the establishment of uniform diagnostic criteria for posttransplant diabetes.

Highly Active Antiretroviral Therapy

The prognosis for HIV-positive patients improved dramatically after the introduction of highly active antiretroviral therapy (HAART) in the mid-1990s. However, significant metabolic and somatic abnormalities, grouped under the denomination of lipodystrophy syndrome, have been described as a consequence of the use of the protease inhibitors and nucleoside reverse transcriptase inhibitors that are part of HAART. Acting via immunologic (increased levels of proinflammatory cytokines) and endocrine (activation of the hypothalamic-pituitary-adrenal axis) mechanisms, viral burden and stress may exert a deleterious effect on glucose metabolism. Since the introduction of HAART disruptions in glucose homeostasis resulting from insulin resistance associated with fat redistribution and increased lipolysis and with dysadipocytokinemia as well have resulted in a clear-cut increase in the prevalence of glucose intolerance and diabetes mellitus (increases have been in the range of

100%–400%) (Brown et al. 2005; Ledergerber et al. 2007). According to the Swiss HIV Cohort Study, factors such as male gender, ethnicity (blacks and Asians being disfavored), disease stage (Centers for Disease Control and Prevention disease stage C), and obesity were associated with an increased incidence rate of diabetes mellitus (Ledergerber et al. 2007).

Because long-term HAART has been highly successful in controlling HIV infection and disease progression as well as AIDS-associated morbidity and mortality in affected patients, it would be desirable to decrease the magnitude and the frequency of HAART-induced adverse effects that put these individuals at higher risk of premature cardiovascular disease. Fortunately, treatment with metformin or rosiglitazone has proven effective in lowering insulin resistance in HIV-infected individuals with lipodystrophy and abnormal glucose homeostasis (Hadigan et al. 2000, 2004).

Antipsychotic Drugs

Repeated observations originating in the past 150 years have demonstrated an increased prevalence of deranged glucose metabolism in untreated patients with schizophrenia (Redlich 1903); according to studies performed in the last 40 years, the prevalence of diabetes in these patients varies between 10% and 36% (Balter 1961; Dixon et al. 2000). Neuroleptics were first used for the treatment of schizophrenia in the early 1950s; shortly thereafter, they were shown to increase the prevalence of hyperglycemia (Hiles 1956; Thonnard-Neumann 1968). Newer drugs introduced in the 1990s, called atypical or second-generation antipsychotics, induce fewer extra-pyramidal and anticholinergic effects, but they still retain a significant diabetogenic effect (Bettinger et al. 2000). Causative mechanisms for hyperglycemia are associated with increased insulin resistance due to weight gain and/or fat redistribution or to a direct effect on target tissues; however, a direct effect on insulin secretion has been postulated (Bettinger et al. 2000). During the late 1990s concerns were raised regarding an increased prevalence of hyperglycemia during treatment with novel antipsychotics, and soon afterwards these suspicions were confirmed in pharma-coepidemiologic studies (Carlson et al. 2006). As reviewed recently, in most studies clozapine and olanzapine have been shown to pose the greater risk of developing hyperglycemia and dyslipidemia (Lean et al. 2003). In general elevated glycemic levels found during atypical antipsychotic treatment returned to normal soon after the medication was discontinued; in some patients diabetes persisted but was attenuated after a switch to another antipsychotic. Hence, patients on atypical antipsychotics should count as a high-risk group for diabetes and vascular disease.

Diabetes Related to Other Genetic Syndromes

Many genetic syndromes, including Down, Turner, Klinefelter, and Wolfram syndromes, are accompanied by an increased incidence of diabetes mellitus (American Diabetes Association 2007). Turner syndrome, which is associated with abnormalities of the X chromosome, has an estimated prevalence, based on a number of cytogenetic studies, that ranges from 25 to 210 per 100,000 females, with an estimated proportion of about 50 per 100,000 females in white populations (Hierrild, Mortensen, and Gravholt 2008). The relative risk of diabetes in these patients seems to be significantly increased. Data from a study in Denmark that relied on the Danish Cytogenetic Central Register and the Danish National Registry of Patients showed a relative risk of 11.6 and 4.4 for type 1 and type 2 diabetes, respectively (Gravholt et al. 1998). However, this finding has not been confirmed by others (Gravholt 2005). The primary pathogenic event is thought to be β-cell dysfunction (with no clear evidence of autoimmunity), but insulin resistance also plays a central role. Klinefelter syndrome is the most common sex chromosome disorder, affecting 1 in every 600 males (Bojesen et al. 2003); this syndrome has been associated with an increased risk of diabetes and with the metabolic syndrome. Epidemiologic studies on Klinefelter syndrome have shown an increased risk of dying from diabetes or being admitted to the hospital with diabetes (Bojesen et al. 2006). Wolfram syndrome is an autosomal recessive disorder characterized by insulin-deficient diabetes and the absence of β-cells at autopsy. Additional manifestations include diabetes insipidus, hypogonadism, optic atrophy, and neural deafness (American Diabetes Association 2007).

Down syndrome is an important public health problem, and this common genetic defect (1 in 700 live births) affects over 300,000 people in the United States (Korenberg et al. 1994). A considerably increased risk of diabetes has been consistently reported in children with the condition. As early as 1968 an increased prevalence of diabetes mellitus in persons with Down syndrome was reported, but the types were not differentiated (Milunsky and Neurath 1968). In the 1990s the second Dutch nationwide study on the incidence of type 1 diabetes in children (age range 1–14 years) reported five cases of Down syndrome. The authors estimated an annual incidence of diabetes mellitus (per 100,000 population with the syndrome) of 50 (95% CI 16 to 116), versus 12.4 (95% CI 12.1 to 12.7) in the general population. They also estimated the prevalence of diabetes mellitus in a population-based study that included 893 children with Down syndrome aged 0–9 years who were born between 1986 and 1994 and found it to be 335 per 100,000 (95% CI 87 to 980/100,000) (Van Goor, Massa, and Hirasing 1997).

A more recent study from England, using the Oxford Record Linkage Study (ORLS), found that diabetes mellitus under the age of 30 years was significantly more common in the population with Down syndrome than in the reference cohort (rate ratio 2.8, 95% CI 1.0 to 6.1) (Goldacre et al. 2004). A more recent population-based study of the prevalence of type 1 diabetes in Down syndrome in Denmark demonstrated a fourfold increased risk of type 1 diabetes in children with this condition. In a questionnaire-based study of 20,362 patients with Down syndrome in the United Kingdom and the United States the prevalence of diabetes diagnosed before age 20 years was some six times as high as expected. Although the children in these studies appear to have had type 1 diabetes, only one study has examined the immunogenetic characteristics of diabetes in subjects with Down syndrome. That study showed an excess of diabetes-associated HLA class II genotypes in children with Down syndrome and type 1 diabetes compared with age- and gender-matched healthy control subjects. Islet autoimmunity was also increased in children with Down syndrome compared with healthy schoolchildren (Bergholdt et al. 2006).

■ Current and Future Challenges

The last few decades have brought a major understanding of the different types of diabetes and their public health impact. Continuous monitoring across populations and time using standardized criteria and international collaboration has been critical to assessing the burden of the disease. Although type 2 accounts for the majority of cases worldwide, type 1 is still the most prevalent form of the disease in childhood, and its incidence continues to rise. A greater understanding of pathophysiology and genetics has increased our knowledge of other causes of diabetes mellitus. Surveillance is imperative for evaluating trends, identifying risk factors, generating hypotheses, and allocating resources. This is particularly true in view of the rising prevalence of the disease and the need for assessing intervention strategies at a population level. Initiatives should take into account recent challenges, which have included a widened spectrum of diabetes etiologies and an overlap of risk factors and phenotypes (e.g., children with autoimmunity who also present with obesity and acanthosis nigricans). Updated diagnostic criteria and standardized methods of ascertainment and classification need to be discussed to address these challenges and assure that surveillance is effective. Mandated case reporting should be considered.

■ References

Abiru N, Kawasaki E, Eguch K (2002). Current knowledge of Japanese type 1 diabetic syndrome. *Diabetes/Metabolism Research and Reviews* **18**, 357–66.

Akerblom HK et al. (2005). Dietary manipulation of beta cell autoimmunity in infants at increased risk of type 1 diabetes: a pilot study. *Diabetologia* **48**, 829–37.

Amdisen A (1968). Changes of the oral glucose tolerance test during long-term treatment with neuroleptics. *Acta Psychiatrica Scandinavica* **203**, 95–6.

American Diabetes Association (n.d.). The Dangerous Toll of Diabetes. Available at: http://diabetes.org/diabetes-statistics/dangerous-toll.jsp. Accessed April 8, 2007.

American Diabetes Association (2007). Diagnosis and classification of diabetes mellitus. *Diabetes Care* **30** (Suppl. 1), s42–7.

Araki M et al. (2006). Posttransplant diabetes mellitus in kidney transplant recipients receiving calcineurin or mTOR inhibitor drugs. *Transplantation* **81**, 335–41.

Balaji LN et al. (1993). Prevalence and clinical features of chronic pancreatitis in Southern India. *International Journal of Pancreatology* **15**, 29–34.

Balter AM (1961). Glucose intolerance curves in neuropsychiatric patients. *Diabetes* **10**, 100–4.

Banks S, Marks IN, Vinik AL (1975). Clinical and hormonal aspects of pancreatic diabetes. *American Journal of Gastroenterology* **6**, 13–22.

Bell DS (2004). Advantages of a third-generation beta-blocker in patients with diabetes mellitus. *American Journal of Cardiology* **93**, 49B–52B.

Bergholdt R et al. (2006). Increased prevalence of Down's syndrome in individuals with type 1 diabetes in Denmark: a nationwide population-based study. *Diabetologia* **49**, 1179–82.

Bettinger TL et al. (2000). Olanzapine-induced glucose dysregulation. *Annals of Pharmacotherapy* **34**, 865–7.

Blackburn D et al. (2002). Quantification of the risk of corticosteroid-induced diabetes mellitus among the elderly. *Journal of General Internal Medicine* **17**, 717–20.

Bojesen A, Juul S, Gravholt CH (2003). Prenatal and postnatal prevalence of Klinefelter syndrome: a national registry study. *Journal of Clinical Endocrinology and Metabolism* **88**, 622–6.

Bojesen A et al. (2006). The metabolic syndrome is frequent in Klinefelter's syndrome and is associated with abdominal obesity and hypogonadism. *Diabetes Care* **29**, 1591-8.

Brown TT et al. (2005). Antiretroviral therapy and the prevalence and incidence of diabetes mellitus in the multicenter AIDS cohort study. *Archives of Internal Medicine* **165**, 1179-84.

Cario H et al. (2003). Insulin sensitivity and beta-cell secretion in thalassemia major with secondary hemochromatosis. Assessment by oral glucose tolerance test. *European Journal of Pediatrics* **162**, 139-46.

Carlson C et al. (2006). Diabetes mellitus and antipsychotic treatment in the United Kingdom. *European Neuropsychopharmacology* **16**, 366–75.

Casu A et al. (2004). Type 1 diabetes among Sardinian children is increasing: the Sardinian diabetes register for children aged 0–14 years (1989–1999). *Diabetes Care* **27**, 1623–9.

Chong JW et al. (2007). Marked increase in type 1 diabetes mellitus incidence in children aged 0–14 yr in Victoria, Australia, from 1999 to 2002. *Pediatric Diabetes* **8**, 67–73.

Copenhagen Pancreatic Study Group (1981). An interim report from a prospective epidemiological multicenter study. *Scandinavian Journal of Gastroenterology* **16**, 305–12.

Cox RD et al. (1999). UKPDS 31: hepatocyte nuclear factor-1 alpha (the MODY3 gene) mutations in late-onset type II diabetic patients in the United Kingdom. *Diabetologia* **42**,120–1.

Cudworth AG (1976). The aetiology of diabetes mellitus. *British Journal of Hospital Medicine* **16**, 207–16.

Dahlquist GG, Patterson C, Soltesz G; for the EURODIAB Substudy 2 Study Group (1999). Perinatal risk factors for childhood type 1 diabetes in Europe. *Diabetes Care* **22**, 1698–702.

Daneman D (2006). Type 1 diabetes. *Lancet* **367**, 847–58.

David R et al. (2006). Clinical review: Type 1 diabetes and latent autoimmune diabetes in adults: one end of the rainbow. *Journal of Clinical Endocrinology and Metabolism* **91**, 1654–9.

Del Prato S, Coppelli A, Tiengo A (2004). Diabetes secondary to acquired disease of the pancreas. In: DeFronzo RA et al., eds. *International textbook of diabetes mellitus*, 3rd edn., pp 533–61. John Wiley & Sons Ltd., Chichester, UK

DeStefano F et al. (2001). Childhood vaccinations, vaccination timing and risk of type 1 diabetes mellitus. *Pediatrics* **108**, E112.

Diabetes Epidemiology Research International Group (1988). Geographic patterns of childhood insulin-dependent diabetes mellitus. *Diabetes* **37**, 1113–9.

DIAMOND Project Group (2006). Incidence and trends of childhood Type 1 diabetes worldwide 1990–1999. *Diabetic Medicine* **23**, 857–66.

Dixon L et al. (2000). Prevalence and correlates of diabetes in national schizophrenia samples. *Schizophrenia Bulletin* **26**, 903–12.

Dokheel T, the Pittsburgh Diabetes Epidemiology Research Group (1993). An epidemic of childhood diabetes in the United States? Evidence from Allegheny County, Pennsylvania. *Diabetes Care* **16**, 1606–11.

Ehtisham S, Hattersley AT, Dunger DB (2004). First UK survey of paediatric type 2 diabetes and MODY. *Archives of Disease in Childhood* **89**, 526–9.

EURODIAB Substudy 2 Study Group (1999). Vitamin D supplement in early childhood and risk for type 1 (insulin-dependent) diabetes mellitus. *Diabetologia* **42**, 51–4.

EURODIAB Substudy 2 Study Group (2000). Infections and vaccinations as risk factors for childhood type I (insulin-dependent) diabetes mellitus: a multicentre case-control investigation. *Diabetologia* **43**, 47–53.

EURODIAB Substudy 2 Study Group (2002). Rapid early growth is associated with increased risk of childhood type 1 diabetes in various European populations. *Diabetes Care* **25**, 1755–60.

European Diabetes Epidemiology Group (1998). Epidemiological considerations related to the new diagnostic criteria for diabetes mellitus. *Diabetologia* **41**, 51–2.

Fajans SS, Bell GI, Polonsky K (2001). Molecular mechanisms and clinical pathophysiology of maturity-onset diabetes of the young. *New England Journal of Medicine* **345**, 971–80.

Fajans SS, Conn JW (1960). Tolbutamide-induced improvement in carbohydrate tolerance of young people with mild diabetes mellitus. *Diabetes* **99**, 83–8.

Ferrannini E (2000). Insulin resistance, iron, and the liver. *Lancet* **355**, 2181–2.

FitzSimmons S (1993). The changing epidemiology of cystic fibrosis. *Journal of Pediatrics* **122**, 1–9.

Gale EA (2001). The discovery of type 1 diabetes. *Diabetes* **50**, 217–26.

Gale EA (2002a). The rise of childhood type 1 diabetes in the 20th century. *Diabetes* **51**, 3353–61.

Gale EA (2002b). A missing link in the hygiene hypothesis? *Diabetologia* **45**, 588–94.

Gale EA, Gillespie KM (2001). Diabetes and gender. *Diabetologia* **44**, 3–15.

Ganda OP (1995). Prevalence and incidence of secondary and other types of diabetes. In: Harris MI, ed. *Diabetes in America*, 2nd ed., pp 69–84. Bethesda: National Institutes of Health/National Institute of Diabetes and Digestive and Kidney Diseases. NIH Publication No. 95-1468.

Gerstein HC (1994). Cow's milk exposure and type 1 diabetes mellitus. A critical overview of the clinical literature. *Diabetes Care* 17, 13–9.

Ghadirian P, Lynch HT, Krewski D (2003). Epidemiology of pancreatic cancer: an overview. *Cancer Detection and Prevention* 27, 87–93

Goldacre MJ et al. (2004). Cancers and immune related diseases associated with Down's syndrome: a record linkage study. *Archives of Disease in Childhood* 89, 1014–7.

Gorwitz K, Howen GG, Thompson T (1976). Prevalence of diabetes in Michigan school-aged children. *Diabetes* 25, 122–7.

Gravholt CH (2005). Clinical practice in Turner syndrome. *Nature Clinical Practice. Endocrinology & Metabolism* 1, 41–52.

Gravholt CH et al. (1998). Morbidity in Turner syndrome. *Journal of Clinical Epidemiology* 51, 147–58.

Green A et al.(1981). Epidemiological studies of diabetes mellitus in Denmark. II. A prevalence study based on insulin prescriptions. *Diabetologia* 20, 468–70.

Green A, Patterson CC; on behalf of the EURODIAB TIGER Study Group (2001). Trends in the incidence of childhood-onset diabetes in Europe 1989–1998. *Diabetologia* 44 (Suppl. 3), B3–B8.

Greening A (2000). Cystic fibrosis. In: Seaton A, Seaton D, Letich G, eds. *Crofton and Douglas's Respiratory Diseases*, vol. 2, 5th ed., pp 839–76. London: Blackwell Science.

Gujral JS et al. 1994). Childhood-onset diabetes in the white and South Asian population in Leicestershire, UK. *Diabetic Medicine* 11, 570–2.

Gurwitz JH et al. (1993). Antihypertensive drug therapy and the initiation of treatment for diabetes mellitus. *Annals of Internal Medicine* 118, 273–8.

Gurwitz JH et al. (1994). Glucocorticoids and the risk for initiation of hypoglycemic therapy. *Archives of Internal Medicine* 154, 97–101.

Hadigan C et al. (2000). Metformin in the treatment of HIV lipodystrophy syndrome: a randomized controlled trial. *JAMA* 284, 472–7.

Hadigan C et al. (2004). Metabolic effects of rosiglitazone in HIV lipodystrophy: a randomized controlled trial. *Annals of Internal Medicine* 140, 786–94.

Hagopian WA et al. (2006). TEDDY—The Environmental Determinants of Diabetes in the Young: an observational clinical trial. *Annals of the New York Academy of Sciences* 1079, 320–6.

Hardin DS, Moran A (1999). Diabetes mellitus in cystic fibrosis. *Endocrinology and Metabolism Clinics of North America* 28, 787–800.

Hierrild BE, Mortensen KH, Gravholt CH (2008). Turner syndrome and clinical treatment. *British Medical Bulletin* 86, 77–93.

Hiles BW (1956). Hyperglycemia and glycosuria following chlorpromazine therapy. *Journal of the American Medical Association* 162, 1651–8.

Hoffmeister PA, Storer BE, Sanders JE (2004). Diabetes mellitus in long-term survivors of pediatric hematopoietic cell transplantation. *Journal of Pediatric Hematology and Oncology* **26**, 81–90.

Hyoty H (2004). Environmental causes: viral causes. *Endocrinology and Metabolism Clinics of North America* **33**, 27–44.

Hypponen E, Kenward MG, Virtanen S (1999). Infant feeding, early weight gain and risk of type 1 diabetes. Childhood Diabetes in Finland (DiMe) Study Group. *Diabetes Care* **22**, 1961–5.

Johansson N, Samuelsson U, Ludvigsson J (1994). A high weight gain early in life is associated with an increased risk of type 1 (insulin-dependent) diabetes mellitus. *Diabetologia* **37**, 91–4.

Jun HS, Yoon JW (2003). A new look at viruses in type 1 diabetes. *Diabetes/ Metabolism Research and Reviews* **19**, 8–31.

Kadiki OA, Moawad SE (1993). Incidence and prevalence of type 1 diabetes in children and adolescents in Benghazi, Libya. *Diabetic Medicine* **10**, 866–9.

Kaila B, Taback SP (2002). The effect of day care exposure on the risk of developing type 1 diabetes: a meta-analysis of case-control studies. *Diabetes Care* **24**, 1353–8.

Kalits I, Podar T (1990). Incidence and prevalence of type 1 (insulin-dependent) diabetes in Estonia in 1988. *Diabetologia* **33**, 346–9.

Karvonen M et al.(1999). The onset of type 1 diabetes in Finnish children has become younger. *Diabetes Care* **22**, 1066–70.

Kasiske BL et al. (2003). Diabetes mellitus after kidney transplantation in the United States. *American Journal of Transplantation* **3**, 178–85.

Kiberd M, Panek R, Kiberd BA (2006). New onset diabetes mellitus post–kidney transplantation. *Clinical Transplantation* **20**, 634–9.

Korenberg JR et al. (1994). Down syndrome phenotypes: the consequences of chromosomal imbalance. *Proceedings of the National Academy of Sciences of the United States of America* **91**, 4997–5001.

Kyllo CJ, Nuttall FQ (1978). Prevalence of diabetes mellitus in school-age children in Minnesota. *Diabetes* **27**, 57–60.

Lambert AP et al. (2003). Identifying hepatic nuclear factor 1a mutations in children and young adults with a clinical diagnosis of type 1 diabetes. *Diabetes Care* **26**, 333–7.

Laron Z et al. (2005). Seasonality of month of birth of children and adolescents with type 1 diabetes mellitus in homogeneous and heterogeneous populations. *Israel Medical Association Journal* **77**, 381–4.

Lean ME, Pajonk FG (2003). Patients on atypical antipsychotic drugs: another high-risk group for type 2 diabetes. *Diabetes Care* **26**, 1597–605.

Ledergerber B et al. (2007). Factors associated to the incidence of type 2 diabetes mellitus in HIV-infected participants in the Swiss HIV Cohort Study. *Clinical Infectious Diseases* **45**, 111–9.

Levy-Marchal C, Patterson C, Green A; on behalf of the EURODIAB ACE Study Group (1995). Variation by age group and seasonality at diagnosis of childhood IDDM in Europe. *Diabetologia* **38**, 823–30.

Libman IM et al. (1998). Was there an epidemic of diabetes in nonwhite adolescents in Allegheny County, Pennsylvania? *Diabetes Care* **21**, 1278–81.

Libman IM et al. (2003). Changing prevalence of overweight children and adolescents at onset of insulin-treated diabetes. *Diabetes Care* **26**, 2871–5.

Libman I, LaPorte R (2005). Changing trends in epidemiology of type 1 diabetes mellitus throughout the world: how far have we come and where do we go from here. *Pediatric Diabetes* **6**, 119–21.

Malka D et al. (2000). Risk factors for diabetes mellitus in chronic pancreatitis. *Gastroenterology* **119**, 1324–32.

Marshall BC et al. (2005). Epidemiology of cystic fibrosis-related diabetes. *Journal of Pediatrics* **146**, 681–7.

Marti ML et al. (1994). Diabetes prevalence in a school population of Avellaneda, Argentina. *Medicina (Buenos Aires)* **54**, 110–6 (in Spanish).

McKinney PA, EURODIAB Seasonality of Birth Group. Europe and Diabetes (2001). Seasonality of birth in patients with childhood type 1 diabetes in 19 European regions. *Diabetologia* **39**, 1063–9.

Metz C et al. (2002). Neonatal diabetes mellitus: chromosomal analysis in transient and permanent cases. *Journal of Pediatrics* **141**, 483–9.

Milman N et al. (2001). Clinically overt hemochromatosis in Denmark 1948–1985: epidemiology, factors of significance for long-term survival, and causes of death in 179 patients. *Annals of Hematology* **80**, 737–44.

Milunsky A, Neurath PW (1968). Diabetes mellitus in Down's syndrome. *Archives of Environmental Health* **17**, 372–6.

Molbak AG et al. (1994). Incidence of insulin-dependent diabetes mellitus in age groups over 30 years in Denmark. *Diabetic Medicine* **11**, 650–5.

Montori VM et al. (2002). Posttransplantation diabetes. A systematic review of the literature. *Diabetes Care* **25**, 583–92.

Moussa MA et al. (2005). Prevalence of type 1 diabetes among 6- to 18-year-old Kuwaiti children. *Medical Principles and Practice* **14**, 87–91.

Nakamura M, House DV, Winter WE (1997). Novel mutation identified in the glucokinase (GCK) genes of a patient with atypical diabetes mellitus (ADM) of African Americans (AA). *Diabetes* **46** (Suppl. 1), 175A.

National Diabetes Data Group (1979). Classification and diagnosis of diabetes mellitus and other categories of glucose intolerance. *Diabetes* **28**, 1039–57.

Njolstad P, Molven A, Sovik O (2005). Diagnosis, and management of MODY in a pediatric setting. In: Chiarelli F, Dahl-Jørgensen K, Kiess W, eds., *Diabetes in Childhood and Adolescence. Pediatric and Adolescent Medicine* **10**, pp 84–93. Basel, Switzerland: Karger.

Norris JM, Scott FW (1996). A meta-analysis of infant diet and insulin-dependent diabetes mellitus: do biases play a role? *Epidemiology* **7**, 87–92.

Norris JM et al. (2003). Timing of initial cereal exposure in infancy and risk of islet autoimmunity. *JAMA* **290**, 1713–20.

Onkamo P et al. (1999). Worldwide increase in incidence of type 1 diabetes: the analysis of the data in published incidence trends. *Diabetologia* **42**, 1395–403.

Owen KR et al. (2002). Heterogeneity in young adult onset diabetes: aetiology alters clinical characteristics. *Diabetic Medicine* **19**, 758–61.

Penfornis A, Kury-Paulin S (2006). Immunosuppressive drug-induced diabetes. *Diabetes and Metabolism* **32**, 539–46.

Pfeffer F et al. (1999). Secondary diabetes in pancreatic carcinoma and after pancreatectomy. *Zeitschrift fur Gastroenterologie* (June, Suppl. 1), 10–14 (in German).

Platis O et al (2004). Glucose metabolism disorders improvement in patients with thalassaemia major after 24–36 months of intensive chelation therapy. *Pediatric Endocrinology Reviews* **2** (Suppl. 2), 279–81.

Podar T et al. (1982). Prevalence and ten-year (1970–1979) incidence of insulin-dependent diabetes mellitus in children and adolescents in Finland. *Acta Pediatrica Scandinavica* 71, 893–9.

Porter JR et al. (2006). Asian MODY: are we missing an important diagnosis? *Diabetic Medicine* **23**, 1257–60.

Redlich E (1903). Zur Frage der Beziehungen zwischen Diabetes mellitus und Psychosen. *Wiener Medizinische Wochenshrift* **53**, 1041–6 (in German).

Reunanen A, Tuomilehto J (2001). Increasing incidence of childhood-onset type 1 diabetes in 3 Baltic countries and Finland 1983–1998. *Diabetologia* **44** (Suppl. 3), B17–20.

Riggs AC, Seaquist ER, Moran A (1999). Guidelines for the diagnosis and therapy of diabetes mellitus in cystic fibrosis. *Current Opinion in Pulmonary Medicine* **5**, 378–82.

Saruc M, Pour PM (2003). Diabetes and its relationship to pancreatic carcinoma. *Pancreas* **26**, 381–7.

Schoenle E et al. (2001). Epidemiology of type 1 diabetes mellitus in Switzerland: steep rise in incidence in under 5 year old children in the past decade. *Diabetologia* **44**, 286–9.

SEARCH for Diabetes in Youth Study Group (2006). The burden of diabetes mellitus among US youth: prevalence estimates from the SEARCH for Diabetes in Youth Study. *Pediatrics* **118**, 1510–8.

Shepherd M et al. (2001). Predictive genetic testing in maturity-onset diabetes of the young (MODY). *Diabetic Medicine* **18**, 417–21.

Soltesz G, Patterson CC, Dalquist G; on behalf of EURODIAB Study Group (2007). Worldwide childhood type 1 diabetes incidence—what can we learn from epidemiology? *Pediatric Diabetes* **8** (Suppl. 6), 6–14.

Sperling MA (2006a). ATP-sensitive potassium channels—neonatal diabetes mellitus and beyond. *New England Journal of Medicine* **355**, 507–10.

Sperling MA (2006b). The genetic basis of neonatal diabetes mellitus. *Pediatric Endocrinology Reviews* **4** (Suppl. 1), 71–5.

Steinberg KK et al. (2001). Prevalence of C282Y and H63D mutations in the HFE gene in the United States. *JAMA* **285**, 2216–22.

Tattersall RB, Fajans SS (1975). A difference between the inheritance of classical juvenile-onset and maturity-onset type diabetes of young people. *Diabetes* **24**, 44–53.

The Expert Committee on the Diagnosis and Classification of Diabetes Mellitus (1997). Report of the Expert Committee on the Diagnosis and Classification of Diabetes Mellitus. *Diabetes Care* **20**, 1193–7.

The Writing Group for the SEARCH for Diabetes in Youth Study Group (2007). Incidence of diabetes in youth in the United States. *JAMA* **297**, 2716–24.

Thonnard-Neumann E (1968). Phenothiazines and diabetes in hospitalized women. *American Journal of Psychiatry* **124**, 138–42.

Van Goor JC, Massa GG, Hirasing R (1997). Increased incidence and prevalence of diabetes mellitus in Down's syndrome. *Archives of the Diseases of Children* **772**, 186.

Vaxillaire M, Froguel P (2006). Genetic basis of maturity-onset diabetes of the young. *Endocrinology and Metabolism Clinics of North America* **35**, 371–84.

Velho G. Froguel F (1998). Genetic, metabolic and clinical characteristics of maturity onset diabetes of the young. *European Journal of Endocrinology* **138**, 233–9.

West KM. *Epidemiology of Diabetes and Its Vascular Lesions*. New York: Elsevier, 1978.

Wilkin TJ (2001). The accelerator hypothesis: weight gain as the missing link between type I and type II diabetes. *Diabetologia* **44**, 914–22.

Yoon JW (1995). A new look at viruses in type 1 diabetes. *Diabetes/Metabolism Reviews* **11**, 83–107.

Ziegler AG et al. (2003). Early infant feeding and risk of developing type 1 diabetes-associated autoantibodies. *JAMA* **290**, 1721–8.

Zillich AJ et al (2006). Thiazide diuretics, potassium, and the development of diabetes: a quantitative review. *Hypertension* **48**, 219–2.

SECTION 2

COMPLICATIONS OF DIABETES: EPIDEMIOLOGY AND RISK FACTORS

5. Diabetes and Acute Metabolic Complications, Infections, and Inflammation

Leonard E. Egede and Jeremy B. Soule

Main Public Health Messages

- Diabetes is complicated by two forms of hyperglycemic crisis: diabetic ketoacidosis (DKA) and the hyperglycemic hyperosmolar state (HHS).
- DKA typically occurs in type 1 diabetes. When DKA does complicate type 2 diabetes, it usually occurs in ethnic minorities or those with a profound acute primary illness.
- HHS presents in type 2 diabetes and is characterized by profound hyperglycemia, dehydration, change in mental status, and the absence of ketoacidosis.
- Hypoglycemia is a common complication of diabetes therapy. Severe hypoglycemia more commonly occurs with insulin therapy, but infrequently it can complicate sulfonylurea therapy.
- Patients with diabetes face greater risk of certain infections, including influenza, pneumonia, and foot infections. These infections are associated with increased morbidity and mortality, and treatment is associated with improved health outcomes.
- High-sensitivity C-reactive protein (hs-CRP) is a marker of low-grade chronic inflammation and may be a valuable predictor of cardiovascular disease.

Diabetic Ketoacidosis

Introduction

Patients with type 1 diabetes, who generally are completely deficient in insulin, are prone to diabetic ketoacidosis (DKA). Deficiency in insulin leads to excessive release

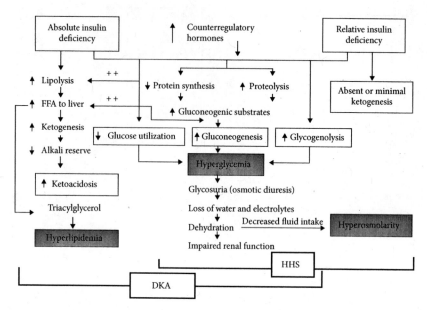

FIGURE 5.1. Pathogenesis of DKA and HHS, stress, infection, and/or insufficient insulin. (Reprinted with permission from Kitabchi et al., *Diabetes Care* 2006.)

of glucose from the liver. Lack of insulin also catabolizes muscle protein into amino acids, some of which the liver converts to glucose, thereby further increasing hyperglycemia. With complete or nearly complete lack of insulin, especially in the setting of severe illness, adipose tissue is catabolized into fatty acids. In turn fatty acids are converted into ketones, and ultimately ketoacids, thus producing the ketosis and acidosis that typify DKA (Kitabchi et al. 2006). Figure 5.1 shows the pathogenesis of DKA.

Background

Patients with DKA present with severe thirst, increased urination, dehydration, gastrointestinal complaints, and varying degrees of obtundation. Indeed DKA may complicate existing diabetes or be the initial manifestation of the disease. Discovering the precipitating causes of a DKA episode is crucial for prompt initiation of appropriate therapies. Infection, inadequate insulin treatment or nonadherence to such treatment, concomitant cardiovascular disease, and substance abuse are common precipitating factors (Kitabchi et al. 2006).

Epidemiology

According to U.S. hospital discharge data from the Centers for Disease Control and Prevention (CDC), the listing of DKA as the first diagnosis increased from 62,000 in 1980 to 115,000 in 2003 (CDC 2008). This trend reflects a large increase in the population of people with diabetes rather than an increase in the rate of DKA among people with diabetes. Indeed, over the same 1980–2003 time period, the number of persons diagnosed with diabetes in the United States increased from 5.6 to 14.3 million (CDC 2008). Based on discharge data estimates, the 100,000 DKA admissions in the United States in 2000 generated over $1 billion in medical charges (Kitabchi et al. 2006).

Mortality

Although DKA is life threatening, mortality rates are less than 5% in experienced centers (Kitabchi et al. 2006). Mortality is related to the nature and severity of the precipitating factor(s), such as infection; DKA mortality also increases with age, likely reflecting comorbid conditions (Kitabchi et al. 2006), but recent data show improved mortality rates in the elderly (CDC 2008). Males suffer higher DKA mortality than females, and this gender difference is particularly pronounced in African Americans (CDC 2008). Cerebral edema is an often fatal complication of DKA treatment (Kitabchi et al. 2006). Rarely reported in adults, cerebral edema complicates as many as 1% of DKA cases in children.

Diabetic Ketoacidosis in Ethnic Minorities

Ketoacidosis is also increasingly recognized among blacks and other minorities with type 2 diabetes and has been termed ketosis-prone type 2 diabetes, atypical diabetes, and Flatbush diabetes (Egede and Willi 2000). Such patients present with DKA but lack the autoimmunity-mediated attack of the insulin-producing cells in the pancreas. Variable recovery of insulin production occurs once glucose levels are controlled. Most widely described in black populations, ketosis-prone type 2 diabetes also occurs more frequently among Asians, Native Americans, and populations of Hispanic descent than among whites (Egede and Willi 2000). In these minority populations, approximately half of adult patients presenting with features of DKA will have type 2, not type 1, diabetes (Egede and Willi 2000; Kitabchi et al. 2006). In contradistinction to the absolute insulin requirement in patients with type 1 diabetes, approximately half of the patients presenting with DKA in the setting of type 2 diabetes will not require insulin therapy after initial glucose stabilization (Balasubramanyam et al. 2008; Egede and Willi 2000; Kitabchi et al. 2006).

Social, Economic, and Ethnic Disparities in Prevalence

Significant differences in DKA epidemiology have been found by demographic group. Discharge data from the 1980s showed that a DKA diagnosis was twice as prevalent in blacks with diabetes as in their white counterparts (CDC 2008), but more recent data show a decrease in the gap between the races. In 2003 the DKA rate among blacks with diabetes was 28.6/1000 discharges, versus 21.4/1000 among whites (CDC 2008). Using 1993–2003 emergency room (ER) data from the U.S. National Hospital

Ambulatory Medical Care Survey sample, DKA rates were 9.2/1000 ER patients with diabetes among blacks and 5.9/1000 among whites (Ginde, Pelletier, and Camargo 2006). The authors of this study suggested that this difference reflects ketosis-prone type 2 diabetes, which is more common in African Americans (Ginde, Pelletier, and Camargo 2006). Recent investigations show that DKA predominantly affects youth and the middle-aged (CDC 2008; Ginde, Pelletier, and Camargo 2006). Predilection by gender has varied with time, with males now being slightly more prone to DKA than females (CDC 2008). Socioeconomic data are missing from most published databases, but DKA at first presentation of type 1 diabetes is more common in children without private health insurance, implying less timely diagnosis in the underinsured (Maniatis et al. 2005).

Public Health Preventive or Intervention Strategies

By preventing diabetes, DKA might be fully prevented. Unfortunately, however, diabetes is increasing, and no current clinical trials have succeeded in completely preventing either type 1 or type 2 diabetes. Increasing the awareness of early symptoms of diabetes, however, has been demonstrated to prevent the development of full-blown DKA at the time that type 1 diabetes is diagnosed, and such greater awareness decreases the morbidity, mortality, and cost associated with DKA (Kitabchi et al. 2006). After diagnosis, interruption of insulin therapy is linked to economic constraints, lack of appropriate self-management behaviors, and substance abuse (Kitabchi et al. 2006). Allocating additional resources to preventive measures might reduce the approximate 25% of total direct medical expenditures in type 1 diabetes spent on treating DKA (Kitabchi et al. 2006).

■ Hyperosmolar Hyperglycemic State

Introduction

Hyperosmolar hyperglycemic state (HHS) is a syndrome of profound hyperglycemia without ketoacidosis that occurs in type 2 diabetes. Osmolarity is a measure of solutes, such as glucose or salt, dissolved in a fluid, such as blood serum. In the absence of insulin action, fat tissue releases fatty acids that are converted to ketoacids. Decreased insulin causes muscle and the liver to increase plasma glucose. Fat is more sensitive to low-level insulin activity than is muscle or the liver. In HHS, insulin is insufficient to stem glucose output by muscle or the liver but is sufficient to prevent breakdown of fat and the resultant formation of ketoacids.

Hyperglycemia leads to loss of glucose and water in the urine, which lowers plasma glucose but leads to dehydration. In DKA or in hyperglycemia without HHS, thirst increases with dehydration. This thirst increases the intake of water to offset dehydration and allows continued loss of glucose in the urine. Patients with

HHS have an inappropriately low thirst drive (often due to age or medications) or an inability to drink water despite thirst (e.g., bed-bound status). As dehydration becomes profound, the ability to lose glucose in urine is diminished because blood flow to the kidneys is decreased. This compounds hyperglycemia, leading to severe elevations in plasma glucose. These changes partially account for the higher plasma glucose levels in HHS (>600 mg/dL) than in DKA (≤500 mg/dL). Figure 5.1 shows the pathogenesis of HHS.

Clinical Presentation and Risk Factors

The identification and treatment of precipitating factors are essential to appropriate therapy. As in DKA, infection is a major precipitator of HHS. Other important precipitating factors include medications that increase glucose levels (e.g., glucocorticoids or diuretics), an inability to access water because of a bedridden state, and profound medical illnesses, which are often cardiovascular (Kitabchi et al. 2006). In up to 40% of patients, HHS may be the initial presentation of type 2 diabetes.

Epidemiology

Prevalence and Incidence

The prevalence and incidence of HHS are difficult to establish because of a paucity of population-level data. In general HHS is thought to account for less than 1% of diabetes admissions to the hospital, well below the 4–9% of admissions due to DKA (Kitabchi et al. 2006). The mortality rate for HHS is approximately 15%, versus less than 5% for DKA (Kitabchi et al. 2006). Mortality from HHS increases with age and concomitant medical illness (Kitabchi et al. 2006), and the condition has largely been confined to the elderly. However, a recent case series in pediatric patients reported HHS in teenage boys of African American descent (Cochran, Walters, and Losek 2006). Obesity and acanthosis nigricans, findings indicative of insulin resistance, were common in this case series. Morbidity and mortality in these patients were tragically high, with 72% of the children in this series dying after a course of fever, renal failure, arrhythmias, and rhabdomyolysis.

Public Health Preventive or Intervention Strategies

Presumably, measures successful in reducing the incidence of type 2 diabetes would decrease episodes of HHS overall, but little data exist to support this notion. Similarly, increased patient education about the symptoms of diabetes is likely to be effective, but well-designed studies are needed to confirm this assumption. Population-based studies are needed to test effective interventions for preventing the development of HHS in patients with type 2 diabetes.

■ Hypoglycemia

Introduction

Hypoglycemia, or abnormally low blood sugar, usually occurs as an unintentional consequence of therapy intended to lower blood sugar. Over the last two decades, multiple randomized clinical trials have documented the clinical benefit of intensive glycemic control to near-normal levels in patients with diabetes. However these studies have also shown that with attempts to lower blood sugars to near-normal levels, hypoglycemia becomes more common (Cryer, Davis, and Shamoon 2003).

Clinical Presentation and Risk Factors

Initially, patients with diabetes who are facing hypoglycemia (plasma glucose ≤60 mg/dL) mount defense mechanisms that raise glucose levels, including activation of the autonomic nervous system and secretion of glucagon and cortisol (Cryer, Davis, and Shamoon 2003). As a result of autonomic nervous system activation, patients experience tremors, palpitations, sweating, and hunger. With time and repeated episodes of hypoglycemia, counterregulatory mechanisms, including autonomic activity, are lost. Absence of autonomic response to hypoglycemia leads to unperceived low blood sugars, a phenomenon termed hypoglycemic unawareness. When blood sugars fall below about 50 mg/dL, the central nervous system's function is impaired and neuroglycopenic symptoms develop. These range from fatigue, tingling, confusion, and decreased vision to loss of consciousness, seizures, and death. Hypoglycemic unawareness can lead to more frequent profound hypoglycemia, including neuroglycopenia (Cryer, Davis, and Shamoon 2003).

People with diabetes may have multiple risk factors for hypoglycemia, including excessive insulin dose, decreased exogenous glucose delivery (e.g., because of missed meals), decreased endogenous glucose production (e.g., following alcohol ingestion), increased insulin sensitivity (e.g., from exercise or weight loss), and decreased insulin clearance (e.g., progressive renal failure) (Cryer, Davis, and Shamoon 2003). An even more important risk factor is compromised glucose counterregulation in type 1 and advanced type 2 diabetes (Cryer, Davis, and Shamoon 2003).

Epidemiology

Prevalence and Incidence

Studies suggest that hypoglycemia is 10 times more common in type 1 than in type 2 diabetes (Cryer, Davis, and Shamoon 2003). Hypoglycemia is life threatening, especially in type 1 diabetes, where it is associated with 4% mortality (Cryer, Davis, and Shamoon 2003). Hypoglycemia can severely impede occupational and social functioning and greatly decrease quality of life for patients and their families.

The incidence of severe hypoglycemia in individuals with type 1 diabetes ranges from 62 to 170 episodes per 100 patient-years (Cryer, Davis, and Shamoon 2003). In the Diabetes Control and Complications Trial (DCCT), 65% of participants in the intensively treated group experienced severe hypoglycemia at least once over 6.5 years of follow-up (Cryer, Davis, and Shamoon 2003). In this study patients experiencing severe hypoglycemia were at high risk for subsequent episodes (The DCCT Research Group 1997). Among DCCT subjects in the intensive arm, 22% experienced five or more severe hypoglycemia episodes over the first 5 years of follow-up (The DCCT Research Group 1997).

Numerous observational studies raise concern that frequent and severe hypoglycemia can negatively affect cognition, especially in children and those with complicated, long-standing diabetes. Fortunately, in adults with type 1 diabetes, the prospective DCCT/EDIC (Epidemiology of Diabetes Interventions and Complications) study found that more frequent hypoglycemia had little long-term effect on function of the central nervous system (Jacobson et al. 2007). Similar prospective studies in older and younger patients and in patients with more advanced diabetes are lacking.

The specific incidence of severe hypoglycemia in type 2 diabetes is debated, with concern that rates in the general community are higher than those seen in clinical trials (Cryer, Davis, and Shamoon 2003). In larger clinical trials of type 2 diabetes, severe hypoglycemia occurs in 2%–4% of patients per annum. However, other studies, primarily population-based and retrospective chart reviews, show rates of severe hypoglycemia ranging between 3 and 73 episodes per 100 patient-years (Cryer, Davis, and Shamoon 2003).

Public Health Preventive or Intervention Strategies

Prevention, early recognition, and appropriate treatment of hypoglycemia are important goals in persons at risk for this problem. Blood Glucose Awareness Training (BGAT) and Hypoglycemia Anticipation, Awareness, and Treatment Training (HAAT) are validated educational programs of comparable efficacy designed to improve detection and response to hypoglycemia (Cox et al. 2006). Both of these programs were developed at the University of Virginia; the HAAT program was devised to aid individuals with recurrent hypoglycemia (Cox et al. 2006). Availability of BGAT and HAAT has been limited. Previously, a third edition of BGAT, which incorporates aspects of HAAT, was available online and supported by a grant from the American Diabetes Association. Results of this online program are promising; however, this program is not currently available (Cox et al. 2008). More information may be found at http://www.healthsystem.virginia.edu/bmc/bgathome/flash/index2.htm. Studies of

BGAT have focused on white adults with type 1 diabetes, but researchers in the field are pursuing studies in type 2 diabetes, in children, and in other racial groups (Cox et al. 2006).

Several technological approaches offer hope for hypoglycemia. Newer insulin analogs, both rapid acting (aspart, lispro, glulisine) and longer acting (glargine, detemir), improve control with lower risk of hypoglycemia. The trade-off is higher cost and limited long-term data (especially in pregnancy). Insulin pump therapy is generally associated with less hypoglycemia, but data are largely observational and mostly from type 1 patients. Finally, continuous glucose monitoring systems, which give real-time interstitial tissue glucose readings, have come to market. Ultimately, these devices may offer significant benefit to those with hypoglycemia unawareness, but the technologies are costly and suffer some limitations in accuracy.

■ Infections and Diabetes

Introduction

There is considerable controversy concerning the presumed link between diabetes and the incidence of serious infections. Although experimental literature supports this theory, strong epidemiologic evidence linking diabetes and serious infections is lacking. However, there is some evidence that patients with diabetes are at greater risk for infection with certain microorganisms and that adults with diabetes are at relatively greater risk for infection-related mortality (Joshi et al. 1999). Table 5.1 summarizes the clinical features, diagnosis, and causative organisms of common infections in people with diabetes (Joshi et al. 1999).

Influenza and Pneumonia

Until the 20th century, information was limited on the risks of influenza in persons with diabetes. In the late 1970s, however, reports began to surface that patients with diabetes might be at greater risk for influenza during both epidemic and non-epidemic control periods. More recent studies have shown that individuals with diabetes are indeed more susceptible to influenza and pneumonia and have greater morbidity and mortality than persons without diabetes (Smith and Poland 2003).

Public Health Preventive or Intervention Strategies

Effectiveness of vaccination. The efficacy of both the influenza and pneumococcal vaccines in decreasing infection-related complications and deaths in the general

TABLE 5.1 *Clinical Features, Diagnosis, and Causative Organisms of Selected Infections in Patients with Diabetes*

Infection	Clinical Features	Diagnostic Procedure*	Organisms	Comments
Respiratory tract				
Community-acquired pneumonia	Cough, fever	Chest radiography	*Streptococcus pneumonia, Staphylococcus aureus, Haemophilus influenzae,* other gram-negative bacilli, atypical pathogens	Pneumococcal infection carries a higher risk of death in people with diabetes than in people without diabetes.
Urinary tract				
Acute bacterial Cystitis	Increased urinary frequency, dysuria, suprapubic pain	Urine culture	*Escherichia coli, Proteus* species	Bacteriuria is more common in women with diabetes than in women without diabetes.
Acute pyelonephritis	Fever, flank pain	Urine culture	*E. coli, Proteus* species	Emphysematous infection should be considered.
Emphysematous pyelonephritis	Fever, flank pain, poor response to antibiotics	Radiography or CT scanning	*E. coli,* other gram-negative bacilli	Emergency nephrectomy often required.
Perinephric abscess	Fever, flank pain, poor response to antibiotics	Ultrasonography or CT scanning	*E. coli,* other gram-negative bacilli	Surgical drainage usually required.
Fungal cystitis	Same as for acute bacterial cystitis	Urine culture	*Candida* species	Difficult to distinguish colonization from infection.

(continued)

TABLE 5.1 *(continued)*

Infection	Clinical Features	Diagnostic Procedure*	Organisms	Comments
Soft tissue†				
Necrotizing fasciitis	Local pain, redness, crepitus, bullous skin lesions	Radiography or CT scanning	Gram-negative bacilli, anaerobes (type I), or group A streptococci (type II)	High mortality; emergency surgery required.
Other				
Invasive otitis externa	Ear pain, otorrhea, hearing loss, cellulitis	Clinical examination, magnetic resonance imaging	*Pseudomonas aeruginosa*	Prompt otolaryngologic consultation recommended.
Rhinocerebral mucormycosis	Facial or ocular pain, fever, lethargy, black nasal eschar	Clinical examination, magnetic resonance imaging, pathological findings	*Mucor* and *rhizopus* species	Strong association with keto acidosis; emergency surgery required.
Abdomen				
Emphysematous cholecystitis	Fever, right-upper-quadrant abdominal pain, systemic toxicity	Radiography	Gram-negative bacilli, anaerobes	High mortality; gallstones in 50%; emergency cholecystectomy required.

*CT denotes computed tomography.
†Foot infections are described in detail in Table 5.2.
Source: Reproduced with permission from Joshi et al. 1999.

population is well established (Smith and Poland 2003). Although there is evidence that individuals with diabetes have appropriate humoral immune response to vaccinations in general (Smith and Poland 2003), there are few clinical trials on the effectiveness of vaccination for influenza and pneumococcal disease in people with diabetes (Smith and Poland 2003). Thus, definitive proof of the efficacy of influenza and pneumococcal vaccination is lacking for people with diabetes. However studies that include diabetics as one of the patient groups who are "at risk" support immunization in people with diabetes (Smith and Poland 2003).

Guidelines for vaccination. Although the efficacy of the pneumococcal/influenza vaccine in preventing non-bacteremic disease is uncertain, there is good evidence that vaccination is effective in reducing life-threatening bacteremic disease (Smith and Poland 2003). Therefore, the Advisory Committee on Immunization Practices (ACIP) recommends that influenza vaccinations be given yearly and that they begin each September for individuals with diabetes who are aged ≥6 months (Smith and Poland 2003). The ACIP also recommends that the pneumococcal vaccine be given to all persons with diabetes to reduce invasive disease from pneumococcus (Smith and Poland 2003). A one-time revaccination is recommended for persons more than 64 years old and those with nephritic syndrome, chronic renal disease, and other immunocompromised states such as status post-organ transplantation (Smith and Poland 2003).

The ACIP also recommends that vaccination be considered for patients with diabetes who: (1) are aged 64 or older, (2) are residents of nursing homes or other chronic care facilities, (3) have frequent medical visits or hospitalization, or (4) have chronic disorders of the cardiopulmonary system (Smith and Poland 2003). Because influenza can be transmitted from person to person it is also recommended that health care workers and the family members of patients with diabetes be vaccinated.

Lower-Extremity Infections

More than 60% of nontraumatic lower-extremity amputations (LEAs) occur in people with diabetes (CDC 2008). In 2004, about 71,000 nontraumatic LEAs were performed in people with diabetes (CDC 2008). Annual incidence rates for LEA range from 5.3 to 8.1 per 1000 individuals with diabetes (Moss, Klein, and Klein 1992). A foot ulcer often begins the chain of events that lead to an LEA. Table 5.2 shows the organisms commonly associated with foot ulcers in individuals with diabetes (Joshi et al. 1999). An estimated 15% of persons with diabetes will develop foot ulcers, with 15%–20% of these persons eventually requiring LEA (Ollendorf et al. 1998). Estimated direct costs for LEAs range from $20,000 to $60,000, but perhaps as many as half of all LEAs could have been prevented by modifying risk factors such as high blood pressure, dyslipidemia, smoking, and inadequate glycemic control and by improving foot care in persons with diabetes (Ollendorf et al. 1998).

TABLE 5.2   *Foot Infections in Patients with Diabetes*

Infection	Clinical Features	Diagnostic Procedure*	Causative Organisms	Initial Management
Mild, not limb threatening	Shallow ulcer; less than 2 cm cellulitis, no evidence of fasciitis, abscess, or osteomyelitis; no evidence of ischemia; good metabolic control	Plain radiography, possibly culture*	Primarily aerobic gram-positive cocci (e.g., *Staphylococcus aureus,* streptococci)	Oral antibiotics[†]; wound care[‡]; outpatient management if there is good home support
Limb threatening	Deep ulcer, more than 2 cm cellulitis; suspected deep infection; ischemia; poor metabolic control	Plain radiography; deep cultures, "probe to bone" test[§]	Polymicrobial; aerobic gram-positive cocci, strict anaerobes (e.g., *Bacteroides fragilis*), and gram-negative bacilli (e.g., *Escherichia coli*)	Immediate hospitalization and surgical consultation; broad-spectrum intravenous antibiotics[¶]; wound care[‡]

*Because gram-positive cocci are the anticipated pathogens, cultures are not clearly required in each case.

[†] Recommended oral antibiotics include cephalexin, clindamycin, and amoxicillin-clavulanate.

[‡] Wound care includes sharp débridement of devitalized tissue and callus, sterile dressings, and relief of pressure at the ulcer.

[§] The ability to touch bone when the wound is gently probed with a sterile surgical probe is predictive of underlying osteomyelitis.

[¶] Recommended intravenous antibiotics include a beta-lactam plus a beta-lactamase inhibitor (e.g., ampicillin-sulbactam) or clindamycin plus a gram-negative drug (e.g., a third-generation cephalosporin, a fluoroquinolone, or aztreonam). Vancomycin plus impipenem-cilastin is recommended for life-threatening infections.

Source: Reproduced with permission from Joshi et al. 1999.

Because of the high personal and societal cost of amputations, several attempts have been made to develop and implement preventive strategies to prevent the need for this procedure. Currently, available data support three strategic methods: educational interventions for patients and providers, multidisciplinary clinics, and insurance coverage for therapeutic shoes (Ollendorf et al. 1998). According to available data, up to a 50%–85% reduction in LEAs can be attained by implementing a combination of these interventions (Ollendorf et al. 1998).

Mucormycosis and Malignant Otitis Externa

Mucormycosis and malignant otitis externa are rare severe life-threatening infections that can occur in people with diabetes and are associated with high rates of morbidity and mortality (Joshi et al. 1999); these infections tend to occur in patients whose diabetes is very poorly controlled. Mucormycosis is a fungal infection of the sinuses, brain, or lungs that is attributed to immune suppression that occurs in diabetes. Rhinocerebral mucormycosis is a severe and potentially fatal infection of the sinuses and brain (Joshi et al. 1999) that is treated by surgical debridement of infected tissue and drainage of infected sinuses. Crucial adjunctive therapies for rhinocerebral mucormycosis involve controlling blood sugar levels in people with diabetes and the institution of amphotericin B therapy.

Malignant otitis externa is a potentially life-threatening infection of the external auditory canal and skull. When it affects people with diabetes, it is more commonly seen in elderly persons with type 2 disease (Joshi et al. 1999). In the vast majority of patients, *Pseudomonas aeruginosa* is the pathogen involved. Symptoms include unrelenting pain, otorrhea, and hearing loss without fever (Joshi et al. 1999). The goal of treatment is to cure the infection. Treatment takes several months because of the difficulties of treating the bacteria and reaching infection that is housed within bone tissue. Strict control of the patient's diabetes is mandatory but can be difficult to achieve during acute illness.

■ Inflammation and Diabetes

Introduction

Inflammatory Markers

The role of inflammatory markers in the pathogenesis of diabetes and associated cardiovascular complications is controversial. Support for a role for inflammation comes from recent studies suggesting that subclinical chronic inflammation may be an important pathogenetic factor in the development of insulin resistance and type 2 diabetes. Surrogate markers for this low-grade chronic inflammation include high-sensitivity C-reactive protein (hs-CRP), interleukin-1 (IL-1), interleukin-6 (IL-6), and tumor necrosis factor α (TNF-α) (Sjoholm 2006).

C-Reactive Protein and Risk of Diabetes

The most widely studied inflammatory marker is hs-CRP. Available data indicate that, at least in women, elevated hs-CRP levels predict development of the metabolic syndrome (often defined as an individual having three or more of the following: abdominal obesity, hypertriglyceridemia, low HDL [high-density lipoprotein] cholesterol, hypertension, elevated fasting glucose).

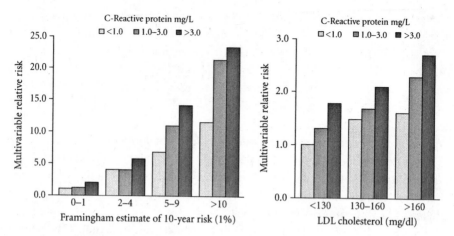

FIGURE 5.2. Multivariable-adjusted relative risks of cardiovascular disease according to levels of C-reactive protein and the estimated 10-year risk based on the Framingham Risk Score as currently defined by the National Cholesterol Education Program and according to levels of C-reactive protein and categories of LDL cholesterol. (Reproduced with permission from Ridker et al., *New England Journal of Medicine*, 2002.)

In a 6-year follow-up to the Mexico City Diabetes Study that included 729 women, baseline hs-CRP was significantly correlated with the development of the metabolic syndrome. Versus the lowest tertile, women in the highest tertile of baseline hs-CRP levels had a relative risk of 4.0 for developing the metabolic syndrome (Han et al. 2002). Elsewhere, in the Insulin Resistance Atherosclerosis Study (IRAS), 1047 subjects without diabetes were followed over 5 years. The investigators found a significant linear association between the incidence of new-onset diabetes and increasing quartiles of fibrinogen, hs-CRP, and plasminogen activator inhibitor-1 (PAI-1) (Festa et al. 2002).

C-Reactive Protein and Risk of Cardiovascular Events

Recent data suggest that inflammatory markers such as CRP add significant information to conventional measures of cardiovascular risk in individual patients. In a recent study that followed 27,939 healthy American women, CRP was found to be a stronger predictor of cardiovascular events than LDL cholesterol (see Fig. 5.2) (Ridker et al. 2002), which has long been recognized as a cardiovascular risk factor and is the focus for current guidelines on the assessment of cardiovascular risk. The same study examined the addition of CRP to the Framingham risk score and to LDL cholesterol categories of <130, 130–160, and >160 mg/dL in predicting cardiovascular events; the authors found that increasing levels of CRP were associated with increased risk of cardiovascular events at all levels of estimated 10-year Framingham risk scores and at all levels of LDL cholesterol (<130, 130–160, and >160 mg/dL) (Ridker et al. 2002).

■ Future Directions

In a recent consensus statement for health professionals jointly sponsored by the CDC and the American Heart Association (AHA), the two groups concluded that hs-CRP may be a valuable marker to add to traditional risk factors in predicting the risk of cardiovascular disease (Pearson et al. 2003). The CDC and the AHA jointly recommend that CRP measurements be considered for patients at intermediate risk (10-year risk of coronary heart disease of 10%–20%), in whom the results may be of value in guiding further assessments and treatment decisions (Pearson et al. 2003).

Although it remains unclear whether hs-CRP should be a treatment target, recent studies found that treatment with a statin (Nissen et al. 2004) and treatment with metformin and lifestyle changes in the Diabetes Prevention Program led to significant reductions in hs-CRP levels (Haffner et al. 2005). Future clinical trials are needed to validate these early findings and recommendations.

■ References

Balasubramanyam A et al. (2008) Syndromes of ketosis-prone diabetes mellitus. *Endocrine Reviews* **29**, 292–302.

Centers for Disease Control and Prevention (2008). National diabetes fact sheet: general information and national estimates on diabetes in the United States, 2007. Atlanta, GA: U.S. Department of Health and Human Services, Centers for Disease Control and Prevention, 2008. Available at: http://www.cdc.gov/diabetes/statistics. Accessed September 18, 2008.

Cochran JB, Walters S, Losek JD (2006). Pediatric hyperglycemic hyperosmolar syndrome: diagnostic difficulties and high mortality rate. *American Journal of Emergency Medicine* **24**, 297–301.

Cox DJ et al. (2006). Blood Glucose Awareness Training (BGAT): what is it, where is it, and where is it going? *Diabetes Spectrum* **19**, 43–9.

Cox DJ et al. (2008). Blood Glucose Awareness Training delivered over the Internet. *Diabetes Care* **31**, 1527–8.

Cryer PE, Davis SN, Shamoon H (2003). Hypoglycemia in diabetes. *Diabetes Care* **26**, 1902–12.

The DCCT Research Group (1997). Hypoglycemia in the Diabetes Control and Complications Trial. *Diabetes* **46**, 271–86.

Egede LE, Willi SM (2000). Atypical diabetes mellitus: time for a consensus? *Pediatric Diabetes* **1**, 226–32.

Festa A et al. (2002). Elevated levels of acute-phase proteins and plasminogen activator inhibitor-1 predict the development of type 2 diabetes: the insulin resistance atherosclerosis study. *Diabetes* **51**, 1131–7.

Ginde AA, Pelletier AJ, Camargo CA Jr (2006). National study of U.S. emergency department visits with diabetic ketoacidosis, 1993–2003. *Diabetes Care* **29**, 2117–9.

Haffner S et al. (2005). Intensive lifestyle intervention or metformin on inflammation and coagulation in participants with impaired glucose tolerance. *Diabetes* **54**, 1566–72.

Han TS et al. (2002). Prospective study of C-reactive protein in relation to the development of diabetes and metabolic syndrome in the Mexico City Diabetes Study. *Diabetes Care* **25**, 2016–21.

Jacobson AM et al. (2007). Long-term effect of diabetes and its treatment on cognitive function. *New England Journal of Medicine* **356**, 1842–52.

Joshi N et al. (1999). Infections in patients with diabetes mellitus. *New England Journal of Medicine* **341**, 1906–12.

Kitabchi AE et al. (2006). Hyperglycemic crises in adult patients with diabetes: a consensus statement from the American Diabetes Association. *Diabetes Care* **29**, 2739–48.

Maniatis AK et al. (2005). Increased incidence and severity of diabetic ketoacidosis among uninsured children with newly diagnosed type 1 diabetes mellitus. *Pediatric Diabetes* **6**, 79–83.

Moss SE, Klein R, Klein BE (1992). The prevalence and incidence of lower extremity amputation in a diabetic population. *Archives of Internal Medicine* **152**, 610–6.

Nissen SE et al. (2004). Effect of intensive compared with moderate lipid-lowering therapy on progression of coronary atherosclerosis: a randomized controlled trial. *JAMA* **291**, 1071–80.

Ollendorf DA et al. (1998). Potential economic benefits of lower-extremity amputation prevention strategies in diabetes. *Diabetes Care* **21**, 1240–5.

Pearson TA et al. (2003). Markers of inflammation and cardiovascular disease: application to clinical and public health practice: a statement for healthcare professionals from the Centers for Disease Control and Prevention and the American Heart Association. *Circulation* **107**, 499–511.

Ridker PM et al. (2002). Comparison of C-reactive protein and low-density lipoprotein cholesterol levels in the prediction of first cardiovascular events. *New England Journal of Medicine* **347**, 1557–65.

Sjoholm A, Nystrom T (2006). Inflammation and the etiology of type 2 diabetes. *Diabetes/Metabolism Research and Reviews* 22(1), 4-10.

Smith SA, Poland GA (2003). Immunization and the prevention of influenza and pneumococcal disease in people with diabetes. *Diabetes Care* **26** (Suppl. 1), S126–8.

6. DIABETES AND VISION

Ronald Klein, Jinan B. Saaddine, and Barbara E. K. Klein

■ Main Public Health Messages

- Diabetic retinopathy, a leading cause of visual impairment, is a frequent complication of diabetes.
- Inadequate blood glucose and blood pressure control are important risk factors for diabetic retinopathy.
- The early detection and timely treatment of diabetic retinopathy can prevent loss of vision.
- Many people are not receiving recommended eye care for diabetic retinopathy.
- Various public health programs have been developed to overcome barriers to optimal eye care.

■ Introduction

A primary function of the eye is to provide sharp vision for both near and distant activities. To achieve this, the ocular media of the eye (cornea, lens, vitreous gel) must be clear, and the structure and function of the retina and optic nerve must be undisturbed. Visual acuity may be reduced by changes in lens clarity (cataract) and by damage to the retinal nerve fiber layer from relatively high intraocular pressure (glaucoma). Vision may also be lost due to abnormalities in the structure and function of small retinal blood vessels (retinopathy). Progression of diabetic retinopathy may result in swelling of the central portion of the retina or of the macula (macular edema) and/or lead to the growth of fragile retinal new blood vessels (proliferative diabetic retinopathy [PDR]) with bleeding into the vitreous gel in front of the retina (vitreous hemorrhage) and traction on the macula. Loss of vision from these advanced stages of diabetic retinopathy can be prevented with timely detection and treatment before bleeding or traction has occurred. The purpose of this chapter is to review the epidemiology of visual loss associated with early and advanced stages of these ocular complications and to briefly discuss public health interventions.

■ Background/Historical Perspective

Visual Impairment in Persons with Diabetes

Data from epidemiologic studies in the early 1980s (e.g., the Wisconsin Epidemiologic Study of Diabetic Retinopathy [WESDR]) showed a relatively high prevalence (8.3% in younger-onset type 1 and 12.3% in older-onset type 2 diabetes) of any visual impairment (visual acuity in best-corrected better eye of 20/40 or worse) (Klein R, Klein B, and Moss 1984) in persons with diabetes. Severe loss of vision (visual acuity best corrected in better eye of 20/200 or worse) was present in 3.2% of the younger-onset group; in 85.7% of these the cause was severe retinopathy. In older-onset persons severe loss of vision was present in 1.6%; in 33.0% the cause was severe retinopathy, and in 50% the causes included cataract, glaucoma, or other problems.

In a compilation of data from population-based epidemiologic studies done 10–20 years after the WESDR, the prevalence of severe visual impairment attributed to diabetic retinopathy was lower (Congdon et al. 2004). In one of the studies, the Beaver Dam Eye Study, in people aged 43–86 years at baseline, PDR or macular edema was the cause of incident severe visual impairment in only 3%, versus 33% in WESDR participants with type 2 diabetes seen approximately 10 years earlier (Klein R et al. 2006). It was assumed that better control of glycemia and blood pressure and earlier detection and timely treatment of PDR and macular edema by laser photocoagulation had led to less severe loss of vision than in the past.

In the WESDR in persons with type 1 disease the estimated annual incidence of severe visual impairment due to diabetic retinopathy was lower in successive follow-up periods. Furthermore, for any given duration of diabetes, type 1 diabetic persons diagnosed earlier were more likely to have visual impairment than those whose diagnosis was in later years (R. Klein unpublished data). In a clinic-based study in Denmark in 2004, the prevalence of visual impairment was also lower than anticipated from the existing literature (Hovind et al. 2003). With continued changes in medical care leading to changes in prevalence and incidence of diabetic retinopathy, ongoing surveillance will be needed to estimate visual loss due to diabetes in the U.S. population. Most of these data on visual loss in persons with diabetes are from studies of persons of European ancestry, and there is a need to examine racial/ethnic disparities regarding loss of vision due to diabetic retinopathy.

Natural History of Diabetic Retinopathy

Micronaneurysms (MAs), the earliest clinically apparent abnormality in the retina, are found in about 20%–30% of persons with type 2 diabetes at the time of diagnosis but are rarely seen in persons with type 1 diabetes until 5 years after diagnosis.

By themselves, retinal MAs are not a threat to vision, but as retinopathy progresses, there may be leakage of blood and lipoproteins from retinal capillaries or MAs, leading to the appearance of blot hemorrhages (BHs) and hard exudates (HEs), respectively. Eyes with only retinal MAs and BHs and/or HEs are classified as having mild nonproliferative diabetic retinopathy. These exudative changes are often accompanied by reduced blood flow due to closure of the retinal capillaries and arterioles. This results in various signs of lack of oxygenation of the retinal tissue ("cotton wool spots" or "soft exudates"), dilated retinal capillaries (intraretinal microvascular abnormalities); large, dark, intraretinal hemorrhages; and venous beading and duplication. These changes have been called the "preproliferative phase" and are a warning sign of impending growth of abnormal new retinal vessels. Patients are classified as having moderate to severe nonproliferative diabetic retinopathy, and it is not unusual for them to be asymptomatic.

The appearance of abnormal, fragile new blood vessels and fibrous tissue from the inner retinal surface defines the onset of the proliferative phase of diabetic retinopathy; at this point, patients have PDR. Screening programs using ophthalmoscopy through dilated pupils or examination of fundus photographs are designed to detect PDR before vitreous hemorrhage or traction on the macular occurs and affects vision.

Macular Edema

Increased leakage from the retinal capillaries and MAs may result in macular edema, seen as a thickening of the normally compact macular tissue. If the fovea is involved, visual acuity may decrease. Screening is designed to detect macular edema before the fovea is affected.

Pathogenesis

Data from epidemiologic studies have demonstrated strong dose-response relationships between hyperglycemia and the incidence and progression of diabetic retinopathy (Klein R et al. 1994a). Fortunately, randomized controlled clinical trials such as the Diabetes Control and Complications Trial (DCCT) and United Kingdom Prospective Diabetes Study (UKPDS) (Diabetes Control and Complications Trial Research Group 1993; UK Prospective Diabetes Study [UKPDS] Group 1998a) have demonstrated that intensive treatment and reduction of hyperglycemia reduce the incidence and progression of retinopathy.

■ Epidemiology

Prevalence of Diabetic Retinopathy

The overall prevalence of diabetic retinopathy found in 1980–1982 in the WESDR among whites was 71% in persons with younger-onset type 1 diabetes and 50% in persons with older-onset type 2 diabetes. The prevalence of PDR was highest

TABLE 6.1   *Prevalence and Severity of Retinopathy and Macular Edema at Baseline Examination in the Wisconsin Epidemiologic Study of Diabetic Retinopathy (WEDRS)*

Retinopathy Status	Younger-Onset, Taking Insulin (n = 996)	Older-Onset, Taking Insulin (n = 673)	Older-Onset, Not Taking Insulin (n = 673)
None	29	30	61
Early nonproliferative	30	31	27
Moderate to severe nonproliferative	18	26	9
Proliferative without DRS high-risk characteristics	13	9	1
Proliferative with DRS high-risk characteristics or worse	10	5	1
Clinically significant macular edema	6	12	4

DRS, Diabetic Retinopathy Study.

Source: Modified from Klein R (1995). Copyright 1995; Elsevier.

in the younger-onset group, whereas the prevalence of macular edema was similar in younger-onset (type 1) persons and older-onset persons not taking insulin (Table 6.1). The frequency of any retinopathy was associated with duration in all three groups (younger-onset, taking insulin; older-onset, taking insulin; older-onset, not taking insulin) (see Figs. 6.1A,B). The finding of vision-threatening PDR in older-onset persons at the time of diagnosis was one reason for the development of guidelines for dilated ophthalmoscopic examination in these persons by skilled ophthalmoscopists because they were often asymptomatic and unlikely to be detected by a primary care physician or diabetologist.

Period Cohort Effect

Lower prevalence of any retinopathy and of PDR has been reported in more recent years in diabetic persons of European ancestry than had previously been reported in the WESDR (Kempen et al. 2004). In the WESDR, for any given duration of diabetes, persons with type 1 diabetes whose year of diagnosis was in earlier years were more likely to have PDR than those diagnosed in later years. For example among type 1 patients with disease duration of 25 to 29 years, prevalence of PDR was 25% among those diagnosed in 1953–1957; 18% among those diagnosed in 1958–1962; 8% among those diagnosed in 1963–1967; and 2% among those diagnosed in 1968–1972. In a clinic-based study in

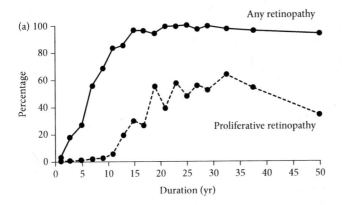

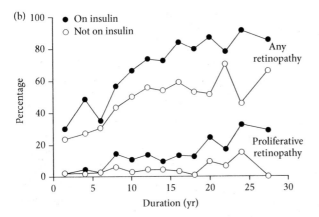

FIGURE 6.1. (a) Prevalence of any retinopathy and of proliferative diabetic retinopathy in patients diagnosed with diabetes at age 30 years or older, by duration of diabetes. Data are from Wisconsin Epidemiologic Study of Diabetic Retinopathy 1980–1982. (Reproduced with permission from Klein, Klein, and Moss 1992.) (b) Prevalence of any retinopathy and of proliferative diabetic retinopathy in patients diagnosed with diabetes at age 30 years or older, by duration of diabetes. Data are from Wisconsin Epidemiologic Study of Diabetic Retinopathy 1980–1982. (Reproduced with permission from Klein, Klein, and Moss 1992.)

Denmark in 2004, for persons with similar durations of diabetes, the prevalence of PDR was also lower in later than in earlier periods (Hove et al. 2004). However, this was not found in a cohort studied in Allegheny County, Pennsylvania (Pambianco et al. 2006).

Incidence of Diabetic Retinopathy

The overall 10-year incidence of diabetic retinopathy found in the WESDR was 89% in persons with younger-onset type 1 diabetes, 79% in persons with older-onset type 2 taking insulin, and 67% in persons with type 2 not taking insulin (Klein R et al. 1994b). Incidence of PDR was highest in the younger-onset group, while the 4-year incidence of macular edema was similar in younger-onset persons and older-onset persons taking insulin (Table 6.2).

TABLE 6.2   *Ten-Year Incidence of Progression of Diabetic Retinopathy and Clinically Significant Macular Edema in the Wisconsin Epidemiologic Study of Diabetic Retinopathy (WESDR), 1980–1982 to 1990–1992*

	Younger-Onset (%)	Older-Onset Taking Insulin (%)	Older-Onset Not Taking Insulin (%)
Incidence of any retinopathy	89	79	67
Progression of two or more steps	76	69	53
Progression to PDR	30	24	10
Incidence of CSME	14	18	9

PDR, proliferative diabetic retinopathy; CSME, clinically significant macular edema.

Source: Reprinted with permission from The American Diabetes Association. Modified from: Klein R et al. (1994b). Copyright 1994 American Diabetes Association.

Race/Ethnicity

The reported prevalence of diabetic retinopathy among persons with type 2 disease was higher in African Americans and Mexican Americans than in whites in the Multi-Ethnic Study of Atherosclerosis (MESA) (Wong et al. 2006). In MESA, however, the differences by racial/ethnic group were attenuated when analyses were adjusted for glycemic levels, waist-to-hip ratios, and diabetes duration, suggesting that these factors might explain the higher rates found in blacks and Hispanics in that study (in MESA, Mexican Americans and Puerto Ricans constituted the Hispanic group) (Wong et al. 2006). Similar findings have been observed in other population-based studies comparing whites with Hispanics and blacks. Also, in MESA, the prevalence of retinopathy was similar in Chinese Americans and whites (Wong et al. 2006).

Among patients with type 2 disease the frequency and severity of retinopathy in Native Americans has been thought to be higher than in whites (Lee et al. 2001). In one comparison, however, a lower duration-adjusted 4-year cumulative incidence of retinopathy was found in one Native American group, the Pima, compared with that found in whites with type 2 diabetes in the WESDR (Diabetes Control and Complications Research Group 2002).

Risk Factors for Diabetic Retinopathy

Glycemia

Data from almost all epidemiologic studies have shown hyperglycemia to be the strongest risk factor for the incidence and progression of diabetic retinopathy and the incidence of macular edema, regardless of duration of disease or level of retinopathy prior to the development of PDR (Klein et al. 1994a; Klein B and Klein R 1995). The WESDR data showed that the level of glycemia and not the type of diabetes was associated with progression of retinopathy (see Fig. 6.2) (Klein R et al. 1994). Reduction of hyperglycemia was associated with a reduced risk of progression of retinopathy at all levels of hyperglycemia, suggesting there was no threshold below which there was no benefit of controlling hyperglycemia.

Both the DCCT and the UKPDS showed the efficacy of intensive glycemic control in reducing the incidence and progression of retinopathy in persons with type 1 and 2 diabetes, respectively (Diabetes Control and Complications Trial Research Group 1993; UK Prospective Diabetes Study [UKPDS] Group 1998a). The DCCT examined both primary prevention (preventing diabetic retinopathy in patients with no retinopathy) and secondary prevention (preventing the progression of early retinopathy) in a study involving 1441 persons aged 13–39 years who were randomized to either conventional or intensive insulin therapy (Diabetes Control and Complications Trial Research Group 1993).

Intensive treatment reduced by 76% the adjusted mean risk of incident diabetic retinopathy among persons with no retinopathy. In the secondary-intervention group, patients assigned to intensive therapy reduced their average risk of progression by 54% during the entire study period when compared with patients assigned to conventional therapy. With both cohorts combined the intensive-therapy group also had a reduction in risk for development of severe nonproliferative retinopathy or PDR by 47% and of treatment with photocoagulation by 51% compared with the conventional therapy group. The beneficial effects became apparent after 3 years.

In the UKPDS, newly diagnosed patients with type 2 diabetes were randomly assigned to intensive glycemic control with either insulin, a sulfonylurea, or metformin and then compared to patients given conventional glycemic control (UK Prospective Diabetes Study [UKPDS] Group 1998a). The 1704 patients given metformin were all overweight, and analyses included comparison of the effect of metformin against conventional therapy in these patients. There was a 21% reduction in the 12-year rate of progression of diabetic retinopathy and a 29% reduction in need for laser photocoagulation in the intensive versus the conventional treatment group.

Evidence from epidemiologic studies and clinical trials has led to making the reduction of hyperglycemia through intensive treatment the primary public health care strategy for reducing the risk of visual loss from diabetic retinopathy in persons with type 1 or type 2 diabetes. Correspondingly in 1994 the American Diabetes Association (ADA) established a target goal of 7% for glycosylated hemoglobin among persons with diabetes (American Diabetes Association 1994). However, data from epidemiologic studies show that, despite some recent improvement in glycemic control, only 56% of adults with diabetes achieve this level of glycemic control, suggesting the need for new intervention strategies (Hoerger et al. 2008).

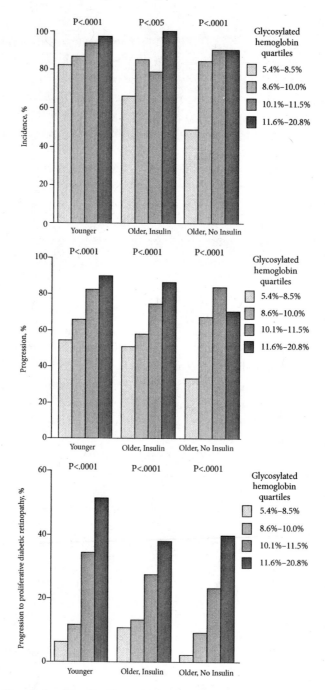

FIGURE 6.2. The relationship of incidence (top), progression (center), and progression to proliferative retinopathy (bottom) in persons with younger-onset diabetes, persons with older-onset diabetes taking insulin, and persons with older-onset diabetes not taking insulin over a 10-year period to Glycosylated Hemoglobin levels by quartiles for the whole population at baseline. The p values are based on the Mantel-Haenszel test of trend. Definitions: "Younger" = less than age 30 years when diagnosed, and "Older" = age 30 years or more when diagnosed with diabetes. (Reprinted with permission from the American Medical Association. Klein R et al. 1994. Copyright 1994, American Medical Association.)

Blood Pressure

High blood pressure damages the small blood vessels of the retina and clinically has been thought to increase the risk of retinopathy. In the WESDR, higher blood pressure at baseline was associated with the 14-year incidence of diabetic retinopathy in people with type 1 diabetes and an increase in the risk of macular edema in people with type 2 diabetes (Klein R et al. 1995; Klein R et al. 1998). Similarly, epidemiologic data from the UKPDS showed that for each 10 mm Hg decrease in mean systolic blood pressure there was a 13% reduction in microvascular complications, including retinopathy in persons with newly diagnosed type 2 diabetes (Adler et al. 2000). There was also a reported risk reduction in the UKPDS of microvascular complications, including an 11% drop in retinopathy per decrement of 10 mm Hg systolic blood pressure.

In contrast to the epidemiologic studies, randomized controlled clinical trials have not consistently shown that reductions in blood pressure result in reductions in the incidence and progression of retinopathy. In one such trial, The EURODIAB Controlled Trial of Lisinopril in Insulin-Dependent Diabetes Mellitus (EUCLID), in a group of largely normo-albuminuric normotensive type 1 diabetic patients, those randomized to lisinopril, an angiotensin-converting enzyme (ACE) inhibitor, had a 50% reduction in the progression of retinopathy over a 2-year period (Chaturvedi et al. 1998). However, when other factors were controlled for, the relationship did not reach significance ($p = 0.06$). Progression to PDR was also reduced, although again the relation was not significant.

In the UKPDS, 1048 patients with hypertension (mean blood pressure 160/94 mm Hg) were randomized to a regimen of tight control with either captopril (an ACE inhibitor) or atenolol (a beta blocker), while another 390 patients were randomized to less tight control (UK Prospective Diabetes Study [UKPDS] Group 1998b). At 4.5 years, those randomized to tight control had a highly significant 30% reduction in the number of subjects with five or more retinal MAs compared with those randomized to less tight control. There was also a 47% reduction in HEs and cotton wool spots, a 25% reduction in the progression of retinopathy, a 42% reduction in photocoagulation for diabetic macular edema, and a 24% reduction in risk of legal blindness in the tightly controlled group versus the less tightly controlled group. The effects of blood pressure control were independent of those of glycemic control. These findings support the recommendations for blood pressure control in patients with type 2 diabetes as a means of preventing visual loss from diabetic retinopathy.

The Appropriate Blood Pressure Control in Diabetes (ABCD) Trial involved two randomized masked clinical trials comparing intensive and moderate blood pressure control in persons with type 2 diabetes (Estacio et al. 2000; Schrier et al. 2002). Unlike the UKPDS, there was no difference between the intensive and moderate groups with regard to progression of diabetic retinopathy in hypertensive subjects in the first trial. However, in a second trial a significant reduction in the progression but not the incidence of retinopathy was found in normotensive patients.

The ADA guidelines recommend blood pressure level targets of <130/85 mm Hg based on the above clinical trial data (American Diabetes Association 1994). In the U.S. National Health and Nutrition Examination Survey (NHANES), among adults with diabetes in 1999–2002, only 40% met the ADA's recommendations (Resnick et al. 2006). These data show the difficulty of achieving recommendations based on findings from clinical trials in actual practice and the need for new approaches.

Lipid Levels

Epidemiologic data have shown that higher levels of serum lipids are associated with a higher frequency and incidence of retinal hard exudates (HEs) in persons with diabetes (Chew et al. 1996; Klein B et al. 1991). In the WESDR, independent of other risk factors, persons with higher serum total cholesterol were more likely to have retinal HEs (in those with type 1 diabetes, odds ratio [OR] per 50 mg/dL 1.65, 95% confidence interval [CI] 1.24 to 2.18, and in those with type 2 taking insulin, OR 1.50, 95% CI 1.01 to 2.22) (Klein B et al. 1991). Higher serum triglycerides, low-density lipoproteins (LDL), and very-low-density lipoproteins at baseline were associated with prevalent and incident retinal HEs and incident visual loss in the ETDRS (Early Treatment Diabetic Retinopathy Study) (Chew et al. 1996). Similar associations have been reported in other epidemiologic studies.

To date, there have been no completed large clinical trials showing the efficacy of lipid- lowering agents such as statins in reducing the progression of retinopathy, the incidence of macular edema, or loss of vision.

Smoking and Alcohol Consumption

Most epidemiologic data do not show a relationship between cigarette smoking or alcohol consumption and diabetic retinopathy (Klein R and Klein B 1995; Moss, Klein R, and Klein B 1994).

Use of Hormones and Reproductive Exposures

The use of oral contraceptives, which contain estrogens as well as progestins, or use of hormone replacement therapy after menopause, does not appear to increase the risk of retinopathy (Klein B, Klein R, and Moss 1999).

Progression of retinopathy in pregnancy is related to glycemia, blood pressure level, and prior duration of diabetes. However, pregnancy has been shown to be associated with more rapid progression of retinopathy independent of the level of glycemia and blood pressure (Klein B, Moss, and Klein R 1990; Chew et al. 1995). Even so, the number of past pregnancies has been reported to be unrelated to the severity of diabetic retinopathy in women with type 1 diabetes (Klein B, Klein R, and Moss 1999). Close observation of women with type 1 diabetes, especially those with retinopathy, is indicated during pregnancy and after delivery.

Genetics

The reader is referred to recent reviews that describe the genetics of diabetic retinopathy (Hanis and Hallman 2006). As of this writing few genes have been consistently found to be associated with diabetic retinopathy. This is likely to change with the advent of new technologies now being used to identify disease- and complication-specific genes.

Cataract

Cataract is the most common cause of visual impairment and blindness worldwide (Thylefors et al. 1995), and persons with diabetes are at increased risk of cataract (Ederer, Hiller, and Taylor 1981). The increased risk seems to be primarily due to cortical cataract and is also reflected in a higher prevalence of posterior subcapsular cataract and cataract surgery (Klein B et al. 1995).

Early data regarding the increased risk of cataract in those with diabetes were reported in the NHANES (Klein R and Klein B 1995). In addition, in those who had previously undiagnosed diabetes the rates of cataract were higher than for those who did not have diabetes (Klein R and Klein B 1995). Similar findings were reported for the Framingham Eye Study, but here the effect was more pronounced in younger persons (Ederer, Hiller, and Taylor 1981). Cataracts were more common in women than in men with diabetes in the WESDR (Klein B, Klein R, and Moss 1985). Age and duration of diabetes (Klein B et al. 1995) and triglyceride levels appear to increase the risk (Chen et al. 2008), and data suggest that the level of glycemia is important in determining the age at incidence of cataract (Klein B, Klein R, and Moss 1985; Klein B et al. 1995). The relationship of glycemia with cataract prompted the UKPDS to include cataract as an adverse endpoint in the clinical trial aimed at reducing diabetes complications (UK Prospective Diabetes Study [UKPDS] Group 1998a; Clarke et al. 2003). At this time it is unclear whether there is any substantial difference by race or ethnicity in risk of cataract among those with diabetes. The rate of cataract formation, however, is higher in persons who have had treatment for diabetic retinopathy (i.e., laser treatment, vitrectomy) and diabetic macular edema (i.e., periorbital or intraocular steroids) (Cardillo et al. 2005).

There is no treatment known to be successful in preventing cataract in those with diabetes except for the inferred benefit accrued from decreased hyperglycemia. Cataract surgery is currently the only known treatment for visually disabling cataract in those with or without diabetes. Cataract surgery is about twice as common in those with diabetes as in those without it (Klein B et al. 1995). Although cataract surgery in those with diabetes tends to be associated with increased complications (Ivancic et al. 2005), it is still usually successful in restoring visual acuity. It seems likely that despite glycemic control, cataract will still occur somewhat "prematurely" in those with diabetes. Therefore, health care planners need to provide sufficient support for surgery, follow-up care, and refractive services earlier in life for those with diabetes.

The pathophysiologic mechanisms responsible for cataracts in those with or without diabetes are poorly understood. Oxidative stress associated with hyperglycemia has been postulated as a cause of cataracts in those with diabetes (Osawa and Kato 2005), as have low levels of aldose reductase (Hegde and Varma 2005), activated polyol pathways, and glycosylation of lens proteins (Kyselova, Stefek, and Bauer 2004). There has been some research into the possibility of altering these pathophysiologic mechanisms in the lens in order to prevent cataract (Kyselova, Stefek, and Bauer 2004), but at this time, there is no proven medical therapy arising from this research.

Primary Open-Angle Glaucoma

Glaucoma manifests as loss of the visual field attributable to pressure on the optic nerve, resulting in loss of nerve fibers. Although there is always pressure within the globe (intraocular pressure), the level of pressure that leads to loss of nerve fibers varies from person to person, and the risk of glaucoma increases with increasing pressure. There are many types of glaucoma, but the vast majority of cases are primary open-angle glaucoma. The prevalence (and incidence) of this form of glaucoma rises with increasing age. In the NHANES II, which relies on self-reports, among persons aged ≥35 years there was a higher prevalence of glaucoma in those without diabetes (Klein R, Klein B 1995). Similar relationships were found from the National Health Interview Survey (Klein R, Klein B 1995). Many other studies have reported increased rates of glaucoma in persons with diabetes (Klein B, Klein R, and Jensen 1994; Klein R, Klein B 1995; Mitchell et al. 1997; Perruccio, Badley, and Trope 2007). A meta-analysis indicates that the relationship is consistent across many different studies representing different ethnic groups (Bonovas, Peponis, and Filioussi 2004). Duration of diabetes may increase the risk of glaucoma (in those with type 2 diabetes), but this association may be due to age (Klein R and Klein B 1995).

The physiologic cause of increased risk of glaucoma in those with diabetes is not certain, although some investigators suggest that it may reflect the slightly higher intraocular pressures in persons with diabetes (Klein B, Klein R, and Moss 1984; Leske and Podgor 1983).

Neovascular glaucoma results from the new growth of blood vessels in the front of the eye, where the normal fluid that is produced normally drains from the eye to the venous system. This form of glaucoma is associated with pain, often very elevated intraocular pressure, and profound loss of vision. It occurs most often in the presence of diabetes of long duration and in those who have had PDR. The loss of vision is thought to be due to the extreme elevation in intraocular pressure.

Corneal Disease

Recent studies have shown that changes in the corneal nerve plexus occur in persons with diabetes (Midena et al. 2006; Mocan et al. 2006). Whether this is associated with symptoms such as dry eye (as occurs with Sjogren disease) (Zhang et al. 2005) is not certain (Benitez-Del-Castillo et al. 2007). Changes in corneal nerves in those with diabetes are associated with peripheral neuropathy (Midena et al. 2006). Changes in the ocular surface appear to be particularly exacerbated in the presence of poor glycemic control (Yoon, Im, and Seo 2004). These problems may be an important consideration when considering refractive surgery (Yoon et al. 2004). Wound healing is likely delayed in the presence of diabetes (Wakuta et al. 2007). Diabetes seems to alter hydration control of the cornea, which may affect the ability to tolerate contact lenses (O'Donnell and Efron 2006). Neurotropic keratopathy is an uncommon complication of diabetes, but when it occurs it may be severe enough to cause corneal ulceration (Lockwood, Hope-Ross, and Chell 2006). Persons with diabetes may have a more prolonged recovery of optimal vision after cataract surgery (Morikubo et al. 2004; Lee et al. 2005). A clinical trial of a topical aldose reductase inhibitor has been shown to improve some of the corneal epithelial dysfunction in persons with diabetes (Nakahara et al. 2005).

Refraction

Refractive errors (often necessitating the use of spectacles or contact lenses for good vision) have been reported to be more common in persons with diabetes (Sonmez et al. 2005; Tarczy-Hornoch, Ying-Lai, and Varma 2006). Refractive error in the face of relatively poorly controlled glycemia is usually reversed or attenuated when better glycemic control is achieved. Refractive surgeons need to be aware of the glycemic control of their diabetic patients as they plan for such surgery (Sonmez et al. 2005, Tarczy-Hornoch, Ying-Lai, Varma 2006). Finally, eye care providers who refract for the prescription of spectacles or contact lenses should be aware of the variability in refraction due to levels of glycemia.

■ Public Health Preventive or Intervention Strategies

Effective primary and secondary interventions are available to reduce the incidence and progression of diabetic retinopathy, but implementation of these interventions has been suboptimal.

Rationale for Early Detection and Treatment of Diabetic Retinopathy

An important impetus for screening for diabetic retinopathy is the established efficacy of laser photocoagulation surgery in preventing visual loss. Two large randomized controlled clinical trials sponsored by the National Eye Institute, the Diabetes Retinopathy Study (DRS), and the ETDRS, provide strong support for the therapeutic benefit of retinal photocoagulation surgery in preventing visual loss due to diabetic retinopathy (Diabetic Retinopathy Study Research Group 1981; Early Treatment Diabetic Retinopathy Study Research Group 1991). The DRS showed that panretinal photocoagulation significantly reduced the risk of severe vision loss (best corrected visual acuity of 5/200 or worse) from PDR (rates were 15.9% in untreated and 6.4% in treated eyes). The ETDRS established the benefit of focal or grid laser photocoagulation in the macular area in eyes with clinically significant macular edema (20% of untreated eyes had a doubling of the visual angle [e.g., 20/20 to 20/40, 20/50 to 20/100] compared with 8% of treated eyes after 2 years of follow-up).

Both the DRS and the ETDRS showed the efficacy of photocoagulation in reducing progression of diabetic retinopathy before vision is lost. This and the fact that patients with PDR or macular edema may be asymptomatic highlight the importance of regular dilated eye examinations. In addition, from a societal or governmental viewpoint, annual dilated eye examinations (screening) and timely treatment for vision-threatening retinopathy (PDR and clinically significant macular edema) are cost effective and could be cost saving (Javitt, Canner, and Sommer 1989; Dasbach et al. 1991; James et al. 2000).

Guidelines and Barriers to Quality Eye Care

The ADA, the American College of Physicians, and the American Academy of Ophthalmology have recommended that patients with type 1 diabetes have a dilated and comprehensive eye examination by an ophthalmologist or optometrist within 5 years after the onset of diabetes (Fong et al. 2004). Patients with type 2 diabetes should have an initial dilated and comprehensive eye examination by an ophthalmologist or optometrist shortly after diagnosis. Subsequent examinations for type 1 and type 2 patients should be repeated at least annually by an ophthalmologist or optometrist who is knowledgeable and experienced in diagnosing the presence of diabetic retinopathy and is aware of its management. Examinations are required more frequently if retinopathy is present or progressing. Alternatively when eye care professionals are not available, retinal photography (with or without dilation of the pupil) with readings of the retinal images by experienced experts in this field may be performed. Results of eye examinations should be documented and transmitted to the referring health care professional (Javitt, Canner, and Sommer 1989). In-person exams are still necessary when the retinal photographs are unacceptable and for follow-up when abnormalities are detected.

A large proportion of people with diabetes (35%–79%) do not receive recommended care. Two studies showed that 32%–50% of the people with diabetes had minimal or no ophthalmologic eye examinations and subsequently were at high risk for unrecognized diabetic eye disease (Brechner et al. 1993; Moss, Klein R, and Klein B 1995). Brown and colleagues found high rates of unrecognized and untreated eye diseases among Medicare beneficiaries who were enrolled in fee-for-service or in Medicare Plus Choice (Brown et al. 2005). Moreover, population-based studies found that at least 25% of type 1 patients developed PDR by the time they had had diabetes for 15 years (up to 71% in a lifetime), and 46% of such patients had not received timely photocoagulation (Klein R et al. 1984). Slight improvements in the age-adjusted rates of annual dilated eye examinations have occurred in the last 10 years; the largest increase occurred among those aged 45 to 64 (from 58.0% in 1994 to 69.1% in 2005) (CDC 2007). One of the national health objectives is to increase the proportion of people with diabetes examined yearly for diabetic retinopathy to 75% by 2010.

Data from some studies suggest that less frequent dilated eye exams (every 2–3 years) may be considered with the advice of an eye care professional in the setting of a normal eye exam (Vijan, Hofer, and Hayward 2000; Olafsdottir and Stefansson 2007). Biennial dilated eye examinations would reduce screening visits more than 25% and in turn reduce health costs and patient burden from unnecessary examinations.

Several studies have investigated barriers to dilated eye examinations and factors associated with such barriers in efforts to explain the low percentage of persons with diabetes receiving recommended eye care. These studies addressed factors at several levels, including the patient, provider, and health care system as well as public health policies.

In the WESDR cohort, diabetic persons who had not received an annual dilated eye examination were less educated, had lower income, were less likely to have health insurance covering eye examinations, were more likely to be unable to afford the examination, and were more likely to report no visual symptoms than were persons receiving such care (Moss, Klein R, and Klein B 1995). In another study, investigators found that, among their indigent diabetic population, patients' and physicians' perceptions of barriers differed in ranking of importance and in theme (Hartnett et al. 2005). From the patients' perspective, cost and access were major barriers to diabetes care. Additionally more than half of the diabetic patients knew the recommendation for annual dilated eye examinations from their providers but lacked understanding of the rationale for this recommendation. In this study although patients believed that they received adequate education about their diabetes and its complications, only one-third knew that diabetes could cause blindness. Patients stated that the burden of diabetes and its treatment overshadowed concern about eye disease and the need for an annual dilated eye examination. On the other hand, medical providers of care for diabetic patients ranked education and access as major barriers and did not mention cost as a barrier to receiving optimal eye care. In addition, poor communication between primary care physicians and ophthalmologists was cited as a barrier to quality diabetes eye care.

■ Implications for Health Policy

Programs to Overcome Barriers to Care

A number of ongoing retinal screening and preventive treatment programs for persons with diabetes have been established in northern Europe, with positive outcomes (Stefansson et al. 2000; Younis et al. 2002; Olafsdottir and Stefansson 2007; Zoega et al. 2008). In most of these programs both the prevalence and incidence of blindness associated with diabetic retinopathy have decreased. The Iceland systematic screening program, in place for 25 years, has shown a significant decrease in the prevalence of diabetic blindness, from 2.4% in 1980 to 0.5% in 2005 (Stefansson et al. 2000; Zoega et al. 2008).

Other examples of public health preventive approaches in the United States include the National Eye Health Education Program (NEHEP), the National Diabetes Education Program (NDEP), and the diabetes prevention and control programs sponsored by the Centers for Disease Control and Prevention (CDC) (CDC 2007; National Institutes of Health 1990). The focus of the NEHEP is on public and professional education programs that encourage early detection and timely treatment of diabetic eye disease, with the ultimate goal of behavior change in diabetic patients. The NEHEP also aims to increase awareness among health care providers of the need for regular, comprehensive eye examinations with dilation of pupils for those at risk for diabetic eye disease. The NDEP, through its Pharmacy, Podiatry, Optometry, and Dentistry Workgroup (PPOD), uses its respective organizations and providers to promote increased awareness of and access to quality care for people with diabetes. It also provides information and educational materials to assist in diabetes self-management and recommendations for referral. The CDC has promoted dilated eye examinations as a national objective for the State-Based Diabetes Prevention & Control Programs, which are located in every state in the United States and its eight territories. Although there are data suggesting an increase in annual dilated eye examinations, the effectiveness of these U.S. programs in reducing visual loss by timely detection and treatment of vision-threatening retinopathy has not been demonstrated.

Economic Issues and Implications

In 2004, the societal economic burden and the governmental budgetary impact of diabetic retinopathy among U.S. adults aged 40 and older reached approximately $500 million, including direct medical costs, other direct costs, and productivity losses (Rein et al. 2006). Screening for diabetic eye disease is demonstrated to be cost saving or cost effective. In 2007 screening and treatment of eye disease in patients with diabetes cost just $6900 to buy an additional year of life in full health or $3800 per life-year of sight gained (Javitt and Aiello 1996). Indeed, screening for diabetic retinopathy is more cost effective than are many routinely provided health interventions.

■ Areas of Uncertainty or Controversy

It remains unclear why some people with good glycemic control or who are either normotensive or have only modestly elevated blood pressure develop severe diabetic retinopathy whereas others with poor glycemic control or who have elevated blood pressure do not. Controversy remains regarding the optimal frequency of subsequent screening in diabetic patients found not to have retinopathy on dilated eye examination. Some authorities like the American Diabetes Association recommend less frequent exams (every 2–3 years) to be considered following one or more normal eye examinations. However, examinations will be needed more frequently if retinopathy is progressing to more severe stages.

■ Developments over the Next 5 to 10 Years

Detection of Retinopathy Using New Technologies

The use of telemedicine with centralized grading facilities for the detection and treatment of diabetic retinopathy has been advocated as a new approach to caring for patients with diabetes (Wilson et al. 2005; Chow et al. 2006). Several studies have shown how sound, effective, and cost effective this technology is while not compromising the care of patients with diabetes. In any case telemedicine is not meant to replace clinic-based eye examination, but it can be used to deliver routine eye care for people with diabetes (Lee 1999; Cavallerano et al. 2004; Whited 2006).

Future Research

Future research should be aimed at developing new approaches for primary prevention of diabetes. Research identifying genes associated with both rapid and slow progression of retinopathy and their interactions with glycemia and other risk factors is needed. Research studies are needed to examine the effects of a combination of intensive control of glycemia, blood pressure, and lipids in minimizing macrovascular and microvascular complications. Research is needed on new approaches for successfully translating findings from clinical trials (e.g., DRS, ETDRS) into clinical practice to achieve timely detection and treatment of vision-threatening diabetic retinopathy. This might include the development, implementation, and testing of new strategies (e.g., telemedicine, changing the intervals between dilated eye examinations). Also, new research on nonsurgical approaches to induce regression of retinal new vessels and macular edema in persons not successfully treated with photocoagulation is needed. The Diabetic Retinopathy Clinical Research Network has ongoing studies of treatment options for diabetic retinopathy, which include drug therapies targeting vascular endothelial growth factors, vitrectomy, and combined treatment with pharmacotherapy and laser. These study results may have a tremendous impact on reducing visual loss associated with advanced diabetic retinopathy. Taking into account the fact that 50%–90% of blindness related to diabetic retinopathy is preventable and that there is ample information on how to detect and treat diabetic retinopathy, studies are needed in operations research and in health services to reduce the burden of blindness in persons with diabetes.

■ References

Adler AI et al. (2000). Association of systolic blood pressure with macrovascular and microvascular complications of type 2 diabetes (UKPDS 36): prospective observational study. *British Medical Journal* **321**, 412–9.

American Diabetes Association (1994). Standards of medical care for patients with diabetes mellitus. *Diabetes Care* **17**, 616–23.

Benitez-Del-Castillo JM et al. (2007). Relation between corneal innervation with confocal microscopy and corneal sensitivity with noncontact esthesiometry in patients with dry eye. *Investigative Ophthalmology & Visual Science* **48**, 173–81.

Bonovas S, Peponis V, Filioussi K (2004). Diabetes mellitus as a risk factor for primary open-angle glaucoma: a meta-analysis. *Diabetic Medicine* **21**, 609–14.

Brechner RJ et al. (1993). Ophthalmic examination among adults with diagnosed diabetes mellitus. *Journal of the American Medical Association* **270**, 1714–8.

Brown AF et al. (2005). Need for eye care among older adults with diabetes mellitus in fee-for-service and managed Medicare. *Archives of Ophthalmology* **123**, 669–75.

Cai J, Boulton M (2002). The pathogenesis of diabetic retinopathy: old concepts and new questions. *Eye* **16**, 242–60.

Cardillo JA et al. (2005). Comparison of intravitreal versus posterior sub-Tenon's capsule injection of triamcinolone acetonide for diffuse diabetic macular edema. *Ophthalmology* **112**, 1557–63.

Cavallerano J et al. (2004). Telehealth practice recommendations for diabetic retinopathy. *Telemedicine Journal and E-Health* **10**, 469–82.

Centers for Disease Control and Prevention (2007). Data from the Centers for Disease Control and Prevention Behavioral Risk Factor Surveillance System. Age-adjusted rates of annual dilated eye exam per 100 adults with diabetes, United States, 1994–2005. Available at: http://www.cdc.gov/diabetes/statistics/preventive/fX_eye.htm. Accessed October 5, 2007.

Chaturvedi N et al. (1998). Effect of lisinopril on progression of retinopathy in normotensive people with type 1 diabetes. The EUCLID Study Group. EURODIAB controlled trial of lisinopril in insulin-dependent diabetes mellitus. *Lancet* **351**, 28–31.

Chen SJ et al. (2008). Prevalence and associated factors of lens opacities among Chinese type 2 diabetics in Kinmen, Taiwan. *Acta Diabetologica* **45**, 7–13.

Chew EY et al. (1995). Metabolic control and progression of retinopathy. The Diabetes in Early Pregnancy Study. National Institute of Child Health and Human Development Diabetes in Early Pregnancy Study. *Diabetes Care* **18**, 631–7.

Chew EY et al. (1996). Association of elevated serum lipid levels with retinal hard exudate in diabetic retinopathy. Early Treatment Diabetic Retinopathy Study (ETDRS) Report 22. *Archives of Ophthalmology* **114**, 1079–84.

Chow SP et al. (2006). Comparison of nonmydriatic digital retinal imaging versus dilated ophthalmic examination for nondiabetic eye disease in persons with diabetes. *Ophthalmology* **113**, 833–40.

Clarke P et al. (2003). The impact of diabetes-related complications on healthcare costs: results from the United Kingdom Prospective Diabetes Study (UKPDS Study No. 65). *Diabetic Medicine* **20**, 442–50.

Congdon N et al. (2004). Causes and prevalence of visual impairment among adults in the United States. *Archives of Ophthalmology* **122**, 477–85.

Dasbach EJ et al. (1991). Cost-effectiveness of strategies for detecting diabetic retinopathy. *Medical Care* **29**, 20–39.

Diabetes Control and Complications Research Group (2002). Effect of intensive therapy on the microvascular complications of type 1 diabetes mellitus. *Journal of the American Medical Association* **287**, 2563–69.

Diabetes Control and Complications Trial Research Group (1993). The effect of intensive treatment of diabetes on the development and progression of long-term complications in insulin-dependent diabetes mellitus. *New England Journal of Medicine* **329**, 977–86.

Diabetic Retinopathy Study Research Group (1981). Photocoagulation treatment of proliferative diabetic retinopathy. Clinical application of Diabetic Retinopathy Study (DRS) findings, DRS Report Number 8. *Ophthalmology* **88**, 583–600.

Early Treatment Diabetic Retinopathy Study Research Group (1991). Effects of aspirin treatment on diabetic retinopathy. ETDRS report number 8. *Ophthalmology* **98**, 757–65.

Ederer F, Hiller R, Taylor HR (1981). Senile lens changes and diabetes in two population studies. *American Journal of Ophthalmology* **91**, 381–95.

Estacio RO et al. (2000). Effect of blood pressure control on diabetic microvascular complications in patients with hypertension and type 2 diabetes. *Diabetes Care* **23** (Suppl. 2), B54–64.

Fong DS et al. (2004). Retinopathy in diabetes. *Diabetes Care* **27** (Suppl. 1), S84–7.

Hanis CL, Hallman D (2006). Genetics of diabetic retinopathy. *Current Diabetes Reports.* **6**, 155–61.

Hartnett ME et al. (2005). Perceived barriers to diabetic eye care: qualitative study of patients and physicians. *Archives of Ophthalmology* **123**, 387–91.

Hegde KR, Varma SD (2005). Cataracts in experimentally diabetic mouse: morphological and apoptotic changes. *Diabetes, Obesity & Metabolism* **7**, 200–204.

Hoerger TJ et al. (2008). Is glycemic control improving in U.S. adults? *Diabetes Care* **31**, 81–6.

Hove MN et al. (2004). The prevalence of retinopathy in an unselected population of type 2 diabetes patients from Aarhus County, Denmark. *Acta Ophthalmologica Scandinavica* **82**, 443–8.

Hovind P et al. (2003). Decreasing incidence of severe diabetic microangiopathy in type 1 diabetes. *Diabetes Care* **26**, 1258–64.

Ivancic D et al. (2005). Cataract surgery and postoperative complications in diabetic patients. *Collegium Antropologicum* **29** (Suppl. 1), 55–8.

James M et al. (2000). Cost effectiveness analysis of screening for sight threatening diabetic eye disease. *British Medical Journal* **320**, 1627–31.

Javitt JC, Aiello LP (2006). Cost-effectiveness of detecting and treating diabetic retinopathy. *Annals of Internal Medicine* **124**, 164–9.

Javitt JC, Canner JK, Sommer A (1989). Cost effectiveness of current approaches to the control of retinopathy in type I diabetics. *Ophthalmology* **96**, 255–64.

Kempen JH et al. (2004). The prevalence of diabetic retinopathy among adults in the United States. *Archives of Ophthalmology* **122**, 552–63.

Klein BE, Klein R, Jensen SC (1994). Open-angle glaucoma and older-onset diabetes. The Beaver Dam Eye Study. *Ophthalmology* **101**, 1173–77.

Klein BE, Klein R, Moss SE (1984). Intraocular pressure in diabetic persons. *Ophthalmology* **91**, 1356–60.

Klein BE, Klein R, Moss SE (1985). Prevalence of cataracts in a population-based study of persons with diabetes mellitus. *Ophthalmology* **92**, 1191–6.

Klein R, Klein BEK, Moss SE (1992). Risk factors for retinopathy. In: Feman SS, ed. *Ocular Problems in Diabetes Mellitus*, p. 39. Boston: Blackwell Publishing.

Klein BE, Klein R, Moss SE (1999). Exogenous estrogen exposures and changes in diabetic retinopathy. The Wisconsin Epidemiologic Study of Diabetic Retinopathy. *Diabetes Care* **22**, 1984–7.

Klein BE, Moss SE, Klein R (1990). Effect of pregnancy on progression of diabetic retinopathy. *Diabetes Care* **13**, 34–40.

Klein BE et al. (1991). The Wisconsin Epidemiologic Study of Diabetic Retinopathy. XIII. Relationship of serum cholesterol to retinopathy and hard exudate. *Ophthalmology* **98**, 1261–5.

Klein BE et al. (1995). Older-onset diabetes and lens opacities. The Beaver Dam Eye Study. *Ophthalmic Epidemiology* **2**, 49–55.

Klein R (1995). Diabetes mellitus: oculopathy. In: De Groot LJ, Jameson JL, eds. *Endocrinology* 4th ed., pp 857–67. Philadelphia: WB Saunders.

Klein R, Klein BE (1995). Vision disorders in diabetes. In: Harris MI et al., eds. *Diabetes in America*, 2nd ed., pp 293–338. Bethesda: National Institutes of Health. National Institute of Diabetes and Digestive and Kidney Diseases. NIH Publication No. 95-1468.

Klein R, Klein BE, Moss SE (1984). Visual impairment in diabetes. *Ophthalmology* **91**, 1–9.

Klein R et al. (1984). The Wisconsin Epidemiologic study of Diabetic Retinopathy. II. Prevalence and risk of diabetic retinopathy when age at diagnosis is less than 30 years. *Archives of Ophthalmology* **102**, 520–6.

Klein R et al. (1994a). Relationship of hyperglycemia to the long-term incidence and progression of diabetic retinopathy. *Archives of Internal Medicine* **154**, 2169–78.

Klein R et al. (1994b). The Wisconsin Epidemiologic Study of Diabetic Retinopathy. XIV. Ten-year incidence and progression of diabetic retinopathy. *Archives of Ophthalmology* **112**, 1217–28.

Klein R et al. (1995). The Wisconsin Epidemiologic Study of Diabetic Retinopathy. XV. The long-term incidence of macular edema. *Ophthalmology* **102**, 7–16.

Klein R et al. (1998). The Wisconsin Epidemiologic Study of Diabetic Retinopathy: XVII. The 14-year incidence and progression of diabetic retinopathy and associated risk factors in type 1 diabetes. *Ophthalmology* **105**, 1801–15.

Klein R et al. (2006). Changes in visual acuity in a population over a 15-year period: the Beaver Dam Eye Study. *American Journal of Ophthalmology* **142**, 539–49.

Kumar PA et al. (2005). Modulation of alpha-crystallin chaperone activity in diabetic rat lens by curcumin. *Molecular Vision* **11**, 561–8.

Kyselova Z, Stefek M, Bauer V (2004). Pharmacological prevention of diabetic cataract. *Journal of Diabetes Complications* **18**, 129–40.

Lee ET et al. (2001). Vascular disease in younger-onset diabetes: comparison of European, Asian and American Indian cohorts of the WHO Multinational Study of Vascular Disease in Diabetes. *Diabetologia* **44** (Suppl. 2), S78–81.

Lee JS et al. (2005). Corneal endothelial cell change after phacoemulsification relative to the severity of diabetic retinopathy. *Journal of Cataract and Refractive Surgery* **31**, 742–9.

Lee P (1999). Telemedicine: opportunities and challenges for the remote care of diabetic retinopathy. *Archives of Ophthalmology* **117**, 1639–40.

Leske MC, Podgor MJ (1983). Intraocular pressure, cardiovascular risk variables, and visual field defects. *American Journal of Epidemiology* **118**, 280–287.

Lockwood A, Hope-Ross M, Chell P (2006). Neurotrophic keratopathy and diabetes mellitus. *Eye* **20**, 837–39.

Midena E et al. (2006). Corneal diabetic neuropathy: a confocal microscopy study. *Journal of Refractive Surgery* **22**, S1047–52.

Mitchell P et al. (1997). Open-angle glaucoma and diabetes: the Blue Mountains eye study, Australia. *Ophthalmology* **104**, 712–18.

Mocan MC et al. (2006). Morphologic alterations of both the stromal and subbasal nerves in the corneas of patients with diabetes. *Cornea* **25**, 769–73.

Morikubo S et al. (2004). Corneal changes after small-incision cataract surgery in patients with diabetes mellitus. *Archives of Ophthalmology* **122**, 966–9.

Moss SE, Klein R, Klein BE (1994). The association of alcohol consumption with the incidence and progression of diabetic retinopathy. *Ophthalmology* **101**, 1962–68.

Moss SE, Klein R, Klein BE (1995). Factors associated with having eye examinations in persons with diabetes. *Archives of Family Medicine* **4**, 529–34.

Nakahara M et al. (2005). A randomised, placebo controlled clinical trial of the aldose reductase inhibitor CT-112 as management of corneal epithelial disorders in diabetic patients. *British Journal of Ophthalmology* **89**, 266–8.

O'Donnell C, Efron N (2006). Corneal hydration control in contact lens wearers with diabetes mellitus. *Optometry and Vision Sciences* **83**, 22–26.

Olafsdottir E, Stefansson E (2007). Biennial eye screening in patients with diabetes without retinopathy: 10-year experience. *British Journal of Ophthalmology* **91**, 1599–601.

Osawa T, Kato Y (2005). Protective role of antioxidative food factors in oxidative stress caused by hyperglycemia. *Annals of the New York Academy of Sciences* **1043**, 440–451.

Pambianco G et al. (2006). The 30-year natural history of type 1 diabetes complications: the Pittsburgh Epidemiology of Diabetes Complications Study experience. *Diabetes* **55**, 1463–69.

Perruccio AV, Badley EM, Trope GE (2007). Self-reported glaucoma in Canada: findings from population-based surveys, 1994–2003. *Canadian Journal of Ophthalmology* **42**, 219–26.

Rein DB et al. (2006). The economic burden of major adult visual disorders in the United States. *Archives of Ophthalmology* **124**, 1754–60.

Resnick HE et al. (2006). Achievement of American Diabetes Association clinical practice recommendations among U.S. adults with diabetes, 1999–2002: the National Health and Nutrition Examination Survey. *Diabetes Care* **29**, 531–7.

Schrier RW et al. (2002). Effects of aggressive blood pressure control in normotensive type 2 diabetic patients on albuminuria, retinopathy and strokes. *Kidney International* **61**, 1086–97.

Singer GM, Izhar M, Black HR (2002). Goal-oriented hypertension management: translating clinical trials to practice. *Hypertension* **40**, 464–69.

Sonmez B et al. (2005). Effect of glycemic control on refractive changes in diabetic patients with hyperglycemia. *Cornea* **24**, 531–37.

Stefansson E et al. (2000). Screening and prevention of diabetic blindness. *Acta Ophthalmologica Scandinavica* **78**, 374–85.

Tarczy-Hornoch K, Ying-Lai M, Varma R (2006). Myopic refractive error in adult Latinos: the Los Angeles Latino Eye Study. *Investigative Ophthalmology & Visual Science* **47**, 1845–52.

The National Institutes of Health (1990). *The National Eye Health Education Program: from vision research to health education; planning the partnership*. Bethesda: National Institutes of Health.

Thylefors B et al. (1995). Global data on blindness. *Bulletin of the World Health Organization* **73**, 115–21.

UK Prospective Diabetes Study (UKPDS) Group (1998a). Intensive blood-glucose control with sulphonylureas or insulin compared with conventional treatment and risk of complications in patients with type 2 diabetes (UKPDS 33). *Lancet* **352**, 837–53.

UK Prospective Diabetes Study (UKPDS) Group (1998b). Tight blood pressure control and risk of macrovascular and microvascular complications in type 2 diabetes: UKPDS 38. *British Medical Journal* **317**, 703–13.

Vijan S, Hofer TP, Hayward RA (2000). Cost-utility analysis of screening intervals for diabetic retinopathy in patients with type 2 diabetes mellitus. *Journal of the American Medical Association* **283**, 889–96.

Wakuta M et al. (2007). Delayed wound closure and phenotypic changes in corneal epithelium of the spontaneously diabetic Goto-Kakizaki rat. *Investigative Ophthalmology & Visual Science* **48**, 590–596.

Whited JD (2006). Accuracy and reliability of teleophthalmology for diagnosing diabetic retinopathy and macular edema: a review of the literature. *Diabetes Technology & Therapeutics.* **8**, 102–11.

Wilson C et al. (2005). Addition of primary care-based retinal imaging technology to an existing eye care professional referral program increased the rate of surveillance and treatment of diabetic retinopathy. *Diabetes Care* **28**, 318–22.

Wong TY et al. (2006). Diabetic retinopathy in a multi-ethnic cohort in the United States. *American Journal of Ophthalmology* **141**, 446–55.

Yoon KC, Im SK, Seo MS (2004). Changes of tear film and ocular surface in diabetes mellitus. *Korean Journal of Ophthalmology* **18**, 168–74.

Younis N et al. (2002). Current status of screening for diabetic retinopathy in the UK. *Diabetic Medicine* **19** (Suppl. 4), 44–9.

Zhang M et al. (2005). Altered corneal nerves in aqueous tear deficiency viewed by in vivo confocal microscopy. *Cornea* **24**, 818–24.

Zoega GM et al. (2005). Screening compliance and visual outcome in diabetes. *Acta Ophthalmologica Scandinavica* **83**, 687–90.

7. Diabetes and Chronic Kidney Disease

Meda E. Pavkov, Nilka R. Burrows, William C. Knowler,
Robert L. Hanson, and Robert G. Nelson

■ Main Public Health Messages

- In the United States, over 15% of the population has chronic kidney disease (CKD), and more than 90% of those with CKD also have diabetes, hypertension, or both.
- In 1980, diabetes accounted for only 18% of prevalent end-stage renal disease (ESRD) in the United States, but by 2004 the proportion of ESRD patients with a primary diagnosis of diabetes had risen to 45%.
- An increasing prevalence of diabetes and improved survival in patients with cardiovascular disease are responsible, in part, for the growth in diabetes as a cause of ESRD.
- The projected 65% increase in the prevalence of diabetes in the U.S. adult population between 2001 and 2031 is expected to lead to a further rise in diabetes and CKD. Current projections indicate that patients with ESRD caused by diabetes will account for 47% of the incident ESRD population and 37% of the prevalent population by 2020.
- The rise in type 2 diabetes among children and adolescents and the appearance of end-stage diabetes complications, including CKD, in midlife among those who develop type 2 diabetes in youth is of great concern.
- Significant therapeutic advances have been made in recent years that successfully slow the progression of diabetic CKD. Timely application of appropriate therapy requires early recognition of CKD, which requires improved methods for estimating the glomerular filtration rate and could benefit by the identification of more sensitive and specific biomarkers of kidney damage.
- The Centers for Disease Control and Prevention (CDC) Chronic Kidney Disease Initiative is developing state-level screening programs for kidney disease, assessing the burden of kidney disease, documenting the direct and indirect costs of kidney disease, and developing models that will both predict the progression of kidney disease and test the effectiveness of public health intervention strategies.

■ Introduction

Reduced kidney function or the presence of kidney damage for at least 3 months, regardless of kidney function, defines chronic kidney disease (CKD)—a condition affecting over 15% of the U.S. population. Kidney function is assessed by either measuring or estimating the glomerular filtration rate (GFR), which is the rate at which the kidneys filter blood to produce urine, and kidney damage is ascertained by increased urinary markers, such as albuminuria, or by abnormal urinary sediment, abnormal imaging studies, or kidney biopsy (National Kidney Foundation 2002). Diabetes mellitus is the leading cause of CKD in the United States and in other developed countries and is rapidly becoming the leading cause of CKD worldwide as a consequence of the global increase in type 2 diabetes (Zimmet, Alberti, and Shaw 2001). This chapter describes the frequency, course, and risk factors for diabetic kidney disease (DKD). Current management strategies are reviewed, and the impact of management on progression of kidney disease is discussed. The chapter concludes with a description of public health programs under development at the Centers for Disease Control and Prevention (CDC) to address diabetes and CKD.

■ Background

Albuminuria

Elevated albuminuria is the earliest marker of DKD, and the urinary albumin-to-creatinine ratio (ACR) is the preferred screening method for identifying this condition. Patients are classified as having elevated albuminuria if at least two urine samples collected within 3 to 6 months contain $\geq$30 mg albumin/g creatinine in the absence of clinical or laboratory evidence of urinary-tract infection (National Kidney Foundation 2007). Exercise within 24 hours before urine testing or the presence of infection, fever, congestive heart failure, poor glycemic or blood pressure control, pregnancy, extreme obesity, or hematuria may increase urinary albumin excretion in the absence of DKD. Caution is also required in interpreting the ACR in patients with very low or high muscle mass because muscle mass affects creatinine excretion (Mattix et al. 2002).

The diagnosis of DKD is based largely on the finding of elevated excretion of urinary albumin. Elevated albuminuria is associated with a progressive decline in kidney function, an increase in systemic blood pressure, and a high risk for kidney failure. It is also associated with nonfatal and fatal cardiovascular events independent of other cardiovascular risk factors (Gerstein et al. 2001; Ibsen et al. 2006; Xu et al. 2007). High normal levels of albuminuria also predict nonfatal and fatal cardiovascular events independent of other cardiovascular risk factors (Gerstein et al. 2001; Xu et al. 2007). Although albuminuria is a continuous risk factor, it is arbitrarily divided into microalbuminuria (ACR between 30 and 299 mg/g) and macroalbuminuria (ACR ≥ 300 mg/g).

Glomerular Filtration Rate

Reduced kidney function is defined by a GFR < 60 ml/min/1.73 m^2. Measuring GFR requires infusion of special markers (e.g., inulin, iothalamate, iohexol, or ^{51}Cr-EDTA) into the bloodstream and measurement of their disappearance from the blood or their appearance in the urine; such testing is time consuming, cumbersome, and expensive. Accordingly the National Kidney Foundation (2002) recommends using equations to estimate GFR that include easily obtained variables. The best validated and currently most widely used equation for adult patients in the office setting is the Modification of Diet in Renal Disease (MDRD) study equation, which estimates GFR from the measured serum creatinine concentration after standardizing for age, gender, and race (Levey et al. 2006). A cross-sectional analysis comparing estimated GFR (eGFR) by the MDRD equation with GFR measured by the urinary clearance of iothalamate found that eGFR is unbiased and reasonably accurate for use in clinical practice when the estimate is less than 60 ml/min/1.73 m^2 (Stevens et al. 2007). Precision is lower and bias is higher, however, at higher eGFR values. Therefore, the clinical context should be considered when diagnosing reduced kidney function by eGFR.

During infancy and through the first 12 to 18 months of life GFR increases with physical maturation, and at about 2 years it reaches the level found in adults. Several formulas for estimating GFR in children aged less than 18 years have been developed; the Schwartz and Counahan-Barratt formulas are the most frequently used in clinical practice, providing an improved estimate of GFR over serum creatinine alone (Hogg et al. 2003).

In most diabetic patients, careful screening is sufficient for identifying those with DKD. Nevertheless evaluation of diabetic persons with elevated albuminuria who present with atypical features should include additional diagnostic testing. Atypical features include absence of diabetic retinopathy, presence of casts or red cells in the urine, or a particularly rapid decline in kidney function. On the other hand DKD may develop in the absence of elevated albuminuria and may be identified only by a reduction in GFR, reflecting the value of the current screening strategy, which involves both measurement of albuminuria and estimation of GFR (National Kidney Foundation 2007).

■ The Burden of Diabetic Kidney Disease

In the United States 15.5% of the population has CKD, with 8.4% of this group having an eGFR less than 60 ml/min/1.73 m^2 (U.S. Renal Data System 2008). The elderly have a higher CKD prevalence, due in large part to the higher prevalence of

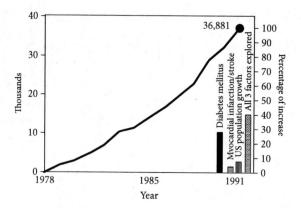

FIGURE 7.1. Increase in number of incident treated ESRD cases from 1978 to 1991 (line), and number/percentage of total increase in ESRD attributable to improved survival following myocardial infarction and stroke, increased prevalence of diabetes, and a larger U.S. population in 1991 (bars). the study used data from respondents aged ≥ 30 years participating in NHANES II and NHANES III, from the USRDS, and from the U.S. census. (Source: Muntner et al. 2003.)

eGFR <60 ml/min/1.73m^2 in this age group. This suggests that the current definition of CKD based on the MDRD estimate of GFR is overestimating CKD prevalence because of the effect of population age distribution on eGFR. Because age is part of the formula for estimating GFR, as the population ages, the prevalence of CKD would rise as well. Nevertheless, in more than 90% of those with CKD, kidney disease is accompanied by diabetes, hypertension, or both. In 1980, diabetes accounted for only 18% of prevalent end-stage renal disease (ESRD) in the United States, but by 2004 the proportion of ESRD patients with a primary diagnosis of diabetes had risen to 45%. An increasing prevalence of diabetes and improved cardiovascular disease (CVD) survival are responsible, in part, for this growth (Muntner 2003) (see Fig. 7.1). The projected doubling in the prevalence of diabetes in the U.S. population between 2005 and 2050 (Narayan et al. 2006) is expected to lead to a further rise in diabetic ESRD. Current projections indicate that patients with ESRD caused by diabetes will account for 47% of the incident ESRD population and 37% of the prevalent population by 2020 (U.S. Renal Data System 2007). There are currently no projections for the future prevalence and incidence of CKD itself.

Twenty percent to 40% (CDC n.d.a; Molitch et al. 2004) of patients with diabetes develop CKD. Because of their increased comorbidity, DKD patients have higher hospitalization rates than those without DKD but are 5 to 11 times more likely to die from other causes, primarily CVD, than to progress to ESRD (Collins et al. 2003). Certain ethnic groups, including African Americans, Hispanics, and Native Americans, are particularly predisposed to kidney disease as a complication of diabetes. Moreover, while the incidence of diabetic ESRD declined after 1994 in whites younger than 40 years, it continued to rise in blacks of similar age and remained unchanged in Hispanics (U.S. Renal Data System 2008). Nonetheless, among American Indians/Alaska Natives and Asians/Pacific Islanders (CDC n.d.b), the overall incidence of

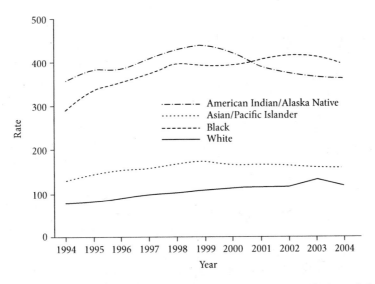

FIGURE 7.2. Age-adjusted annual incidence rates of ESRD per million population with diabetes as the primary diagnosis, by race, in the U.S. 1994–2004. Age-adjusted to the 2000 U.S. standard population. Race-specific estimates include persons of both Hispanic and non-Hispanic origin. (Source: http://www.cdc.gov/mmwr/preview/mmwrhtml/mm5443a2.htm. Accessed January 23, 2009.)

diabetic ESRD declined between 1999 and 2004 despite an increasing prevalence of diabetes in these populations, suggesting that current diabetes management practices effectively slow progression of the disease (see Fig. 7.2).

Youth

Type 2 diabetes accounts currently for up to 45% of new-onset cases of diabetes among adolescents (ADA 2000). Many children with type 2 diabetes are obese at diagnosis, they often have a strong family history of type 2 diabetes, and some are the offspring of mothers with gestational diabetes. Those who develop diabetes in childhood and adolescence are affected disproportionately in early adulthood by the microvascular and macrovascular complications of diabetes, including DKD (Nelson et al. 2008).

In the SEARCH for Diabetes in Youth study, the prevalence of elevated ACR in youth aged <20 years was 9.2% in type 1 and 22.2% in type 2 diabetes (prevalence ratio 2.4, 95% confidence interval [CI] 1.9–3.0) (Maahs et al. 2007). About half of those with type 1 diabetes who develop microalbuminuria subsequently regress to normal albuminuria (Amin et al. 2008; Pinhas-Hamiel and Zeitler 2007). Higher levels of hemoglobin A1C increase the risk of persistent elevated albuminuria beyond puberty and potentially the risk for early CVD (Writing Team for the DCCT/EDIC Research Group 2003). The long-term significance of elevated albuminuria in young type 2 patients is essentially unknown because of the lack of longitudinal studies.

In Pima Indians, diabetes duration-specific incidence rates of proteinuria were similar with onset of diabetes before and after age 20. By contrast, the frequency of retinopathy was lower in youth- than adult-onset type 2 diabetes, suggesting that youth does not offer the same protection from progressive DKD as it does from diabetic retinopathy (Krakoff et al. 2003). Onset of diabetes during childhood or adolescence leads to substantially increased ESRD rates in midlife (Nelson et al. 2008). The age-gender–adjusted incidence of diabetic ESRD in Pima Indians diagnosed with type 2 diabetes before age 20 was nearly five times as high as in those of the same age but with older-onset diabetes. In that study the longer duration of diabetes by middle age in those diagnosed during childhood or adolescence largely accounted for the higher incidence of ESRD. The World Health Organization Multinational Study of Vascular Disease in Diabetes (Lee et al. 2001) reported that Native Americans from Arizona and Oklahoma diagnosed with diabetes before age 30 had a higher age-adjusted incidence rate of kidney failure during a mean follow-up of 9.5 years than European or Asian populations with early-onset diabetes. Although susceptibility to DKD differs by ethnicity, the rise in childhood type 2 diabetes in different ethnic groups is likely to increase the frequency of kidney disease in these populations. Furthermore, the higher rates of DKD in young and middle-aged adults with youth-onset diabetes may contribute to a rise in cardiovascular complications in these age groups (Nelson et al. 2008; Pavkov et al., 2004). These complications have potential economic and public health impact because they will affect those with youth-onset diabetes during their peak productive years.

Pregnancy

Between 30% and 40% of women with a preconception serum creatinine above 1.4 mg/dL will experience acceleration of kidney disease during pregnancy, with many of these women progressing to ESRD within 15 years of delivery (Davison 2001; Jones and Hyslett 1996). A case-control study in type 1 diabetic women with DKD who were followed for up to 26 years found a high prevalence of low birth weight, short gestational age, neonatal deaths, congenital abnormalities, and cesarean sections, reflecting the often difficult course of these pregnancies. Ten years after their last delivery, morbidity and mortality remained higher in these women than in those without pregnancies (Rossing K et al. 2002).

The offspring of diabetic mothers have a much higher risk of obesity and diabetes during childhood or as young adults than do the offspring of nondiabetic mothers (Knowler et al. 1990). In addition to obesity and the transmission of diabetes-susceptibility genes to the next generation, intrauterine exposure to gestational diabetes can lead to increased risk for long-term complications of diabetes (Nelson 2003).

Elderly

The greater frequency of comorbid conditions in the elderly with diabetes is responsible for a greater prevalence of elevated albuminuria unrelated to DKD. Between 13% and 42% of diabetic patients with advanced CKD have normal excretion of urinary albumin; the patients presenting this way most often are elderly women and those on renin-angiotensin–system (RAS) inhibitors (Rigalleau 2007). Accordingly, changes in GFR may be a more specific marker of DKD progression in the elderly than is elevated albuminuria, even in those with diabetes of long duration, although the significance of a moderate reduction in GFR in the absence of elevated albuminuria is uncertain (Garg et al. 2002; Wasen et al. 2004). In the United States in 1999–2004, 26% of diabetic patients aged ≥65 years had microalbuminuria, 10% had macroalbuminuria, and 31% had a GFR <60 ml/min/1.73 m^2 (Suh et al. 2008). Since 2001 adjusted incidence rates of diabetic ESRD among patients aged 65–74 have fallen by 2.0%, somewhat below the 4.5% decrease seen in those aged 45 to 64. By contrast in patients aged ≥75 years, the incidence rate of ESRD due to diabetes increased by 11.2% between 2001 and 2006 (U.S. Renal Data System 2008). During the same time, use of RAS inhibitors and lipid-lowering medicines in patients with CKD and diabetes was similar across these age groups and remained stable over time (U.S. Renal Data System 2008), suggesting that CKD management may be more difficult or less effective in the elderly than in the younger diabetic population or that other factors may be involved in the progression of kidney disease in the elderly. Development of diabetic complications, including DKD, is strongly associated with mortality in elderly persons (Otiniano et al. 2003; Kuo et al. 2003). Excess death, assessed by the standardized mortality ratio, declines with older age but is higher in patients with ESRD due to diabetes than to other causes (Villar et al. 2007).

The elderly are particularly prone to other complications of diabetes if they have DKD. Ninety percent of patients aged 75 years and older with ESRD and diabetes have CVD before initiation of kidney replacement therapy. Congestive heart failure is the most common cardiac condition among elderly patients with diabetes and kidney failure, affecting 71% of these patients, with 67% affected by ischemic heart disease (U.S. Renal Data System 2008). Other comorbidities are also more prevalent in elderly patients with DKD, and intensive management may pose relatively greater risks because hypotension and hypoglycemia are more common in this group. Because of these risks, medicines for hyperglycemia, hypertension, and dyslipidemia should be started at lower doses in the elderly and carefully titrated while monitoring for responses and side effects (National Kidney Foundation 2007). In addition, some medicines such as metformin and many sulfonylureas and the α-glucosidase inhibitors should be avoided in those with more advanced kidney disease because of their reduced renal clearance and enhanced toxicity.

■ Economic Burden

Managing DKD is costly, imposing a heavy economic burden on patients, the health system, and society. In a Michigan study, among patients with type 2 diabetes, microalbuminuria increased costs by 20%, proteinuria by 30%, and dialysis by 950% versus those with normal urinary albumin excretion (Brandle et al. 2003). Although CKD patients without ESRD represent 8.7% of the Medicare population, they claim 25% of the total costs. In 2006, predialysis per patient per month (PPPM) Medicare expenditures were approximately $1300 for patients with CKD and diabetes and nearly $3000 for patients who were also diagnosed with congestive heart failure (U.S. Renal Data System 2008). Transition to ESRD is associated with a spike in health care expenditures during the month following initiation of dialysis, with costs remaining higher compared with predialysis or transplant patients (U.S. Renal Data System 2008). A cost-effectiveness model simulating lifetime CKD progression, health care costs, quality-adjusted life-years (QALYs), and incremental cost-effectiveness ratios in patients 50 years and older, showed that relative to no screening, targeted annual screening for microalbuminuria heralds cost effectiveness ratios of $21,000/QALY, $55,000/QALY, and $155,000/QALY for persons with diabetes, those with hypertension, and those with neither diabetes nor hypertension, respectively. The study thus suggests that microalbuminuria screening is highly cost-effective for patients with diabetes or hypertension, whereas in those with neither disease it is most cost-effective when screening is conducted as part of standard physician visits (*Am J Kidney Dis* 55:463–473).

■ Epidemiology

The prevalence, incidence, and cumulative incidence of microalbuminuria and macroalbuminuria in type 1 and type 2 diabetes are presented in Table 7.1 (Parving, Mauer, and Ritz 2007). Depending on the population, the prevalence of microalbuminuria varies between 17% and 21% in type 1 diabetes and between 9% and 46% in type 2. The prevalence of microalbuminuria by age and gender in the U.S. diabetic population is presented in Figure 7.3 (Jones et al. 2002). The odds of elevated albuminuria are 1.4 to 2.8 times as high in persons with diabetes as in those without diabetes across ethnic groups (Bryson et al. 2006). In type 1 diabetes DKD rarely develops in the first 10 years after diagnosis. The rate of progression to macroalbuminuria is highest between 10 and 20 years (3% per year), and subsequently the incidence rate declines (Parving, Mauer, and Ritz 2007). Hence, the risk of developing DKD for a normoalbuminuric type 1 patient who has had diabetes for more than 30 years is very low. Unfortunately, without specific interventions, 60%–85% of type 1 patients with sustained microalbuminuria will progress to macroalbuminuria over a period of 10 to 15 years, with hypertension and proliferative retinopathy also developing along the way. Once overt nephropathy occurs, the GFR falls at a variable rate (from 2 to 20 ml/min/year) (Parving, Mauer, and Ritz 2007).

In type 2 diabetes the development and progression of DKD are more heterogeneous and therefore more difficult to characterize, in part reflecting a greater heterogeneity of kidney lesions and the relatively high prevalence of nondiabetic kidney disease, a consequence of the older age at onset of diabetes. Approximately 3% of newly diagnosed type 2 patients have overt nephropathy (Parving, Mauer, and Ritz 2007), largely because of delayed diabetes diagnosis. By 10 years after diagnosis about 25% of type 2 patients have microalbuminuria. Half of those who develop

TABLE 7.1 *Prevalence, Incidence, and Cumulative Incidence of Elevated Albuminuria in Persons with Type 1 or Type 2 Diabetes*

	Clinic-Based Studies		Population-Based Studies
Prevalence (%)	Type 1	Type 2	Type 2
Microalbuminuria	13 (9–20)	25 (13–27)	20 (17–21)
Macroalbuminuria	15 (8–22)	14 (5–48)	16 (9–46)
Incidence of macroalbuminuria (% per year)	1.2 (0–3)	1.5 (1–2)	—
Cumulative incidence of macroalbuminuria (% per 25 years)	31 (28–34)	28 (25–31)	—

Values are indicated as median and range.

Source: Adapted from Parving, Mauer, and Ritz (2007).

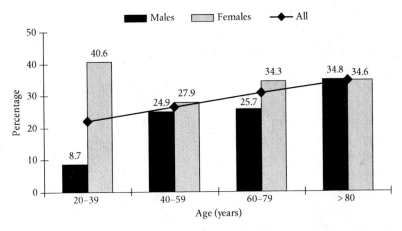

FIGURE 7.3. Age- and sex-specific prevalence of microalbuminuria in the U.S. population with self-reported diabetes, NHANES III 1988–1994. (Adapted from Jones et al. 2002.)

microalbuminuria do so within 20 years of diagnosis. The natural history of kidney disease in patients with newly diagnosed type 2 diabetes is presented in Figure 7.4 (Adler et al. 2003). From any level of nephropathy, the rate of progression to the next level of severity is 2%–3% per year. In addition to kidney failure, elevated albuminuria and declining kidney function predict CVD. In the Framingham Heart Study (Foster et al. 2007) patients with reduced eGFR and elevated ACR were 1.6 times as likely to die from CVD (95% CI 1.0–2.5) as patients with eGFR $\geq$ 60 ml/min/1.73 m² without elevated ACR, after adjusting for multiple risk factors. Patients with elevated ACR were more likely to have hypertension, diabetes, and CVD than those

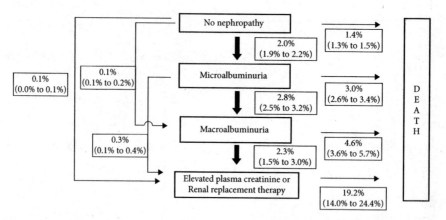

FIGURE 7.4. Estimated annual percentage of patients with type 2 diabetes (95% confidence interval) transitioning from normal albuminuria to microalbuminuria and macroalbuminuria and to death from any level of albuminuria or elevated serum creatinine. Estimates are unadjusted for kidney disease risk factors. (Source: Adler et al. 2003.)

without elevated ACR in any eGFR category, and patients with both reduced eGFR and elevated ACR had the highest prevalence of risk factors.

Improvements in the management of DKD have extended the time course from onset of proteinuria to kidney failure (Nelson et al. 2008). The rate of DKD progression and the cardiovascular risk are considerably lower for persons with diabetes who have tight control of their glucose level and blood pressure early in the course of their diabetes (National Kidney Foundation 2007). Moreover a substantial proportion of persons with type 1 or type 2 diabetes and microalbuminuria spontaneously regress to normoalbuminuria, suggesting that microalbuminuria may represent an initial phase of dynamic and reversible kidney injury rather than the onset of an inevitable progression to ESRD. A 6-year follow-up study of persons with type 1 diabetes and microalbuminuria found that only 19% developed overt proteinuria, while 60% regressed to normal albuminuria (Perkins et al. 2003). Regression of microalbuminuria was associated with lower systolic blood pressure, lower A1C, and lower serum levels of total cholesterol than in those who progressed. The proportion of type 2 patients who regress from microalbuminuria to normoalbuminuria is 30%–54% (Parving, Mauer, and Ritz 2007), while the frequency of progression to overt proteinuria is 12%–36%. Microalbuminuria of short duration, use of RAS inhibitors, lower A1C (<6.9%), and systolic blood pressure <129 mm Hg were independently associated with regression (Parving, Mauer, and Ritz 2007).

■ Risk Factors for the Development and Progression of DKD

In addition to albuminuria, recognized risk factors for the development and progression of DKD include hyperglycemia, hypertension, diabetes duration, age at onset, and smoking (Shoham et al. 2008). Strong familial aggregation of DKD suggests that genetic factors may play an important role.

In describing risk factors for DKD, we must consider socioeconomic factors. Low socioeconomic status is associated with increased prevalence of diabetes and associated morbidity in different populations. In the United States, poverty was found to be associated with higher odds of microalbuminuria than was affluence (Parving et al. 2006). Cumulative exposure to working-class status was positively associated with CKD. Although the mechanisms of these associations are unclear, low socioeconomic status, particularly when combined with low educational achievement, may have a compounding effect on the overall risk profile of those affected. Of concern, exposure to an adverse prenatal environment, including poor dietary habits, smoking, or poor health care, introduces health traits in subsequent generations that may persist in the absence of the initial exposure.

Hyperglycemia

Hyperglycemia is a strong risk factor for the occurrence and progression of microalbuminuria (Mauer et al. 1989; Nosadini et al. 2000; Scott et al. 2001) but has a lesser impact on progression of more advanced stages of kidney dysfunction (Keane et al. 2003), when hypertension, hypercholesterolemia, and genetic factors play a greater role in shaping the outcome (Parving, Mauer, and Ritz 2007). In type 1 diabetes the risk of microalbuminuria increases steeply above an A1C of 8.1%, independent of the duration of diabetes (see Fig. 7.5) (Krolewski et al. 1988). In Pima Indians with type 2 diabetes, 2-hour plasma glucose concentration,

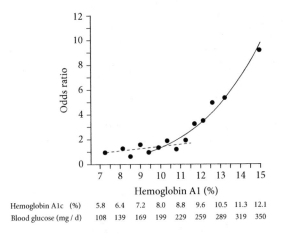

FIGURE 7.5. Association between mean hemoglobin A1C level and the risk of microalbuminuria in patients with type 1 diabetes. Hemoglobin A1C values were modeled in a logistic-regression model of the prevalence of microalbuminuria, adjusted for the age at onset of diabetes, sex, and diabetes duration. the reference was the group with A1C values between 5.9% and 7.9%. A change point model, including the same covariates, was fitted to the logarithm of A1C1 as a continuous variable to estimate the location of the change point and the regression slopes below and above the change point (continuous line). The horizontal axis shows A1C values as well as the equivalent values of A1C and the blood glucose profile. (Source: Krolewski et al. 1995.)

fasting plasma glucose, and A1C each predicted elevated albuminuria, defined as an ACR ≥30 mg/g, after adjustment for age, sex, and duration of diabetes (Nelson et al. 1993).

Blood Pressure

In type 1 diabetes the presence of hypertension generally indicates the presence of DKD, whereas in type 2 disease the onset of hypertension and macrovascular disease generally precedes DKD and is often associated with obesity. Persons with type 1 diabetes and DKD have a higher prevalence of parental hypertension and a higher mean arterial blood pressure during adolescence (Barzilay et al. 1992). Similarly the risk of DKD is three times as high in those with type 1 diabetes who have a hypertensive parent as in those whose parents are not hypertensive (Krolewski et al. 1988). In Pima Indian offspring with type 2 diabetes, the prevalence of proteinuria was similar if neither parent nor only one parent had hypertension (8.9% and 9.4%, respectively) but was significantly higher if both parents had hypertension (18.8%). In addition studies in Pima Indians indicate that higher blood pressure before the onset of type 2 diabetes is related to a higher prevalence of elevated albuminuria after the onset of diabetes, suggesting that blood pressure plays a causal role in the development of DKD (Nelson et al. 1993).

Smoking

Cigarette smoking is an established risk factor for the development of albuminuria in diabetic patients (Chaturvedi et al. 1995; Rossing P et al. 2002; Scott et al. 2001). Nicotine promotes the proliferation of mesangial cells and up-regulates specific molecules involved in extracellular matrix production (Jaimes et al. 2007). Versus nonsmokers, type 1 diabetic smokers had almost three times the risk of albuminuria (Chase et al. 1991). In patients with type 1 or type 2 diabetes and normal or near-normal kidney function, cigarette smoking is also associated with a decrease in the estimated GFR, independent of proteinuria (Orth et al. 2005). Other studies in type 2 diabetes suggest that smoking is associated with DKD progression despite blood pressure control and treatment with RAS inhibitors (Chuahirun et al. 2003; Gambaro et al. 2001).

Obesity

Obesity is a major risk factor for diabetes, hypertension, and CVD, all of which increase the risk for DKD. Animal and human studies indicate that obesity leads to glomerular hyperfiltration, which, in turn, causes proteinuria and focal segmental glomerulosclerosis (Wang et al. 2008). In addition, leptin secreted from excess adipose tissue might lead directly to kidney fibrosis (Wolf et al. 2002). A meta-analysis based on data from 18 cohort studies found that, compared with normal-weight persons, overweight persons have a 40% higher risk for CKD, and obese persons an 80% higher risk (Wang et al. 2008).

Periodontal Disease

Periodontal disease, a frequent complication of diabetes (Taylor and Borgnakke 2008), is a risk factor for development of DKD. Children with diabetes have significantly more frequent and severe periodontal disease than do nondiabetic controls (Lalla et al. 2006). Women with gestational diabetes have nine times the risk of periodontal disease experienced by nondiabetic nonpregnant women in the general U.S. population (Taylor and Borgnakke 2008). Severity of periodontitis and being edentulous predicted macroalbuminuria and ESRD in a dose-dependent manner among Pima Indian adults with type 2 diabetes within a median follow-up of 9 years (Shultis et al. 2007). Control of periodontal infection in diabetic adults has a positive effect on A1C level (Taylor and Borgnakke 2008) and reduces the levels of various markers of inflammation, coagulation, and adhesion.

Dyslipidemia

In addition to its established atherogenic effect in the coronary and peripheral arteries, dyslipidemia might contribute to onset and progression of DKD through similar mechanisms in the kidneys (Cooper and Jandeleit-Dahm 2005). The World Health Organization Multinational Study of Vascular Disease in Diabetes, which included type 1 and type 2 patients, found an association between serum triglycerides and ESRD in type 2 diabetes during 8 years of follow-up (Colhoun et al. 2001). Over a longer period (median follow-up 15 years), low-density lipoprotein (LDL) cholesterol and triglycerides were independent predictors of albuminuria in type 2 diabetes (Retnakaran et al. 2006). In patients with type 2 diabetes in the RENAAL study, total and LDL cholesterol increased the risk of ESRD by 96% per 100 mg/dL and 47% per 50 mg/dL, respectively. Lowering LDL cholesterol was associated with reduced risk of ESRD after 1 year of treatment, but these associations between LDL cholesterol and ESRD were largely mediated by concurrent changes in albuminuria (Tershakovec et al. 2008). Hence, there is no solid evidence from clinical trials of a kidney-protective effect of lipid-lowering treatments in diabetes.

Urinary Tract Infection

Diabetic women with asymptomatic bacteriuria do not have an increased risk for a faster decline in kidney function or the development of hypertension after 6 years of follow-up (Meiland et al. 2006). Although urinary tract infection can severely impair kidney function, the available evidence suggests that this is rare in the absence of a major predisposing factor such as obstruction, calculus, reflux, or abnormalities of the voiding mechanism.

Intrauterine Factors

Exposure to a diabetic intrauterine environment may impair normal embryogenesis (Nelson 2003). Most of the information about the magnitude of this risk comes from longitudinal studies in Pima Indians. Over a 30-year period, the proportion of Pima children exposed to diabetes in utero increased nearly fourfold (Dabelea et al. 1998); this increase was associated with a doubling of the number of cases of diabetes attributable to this exposure. Moreover, the prevalence of DKD in the offspring of diabetic mothers was nearly four times as high as in the offspring of nondiabetic or prediabetic mothers. This association persisted even after adjusting for the effects of parental hypertension and proteinuria, suggesting that the intrauterine exposure to diabetes is a strong and independent risk factor for the development of DKD (Nelson 2003). A likely explanation for this observation is that the diabetic intrauterine environment may have a fuel-mediated teratogenic effect on the developing nephrons that in turn leads to earlier development of kidney disease once diabetes develops (Abrahamson and Steenhard 2008).

A reduction in maternal fuels during pregnancy may manifest as intrauterine growth retardation, defined as birth weight below the 10th percentile for gestational age. Low birth weight is frequent among minority populations, transitional populations, and those with low socioeconomic status, as it is in pregnancies with inadequate maternal weight gain, poor antenatal care, shorter maternal height, maternal hypertension, or smoking. In a population-based screening program of high-risk adults, self-reported birth weight had a U-shaped relationship with CKD among men. The odds of developing CKD later in life were significantly higher among those with a birth weight below 2500 g or above 4500 g compared with men with normal birth weight (Li et al. 2007). Similarly in diabetic Pima Indians, low birth weight was associated with higher prevalence of elevated albuminuria than was normal birth weight after adjustment for age, sex, diabetes duration, A1C, and mean blood pressure (Nelson 2003). Animal models and autopsy studies demonstrate that low birth weight is associated with impaired nephrogenesis, a congenital low number of nephrons, and compensatory increased glomerular size. Increasing evidence suggests that individuals with reduced nephron endowment are prone to develop hypertension, kidney failure, and CVD later in life (Nelson 2003).

Genetics

Diabetic siblings of persons with DKD are at higher risk for nephropathy than are diabetic siblings of diabetic persons without DKD. This familial aggregation is found in various populations with type 1 or type 2 diabetes and reflects an inherited predisposition to the disease. Albuminuria and, to a greater degree, GFR are heritable (Langefeld et al. 2004), but the actual genes responsible for DKD remain elusive. Studies of persons with type 1 diabetes and albuminuria found evidence for linkage around chromosome 3q24 (Chistiakov et al. 2004). Combining the emerging technology of high-density single nucleotide polymorphism (SNP) microarrays with a pooled genomic DNA design, a recent study in Pima Indians with type 2 diabetes provided the first evidence supporting a potential locus for ESRD within the *PVT1* gene (Hanson et al. 2007). The *D* allele of the angiotensin-converting enzyme (ACE) gene is associated with an increased risk of diabetic nephropathy, but the potential for publication bias means this finding should be interpreted with caution (Staessen et al. 1997).

Large multicenter studies such as GoKinD (Genetics of Kidneys in Diabetes) and FIND (Family Investigation of Nephropathy and Diabetes) may facilitate the identification of relevant genes for diabetic nephropathy. GoKinD recruited subjects informative for nephropathy due to type 1 diabetes, and FIND, the largest DKD genetic study to date, collected DNA and cell lines from European American, African American, Native American, and Hispanic American families in whom type 2 diabetes was the predominant cause of DKD (Knowler et al. 2005). For all ethnicities combined, the strongest evidence for linkage to diabetic nephropathy in FIND was on chromosomes 7q21.3, 10p5.3, 14q23.1, and 18q22.3, to ACR on chromosomes 2q14.1, 7q21.1, and 15q26.3, and to GFR on chromosomes 1q43, 7q36.1, and 8q13.3. Additionally, the data suggest that unique DKD alleles cluster within these ethnic groups (Iyengar et al. 2007; Schelling et al. 2008).

■ Trends in Risk Factors Associated with DKD

Between 1971 and 2000 the proportion of noninstitutionalized U.S. adults with diabetes and hypertension declined from 64% to 37%, and smoking prevalence declined from 32% to 17% (Imperatore et al. 2004). Between 1988 and 2002, the proportion of diabetic persons with poor glycemic control (A1C >9%) declined by nearly 4%, while the proportion of persons with A1C between 6% and 8% increased from 34% to 47% (Saaddine et al. 2006). Although these trends are encouraging, one in three persons with diabetes still has uncontrolled hypertension, one in five has poor glycemic control, and one in six is smoking. Among southwestern American Indians, reduction in risk factors for diabetes-related ESRD may have contributed to the decline in ESRD incidence in all age groups in this population between 1993 and 2001 (Burrows et al. 2005). Similarly, the decline in the age- and gender-adjusted incidence of ESRD among Pima Indians with type 2 diabetes coincided with the introduction and widespread use within this community of new hypoglycemic medicines and medicines that block the RAS (Nelson et al. 2008). However, despite improvements in blood pressure and in glycemic and cholesterol control, the incidence of proteinuria remained largely unchanged between 1967 and 2002 in those of similar age, gender, and duration of diabetes. Hence, newer treatments for DKD, although not preventing the development of kidney disease, may slow its progression.

■ Management of Diabetes and CKD

Hyperglycemia

Intensive treatment of hyperglycemia prevents DKD and may slow progression of established kidney disease. Treatment guidelines of the American Diabetes Association (ADA) recommend maintaining fasting plasma glucose values within 90–130 mg/dL and an overall A1C goal of less than 7% for persons with type 1 or type 2 diabetes (ADA 2007).

In the Diabetes Control and Complications Trial (DCCT) (DCCT Research Group 1995), intensive glycemic control with the goal of reducing the A1C to <7% reduced the risk of microalbuminuria by 34% in the primary prevention cohort—which included subjects with type 1 diabetes for less than 5 years, no retinopathy, and a normal urinary albumin excretion rate. After the first year of therapy, the albumin excretion rate was reduced by 15% even though more than half of the subjects in the intensively treated group did not achieve this goal. In the secondary intervention cohort, including subjects with a longer duration of type 1 diabetes, minimal to moderate retinopathy, and elevated albuminuria, intensive insulin therapy reduced the risk of microalbuminuria by 43% to 56% and the risk of clinical albuminuria (ACR ≥208 μg/min) by 56%. These findings suggest that early and intensive treatment to achieve a target A1C of <7% is beneficial for preventing and reducing the progression of DKD.

The Wisconsin Epidemiological Study of Diabetic Retinopathy (Klein, Klein, and Moss 1993) followed patients with onset of diabetes at less than age 30, presumably mostly a type 1 cohort, and patients with onset at age ≥30 years, presumably mostly type 2. After 10 years of follow-up, a consistent exponential increase in the incidence of DKD with worsening glycemic control was found. The relationship was the same in patients with young-onset disease who required insulin as it was in patients with older-onset diabetes for any given level of hyperglycemia and was similar to the relationship found in the DCCT.

In patients with type 2 diabetes, data from the United Kingdom Prospective Diabetes Study (UKPDS) (UKPDS Group 1998) confirmed that improved blood glucose control with sulfonylureas or insulin reduces the risk of DKD and other microvascular complications, although without any impact on macrovascular complications. Except for the concern regarding increased mortality from cardiovascular causes in patients treated with sulfonylurea, there are no data supporting differential effects of insulin- and sulfonylurea-based treatments on diabetes complications.

Hypoglycemia is a major concern for persons with decreased kidney function because of impaired kidney clearance of insulin and some of the oral agents used to treat diabetes. In addition gluconeogenesis is decreased with reduced kidney mass (Gerich et al. 2001), potentially increasing the likelihood that a patient with excessive insulin/oral agent dosage or inadequate food intake will develop hypoglycemia. In persons with advanced CKD, intensive glycemic control may not prevent further deterioration in kidney function, but it may still prevent or slow the progression of retinopathy, neuropathy, and macrovascular disease and also improve survival (Morioka et al. 2001; Yu et al. 1997).

Hypertension

Long-term clinical trials that evaluated the rate of decline in kidney function at a randomized level of blood pressure have demonstrated that the lower the blood pressure, the greater the preservation of kidney function (Hart and Bakris 2004) (see Fig. 7.6). A slower rate of progression of kidney disease was evident even in persons who had greater than 1 g per day of proteinuria and reduced GFR when the blood pressure was less than 125/75 mm Hg (National Kidney Foundation 2007). Control of blood pressure is also essential for reducing risk of CVD. Although earlier retrospective studies suggested a possible J-shaped relation between blood pressure and cardiovascular events (Kaplan 1998), there was no increased risk of cardiovascular or kidney events in subsequent clinical trials that randomized persons with type 2 diabetes and hypertension to a goal of diastolic blood pressure less than 85 mm Hg (Bakris et al. 2003).

The National Kidney Foundation KDOQI™ Guidelines (National Kidney Foundation 2007) recommend a target of <130/80 mm Hg in patients with diabetes and kidney disease. This target must be achieved with a regimen including RAS inhibitors because these agents, which include ACE inhibitors and the newer angiotensin receptor blockers (ARBs), slow the increase in albuminuria and delay the progression from microalbuminuria to macroalbuminuria in diabetic

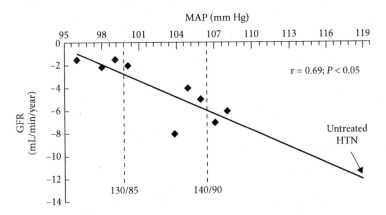

FIGURE 7.6. Relationship between achieved blood pressure control and declines in GFR in clinical trials of diabetic and nondiabetic kidney disease. In the table, the trials marked by an asterisk are those in nondiabetic kidney disease patients. (Source: Hart et al. 2004.)

persons, thus reducing the incidence of ESRD. The superiority of RAS inhibitors over other antihypertensive agents is less well established in the primary prevention of kidney disease in patients with type 2 diabetes. In patients with more advanced kidney disease, that is, macroalbuminuria and reduced GFR, ARBs are more effective than other antihypertensive classes in reducing albuminuria and slowing progression of kidney disease (Brenner et al. 2001). In the RENAAL study, treatment with ARBs reduced by 45% the risk of doubling of serum creatinine or ESRD after a 4-year follow-up. In addition, for every 50% reduction in albuminuria achieved, cardiovascular risk was reduced by 18%, and risk of heart failure by 27%. Similar studies are not available for ACE inhibitors, but ARBs appear similar to ACE inhibitors in reducing proteinuria. In the ONTARGET study (ONTARGET Investigators 2008), the combination of full doses of ARBs and ACE inhibitors had no additional advantage compared with ACE inhibitors alone despite a substantial lowering of blood pressure. Moreover, the two-drug regimen significantly increased the risk of side effects, including kidney dysfunction requiring dialysis.

Dyslipidemia

Recommendations for treatment of dyslipidemia in diabetes and CKD are based on reducing the risk of CVD because the current state of evidence from clinical trials is insufficient to support treatment to preserve kidney function (Tershakovec et al. 2008), even though there is evidence of a relation between hyperlipidemia and kidney disease in observational studies. Current National Kidney Foundation and National Cholesterol Education Project Adult Treatment Panel III (NCEP-ATP-III) guidelines support lowering of LDL cholesterol in patients with diabetes and CKD stages 1 to 4 to reduce risk of CVD. These recommendations, however, are based on post hoc subgroup analyses of clinical trials, and there is no direct evidence for the target level of LDL cholesterol in these patients.

Nutrition

Dietary intake of protein at all stages of CKD appears to have an important effect on persons with diabetes. Nutrition surveys indicate that most Americans consume protein in excess of the recommended daily allowance level of 0.8 g/kg body weight per day (about 10% of total calories) (Wright et al. 2003). In two meta-analyses, low-protein diets reduced risks of progression of albuminuria/proteinuria and loss of GFR, with more pronounced benefits in DKD than in non-DKD (Kasiske et al. 1998). Even a modest limitation to an average dietary protein intake of 0.89 g/kg body weight per day compared with 1.02 g/kg body weight per day was shown to reduce the risk of ESRD or death (relative risk = 0.23, 95% CI 0.07 to 0.72) in a randomized study of persons with type 1 diabetes, eGFR of 60–90 ml/min/1.73 m^2, and elevated albuminuria (National Kidney Foundation 2007). Benefits of limiting dietary protein are more evident in type 1 than type 2 diabetes, but fewer studies have been done in the latter population. Emerging epidemiologic evidence indicates that higher protein intake ($\geq$20% versus 10% of total daily calories) is associated with loss of kidney function in women with mildly decreased GFR and with the development of microalbuminuria in persons with diabetes and hypertension (National Kidney Foundation 2007).

Multifaceted Management

There is growing evidence that intensive, multidisciplinary management of CKD patients, involving multiple drug combinations and behavioral adjustment, has sustained benefits on the progression of kidney disease per se and on the associated microvascular and macrovascular outcomes. In the Steno-2 study, a prospective, randomized, open-label, blinded trial conducted in Denmark (Gæde et al. 2008), mortality was significantly lower with intensive therapy than with usual therapy (hazard ratio = 0.54, 95% CI 0.32 to 0.89). The study assigned 160 patients with type 2 diabetes and persistent microalbuminuria to either intensive therapy or conventional therapy for an average of 7.8 years. Patients were subsequently followed observationally for a mean of 5.5 years. The primary end point at 13.3 years of follow-up was the time to death from any cause. The absolute risk reduction for cardiovascular events was 29% (hazard ratio = 0.41, 95% CI 0.25 to 0.67). Fewer patients developed overt proteinuria (relative risk = 0.44, 95% CI 0.25 to 0.77), and only one patient in the intensive-therapy group progressed to ESRD, as compared with six patients in the conventional-therapy group (p = 0.04) (Gæde et al. 2008). Moreover early intervention in high-risk diabetic patients with microalbuminuria achieved persistent risk reductions after the interventional period, as compared with a late intervention.

■ Current CDC Projects in CKD

Health conditions are regarded as public health issues when they meet a number of criteria, including a high disease burden that is perceived as a threat by the public; the disproportionate distribution of the disease among minority and disadvantaged groups; and the demonstration that public health strategies targeting specific socioeconomic and environmental factors may significantly reduce the disease burden (Schoolwerth et al. 2006). CKD largely meets these criteria and therefore is considered a public health problem.

Nearly all ESRD cases in the United States are captured by the United States Renal Data System (USRDS), a national surveillance data system on ESRD that collects, analyzes, and distributes information from the Medical Evidence Report to the Centers for Medicare & Medicaid Services. Based on this information, USRDS releases the *Annual Data Report* describing the burden of ESRD and associated morbidity, mortality, and costs. In addition, USRDS produces the *Researcher's Guide*, fulfills requests for data, and provides standard analytical files to researchers. Since 2007, the *Annual Data Report* has included information on CKD using different data sources, but there is no current national surveillance system for CKD prior to dialysis unless the patients are aged 65 or older and covered by Medicare. The CDC's National Diabetes Surveillance System (NDSS) is the only surveillance system nationally that collects, analyzes, and disseminates national and state data on the public health burden of diabetes and its complications, including DKD (available from www.cdc.gov/diabetes).

In recognition of the growing problem of CKD, Congress passed legislation in 2006 to develop capacity and infrastructure at CDC for a kidney disease surveillance program. CDC's Chronic Kidney Disease Initiative was thus established to support state-based demonstration projects for CKD prevention and control and to lay the groundwork for a formal Public Health Kidney Disease Action Plan for prevention and control of kidney disease. As part of this initiative CDC is implementing the CKD Surveillance Project and contributing to kidney measures to the National Health and Nutrition Examination Survey (NHANES) and to the Health, Aging, and Body Composition study targeting persons aged 70 years or older. For the CKD Surveillance Project, the CDC is collaborating with the University of Michigan and Johns Hopkins University to comprehensively document the burden and trends of CKD and its risk factors in the United States. In addition CDC is sponsoring two health care cost studies and an ongoing demonstration project for identifying persons at high risk for CKD. The CKD Health Evaluation Risk Information Sharing project (CHERISH), implemented in collaboration with the National Kidney Foundation and Chronic Disease Research Group (CDRG), is a state-based early detection and screening demonstration program with the primary goals of testing the feasibility of a CKD detection program in high-risk groups and examining participants' follow-up within the health care system. The information will be used to develop population screening strategies for early detection of CKD with the goal of reducing the rate of cardiovascular events, death rates from CVD, and progression to ESRD.

In addition to maintaining NDSS, the CDC initiates and collaborates on studies to improve both the methods of surveillance and the efficacy of surveillance data, and it assists state, national, and international partners in the development of diabetes surveillance programs.

■ References

Abrahamson DR, Steenhard BM. (2008). Perinatal nephron programming is not so sweet in maternal diabetes. *Journal of the American Society of Nephrology* **19**, 837–9.

Adler AI et al., on behalf of the UKPDS Group (2003). Development and progression of nephropathy in type 2 diabetes: the United Kingdom Prospective Diabetes Study (UKPDS 64). *Kidney International* **63**, 225–32.

American Diabetes Association (2000). Type 2 diabetes in children and adolescents. *Diabetes Care* **23**, 381–9.

American Diabetes Association (2007). Clinical practice recommendations. *Diabetes Care* **30** (Suppl. 1), S19–20.

Amin R et al. (2008). Risk of microalbuminuria and progression to macroalbuminuria in a cohort with childhood onset type 1 diabetes: prospective observational study. *British Medical Journal* **336**, 697–701.

Bakris GL et al. (2003). Effects of blood pressure level on progression of diabetic nephropathy: results from the RENAAL Study. *Archives of Internal Medicine* **163**, 1555–65.

Barzilay J et al. (1992). Predisposition to hypertension: risk factor for nephropathy and hypertension in IDDM. *Kidney International* **41**, 723–30.

Brandle M et al. (2003). The direct medical cost of type 2 diabetes. *Diabetes Care* **26**, 2300–4.

Brenner BM et al. (2001). Effects of losartan on renal and cardiovascular outcomes in patients with type 2 diabetes and nephropathy. *New England Journal of Medicine* **345**, 861–9.

Bryson CL et al. (2006). Racial and ethnic variations in albuminuria in the US Third National Health and Nutrition Examination Survey (NHANES III) population: associations with diabetes and level of CKD. *American Journal of Kidney Disease* **48**, 720–6.

Burrows NR et al. (2005). End-stage renal disease due to diabetes among Southwestern American Indians, 1990–2001. *Diabetes Care* **28**, 1041–4.

Centers for Disease Control and Prevention (n.d.a). http://www.cdc.gov/mmwr/preview/mmwrhtml/mm5443a2.htm. Accessed January 23, 2009.

Centers for Disease Control and Prevention (n.d.b). http://www.cdc.gov/mmwr/preview/mmwrhtml/mm5608a2.htm. Accessed January 23, 2009.

Chase HP et al. (1991). Cigarette smoking increases the risk of albuminuria among subjects with type 1 diabetes. *Journal of the American Medical Association* **265**, 614–7.

Chaturvedi N et al. (1995). The relationship between smoking and microvascular complications in the EURODIAB IDDM Complications Study. *Diabetes Care* **18**, 785–92.

Chistiakov DA et al. (2004). Confirmation of a susceptibility locus for diabetic nephropathy on chromosome 3q23-q24 by association study in Russian type 1 diabetic patients. *Diabetes Research and Clinical Practice* **66**, 79–86.

Chuahirun T et al. (2003). Cigarette smoking and increased urine albumin excretion are interrelated predictors of nephropathy progression in type 2 diabetes. *American Journal of Kidney Disease* **41**, 13–21.

Colhoun HM et al. (2001). Risk factors for renal failure: the WHO Multinational Study of Vascular Disease in Diabetes. *Diabetologia* **44**, S46–53.

Collins AJ et al. (2003). Chronic kidney disease and cardiovascular disease in the Medicare population. *Kidney International. Supplement* **87**, S24–31.

Cooper ME, Jandeleit-Dahm KA (2005). Lipids and diabetic renal disease. *Current Diabetes Reports* **5**, 445–8.

Dabelea D et al. (1998). Increasing prevalence of type II diabetes in American Indian children. *Diabetologia* **41**, 904–10.

Davison JM (2001). Renal disorders in pregnancy. *Current Opinion in Obstetrics and Gynecology* **13**, 109–14.

Diabetes Control and Complications (DCCT) Research Group (1995). Effect of intensive therapy on the development and progression of diabetic nephropathy in the Diabetes Control and Complications Trial. *Kidney International* **47**, 1703–20.

Foster MC et al. (2007). Cross-classification of microalbuminuria and reduced glomerular filtration rate: associations between cardiovascular disease risk factors and clinical outcomes. *Archives of Internal Medicine* **167**, 1386–92.

Gæde P et al. (2008). Effect of multifactorial intervention on mortality in type 2 diabetes. *New England Journal of Medicine* **358**, 580–9.

Gambaro G et al. (2001). Cigarette smoking is a risk factor for nephropathy and its progression in Type 2 diabetes mellitus. *Diabetes, Nutrition & Metabolism* **14**, 337–42.

Garg AX et al. (2002). Albuminuria and renal insufficiency prevalence guides population screening: results from the NHANES III. *Kidney International* **61**, 2165–75.

Gerich JE et al. (2001). Renal gluconeogenesis: its importance in human glucose homeostasis. *Diabetes Care* **24**, 382–91.

Gerstein HC et al. (2001). Albuminuria and risk of cardiovascular events, death, and heart failure in diabetic and nondiabetic individuals. *JAMA* **286**, 421–6.

Hanson RL et al. (2007). Identification of PVT1 as a candidate gene for end-stage renal disease in type 2 diabetes using a pooling-based genome-wide single nucleotide polymorphism association study. *Diabetes* **56**, 975–83.

Hart PD, Bakris GL (2004). Managing hypertension in the diabetic patient. In: Egan BM, Basile JN, Lackland DT, eds. *Hot Topics in Hypertension*, pp 249–52. Philadelphia: Hanley & Belfus.

Hogg RJ et al. (2003). National Kidney Foundation's Kidney Disease Outcomes Quality Initiative Clinical Practice Guidelines for Chronic Kidney Disease in Children and Adolescents: evaluation, classification, and stratification. *Pediatrics* **111**, 1416–21.

Ibsen H et al. (2006). Does albuminuria predict cardiovascular outcomes on treatment with losartan versus atenolol in patients with diabetes, hypertension, and left ventricular hypertrophy? The LIFE study. *Diabetes Care* **29**, 595–600.

Imperatore G et al. (2004). Thirty-year trends in cardiovascular risk factor levels among US adults with diabetes: National Health and Nutrition Examination Surveys, 1971–2000. *American Journal of Epidemiology* **160**, 531–9.

Iyengar SK et al. (2007). Genome-wide scans for diabetic nephropathy and albuminuria in multiethnic populations: the Family Investigation of Nephropathy and Diabetes (FIND). *Diabetes* **56**, 1577–85.

Jaimes EA et al. (2007). Nicotine: the link between cigarette smoking and the progression of renal injury? *American Journal of Physiology. Heart and Circulatory Physiology* **292**, H76–82.

Jones CA et al. (2002). Microalbuminuria in the US population: third National Health and Nutrition Examination Survey. *American Journal of Kidney Disease* **39**, 445–59.

Jones DC, Hyslett JP (1996). Outcome of pregnancy in women with moderate to severe renal insufficiency. *New England Journal of Medicine* **335**, 226–32.

Kaplan N (1998). J-curve not burned off by HOT study. Hypertension Optimal Treatment. *Lancet* **351**, 1748–9.

Kasiske BL et al. (1998). A meta-analysis of the effects of dietary protein restriction on the rate of decline in renal function. *American Journal of Kidney Disease* **31**, 954–61.

Keane WF et al. (2003). The risk of developing end-stage renal disease in patients with type 2 diabetes and nephropathy: the RENAAL study. *Kidney International* **63**, 1499–507.

Klein R, Klein BE, Moss SE (1993). Prevalence of microalbuminuria in older-onset diabetes. *Diabetes Care* **16**, 1325–30.

Knowler WC et al. (1990). Diabetes mellitus in the Pima Indians: Incidence, risk factors and pathogenesis. *Diabetes/Metabolism Reviews* **6**, 1–27.

Knowler WC et al. (2005). The Family Investigation of Nephropathy and Diabetes (FIND): design and methods. *Journal of Diabetes Complications* **19**, 1–9.

Krakoff J et al. (2003). Incidence of retinopathy and nephropathy in youth-onset compared with adult-onset type 2 diabetes. *Diabetes Care* **26**, 76–81.

Krolewski AS et al. (1988). Predisposition to hypertension and susceptibility to renal disease in insulin-dependent diabetes mellitus. *New England Journal of Medicine* **318**, 140–5.

Krolewski AS et al. (1995). Glycosylated hemoglobin and the risk of microalbuminuria in patients with insulin-dependent diabetes mellitus. *New England Journal of Medicine* **332**, 1251–5.

Kuo YF et al. (2003). Inconsistent use of diabetes medications, diabetes complications, and mortality in older Mexican Americans over a 7-year period: data from the Hispanic established population for the epidemiologic study of the elderly. *Diabetes Care* **26**, 3054–60.

Lalla E et al. (2006). Periodontal changes in children and adolescents with diabetes: a case-control study. *Diabetes Care* **29**, 295–9.

Langefeld CD et al. (2004). Heritability of GFR and albuminuria in Caucasians with type 2 diabetes mellitus. *American Journal of Kidney Disease* **43**, 796–800.

Lee ET et al. (2001). Follow-up of the WHO Multinational Study of Vascular Disease in Diabetes: general description and morbidity. *Diabetologia* **44** (Suppl. 2), S3–13.

Levey AS et al. (2006). Using standardized serum creatinine values in the modification of diet in renal disease study equation for estimating glomerular filtration rate. *Annals of Internal Medicine* **145**, 247–54.

Li S et al. (2007). Low birth weight is associated with chronic kidney disease only in men. *Kidney International* **73**, 637–42.

Maahs DM et al. (2007). Higher prevalence of elevated albumin excretion in youth with type 2 than type 1 diabetes. *Diabetes Care* **30**, 2593–8.

Mattix HJ et al. (2002). Use of the albumin/creatinine ratio to detect microalbuminuria: implications of sex and race. *Journal of the American Society of Nephrology* **13**, 1034–9.

Mauer SM et al. (1989). Long-term study of normal kidneys transplanted into patients with type I diabetes. *Diabetes* **38**, 516–23.

Meiland R et al. (2006). Asymptomatic bacteriuria in women with diabetes mellitus: effect on renal function after 6 years of follow-up. *Archives of Internal Medicine* **166**, 2222–7.

Molitch ME et al. (2004). Nephropathy in diabetes. *Diabetes Care* **27** (Suppl. 1), S79–83.

Morioka T et al. (2001). Glycemic control is a predictor of survival for diabetic patients on hemodialysis. *Diabetes Care* **24**, 909–13.

Muntner P et al. (2003). The contribution of increased diabetes prevalence and improved myocardial infarction and stroke survival to the increase in treated end-stage renal disease. *Journal of the American Society of Nephrology* **14**, 1568–77.

Narayan KM et al. (2006). Impact of recent increase in incidence on future diabetes burden. *Diabetes Care* **29**, 2114–16.

National Kidney Foundation (2002). K/DOQI Clinical Practice Guidelines for Chronic Kidney Disease: evaluation, classification, and stratification. *American Journal of Kidney Disease* **39** (Suppl. 1), S1–266.

National Kidney Foundation (2007). K/DOQI Clinical Practice Guidelines and Clinical Recommendations for Diabetes and Chronic Kidney Disease. *American Journal of Kidney Disease* **49** (Suppl. 2), S12–154.

Nelson RG (2003). Intrauterine determinants of diabetic kidney disease in disadvantaged populations. *Kidney International. Supplement* **83**, 13–6.

Nelson RG et al. (1993). Pre-diabetic blood pressure predicts urinary albumin excretion after the onset of type 2 (non-insulin-dependent) diabetes mellitus in Pima Indians. *Diabetologia* **36**, 998–1001.

Nelson RG et al. (1995). Incidence and determinants of elevated urinary albumin excretion in Pima Indians with NIDDM. *Diabetes Care* **18**, 182–7.

Nelson RG et al. (2008). Changing course of diabetic nephropathy in the Pima Indians. *Diabetes Research and Clinical Practice* **82**(Suppl. 1), S10–4.

Nosadini R et al. (2000). Course of renal function in type 2 diabetic patients with abnormalities of albumin excretion rate. *Diabetes* **49**, 476–84.

ONTARGET Investigators (2008). Telmisartan, Ramipril, or both in patients at high risk for vascular events. *New England Journal of Medicine* **358**, 1547–59.

Orth SR et al. (2005). Effects of smoking on renal function in patients with type 1 and type 2 diabetes mellitus. *Nephrology, Dialysis, Transplantation* **20**, 2414–9.

Otiniano ME et al. (2003). Self-reported diabetic complications and 7-year mortality in Mexican American elders. Findings from a community-based study of five Southwestern states. *Journal of Diabetes Complications* **17**, 243–8.

Parving HH et al. (2006). Prevalence and risk factors for microalbuminuria in a referred cohort of type II diabetic patients: a global perspective. *Kidney International* **69**, 2057–63.

Parving HH, Mauer M, Ritz E (2007). Diabetic nephropathy. In: Brenner BM, ed. *Brenner & Rector's the Kidney*, 8th ed., pp 1265–99. Philadelphia: Saunders Elsevier.

Pavkov ME et al. (2004). An explanation for the increase in heart disease mortality rates in diabetic Pima Indians: effect of renal replacement therapy. *Diabetes Care* **27**, 1132–6.

Perkins BA et al. (2003). Regression of microalbuminuria in type 1 diabetes. *New England Journal of Medicine* **348**, 2285–93.

Pinhas-Hamiel O, Zeitler P (2007). Acute and chronic complications of type 2 diabetes mellitus in children and adolescents. *Lancet* **369**, 1823–31.

Retnakaran R et al. (2006). Risk factors for renal dysfunction in type 2 diabetes: U.K. Prospective Diabetes Study 74. *Diabetes* **55**, 1832–9.

Rigalleau V et al. (2007). Normoalbuminuric renal-insufficient diabetic patients: a lower-risk group. *Diabetes Care* **30**, 2034–9.

Rossing K et al. (2002). Pregnancy and progression of diabetic nephropathy. *Diabetologia* **45**, 36–41.

Rossing P et al. (2002). Risk factors for development of incipient and overt diabetic nephropathy in type 1 diabetic patients: a 10-year prospective observational study. *Diabetes Care* **25**, 859–64.

Saaddine JB et al. (2006). Improvements in diabetes processes of care and intermediate outcomes: United States, 1988–2002. *Annals of Internal Medicine* **144**, 465–74.

Schelling JR et al. (2008). Genome-wide scan for estimated GFR in multi-ethnic diabetic populations: the Family Investigation of Nephropathy and Diabetes. *Diabetes* **57**, 235–43.

Schoolwerth AC et al. (2006). Chronic kidney disease: a public health problem that needs a public health action plan. *Preventing Chronic Disease* **3**(2), A57. Available at: http://www.cdc.gov/pcd/issues/2006/apr/05_0105.htm. Accessed February 8, 2008.

Scott LJ et al. (2001). A nonlinear effect of hyperglycemia and current cigarette smoking are major determinants of the onset of microalbuminuria in type 1 diabetes. *Diabetes* **50**, 2842–9.

Shoham DA et al. (2008). Kidney disease and the cumulative burden of life course socioeconomic conditions: the Atherosclerosis Risk in Communities (ARIC) study. *Social Science & Medicine* **67**, 1311–20.

Shultis WA et al. (2007). Effect of periodontitis on overt nephropathy and end-stage renal disease in type 2 diabetes. *Diabetes Care* **30**, 306–11.

Staessen JA et al. (1997). The deletion/insertion polymorphism of the angiotensin converting enzyme gene and cardiovascular-renal risk. *Journal of Hypertension* **15**, 1579–92.

Stevens LA et al. (2007). Evaluation of the Modification of Diet in Renal Disease Study Equation in a large, diverse population. *Journal of the American Society of Nephrology* **18**, 2749–57.

Suh DC et al. (2008). Comorbid conditions and glycemic control in elderly patients with type 2 diabetes mellitus, 1988 to 1994 to 1999 to 2004. *Journal of the American Geriatrics Society* **56**, 484–92.

Taylor GW, Borgnakke WS (2008). Periodontal disease: associations with diabetes, glycemic control and complications. *Oral Diseases* **14**, 191–203.

Tershakovec AM et al. (2008). Effect of LDL cholesterol and treatment with losartan on end-stage renal disease in the RENAAL Study. *Diabetes Care* **31**, 445–7.

UK Prospective Diabetes Study (UKPDS) Group (1998). Intensive blood-glucose control with sulphonylureas or insulin compared with conventional treatment and risk of complications in patients with type 2 diabetes (UKPDS 33). *Lancet* **352**, 837–53.

U.S. Renal Data System (2007). *USRDS 2007 Annual Data Report. Atlas of Chronic Kidney Disease and End-Stage Renal Disease in the United States.* Bethesda: National Institutes of Health, National Institute of Diabetes and Digestive and Kidney Diseases.

U.S. Renal Data System (2008). *USRDS 2008 Annual Data Report. Atlas of Chronic Kidney Disease and End-Stage Renal Disease in the United States.* Bethesda: National Institutes of Health, National Institute of Diabetes and Digestive and Kidney Diseases.

Villar E et al. (2007). Effect of age, gender, and diabetes on excess death in end-stage renal failure. *Journal of the American Society of Nephrology* **18**, 2125–34.

Wang Y et al. (2008). Association between obesity and kidney disease: a systematic review and meta-analysis. *Kidney International* **73**, 19–33.

Wasen E et al. (2004). Renal impairment associated with diabetes in the elderly. *Diabetes Care* **27**, 2648–53.

Wolf G et al. (2002). Leptin and renal disease. *American Journal of Kidney Disease* **39**, 1–11.

Wright JD et al. (2003). Dietary intake of ten key nutrients for public health, United States: 1999-2000. *Advance Data* **334**, 1–4.

Writing Team for the Diabetes Control and Complications Trial/Epidemiology of Diabetes Interventions and Complications Research Group (2003). Sustained effect of intensive treatment of type 1 diabetes mellitus on development and progression of diabetic nephropathy: the Epidemiology of Diabetes Interventions and Complications (EDIC) study. *JAMA* **290**, 2159–67.

Xu J et al. (2007). Albuminuria within the "normal" range and risk of cardiovascular disease and death in American Indians: the Strong Heart Study. *American Journal of Kidney Disease* **49**, 208–16.

Yu CC et al. (1997). Predialysis glycemic control is an independent predictor of clinical outcome in type II diabetics on continuous ambulatory peritoneal dialysis. *Peritoneal Dialysis International* **17**, 262–8.

Zimmet P, Alberti KG, Shaw J (2001). Global and societal implications of the diabetes epidemic. *Nature* **414**, 782–7.

8. Diabetes and Lower-Extremity Diseases

Andrew J. M. Boulton and Frank L. Bowling

■ Main Public Health Messages

- People with diabetes may have a lifetime risk of developing a foot ulcer as high as 15%–25%, and an estimated 1 million people per year lose a leg through amputation as a consequence of this condition.
- Disorders of the foot account for more hospital admissions than any other long-term medical condition.
- As many as 50% of amputations and foot ulcers could be prevented by early identification and patient education.
- Neuropathy is associated with up to 80% of all new foot ulcers.
- Poor glycemic control is related to neuropathy.
- Peripheral vascular disease, which is more common in people with diabetes, makes a sizable contribution to the pathogenesis of foot ulcers.
- Diabetic neuropathy can be identified by clinical examination and does not necessarily require an expensive assessment.
- Diabetic lower-extremity disease can be diagnosed by a simple clinical examination, but it is frequently missed.

■ Introduction

The lifetime risk that a person with diabetes will develop a foot ulcer may be as high as 15%–25%, and every year an estimated 1 million people lose a leg as a consequence of this condition, equating to one amputation every 30 seconds (Boulton et al. 2005a). Diabetic foot ulceration imposes a significant medical, social, and economic burden. Disorders of the foot account for more hospital admissions than any other long-term medical condition and also increase morbidity and mortality. The most costly and feared consequence of foot ulceration is amputation of a lower limb, which occurs 10 to 30 times more often in persons with diabetes (Trautner et al. 1996). Other long-term complications may include nephropathy, retinopathy, neuropathy, and hypertension. Those at risk of foot problems are also likely to have microvascular and macrovascular complications, and when all these factors are combined, the result is a significant social and economic burden.

In view of the factors described above it is fair to assume that prevention should be the focus of intervention, and there is evidence to suggest that up to 50% of amputations and foot ulcers could be prevented by early identification and patient education (Malone et al. 1989).

A clear understanding of the etiology and pathogenesis of ulceration is essential if the incidence is to be reduced and subsequent amputation prevented. What follows is an overview rather than a definitive account of the pathway to ulceration.

■ Background/Historical Perspective

Origins of Lower-Extremity Disease in Diabetes

Diabetic foot ulcers involve a complex interplay among contributory factors (see Box 8.1). Neuropathy is associated with up to 80% of all new foot ulcers, and a study of 10,000 diabetic patients yielded an annual ulcer incidence of 6% among those with neuropathy as opposed to an incidence of 1% in patients with intact sensation (Young et al. 1994).

The prevalence of neuropathy in the diabetic population increases with age and with the duration of the diabetes. Clinic- and population-based studies indicate distal symmetrical neuropathy affects approximately 30% of all diabetic people at any time and 50% after 15 years of diabetes (Young et al. 1993). Poor glycemic control is thought to be a key mechanism contributing to neuropathy. This relation has been highlighted in both type 1 and type 2 diabetes, with the specific mechanism of nerve-tissue breakdown involving a number of complex biochemical changes initiated by prolonged high glucose levels (Sheetz et al. 2002). Age and duration of diabetes are strongly associated with neuropathy, and other correlates include retinopathy, albuminuria, hypertension, obesity, smoking, and hyperlipidemia (Tesfaye et al. 1996).

Underlying these epidemiologic estimates is a diverse set of clinical presentations. Neuropathy is a general term usually used to describe reduced sensation to pain. The clinical features can vary immensely between painful and painless types,

---

BOX 8.1

Pathway to Ulceration
- Neuropathy
- Peripheral vascular disease
- Alteration in foot architecture
- History of ulceration

with the latter being the more common. Neuropathy is characterized by a progressive loss of nerve fibers affecting both the autonomic and somatic divisions of the nervous system.

Diffuse symmetrical distal sensory-motor neuropathy is the most common form of neuropathy, found in 90% of patients with foot ulceration (Young and Gregory 1997). Painful peripheral neuropathy is usually confined to the lower extremities distal to the knee and is symmetrical in distribution. The classical features are reports of burning pains, shooting pains, sharp pains, pins and needles (paresthesias), alteration of normal perception of pain or an unpleasant sensation (allodynia), and heightened sensitivity (hyperesthesia). There may also be negative symptoms such as numbness or absence of feeling. In most cases the symptoms are worse at night and during rest periods, but exercise can often alleviate the pain. This means that improvement through exercise can be a useful indicator of neuropathy (Reiber et al. 1999). Painful neuropathy will inevitably affect the patient's sleep and is highly associated with depression.

Painless, diffuse, peripheral sensory-motor neuropathy is far more common than its painful counterpart and makes a larger contribution to the formation of diabetic foot lesions. Early symptoms can be subtle, such as alterations in gait, but on closer inspection there are certain characteristics indicative of this type of neuropathy. A high medial arch (cavus foot type) can result in prominent metatarsal heads and increased plantar pressures. The lesser digits may retract in the later stages, causing pressure points over the apices and dorsal interphalangeal joints (Young and Boulton 1999). The body's natural response to increased pressure and force at a specific site is to form callus, but over time the continued exposure to such shear forces can result in the formation of ulcers.

An ulcer in an unsuspecting patient can often be discovered on a routine foot check. The fact that patients may not know they have an ulcer is the reason why screening of asymptomatic diabetic patients should be carried out on a regular basis. Testing for loss of sensation (discussed below) may be carried out, but on a practical level, if a patient can ambulate in the presence of a plantar ulcer and feel no pain, he/she must have neuropathy.

Autonomic neuropathy is also associated with diabetes and affects the cardiovascular, gastrointestinal, and urogenital systems. The symptoms of autonomic dysfunction include excessively dry skin, distended veins in the foot, edema, and demineralization of bone. With reference to the lower extremities, it is the cutaneous system that is affected by a loss of sweating and the abnormal diversion of blood supply away from the tissues.

Peripheral Vascular Disease

The association between diabetes and peripheral vascular disease has been established by large epidemiologic studies from around the world, and peripheral vascular disease makes a sizable contribution to the pathogenesis of foot ulceration

(Krishnan et al. 2004). A reduction in distal vascular supply becomes significant when a foot injury occurs, however minor it may be. Under normal health conditions an increase in blood flow to the affected area is required to deliver the necessary components for healing, but in the absence of sufficient circulatory function, demand exceeds supply, and tissue begins to break down.

The nature of the contribution made by peripheral vascular disease to the pathogenesis of ulcers is not fully understood, and a study examining the characteristics of blood flow in patients with and without ulceration failed to illustrate a causal relationship; that is, patients without ulceration had the same level of microvascular dysfunction as those with ulceration (Abbott et al. 2002). The clinical relevance is that screening for peripheral vascular disease will not necessarily identify those at risk of ulceration. Microvascular anomalies may make a contribution to the impaired healing process that essentially maintains an ulcer, although evidence for this idea is sparse.

■ Public Health Preventive or Intervention Strategies

Screening for Lower-Extremity Disease

The first steps in identifying those at risk for foot ulceration are examining the foot without shoes or socks and obtaining a detailed history from the patient (Singh et al. 2005). The examination will highlight changes in the structure of the foot and areas under abnormal pressure, which includes the presence of callus. A history of ulceration is a strong predictor of future ulcers (Singh, Armstrong, and Lipsky 2005). Diabetic neuropathy can be identified by clinical examination and does not necessarily require the use of expensive and lengthy assessments. Studies of nerve conduction may provide a diagnosis of peripheral neuropathy but offer little information regarding the presence or absence of protective sensation. A loss of sensation equates to a degree of neuropathy that significantly increases the propensity for ulceration.

The most commonly used instrument for detecting sensation loss is the monofilament (Semmes-Weinstein) as recommended in the National Institute for Health and Clinical Excellence (NICE) guidelines on diabetes type 2, foot care. When compared with other assessment tools, it is the least expensive, is quick and easy to administer, and has been validated (Smieja et al. 1999). The nylon filament provides a 10-g force to various test sites, and the patient's perception of this pressure is recorded. Insensitivity indicates the presence of neuropathy and clinically signifies large-fiber neuropathy. The anatomical sites to be tested are the hallux, first, third, and fifth metatarsal heads. The 10-g monofilament is able to identify 90% of patients with an insensate foot (Booth and Young 2000), and prospective trials have recorded a sensitivity between 66% and 91%, a specificity of 34% to 86%, a positive predictive value of 18% to 39%, and a negative predictive value of 94% to 95%. Some filaments are more accurate than others, but as a general rule a filament should be used on no more than 10 patients in any 24-hour period to maintain accuracy (Booth and Young 2000).

The tuning fork and tendon hammer are useful for highlighting decreased ankle reflexes and reduced sensation of vibration. The tuning fork should be placed over the apices of the hallux and allowed to omit a frequency of 128 Hz. A cold tuning fork can also be used to screen for loss of temperature sensation. The tuning fork has been found to be accurate for predicting foot ulceration, although the results are less predictive of ulceration than results from the monofilament (Smieja et al. 1999). Screening for peripheral vascular abnormalities begins with palpation of the posterior tibial and dorsalis pedis pulses. The ankle-brachial index (ABI), which is the ratio of systolic blood pressure in the ankle to that in the brachial artery, can provide additional information but may be less informative in patients with neuropathy than in those without this condition. An ABI of 0.90 or less suggests peripheral vascular disease, whereas an index higher than 1.1 may represent a falsely elevated pressure caused by medial arterial calcinosis. This test is easily performed, objective, and reproducible (Smieja et al. 1999).

The vibration perception threshold (VPT) is the most commonly used measurement for quantitative evaluation. The neurothesiometer, a handheld device that assesses the patient's VPT, is placed over the apices of the hallux and allowed to rest under its own weight without force from the clinician. The vibration stimulus is increased until the patient can feel external stimuli, and the process is then repeated. Carrying out the procedure twice permits a mean to be taken to reduce the coefficient of variation. Two studies have produced a sensitivity between 83% and 86%, a specificity of 57% to 63%, a positive predictive value of 20%–32%, and a negative predictive value of 95%–97% (Smieja et al. 1999). Although the accuracy is comparable to that of the monofilament, the device itself is expensive.

Screening for plantar pressures can identify areas of high pressure, which may have a propensity for ulceration. Devices can range from sophisticated computer systems to simple carbon mats such as Pressure Stat (Bailey Instruments, Manchester, United Kingdom). Ultimately, screening assessments are employed to ensure the early identification of risk factors, with the aim of preventing progression to severe disease complications, such as amputation. The NICE guidelines for type 2 diabetes foot care suggest how the screening process should fit into the overall provision of health care for patients with diabetes.

■ Management of Lower-Extremity Disease in Diabetes

Appropriate treatment depends on accurate diagnosis, and although neuropathy is a well-known complication of diabetes, other etiologies may need to be excluded before a treatment regime is commenced.

Although there are few controlled studies of the effectiveness of multifactorial CVD risk factor control on lower extremity disease outcomes, the observational evidence indicates that hyperglycemia, smoking, blood pressure levels, and prior CVD (Adler et al. 2002) are each associated with risk of PVD. Accordingly, smoking cessation and tight management of hypertension and hyperlipidemia are recommended

---

BOX 8.2

Modifiable
- Glycemic control
- Obesity
- Calluses/fissures
- Plantar pressure
- Smoking

---

practices to prevent lower extremity disease. Key risk factors for PVD (Adler et al. 2002) appear in Box 8.2.

Abnormal distribution of pressure can sometimes be corrected by orthotics from a podiatrist. Modification of the factors identified above not only forms part of a treatment program but can also have a strong role in prevention management.

Treatment of painful diabetic neuropathy can be addressed by using tricyclic compounds from the group of antidepressant medications. There is a solid evidence base for choosing these drugs as a first-line treatment, but they are associated with side effects such as drowsiness, dry mouth, and dizziness (Boulton et al., 2005b). Similarly, the anticonvulsants, such as carbamazepine, phenytoin, pregabalin, and gabapentin, have proven effectiveness in relieving neuropathic pain, but again side effects can be an unwanted complication. Pregabalin and gabapentin appear to be more tolerable than the others (Boulton et al. 2005b).

Infection

An infected foot ulcer precedes approximately 60% of lower-limb amputations in the diabetic population (Pecoraro, Reiber, and Burgess 1990). Substantial evidence suggests that people with diabetes are more susceptible to infection because of an altered immune response and reduced arterial inflow. Accordingly, rapid treatment of infection is key to the management of lower-extremity disease in diabetes. The first step in treating an infected foot ulcer is to recognize infection, which must be defined clinically and is typically manifested by signs or symptoms of inflammation. The clinical presentation will vary according to the extent and depth of the invading bacterial organisms. Unresolved infection leads to tissue loss and infection of underlying bone (osteomyelitis). The duration of antibiotic treatment is currently unknown; soft-tissue infections may require 2–3 weeks of treatment, whereas osseous infections may take 3–6 months of treatment to resolve.

The International Working Group on the Diabetic Foot proposes that first-line treatment should be with a broad-spectrum antibiotic while the results of the culture are awaited, and when specific pathogens have been identified, targeted therapy can be administered (Lipsky 2004). However if a wound is clearly responding well to an empirical drug, there may be little reason to narrow the spectrum. Simple, superficial infections can respond to topical or oral preparations with activity against staphylococci and streptococci. Clinically noninfected neuropathic ulcers do just as well without antibiotics (Chantelau et al. 1996). Cephalosporins, penicillins, and β-lactamase inhibitors, fluoroquinolones, and clindamycin have all been shown to be effective treatments for diabetic foot infections. The severity of infection will determine treatment, and those with systemic involvement require initial treatment with broad-spectrum antibiotics to ensure microbiological impact. Severe infections will often need to be treated with intravenous preparations that can be provided only on an inpatient basis, for example, linezolid and vancomycin treatments for severe MRSA (methicillin-resistant *Staphylococcus aureus*) infections.

The wound itself needs modification to facilitate the effectiveness of other treatments and to promote healing. Debridement in its many guises is intended to remove sloughy, necrotic, nonviable tissue for this purpose. The process of debridement removes nonviable tissue and the products remaining from an abnormal, sustained inflammatory response.

The method of debridement selected will depend on the individual characteristics of the wound. Surgical and autolytic regimes are underpinned by encouraging the body's own healing response, and mechanical techniques such as the Versajet® (Smith & Nephew Healthcare, Hull, United Kingdom) work on a similar principle. Enzymatic debridement products attempt to impersonate natural biology, but their efficacy is yet to be established.

A lower-limb diabetic wound will require protection following debridement, but the evidence base for the use of complex dressings is limited. Cullum and colleagues, in a comprehensive review of trials of dressings for diabetic foot ulcers, found that the samples of the studies they looked at were small, with insufficient evidence of effect (Cullum et al. 2000). Clinicians should therefore question the validity of endpoint studies in wound healing.

The final step in treatment is offloading the ulcer by way of a cast. A number of devices exist, ranging from the removable to a nonremovable cast walker. The gold standard is a total-contact cast fabricated from fiberglass that is minimally padded and molded to the contour of the foot and leg. The cast should redistribute pressure from the ulcer site over the entire plantar surface of the foot. Other devices such as the Aircast Pneumatic Walker (Aircast Inc, Summit, NJ, USA) and the DH Walker (Ossur, Reykjavik, Iceland) can also be used effectively to redistribute pressure (Armstrong et al. 2003). Patient compliance is the key to the effectiveness of the removable cast.

■ Education

There is little doubt that diabetic foot ulcers can be prevented, but the specifics of how to do this remain elusive (see Box 8.3 for variables that cannot be modified). Education of both patients and staff is key, but increased knowledge alone is not

BOX 8.3

Nonmodifiable
- Neuropathy
- Previous ulceration
- Previous amputation
- Age, race, and sex

sufficient to decrease the incidence or severity of foot ulcers. Education of patients is also necessary to increase compliance with specific treatments. The impact of noncompliance can never be underestimated, especially in offloading. A study by Armstrong and colleagues found that time to healing of foot ulcers was significantly faster in patients whose casts were nonremovable rather than removable (Armstrong et al. 2005). Furthermore, there is evidence to suggest that patients with removable casts are noncompliant with advice regarding how long to wear the cast, which ultimately decreases the likelihood that their ulcer will heal (Armstrong et al. 2003).

There is a shortage of studies examining the clinical significance in real terms of education, but there is evidence to suggest that regular sessions over a period of months can reduce the incidence of serious lesions (Litzelman et al. 1993). The format taken depends on the desired endpoint but can include face-to-face teaching sessions specific to foot care, telephone reminders, and reminders using postcards. Education can even be provided in an acute setting, as evidenced by one large-scale randomized study that used graphic visual images during a single educational session lasting 1 hour. Those assigned to the education group had only one-third the rate of subsequent ulcers or amputation as those assigned to the control group (Malone et al. 1989). Despite this encouraging finding, a recent Cochrane review (Valk, Kriegsman, and Assendelft 2005) concluded that the quality of data available for examining the direct impact of education on the incidence of ulcer and amputation is poor, with massive variability. This neither negates nor validates educational programs but does highlight the need for large-scale studies of sound design.

The NICE guidelines for type 2 diabetes, foot care, provide an algorithm for the ideal provision of health care for preventing and/or treating complications of the diabetic foot, and it is clear that a wide variety of professionals are required. Specialist nurses, primary care physicians, podiatrists, dieticians, and others could all play a valuable part in identifying and managing foot complications at an early stage. Prompt identification promotes rapid treatment and should prevent an escalation in symptoms.

A study in the Netherlands demonstrated a 40% reduction in risk of amputation coinciding with a significant increase in podiatry services and provision of a multidisciplinary foot care team (van Houtum et al. 2004). Strong links between the different disciplines involved with a patient will improve communication not only between health professionals but also with the patient. Staff in the community (physicians, nurses, others) require a heightened awareness of risk factors and warning signs that contribute to the development of ulcers, and thus the patient is not the only target of training. Primary care staff are often the first point of contact for patients with diabetes-related complaints, and as such they are likely to be the first to see a potential ulcer. They may hold the key to reducing the incidence of diabetic foot ulcers in the community through early identification and through ongoing education of patients and staff.

■ Implications for Health Policy

This chapter has outlined several key components of the public health approach to prevent lower extremity disease outcomes in the community. These include efficient screening, detection and risk stratification, and referral of high-risk feet into effective clinical management are essential to prevent adverse outcomes of diabetes-related neuropathy and peripheral arterial disease. Education of both patients and providers, along with organized systems to ensure that all of these aspects of care are well integrated for the diabetic population, is essential. Despite the consensus about the importance of these elements, there remains a lack of definitive intervention studies to guide specific strategies. For example, there is a continued need to evaluate different screening tools, strategies, and algorithms, the best important mechanisms and elements of patient and provider education, and the most cost effective disease-management models to optimize prevention. There is also a continued need to examine the degree to which the vulnerable population are receiving adequate access and continuity of care to prevent lower-extremity disease and the related sequelae.

■ References

Abbott CA et al. (2002). The North West Diabetes Footcare Study: incidence of, and risk factors for, new diabetic foot ulcers in a community-based cohort. *Diabetic Medicine* **20**, 377–84.

Adler AI et al. (2002). UKPDS 59: hyperglycemia and other potentially modifiable risk factors for peripheral vascular disease in type 2 diabetes. *Diabetes Care* **25**, 894–9.

Armstrong DG et al. (2003). Activity patterns of patients with diabetic foot ulceration. *Diabetes Care* **26**, 1–4.

Armstrong DG et al. (2005). Evaluation of removable and irremovable cast walkers in the healing of diabetic foot wounds: a randomized controlled trial. *Diabetes Care* **28**, 551–4.

Booth J, Young MJ (2000). Differences in the performance of commercially available 10-g monofilaments. *Diabetes Care* **23**, 984–8.

Boulton AJ et al. (2005a). The global burden of diabetic foot disease. *Lancet.* **366**, 1719–24.

Boulton AJ et al. (2005b). Diabetic neuropathies: a statement by the American Diabetes Association. *Diabetes Care* **28**, 956–62.

Boulton AJM (2006). The pathway to ulceration: aetiopathogenesis. In: Boulton AJM, Cavanagh PR, Rayman G, eds. *The Foot and Diabetes*, 4th ed., pp 51–67. Chichester: John Wiley & Sons.

Chantelau E et al. (1996). Antibiotic treatment for uncomplicated neuropathic forefoot ulcers in diabetes. *Diabetic Medicine* **13**, 156–9.

Cullum C et al. (2000). Use of dressings: is there an evidence base? In: Boulton AJM, Connor H, Cavanagh PR, eds. *The Foot in Diabetes*, 3rd ed., pp 153–63, Chichester: John Wiley & Sons.

Krishnan ST et al. (2004). Comparative roles of microvascular and nerve function in foot ulceration in type 2 diabetes. *Diabetes Care* **27**, 1343–8.

Lipsky BA (2004). A report from the international consensus on diagnosing and treating the infected diabetic foot. *Diabetes/Metabolism Research and Reviews* **20** (Suppl. 1), S68–77.

Litzelman DK et al. (1993). Reduction of lower extremity clinical abnormalities in patients with non-insulin- dependent diabetes mellitus. A randomized, controlled trial. *Annals of Internal Medicine* **119**, 36–41.

Malone JM et al. (1989). Prevention of amputation by diabetic education. *American Journal of Surgery* **158**, 520–3.

Pecoraro RE, Reiber GE, Burgess EM (1990). Pathways to diabetic limb amputation. Basis for prevention. *Diabetes Care* **3**, 513–21.

Reiber GE et al. (1999). Causal pathways for incident lower-extremity ulcers in patients with diabetes from two settings. *Diabetes Care* **22**, 157–62.

Sheetz MJ, King GL. (2002). Molecular understanding of hyperglycemias adverse effects on diabetes complications. *JAMA* **288**, 2579–88.

Singh N, Armstrong DG, Lipsky BA (2005). Preventing foot ulcers in patients with diabetes. *JAMA.* 293,217–28.

Smieja M et al. (1999). Clinical examination for the detection of protective sensation in the feet of diabetic patients. *Journal of General Internal Medicine* **14**, 418–24.

Tesfaye S (2006). Diabetic neuropathy. In: Boulton AJM, Cavannagh PR, Rayman G, eds. *The Foot in Diabetes*, 4th ed., pp 30–40. Chichester: John Wiley & Sons.

Tesfaye S et al. (1996). Prevalence of diabetic peripheral neuropathy and its relation to glycaemic control and potential risk factors: the EURODIAB IDDM Complications Study. *Diabetalogia* **39**, 1377–84.

Trautner C et al. (1996). Incidence of lower limb amputations and diabetes. *Diabetes Care* **19**, 1006–9.

Valk GD, Kriegsman DM, Assendelft WJ (2005). Patient education for preventing diabetic foot ulceration. *Cochrane Database of Systematic Reviews* (1), CD001488.

van Houtum WH et al. (2004). Reduction in diabetes-related lower-extremity amputations in The Netherlands: 1991–2000. *Diabetes Care* **27**, 1042–6.

Young M, Boulton AJM (1999). Peripheral vascular disease. In: Dyck PJ et al., eds. *Diabetic Neuropathy*, pp 105–22. Philadelphia: WB Saunders.

Young MJ et al. (1993). A multicentre study of the prevalence of diabetic peripheral neuropathy in the United Kingdom hospital clinic population. *Diabetalogia* **36**, 150–4.

Young MJ et al. (1994). The prediction of diabetic neuropathic foot ulceration using vibration perception thresholds. A prospective study. *Diabetes Care* **76**, 557–60.

Young MJ, Gregory CJ (1997). Diabetic neuropathy: symptoms, signs and assessment. In: Boulton AJM, ed. *Diabetic Neuropathy*, pp 41–61. Lancashire: Marius Press.

9. DIABETES AND CARDIOVASCULAR DISEASE

Alain G. Bertoni and David C. Goff Jr.

■ Main Public Health Messages

- Most persons with diabetes die of cardiovascular disease (CVD), which includes ischemic heart disease, stroke, and heart failure. Although CVD is the leading cause of morbidity and mortality in the United States and other Western societies, even among people without diabetes, persons with diabetes have rates of CVD two to four times those of people without diabetes.
- The level of diabetes control (as measured by hemoglobin A1C), blood pressure, and blood lipids predict risk of CVD in persons with diabetes. Risk factors that contribute to having type 2 diabetes (specifically, obesity and physical inactivity) also increase risk of CVD.
- The cause of heart failure in diabetes is multifactorial, but hyperglycemia may be an important contributing factor in addition to ischemic heart disease and hypertension.
- Persons with diabetes should be considered to be at high risk for future CVD events estimated at 1.5%–2% per year on average by several equations for predicting risk.
- Subclinical disease (e.g., coronary artery calcium, impaired ventricular function) is more common in adults with diabetes. Subclinical disease increases risk of CVD, but at present these measures do not help to target preventive therapies.
- The major outcomes trial of type 2 diabetes (United Kingdom Prospective Diabetes Study) has supported control of A1C to prevent microvascular disease. Several trials have failed to provide definitive evidence that A1C levels <7.0% prevent CVD. Recently, long-term follow-up of the Diabetes Control and Complications Trial does indicate benefit of glucose control for type 1 diabetes.
- Clinical trials provide clear support for control of blood pressure and lipids, particularly for preventing ischemic heart disease. Other accepted preventive

methods include taking aspirin and quitting smoking. Prevention of heart failure is suggested to be related to good blood pressure control and use of angiotensin-converting enzyme inhibitors; the role of glucose control is less clear, and taking thiazolinediones may increase risk.

■ Introduction

The close relationship between diabetes mellitus and atherosclerosis-related cardio-vascular disease (CVD), especially for those with type 2 diabetes mellitus, has long been recognized. An early Framingham Heart Study (a seminal cohort study prospectively evaluating risk factors for CVD) report from 1979 recognized diabetes as one of the major risk factors for CVD, along with smoking, high cholesterol, elevated blood pressure, and family history, and it noted the increased risk of coronary heart disease, heart failure, and peripheral vascular disease compared with adults without diabetes (Kannel and McGee 1979). The biochemical hallmarks of diabetes (hyperglycemia, increased free fatty acids, and insulin resistance) are postulated to have adverse metabolic effects on the vascular endothelium. The impaired endothelium promotes vasoconstriction, inflammation, and thrombosis, which in turn promote the formation of atheromatous plaques (Beckman, Creager, and Libby 2002). There is also a higher prevalence of traditional risk factors for CVD (i.e., hypertension, dyslipidemia, and obesity) in persons with diabetes (compared with those without diabetes), but these risk factors are estimated to account for less than half the excess mortality from coronary heart disease associated with diabetes (American Diabetes Association 1998).

A direct effect of diabetes on atherosclerosis is postulated to account for a significant proportion of the excess CVD observed. Support for this hypothesis is suggested by data demonstrating that the hemoglobin A1C level is related to risk of coronary heart disease in both type 1 and type 2 diabetes (Selvin et al. 2004). However, there has been a vigorous debate regarding the utility of tight glucose control in preventing both the CVD and non-CVD complications of diabetes. The landmark Diabetes Control and Complications Trial (DCCT), published in 1993, first established that lowering blood glucose was associated with decreased micro-vascular complications in patients with type 1 diabetes (DCCT Research Group 1993). Intensive therapy nonsignificantly reduced the risk of major cardiovascular and peripheral vascular events by 41% (to 5 events per 1000 patient-years vs. 8 per 1000; 95% confidence interval [CI] –10% to 68%). The United Kingdom Prospective Diabetes Study (UKPDS), in which newly diagnosed adults with type 2 diabetes were assigned to either intensive or conventional glucose-lowering therapy, including diet, sulfonylureas and/or metformin, or insulin, also found evidence in favor of tight glucose control for microvascular outcomes and suggested benefit for CVD (UKPDS Group 1998a). These trials, and new therapeutic options including human recombinant insulins and new oral agents, ushered in the current century, where the dominant research and clinical questions have been (1) how tightly to control hyperglycemia and other risk factors to prevent CVD, and (2) how best to investigate the genetic and environmental factors contributing to CVD in persons with diabetes.

Large-vessel atherosclerosis is also related to peripheral vascular disease and lower-extremity complications of diabetes, including poor wound healing, ulceration, and amputation. However, these topics are addressed elsewhere in this book.

■ Background/Historical Perspective

In the 1901 edition of *Osler's Principles and Practice of Medicine*, a distinction was drawn between two types of patients with diabetes: the frequently young, emaciated patient with polyphagia, polydypsia, and glycosuria who frequently succumbed to coma and the generally older, "stout" patient who had a better prognosis but who developed gangrene, pneumonia, neurologic problems, and arteriosclerosis (Osler 1901). What is now labeled type 1 diabetes was a death sentence for those, mostly children, who developed it before the discovery, purification, and commercialization of insulin beginning in 1922 (Bliss 2005). Less than 30 years later, there was increasing evidence that diabetes was associated with more severe atherosclerosis (Barach 1949). In one Pennsylvania hospital from 1930 to 1938, the average age at death of hospitalized patients with diabetes was 61 years; 30% of these patients died of cardiovascular causes. From 1939 to 1950, the average age at death increased to 65 years, but 50.3% of deaths were now related to CVD (Blumberg and Zisserman 1951). Data from the 1970s to the 1990s demonstrated that a majority of deaths among persons with diabetes in the United States were attributable to CVD and that people with diabetes had an increased rate of coronary heart disease and stroke mortality compared with persons without diabetes (Gu, Cowie, and Harris 1998).

■ Epidemiology

Diabetes as a Risk Factor for CVD

Data suggest that the impact of diabetes on the risk of coronary death is significantly greater for women than men. For example, a recent meta-analysis of 37 prospective cohort studies found that the summary relative risk (RR) for fatal coronary heart disease in patients with diabetes (versus no diabetes) was significantly greater among women (RR 3.5, 95% confidence interval [CI] 2.70–4.53) than among men (RR 2.1, 95% CI 1.8–2.3) (Huxley, Barzi, and Woodward 2006).

In the twentieth century CVD rates declined among persons with and without diabetes, according to data from the Framingham studies (see Fig. 9.1) (Fox et al.

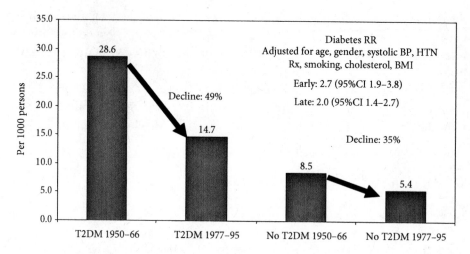

FIGURE 9.1. CVD rates in Framingham studies. BMI, body mass index; BP, blood pressure; HTN, hypertension; Rx, treatment.

2004). In addition the adjusted RR for CVD among persons with diabetes declined from 2.7 (95% CI 1.9–3.8) in the 1950–1966 cohort to 2.0 (95% CI 1.4–1.7) in the 1977–1995 cohort. Because of an increasing prevalence of diabetes, however, these data suggest that the population attributable risk associated with diabetes (for CVD) may have increased despite a decreasing RR.

Diabetes is independently associated with cerebrovascular disease. The RR for stroke among adults with diabetes has been reported to range from 1.5 to 3.0; the excess is largely attributable to an increased risk of ischemic stroke rather than a greater frequency of hemorrhagic strokes (Idris, Thomson, and Sharma 2006). In Saskatchewan, Canada, the age-standardized incidence rate for stroke was 642 per 100,000 person-years in persons with type 1 or type 2 diabetes, compared with 313 per 100,000 person-years in the general population (RR 2.1, 95% CI 1.8–2.3). The excess risk was highest in younger persons (ages 30–44) with diabetes (RR 5.6) and declined with age but remained elevated even in persons aged 75 and older (RR 1.8) (Jeerakathil et al. 2007). Data from the Nurses' Health Study (in women) suggest the increased RR at younger ages may reflect stroke in persons with type 1 diabetes. In multivariate analyses of data from that study, the incidence of total stroke was almost five times as high in women with type 1 diabetes (RR 4.7, 95% CI 3.3– 6.6) and almost twice as high in women with type 2 diabetes (RR 1.8, 95% CI 1.7–2.0) as in nondiabetic women. The multivariable-adjusted RR of ischemic stroke was 6.3 (95% CI 4.0–9.8) in type 1 diabetes and 2.3 (95% CI 2.0–2.6) in type 2 diabetes. Type 1 diabetes was also signifi-cantly associated with the risk of hemorrhagic stroke (3.8, 95% CI 1.2–11.8), but type 2 diabetes was not (RR 1.0, 95% CI 0.7–1.4) (Janghorbani et al. 2007).

Diabetes is an independent risk factor for the development of heart failure (Kannel 2000). The increasing prevalence of diabetes, as well as demographic trends resulting in a large number of elderly persons in the United States (and other

TABLE 9.1   *CVD Incidence Estimates from Samples of Adults with Diabetes*

Study	Population	CVD	MI	CHD	CVA	HF
Kaiser Permanente 1995–98 (Nichols et al. 2004; Karter et al. 2002)	White		13.7		9.8	9.2
	Black		9.1		11.8	10.7
	Asian		9.3		7.4	5.9
	Hispanic		10.1		8	6.3
Framingham 1977–95 (Fox et al. 2004)	Adults aged 45–64	14.7				
ARIC 1987–95 (Saito et al. 2000)	Adults aged 45–64	16.8				
CHS 1989–95 (Kronmal et al. 2006)	Adults aged 65+					
	Without subclinical CVD			19.4	11.3	15.1
	With subclinical CVD			42.6	21.9	23.1

ARIC, Atherosclerosis Risk in Communities; CHS, Cardiovascular Health study; CVD, cardiovascular disease; MI, myocardial infarction; CHD, coronary heart disease; CVA, cerebrovascular accident; HF, heart failure. Rates are per 1000 person-years.

Western societies), suggests that diabetes may emerge as one of the principal causes of heart failure in Western countries.

Descriptive Epidemiology

Estimates of rates of CVD in the population with diabetes come from several sources (see Table 9.1), each with its own set of limitations. Administrative datasets, including Medicare claims or hospital discharge abstracts, rely on accurate ICD-9 (International Classification of Diseases, Ninth Revision) coding and may lead to incorrect statistics either because of misclassification of CVD outcomes or an inaccurate estimation of the denominator (the population with diabetes). Cohort studies, including those using the records of health maintenance organizations (HMOs), have more accurate estimates of the population at risk and outcomes. However, HMO members or other persons within a cohort may not be representative of the general population with diabetes. People who agree to be in a cohort study, and enrollees in an HMO (regardless of membership in a cohort) are likely to be healthier and/or of a higher socioeconomic status than the general population. This may lead to an underestimation of rates of incident complications. However, estimates of the RR associated with diabetes would be less subject to bias, as the comparison group is drawn from the same population.

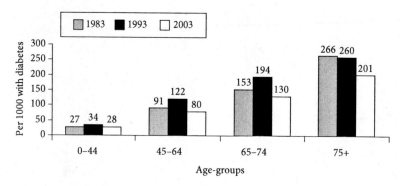

FIGURE 9.2 Rate of CVD hospitalizations

The Centers for Disease Control and Prevention (CDC) maintains diabetes statistics at a publicly accessible Web site (www.cdc.gov/diabetes/statistics/natl_ surveillance_data.htm). Based on data from the National Health Interview Survey (NHIS), which relies on self-reports that are not verified, between 1997 and 2003 an estimated one-fifth of adults with diabetes also had prevalent coronary heart disease, and 8%—9% had had a stroke. In 2003, per the NHIS, the age-adjusted prevalence for persons with diabetes of any CVD condition was 38.7% for white men, 30.7% for white women, 31.3% for black men, 28.9% for black women, 29.9% for Hispanic men, and 23.7% for Hispanic women.

According to combined data from the National Hospital Discharge Survey and NHIS, the annual hospitalization rate for major CVD (ICD-9 codes 410–414, 429.2) with diabetes as a secondary diagnosis in 2003 was 104/1000 population with diabetes. Rates of hospitalization for CVD by age and year are presented in Figure 9.2; two trends are demonstrated. First, in each year graphed (1983, 1993, and 2003) the burden of CVD increased with age. Second, the rate of hospitalization has declined in recent years, especially in the older age groups. These estimates, however, may not fully reflect the impact of CVD in diabetes because of the methodology employed. Putting aside the questions on methodology, the declining rate of hospitalization may reflect improved treatment for CVD, resulting in fewer hospitalizations, or the data may reflect a declining incidence of CVD in this population, as suggested by the Framingham data presented above. In Ontario, Canada, a decline in hospitalization rates for acute myocardial infarction and cerebrovascular accidents (ischemic stroke) was observed using data from the province's health plan between 1992 and 1999. In this population, the decline was mostly seen among those aged <65 years. However, over the same period, the number of diabetes cases increased by 65%. Thus, while CVD rates fell, the absolute number of events occurring in this population rose substantially (acute myocardial infarction: +44.6%; stroke: +26.1%; deaths from acute myocardial infarction: +17.2%, and stroke deaths: +13.2%) (Booth et al. 2006).

Heart failure has become a frequent manifestation of CVD among persons with type 2 diabetes (Bell 2003). In one HMO in Oregon, the overall rate of heart failure among adult patients with diabetes was 30.9/1000 person-years, compared with 12.4/1000 among adults without diabetes. The incidence of heart failure was significantly higher in the population with diabetes (versus those without diabetes) in age categories <85 years (Nichols et al. 2004).

The toll of CVD in persons with diabetes is ultimately reflected in excess mortality. Many studies demonstrate that persons with diabetes suffer excess mortality, in particular, CVD mortality (Gu et al. 1998; Huxley et al. 2006). In the Cardiovascular Health Study 50% of all deaths among those aged 65 and older with pharmacologically treated diabetes were attributed to CVD; the RRs of coronary heart disease mortality and CVD mortality ranged from 2.0 to 2.5 (Kronmal et al. 2006).

Risk Factors for CVD in Diabetes

Among persons with diabetes, the standard risk factors common in the general population (hypertension, dyslipidemia, obesity, and smoking) are also associated with incident coronary heart disease and stroke, but they do not fully explain the excess risk observed in people with diabetes (American Diabetes Association 1998). Nontraditional "novel" risk factors, including measures of thrombosis and inflammation, were also assessed in the Atherosclerosis Risk in Communities (ARIC) study. Levels of albumin, fibrinogen, and von Willebrand factor, factor VIII activity, and leukocyte count were associated with incident coronary heart disease among persons with diabetes, independent of the traditional risk factors (Table 9.2) (Saito et al. 2000).

The "diabetes-specific" risk factor of hyperglycemia is itself a risk factor for CVD. A recent meta-analysis of prospective epidemiologic studies demonstrated that the risk of a CVD event was 18% greater for each increase in A1C of 1 percentage point (e.g., from 7% to 8%) (Selvin et al. 2004). Epidemiologic evidence also suggests that

TABLE 9.2 *Risk Factors for CVD in Diabetes*

Standard	Diabetes-Specific	Novel	Subclinical disease
Cholesterol	A1C	Inflammation	Carotid IMT
Smoking	Diabetic dyslipidemia	Thrombotic factors	Coronary artery calcium
Hypertension			Abnormal ankle-brachial index
Coronary artery disease			Left ventricular hypertrophy
Stroke			Major ECG abnormalities

IMT, intima-medial thickness; ECG, electrocardiography.

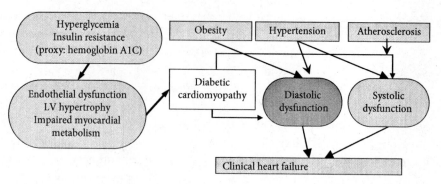

FIGURE 9.3 Mechanisms of heart failure in diabetes mellitus

increased blood pressure, worse glycemic control (higher A1C), increased obesity, and coronary artery disease may be independent risk factors for heart failure among adults with type 2 diabetes (Nichols et al. 2004). Figure 9.3 details the multifactorial nature of heart failure in persons with diabetes. The risk associated with higher A1C is thought to reflect the deleterious effects of chronic hyperglycemia on the heart muscle, the collective effects of which have been labeled "diabetic cardiomyopathy" (Bell 2003).

■ Public Health Preventive or Intervention Strategies

Overview

Strategies for preventing CVD in patients with diabetes include management of glucose, blood pressure, and lipids; smoking cessation; and platelet inhibition (with aspirin). Lifestyle modification, including weight loss and exercise, also may decrease CVD risk, presumably via favorable effects on A1C, blood pressure, and lipids, but direct benefits of exercise on reducing CVD are likely as well. Despite American Diabetes Association (ADA) guidelines suggesting specific targets for A1C (<7.0%), blood pressure (<130/80 mm Hg), low-density lipoprotein cholesterol (LDL-C) (<100 mg/dL or <70 mg/dL if CVD present), and high-density lipoprotein cholesterol (HDL-C) (>40 mg/dL in men, >50 mg/dL in women), much of the evidence supporting these targets comes from epidemiologic analyses or meta-analyses of trials (American Diabetes Association 2007). Large randomized clinical trials are ongoing in North America and elsewhere aimed at determining the optimal strategies to prevent CVD in this population; two such trials (Look AHEAD and ACCORD) are discussed below.

Control of Hyperglycemia

The epidemiologic evidence demonstrating a graded relation between A1C and CVD makes it tempting to conclude that lowering A1C via pharmacologic or lifestyle interventions would decrease the incidence of CVD. Surprisingly, not all clinical trials have yielded results to support the lowering of A1C. In the UPKDS, the group assigned to intensive glycemic control achieved a median A1C of 7.0% over a 10-year period and experienced a 25% reduction in RR in microvascular outcomes and a 12% reduction in RR in all diabetes-related endpoints compared with a policy that achieved a median A1C of 7.9% (United Kingdom Prospective Diabetes Study 1998a). There was a reduced risk of myocardial infarction of borderline statistical significance, with an observed reduction in RR of 16% (95% CI 0%–29%; $p = 0.052$). The Action in Diabetes and Vascular Disease: Preterax and Diamicron MR Controlled Evaluation (ADVANCE) trial assessed the effect of tight glucose control in 11,140 adults with type 2 diabetes. The results demonstrated that after a median of 5 years of follow-up, the mean A1C level was lower in the intensive-control group (6.5%) than in the standard-control group (7.3%). Intensive control did not reduce major CVD events (hazard ratio with intensive control, 0.94; 95% CI 0.84–1.06; $p = 0.32$) (ADVANCE Study Group 2008).

The long-term follow-up of DCCT participants suggests that lowering A1C reduces CVD risk in persons with type 1 diabetes. During the mean 17 years of follow-up, the event rate in the intensive treatment group was 0.38/100 persons-years, versus 0.80/100 person-years in the standard treatment group (difference, $p < 0.01$; number needed to treat 236). The number needed to treat is the number of individuals required to be treated for the outcome under study to be prevented. There was a reduction in risk of first CVD event of 42% (95% CI 9%–63%, $p = 0.02$) and the risk of nonfatal myocardial infarction, stroke, or death from cardiovascular disease of 57% (95% CI 12%–79%, $p = 0.02$) (DCCT/EDIC Study Research Group 2005). The decrease in A1C values during the DCCT was significantly associated with almost all of the positive effects of intensive treatment on the risk of CVD. Microalbuminuria and albuminuria were associated with a significant increase in the risk of CVD, but differences between treatment groups remained significant ($p < 0.05$) after adjusting for these factors.

There are also studies suggesting that intensive glycemic control may worsen CVD outcomes, and achieving tight glycemic control is not without risk from a safety perspective. For example, the 2-year feasibility phase of the VACSDM (Veterans Affairs Cooperative Study on Glycemic Control and Complications in Type II Diabetes) trial found the intensively treated group had a nonsignificant increase in the risk of CVD events (Goff et al. 2007). The ACCORD (Action to Control Cardiovascular Risk in Diabetes) study terminated the tight glycemic control arm (median A1C of 6.4% in that group versus 7.5% in the standard glycemic control group) due to an increase in all-cause mortality of 3/1000 person-years over 4 years (ACCORD Study Group 2008). In ACCORD, intensive therapy was not associated with a decreased risk of the primary outcome (hazard ratio 0.90; 95% CI 0.78–1.04; $p = 0.16$). Potential risks of tight control include serious hypoglycemia and weight gain, and in randomized trials of people with type 2 diabetes, these risks were greatest in insulin-treated individuals. Results from trials suggest that 2%–3% of patients with type 2 diabetes who achieve mean A1C and fasting plasma glucose concentrations approaching normal with intensive insulin therapy will have one or more serious hypoglycemic episodes annually (Goff et al. 2007). In these studies, serious hypoglycemia was usually defined as requiring the assistance of another person (i.e., the patient was unable to self-treat the low blood sugar). In addition to the risks of glucose lowering per se, adverse effects due to the agents used to lower glucose may occur. These effects include the possibility that sulfonylureas will increase the risk of arrhythmias, especially in an ischemic myocardium, that metformin will increase the risk of lactic acidosis and gastrointestinal symptoms, and that the available thiazolinediones will increase the risk of anemia, edema, and possibly congestive heart failure (Smits and Thien 1995; DeFronzo 1999).

Control of Hypertension

High blood pressure is a prevalent comorbidity in patients with type 2 diabetes. Based on the National Health and Nutrition Examination Survey (NHANES) 1999–2000, 43% of women and 31% of men with diabetes in the United States at that time had hypertension (blood pressure 140/90 mm Hg) (Imperatore et al. 2004). In contrast, the prevalence of hypertension in the general U.S. population based on the 1999–2000 NHANES was 28.7% in men and 28.3% in women (Ong et al. 2007). Based on the Behavioral Risk Factor Surveillance System survey, among adults with diabetes (most of which was probably type 2; the survey is based on self-reports that are not corroborated by the investigators), 56% had hypertension, compared with 22% among those without diabetes (Egede and Zheng 2002). Lowering blood pressure pharmacologically has been demonstrated to reduce CVD events in many randomized trials in persons with and without diabetes. The first major trial to do so was UKPDS, which achieved a mean blood pressure of 144/82 mm Hg versus 154/87 in the less intensively treated participants. This difference was associated with a 32% reduction in deaths related to diabetes (13.7/1000 person-years versus 20.3/1000 person-years; number needed to treat 152) and 44% reduction in strokes (6.5/1000 person-years versus 11.6/1000 person-years; number needed to treat 196) (United Kingdom Prospective Diabetes Study 1998b). A meta-analysis by the Blood Pressure Lowering Treatment Trialists' Collaboration reported that in adults with diabetes, having a lower blood pressure goal (versus a higher blood pressure goal—mean differences in goals [in mm Hg] were 6.0 for systolic pressure and 4.6 for diastolic) was associated with a 25% reduction in RR for major CVD events. This analysis also demonstrated significant benefit of angiotensin-converting (ACE) inhibitors versus placebo for both major CVD events and CVD deaths (Blood Pressure Lowering Treatment Trialists' Collaboration 2005). The data also suggested that major CVD events were reduced to a comparable extent in individuals with (and without) diabetes by regimens based on ACE inhibitors, calcium antagonists, angiotensin receptor blockers (ARBs), and diuretics/beta-blockers.

The Appropriate Blood Pressure Control in Diabetes (ABCD) Trial, a prospective, randomized, blinded trial in hypertensive patients with diabetes, compared the effects of moderate control of blood pressure (target diastolic blood pressure 80–89 mm Hg) with those of intensive control (target 75 mm Hg or less) on the incidence of CVD (Estacio et al. 1998). Over 5 years of follow-up the mean blood pressure achieved in the intensive group was 132/78 mm Hg, versus 138/86 mm Hg in the moderate-control group. There were no differences in any microvascular endpoints for the two blood pressure goals. The intensive therapy group had a lower mortality rate (5.5% vs. 10.7%, $p = 0.037$), but there were no significant differences in myocardial infarction, cerebrovascular events, or heart failure to account for the mortality difference. ACCORD tested a goal BP of <120 mm Hg systolic compared to <140 mm Hg in 4733 participants; at 1 year the mean systolic BP was 119 compared to 133.5 in the comparison arm. After 4.7 years of follow-up intensive BP lowering was not associated with a reduced incidence of fatal and nonfatal CVD events (rate 1.87% vs. 2.09%, $p = 0.20$). There was a reduced rate of stroke (0.32% vs. 0.53%, $p = 0.01$); however, serious adverse events attributed to antihypertensive treatment were significantly more frequent in the intensive arm (ACCORD Study Group 2010). The main implication of these trials, especially when compared with the UKPDS results, suggests there may be only limited additional benefits of lowering blood pressure to near normal levels.

The Seventh Report of the Joint National Committee on the Prevention, Detection, Evaluation, and Treatment of High Blood Pressure (JNC 7) recommended beginning drug treatment at lower blood pressures (≥130/80 mm Hg) in patients with diabetes than in patients without diabetes, despite a lack of trial data specifically demonstrating benefit at this threshold and largely on the basis of epidemiologic data suggesting that a lower blood pressure is better in this patient population. According to the JNC 7, in patients with diabetes, treatment to lower blood pressure is recommended when the systolic blood pressure is ≥130 mm Hg or the diastolic blood pressure is ≥80 mm Hg, with treatment goals of <130/80 mm Hg (Chobanian et al. 2003). JNC 7 also suggests that most persons with elevated blood pressure and diabetes will not be controlled by single-agent therapy.

Control of Lipids

The dyslipidemia of diabetes is characterized by mildly to moderately decreased HDL-C, increased triglyceride concentrations, and small, dense LDL particles (Yoshino, Hirano, and Kazumi 1996). The relation between lipoprotein concentrations and risk of CVD is similar in patients with and without diabetes, but the risk at any specific lipoprotein concentration is much greater in patients with diabetes. Diabetes increases the risk of CVD mortality by two to four times at any level of total cholesterol, which strongly suggests an increased CVD risk at any level of LDL-C (Stamler et al. 1993). As a result of these findings, the 2001 ATP III (Adult Treatment Panel III) guideline of the National Cholesterol Education Program declared the presence of diabetes to be equivalent to the presence of CVD and set an LDL-C goal of <100 mg/dL for diabetes patients; a 2004 update suggested an optional LDL-C goal of <70 mg/dL for patients with both diabetes and CVD (Grundy et al. 2004).

Many trials have demonstrated the efficacy of lipid-lowering drugs in reducing the incidence of CVD in persons with or without diabetes. The experiences of participants with diabetes have been addressed by two meta-analyses. The Cholesterol Treatment Trialists' Collaborators included 14 statin (3-hydroxy-3-methyl-glutaryl-CoA *reductase* inhibitors) drug trials; the reported reduction in RR was 21% for major vascular events (major coronary event, nonfatal or fatal stroke, or coronary revascularization) per 1 mmol/L (39 mg/dL) reduction in LDL-C in people with diabetes. The endpoints included in major coronary events were nonfatal myocardial infarction, death from coronary heart disease, and revascularization. One major coronary event might be prevented for every 46 patients with diabetes treated for approximately 4.7 years (the mean duration of the trial), and one major vascular event might be prevented for every 28 patients with diabetes treated (Baigent et al. 2005).

Another meta-analysis of randomized clinical trials with sufficient participants with diabetes considered primary prevention (preventing a first coronary event in persons with no history of coronary heart disease) and secondary prevention (preventing a new coronary event among persons with a history of coronary heart disease) separately. In 10,838 patients with diabetes treated with either statins or gemfibrozil as primary prevention, the risk reduction for a major coronary event was 21% (11% to 30%; $p < 0.001$). Use of these agents for secondary prevention in 5441 diabetes patients resulted in a risk reduction for a major coronary event of 21% (10% to 31%; $p < 0.001$) (Costa et al. 2006). This meta-analysis also included the following numbers needed to treat: for primary prevention of major coronary events, 37 over 4.5 years; secondary prevention of major coronary events, 15 over 5.1 years; and secondary prevention of stroke, 19 over 5.5 years.

Other Preventive Strategies

The use of aspirin is recommended for primary prevention of CVD (American Diabetes Association 2007). Although not specifically evaluated in trials, smoking cessation for patients with diabetes is strongly recommended based on the wealth of epidemiologic data linking tobacco use to CVD. Additional lifestyle measures to reduce CVD risk in patients with diabetes, including exercise, weight loss, and medical nutrition therapy, are generally recommended. Physical activity of moderate or vigorous intensity has beneficial effects on the heart, blood pressure, and lipids in the general population and in those with diabetes may facilitate glycemic control. Weight loss improves glucose control and also contributes to improved blood pressure and lipids. A diet with limited intake of saturated fat, cholesterol, *trans*-unsaturated fatty acids, and sodium and increased fiber may have beneficial effects on lipids and blood pressure. These strategies are detailed in a recent joint position statement of the ADA and American Heart Association (Buse et al. 2007). The impact of weight loss and increased exercise is being evaluated in a major trial (Look AHEAD [Action for Health in Diabetes]) with respect to reducing CVD endpoints (Ryan et al. 2003).

Prediction

Estimation of CVD Risk

There is considerable interest in providing risk estimates for incident CVD in diabetic patients, typically expressed over a 10-year horizon. The 1998 Framingham Risk Score can be used to predict the 10-year risk of coronary heart disease in persons with diabetes, but it does not take into account the degree of control or duration of diabetes (Wilson et al. 1998). The UKPDS risk engine, based on the trial participants with newly diagnosed diabetes in the United Kingdom, does incorporate A1C, years since diabetes was diagnosed, and race (African descent or not). Further description of this tool and software can be obtained at http://www.dtu. ox.ac.uk/index.php?maindoc=/riskengine/. We have demonstrated using a sample of participants from NHANES with diabetes that both the Framingham Risk Score and UKPDS equations predict an average 10-year risk of coronary heart disease of about 20% (Kirk et al. 2007). This estimate is consistent with the ATP III approach of assuming that persons with diabetes are a "coronary heart disease risk-equivalent," and assuming their 10-year risk is 20% without using the Framingham Risk Score. The predicted risk in men under 50 and women under 60 is less than 20%, however (Kirk et al. 2007). The ADA has developed the Diabetes Personal Health Decisions (PHD) risk assessment tool, which is available at http://www.diabetes.org/ diabetesphd/default.jsp. This software asks for similar inputs as UKPDS and additional information including height, weight, physical activity, and whether periodic health evaluations are being received. It provides estimated risks for a variety of diabetes complications, including CVD. This may be of use for individual patients with diabetes but is time-consuming for health care providers to complete for each of their patients.

Subclinical Disease

An active area of research is using measures of subclinical CVD as a means of risk stratification in the general population as well as among those with diabetes. These include measures of carotid atherosclerosis, coronary artery calcification, low ankle-brachial index, electrocardiogram (ECG) abnormalities, and increased ventricular mass/impaired diastolic function. Carotid intima-medial thickness (IMT) assessed by ultrasound is a subclinical measure of atherosclerosis that has been evaluated as a predictor of future CVD events. A systematic review found that in 20 of 21 studies, type 2 diabetes was associated with a greater IMT; meta-analysis suggests the average effect of type 2 diabetes is a 0.13-mm thicker carotid artery IMT (95% CI

0.109–0.131 mm) compared with those without type 2 disease (Brohall, Oden, and Fagerberg 2006). This difference in IMT suggests that the risk of heart attack or stroke is 40% higher in adults with diabetes. Given the increment in IMT associated with aging, another interpretation is that the "vascular age" of an average adult with diabetes is approximately 10 years greater than her/his chronologic age (Brohall et al. 2006).

In the Cardiovascular Health Study, which included participants aged 65 and over, IMT >80th percentile was one of several subclinical CVD measures considered in addition to ankle-brachial index <0.9 and major ECG abnormalities. Among participants with type 2 diabetes (mean age 73 years, 56% female), 44% had subclinical CVD, 40% clinical CVD, and only 16% had no CVD. Among those without type 2 diabetes (mean age 73 years, 57% female), in contrast, 40% had subclinical disease, 26% clinical CVD, and 34% no CVD (comparison $p < 0.001$). There were striking differences in rates of incident clinical CVD events among persons with diabetes between those with subclinical CVD and those who did not have subclinical CVD (see Table 9.3) (Kuller et al. 2000). Rates of incident coronary heart disease, stroke, and heart failure were generally higher in participants with diabetes but without subclinical disease when compared with participants with normal glucose status (glucose <110 mg/dL in this study).

Screening for subclinical atherosclerosis with CT (computed tomographic) scanning for coronary artery calcium (CAC) has become increasingly available. Adults with type 2 diabetes have an increased likelihood of having CAC (Wong et al. 2003). The prevalence of CAC among those with type 1 diabetes increases with age; in one study it increased from 11% among those aged <30 years to 88% among those aged 50–55 years (Olson et al. 2000). The prevalence of any CAC among those with predominantly type 2 diabetes in a population-based multiethnic sample of

TABLE 9.3 *Risk of Incident Cardiovascular Events Associated with Diabetes and Subclinical Cardiovascular Disease in the Cardiovascular Health Study*

	Incident CHD		Incident Stroke		Incident HF	
	Rate	RR	Rate	RR	Rate	RR
Normal	15.1	1	4.4	1	7.1	1
Diabetes	19.4	1.3 (0.8–2.0)	11.3	2.5 (1.3–4.8)	15.1	2.0 (1.2–3.5)
Normal + subclinical	24.1	1.4 (1.1–1.9)	9.1	1.7 (1.1–2.8)	11.8	1.3 (0.9–2.0)
Diabetes + subclinical	42.6	2.5 (1.9–3.4)	21.9	4.1 (2.6–6.7)	23.1	2.7 (1.8–4.0)

CHD, coronary heart disease; HF, heart failure; RR, relative risk.
Source: Data from Kuller et al. (2000).

adults aged 45–84 without CVD was high (62%); 17% had advanced amounts of CAC (Agatston score >400) (Carnethon et al. 2005). Diabetes was also a strong risk factor for incident CAC and the progression of CAC (Kronmal et al. 2007). In fact, in the Multi-Ethnic Study of Atherosclerosis (MESA) population, among the traditional CVD risk factors, diabetes was the strongest risk factor for progression. Whether CAC should be measured in persons with diabetes to further stratify by risk is currently the subject of some debate. Qu and colleagues (2003) did not demonstrate CAC to be independently predictive of incident coronary heart disease for persons with diabetes in models that adjusted for age, gender, body-mass index, exercise, alcohol consumption, systolic blood pressure, and lipids (Qu et al. 2003). Although further data from prospective studies are needed in this area, there are currently no specific medical therapies that would be indicated to specifically target CAC beyond standard risk factor control. There are also no data published from randomized trials assessing whether invasive interventions (such as coronary artery stenting or bypass) performed in asymptomatic persons with diabetes with significant CAC would yield any reductions in CVD morbidity or mortality.

Some have advocated screening echocardiography in patients with diabetes (Bell 2003), but this study is not routinely done, in part due to the considerable cost. Magnetic resonance imaging (MRI) can also be performed to assess cardiac structure and function. The 2005 American Heart Association/ACC Heart Failure Guideline, which places adults with diabetes without clinically evident heart failure in stage A (at high risk for developing heart failure), recommends control of blood pressure, lipids, and glycemia and recommends the use of ACE inhibitors and ARBs as potentially useful preventive drugs (Hunt et al. 2005). These guidelines do not make any recommendations for screening via echocardiography or other imaging modalities or testing for brain natriuretic peptide (BNP) or amino-terminal pro-brain natriuretic peptide (NT-proBNP), two related biomarkers being investigated as possible screening blood tests for heart failure or subclinical left ventricular dysfunction or as a risk marker for future CVD (Bell 2003; Dawson et al. 2005).

Implications for Prevention

Although the risk of CVD can be quantified and estimated via several risk functions, in practice, most adults with diabetes should be presumed to be at a higher risk relative to similarly aged persons without diabetes. The absolute risk of CVD increases with age and approaches 2% per year or greater in those aged 45 and over in the United States and other Western countries, which have the world's highest rates of diabetes. Overall, the evidence is not strong that testing for subclinical CVD is a reasonable strategy to stratify adults with diabetes according to CVD risk. Specifically, no one has yet demonstrated that specific therapies should be targeted differentially on the basis of subclinical parameters, as opposed to assuming all patients with diabetes are at high risk for CVD. Patients with diabetes but no history of CVD may, on average, be subjected to more diagnostic tests for heart disease (e.g., coronary angiography, various cardiac stress tests) and to greater use of revascularization than their counterparts without diabetes, but we are not aware of evidence in favor of "prophylactic" coronary revascularization without demonstration of symptomatic disease.

Control of glycemia, lipids, and hypertension among adults with diabetes would likely decrease their incidence of CVD. And yet there is little evidence that this is being accomplished. NHANES data for 1999–2000 suggests that while 30%–45% of adults with diabetes reached individual goals for A1C, blood pressure, and cholesterol, only 7% of the population had simultaneous control of all three (Saydah, Fradkin, and Cowie 2004). We investigated correlates of controlled risk factors among 5145 overweight adults with diabetes randomized into the Look AHEAD trial during 2001–2004; only 45.8% had A1C <7.0%, just 51.7% had blood pressure <130/80 mm Hg, and only 37.2% had LDL-C <100 mg/dL. All three goals were simultaneously met by only 10.1%. We found consistent evidence for differences in control of risk factors by age, gender, race/ethnicity, degree of obesity, education, income, CVD, source of medical care, and medication use. In multivariable analysis, being African American, having an increased degree of obesity, insulin use, and not using a lipid-lowering agent were associated with simultaneously not meeting all three goals (A1C, blood pressure, and LDL-C) (Bertoni et al. 2008). Improving the care and control of diabetes and related risk factors should clearly be a priority.

■ Other Topics

Health Disparities

Considerable data suggest that African Americans with diabetes have both worse quality of care and less control of risk factors for CVD than whites (Kirk et al. 2005). Worse control of glycemia and blood pressure suggests there should be a higher rate of CVD in African Americans than in whites, and yet an analysis from a large HMO found that risk of CVD among enrollees with diabetes was similar by race or ethnicity (Karter et al. 2002). This finding may be explained by the observation that there is little difference in diabetes-related processes of care by race/ethnicity in the managed care setting (Brown et al. 2005). Many analyses, however, have not considered differential distribution (by race) of other CVD risk factors, such as smoking or lipids. We have demonstrated, using the NHANES 1999–2000 sample, that African Americans do not have a higher predicted risk of coronary heart disease, whether using UKPDS or Framingham Risk Score equations, despite higher A1C and blood pressure, because of more favorable lipid parameters and a lower prevalence of smoking (Kirk et al. 2007).

The available data do not suggest that women with diabetes are at greater risk of CVD than their male counterparts, but they are clearly at greater risk of CVD than women without diabetes, as discussed above. And yet women with diabetes may not be perceived to be as high risk for CVD as they actually are. For example there is some evidence that women with diabetes may be less aggressively treated than men, particularly with respect to lowering LDL-C (Bertoni et al. 2008). These observations might possibly explain the disparity reported for mortality between men and women with diabetes from 1971 to 2000. During this time period all-cause and CVD mortality rates declined for men with diabetes, but there was no decline among women with diabetes (Gregg et al. 2007).

The high burden of CVD in persons with diabetes does contribute to socioeconomic and racial/ethnic disparities of CVD in the overall population. Diabetes is more common in African Americans than in whites, which contributes to the excess CVD experienced by African Americans in general when compared with whites. Similarly diabetes is more common among those in the lower socioeconomic classes, contributing to excess CVD in those groups as well. We have demonstrated that both lower education and lower income are associated with worse control of diabetes, which suggests there may be disparities in CVD outcomes within the population with diabetes by socioeconomic status (Bertoni et al. 2008).

■ Implications for Health Policy

The current epidemic of diabetes mellitus threatens to reverse the population-level improvements in CVD incidence and mortality achieved since the 1960s, a development with important implications for health care costs and policy. The economic impact of the diabetes epidemic is staggering, with the total cost of the disease in the United States estimated to be $174 billion in 2007 (American Diabetes Association 2008). As CVD is the most common complication of diabetes, it is responsible for a large proportion of the direct and indirect costs associated with the disease.

Current policies in the United States tend to favor treatment rather than prevention of CVD, which may help to explain the generally low attainment of goals related to CVD risk factors in the population with diabetes. Policies that promote prevention, such as enhancing access to primary care and the efficiency of this level of care, or improved coverage of medicines used for risk-factor control, or of lifestyle programs, may yield substantial benefits from a health-plan or societal perspective. However, because the majority of persons with diabetes will probably develop CVD at some time in the future, preventing diabetes may be the most effective way of preventing diabetes-related CVD. Interventions to promote weight loss and exercise among the at-risk population may need to be made available via the public-health infrastructure; alternatively, the various states in the United States may need to mandate coverage of these services by health insurers.

■ Areas of Uncertainty or Controversy

The major unanswered question regarding the prevention of CVD in diabetes is how tightly risk factors should be controlled. Although some advocate an A1C of <7.0% and others opt for <6.5%, there is no data from randomized trials for either goal. Similarly, there is limited evidence from randomized trials in favor of a blood pressure goal of <130/80 mm Hg. Finally, it is clear that weight loss and physical activity can have significant beneficial effects on risk factors for CVD in diabetes, but the feasibility and effectiveness of long-term maintenance of these lifestyle changes and their relation to hard endpoints are unclear. A large randomized trial funded by the National Institutes of Health is currently addressing these questions in the United States (Look AHEAD, a lifestyle trial) (Ryan et al. 2003). Follow-up for Look AHEAD is expected to continue until 2012.

■ Developments over the Next 5 to 10 Years

Cardiovascular diseases are likely to remain the leading causes of morbidity and mortality for adults with diabetes in the near future. Absent significant changes in adverse population trends (obesity, physical inactivity) or new advances that might prevent type 2 diabetes, an increasing proportion of the population will burdened by diabetes. This may lead to increased CVD rates overall. Prevention of CVD among persons with diabetes will likely remain a challenging endeavor. The safety of current and future hypoglycemic drugs with respect to CVD outcomes is likely to be an active area of investigation. Efforts to promote control of CVD risk factors among patients with diabetes within the context of the existing health infrastructure (e.g., via enhanced electronic medical records/computerized decision support systems, physician-level quality monitoring with incentives) should be rigorously evaluated and adopted if proven successful. Population-level interventions using public health approaches (e.g., regional diabetes registries, mandatory reporting of A1C to health authorities, publicly supported diabetes education/management programs) may also be necessary to improve the proportions of patients with diabetes who have adequate control of CVD risk factors.

■ Conclusion

Most persons with diabetes will suffer from CVD in their lifetimes, and thus the prevention of CVD in this population is an important public health goal. One immediate challenge is increasing the proportion of adults with diabetes who meet the current standards of diabetes care, which include assessment and control of hyperglycemia, lipids, and blood pressure; smoking cessation; and platelet inhibition. Should tighter control of A1C, blood pressure, or lipids, and/or the use of lifestyle therapy be shown to be successful, this will create new challenges, as multiple drug regimens and/or lifestyle counseling will need to be delivered by a health care system that is already challenged by delivering optimum care as currently defined.

■ References

American Diabetes Association (1998). Consensus development conference on the diagnosis of coronary heart disease in people with diabetes: 10–11 February 1998, Miami, Florida. *Diabetes Care* **21**, 1551–9.

American Diabetes Association (2007). Standards of medical care in diabetes—2007. *Diabetes Care* **30**, S4–41.

American Diabetes Association (2008). Economic costs of diabetes in the U.S. in 2007. *Diabetes Care* **31**, 1–20.

ACCORD Study Group (2010). Effects of Blood-Pressure Control in Type 2 Diabetes Mellitus. *New England Journal of Medicine* 2010 (Epub ahead of print) PMID 20228401

Baigent C et al. (2005). Efficacy and safety of cholesterol-lowering treatment: prospective meta-analysis of data from 90,056 participants in 14 randomized trials of statins. *Lancet* **366**, 1267–78.

Barach JH (1949). Arteriosclerosis and diabetes. *American Journal of Medicine* 7, 617–24.

Beckman JA, Creager MA, Libby P (2002). Diabetes and atherosclerosis: epidemiology, pathophysiology, and management. *JAMA* **287**, 2570–81.

Bell DS (2003). Heart failure: the frequent, forgotten, and often fatal complication of diabetes. *Diabetes Care* **26**, 2433–41.

Bertoni AG et al. (2008). Suboptimal control of glycemia, blood pressure, and LDL cholesterol in overweight adults with diabetes: the Look AHEAD Study. *Journal of Diabetes Complications* **22**, 1–9.

Bliss M (2005). Resurrections in Toronto: the emergence of insulin. *Hormone Research* **64**, 98–102.

Blood Pressure Lowering Treatment Trialists' Collaboration (2005). Effects of different blood pressure-lowering regimens on major cardiovascular events in individuals with and without diabetes mellitus: results of prospectively designed overviews of randomized trials. *Archives of Internal Medicine* **165**, 1410–9.

Blumberg N, Zisserman L (1951). A twenty-year hospital survey of diabetic deaths. *New England Journal of Medicine* **244**, 833–7.

Booth GL et al. (2006). Recent trends in cardiovascular complications among men and women with and without diabetes. *Diabetes Care* **29**, 32–7.

Brohall G, Oden A, Fagerberg B (2006). Carotid artery intima-media thickness in patients with type 2 diabetes mellitus and impaired glucose tolerance: a systematic review. *Diabetic Medicine* **23**, 609–16.

Brown AF et al (2005). Race, ethnicity, socioeconomic position, and quality of care for adults with diabetes enrolled in managed care: the TRIAD Study. *Diabetes Care* **28**, 2864–70.

Buse JB et al (2007). Primary prevention of cardiovascular diseases in people with diabetes mellitus: a scientific statement from the American Heart Association and the American Diabetes Association. *Circulation* **115**, 114–26.

Carnethon MR et al. (2005). Racial/ethnic differences in subclinical atherosclerosis among adults with diabetes: the multiethnic study of atherosclerosis. *Diabetes Care* **28**, 2768–70.

Chobanian AV et al (2003). The Seventh Report of the Joint National Committee on Prevention, Detection, Evaluation, and Treatment of High Blood Pressure: the JNC 7 report. *JAMA* **289**, 2560–72.

Costa J et al. (2006). Efficacy of lipid lowering drug treatment for diabetic and non-diabetic patients: meta-analysis of randomized controlled trials. *British Medical Journal* **332**, 1115–24.

Dawson A et al. (2005). B-type natriuretic peptide as an alternative way of assessing total cardiovascular risk in patients with diabetes mellitus. *American Journal of Cardiology* **96**, 933–4.

DCCT Research Group (1993). The effect of intensive treatment of diabetes on the development and progression of long-term complications in insulin-dependent diabetes mellitus. The Diabetes Control and Complications Trial Research Group [see comments]. *New England Journal of Medicine* **329**, 977–86.

Diabetes Control and Complications Trial/Epidemiology of Diabetes Interventions and Complications (DCCT/EDIC) Study Research Group (2005). Intensive diabetes treatment and cardiovascular disease in patients with type 1 diabetes. *New England Journal of Medicine* **353**, 2643–53.

DeFronzo RA (1999). Pharmacologic therapy for type 2 diabetes mellitus. *Annals of Internal Medicine* **131**, 281–303.

Egede LE, Zheng D (2002). Modifiable cardiovascular risk factors in adults with diabetes: prevalence and missed opportunities for physician counseling. *Archives of Internal Medicine* **162**, 427–33.

Estacio RO et al. (1998). The effect of nisoldipine as compared with enalapril on cardiovascular outcomes in patients with non-insulin-dependent diabetes and hypertension. *New England Journal of Medicine* **338**, 645–52.

Fox CS et al. (2004). Trends in cardiovascular complications of diabetes. *JAMA* **292**, 2495–9.

Gerstein HC et al. (2008). Effects of intensive glucose lowering in type 2 diabetes. *New England Journal of Medicine* **358**, 2545–59.

Goff DC Jr et al (2007). Prevention of cardiovascular disease in persons with type 2 diabetes mellitus: current knowledge and rationale for the Action to Control Cardiovascular Risk in Diabetes (ACCORD) trial. *American Journal of Cardiology* **99**, 4i–20i.

Gregg EW et al. (2007). Mortality trends in men and women with diabetes, 1971 to 2000. *Annals of Internal Medicine* **147**, 149–55.

Grundy SM et al. (2004). Implications of recent clinical trials for the National Cholesterol Education Program Adult Treatment Panel III guidelines. *Circulation* **110**, 227–39.

Gu K, Cowie CC, Harris MI (1998). Mortality in adults with and without diabetes in a national cohort of the U.S. population, 1971–1993. *Diabetes Care* 21, 1138–45.

Hunt SA et al. (2005). ACC/AHA 2005 guideline update for the diagnosis and management of chronic heart failure in the adult--summary article: a report of the American College of Cardiology/American Heart Association Task Force on Practice Guidelines (Writing Committee to Update the 2001 Guidelines for the Evaluation and Management of Heart Failure): Developed in Collaboration with the American College of Chest Physicians and the International Society for Heart and Lung Transplantation: Endorsed by the Heart Rhythm Society. *Circulation* 112, 1825–52.

Huxley R, Barzi F, Woodward M (2006). Excess risk of fatal coronary heart disease associated with diabetes in men and women: meta-analysis of 37 prospective cohort studies. *British Medical Journal* 332, 73–78.

Idris I, Thomson GA, Sharma JC (2006). Diabetes mellitus and stroke. *International Journal of Clinical Practice* 60, 48–56.

Imperatore G et al. (2004). Thirty-year trends in cardiovascular risk factor levels among US adults with diabetes: National Health and Nutrition Examination Surveys, 1971–2000. *American Journal of Epidemiology* 160, 531–9.

Janghorbani M, Hu FB, Willett WC, et al. (2007). Prospective study of type 1 and type 2 diabetes and risk of stroke subtypes: the Nurses' Health Study. *Diabetes Care* 30, 1730–5.

Jeerakathil T et al. (2007). Short-term risk for stroke is doubled in persons with newly treated type 2 diabetes compared with persons without diabetes: a population-based cohort study. *Stroke* 38, 1739–43.

Kannel WB (2000). Vital epidemiologic clues in heart failure. *Journal of Clinical Epidemiology* 53, 229–35.

Kannel WB, McGee DL (1979). Diabetes and cardiovascular disease. The Framingham study. *JAMA* 241, 2035–8.

Karter AJ, Ferrara A, Liu JY, et al. (2002). Ethnic disparities in diabetic complications in an insured population. *JAMA* 287, 2519–27.

Kirk JK et al. (2005). A qualitative review of studies of diabetes preventive care among minority patients in the United States 1993–2003. *American Journal of Managed Care* 11, 349–60.

Kirk JK et al. (2007). Predicted risk of coronary heart disease among persons with type 2 diabetes. *Coronary Artery Disease* 18, 595–600.

Kronmal RA et al. (2006). Mortality in pharmacologically treated older adults with diabetes: the Cardiovascular Health Study, 1989–2001. *PloS Medicine* 3, e400.

Kronmal RA et al. (2007). Risk factors for the progression of coronary artery calcification in asymptomatic subjects: results from the Multi-Ethnic Study of Atherosclerosis (MESA). *Circulation* 115, 2722–30.

Kuller LH et al. (2000). Diabetes mellitus: subclinical cardiovascular disease and risk of incident cardiovascular disease and all-cause mortality. *Arteriosclerosis Thrombosis and Vascular Biology* 20, 823–9.

Nichols GA et al. (2004). The incidence of congestive heart failure in type 2 diabetes: an update. *Diabetes Care* **27**, 1879–84.

Olson JC et al. (2000). Coronary calcium in adults with type 1 diabetes: a stronger correlate of clinical coronary artery disease in men than in women. *Diabetes* **49**, 1571–8.

Ong KL et al. (2007). Prevalence, awareness, treatment, and control of hypertension among United States adults 1999–2004. *Hypertension* **49**, 69–75.

Osler W (1901). *The Principles and Practice of Medicine*, 4th ed. New York: D. Appelton and Company.

Patel A et al. (2008). Intensive blood glucose control and vascular outcomes in patients with type 2 diabetes. *New England Journal of Medicine* **358**, 2560–72.

Qu W et al. (2003). Value of coronary artery calcium scanning by computed tomography for predicting coronary heart disease in diabetic subjects. *Diabetes Care* **26**, 905–10.

Ryan DH et al. (2003). Look AHEAD (Action for Health in Diabetes): design and methods for a clinical trial of weight loss for the prevention of cardiovascular disease in type 2 diabetes. *Controlled Clinical Trials* **24**, 610–28.

Saito I et al. (2000). Nontraditional risk factors for coronary heart disease incidence among persons with diabetes: the Atherosclerosis Risk in Communities (ARIC) Study. *Annals of Internal Medicine* **133**, 81–91.

Saydah SH, Fradkin J, Cowie CC (2004). Poor control of risk factors for vascular disease among adults with previously diagnosed diabetes. *JAMA* **291**, 335–42.

Selvin E et al. (2004). Meta-analysis: glycosylated hemoglobin and cardiovascular disease in diabetes mellitus. *Annals of Internal Medicine* **141**, 421–31.

Smits P, Thien T (1995). Cardiovascular effects of sulphonylurea derivatives. Implications for the treatment of NIDDM? *Diabetologia* **38**, 116–21.

Stamler J et al. (1993). Diabetes, other risk factors, and 12-yr cardiovascular mortality for men screened in the Multiple Risk Factor Intervention Trial. *Diabetes Care* **16**, 434–44.

UK Prospective Diabetes Study (UKPDS) Group (1998a). Intensive blood-glucose control with sulphonylureas or insulin compared with conventional treatment and risk of complications in patients with type 2 diabetes (UKPDS 33). *Lancet* **352**, 837–53.

UK Prospective Diabetes Study (UKPDS) Group (1998b). Tight blood pressure control and risk of macrovascular and microvascular complications in type 2 diabetes (UKPDS 38). *British Medical Journal* **317**, 703–13. [Published erratum appears in *British Medical Journal* 1999, **318**, 29.]

Wilson PW et al. (1998). Prediction of coronary heart disease using risk factor categories. *Circulation* **97**, 1837–47.

Wong ND et al. (2003). The metabolic syndrome, diabetes, and subclinical atherosclerosis assessed by coronary calcium. *Journal of the American College of Cardiology* **41**, 1547–53.

Yoshino G, Hirano T, Kazumi T (1996). Dyslipidemia in diabetes mellitus. *Diabetes Research and Clinical Practice* **33**, 1–14.

10. DIABETES IN PREGNANCY

Adolfo Correa-Villaseñor and Jessica A. Marcinkevage

■ Main Public Health Messages

- The increasing prevalence of obesity, diabetes, and impaired glucose tolerance around the globe is likely to result in more pregnancies complicated by diabetes (diagnosed and undiagnosed) around the world in the next few decades.
- Undiagnosed or poorly managed diabetes in pregnancy is associated with an increased risk for a wide spectrum of acute and long-term effects for the affected mother, her offspring, and the offspring of female offspring of diabetic mothers. However, excess risks for adverse pregnancy outcomes from diabetes in pregnancy can be reduced through glycemic control before and during pregnancy.
- There is a need for population-based surveillance of diabetes in pregnancy and of acute and long-term maternal and fetal complications of diabetes in pregnancy, as well as for population-based research on health services needs and costs, health disparities, and modifiable risk factors for the spectrum of complications associated with diabetes in pregnancy.
- There is a need for a public health framework for translating public health surveillance and research findings on health services needs, health disparities, and modifiable risk factors for complications of diabetes in pregnancy into strategies aimed at the development, implementation, and evaluation of various initiatives, including awareness raising, education, training, health promotion, and development of policies and interventions for the prevention and control of complications associated with diabetes in pregnancy.

■ Introduction

During a normal pregnancy, maternal metabolism undergoes a number of changes in preparation for growth and development of the fetus, including a decrease in insulin sensitivity (or increase in insulin resistance) in the third trimester that results in increased availability of nutrients for fetal growth (Lain and Catalano 2007).

The findings and conclusions in this report are those of the authors and do not necessarily represent the official position of the Centers for Disease Control and Prevention.

During a pregnancy complicated by diabetes, such metabolic changes can complicate the management of diabetes, and diabetes, in turn, can result in a wide range of complications for both the mother and the offspring. An extensive body of literature in recent decades has improved our understanding of the pathophysiology and risk factors underlying such complications and helped to guide the development of approaches for their management in the clinical setting (Kitzmiller and American Diabetes Association 2008). However, the literature of the public health implications of and prevention strategies for diabetes in pregnancy has been more limited, standing in stark contrast to the body of literature on the prevention and control of diabetes and its complications among adults (Knowler et al. 2002; Skyler et al. 2009).

Two recent developments underscore the need for more concerted efforts to develop, implement, and promote a similar a public health translational research agenda targeted to diabetes in pregnancy: (1) the prevalence of diabetes in pregnancy has been increasing in many parts of the world; and (2) a growing awareness that diabetes in pregnancy can result in a wide range of acute and long-term effects for mothers, their offspring, and the offspring of female offspring of diabetic mothers. This chapter provides an overview of current public health aspects of diabetes in pregnancy, including an overview of some of the challenges and opportunities for prevention.

■ Background

Most women with diabetes in pregnancy can be classified into two broad categories: (1) diabetes that predates the pregnancy (i.e., preexisting diabetes, type 1 and type 2); and (2) glucose intolerance that begins or is first diagnosed during pregnancy and usually resolves after delivery (i.e., gestational diabetes mellitus [GDM]). Among women with a diagnosis of gestational diabetes, documenting the resolution of GDM after birth is crucial because some women with previously undiagnosed type 2 diabetes are likely to be initially labeled as having GDM. Because GDM shares some of the same risk factors as other common types of hyperglycemia and often represents an unrecognized stage of preexisting diabetes, the epidemiologic aspects and complications from preexisting diabetes and gestational diabetes are discussed in parallel in this chapter.

Preexisting Diabetes

Most pregnant women with preexisting diabetes fall into one of two broad pathogenetic categories: type 1 and type 2 diabetes. Before the discovery of insulin in 1921, pregnancies complicated by preexisting diabetes were generally associated with high maternal and fetal mortality. By the 1940s, with increasing use of insulin and other advances in obstetrics, maternal mortality among women with preexisting diabetes had decreased (Langer and Langer 2006). However, a number of maternal and fetal complications continued to occur, including preeclampsia, late fetal deaths, birth defects, macrosomia, and neonatal hypoglycemia (Papaspyros 1952). Adoption of an interdisciplinary approach to the care of pregnant women with diabetes demonstrated that long-term follow-up, frequent hospitalizations to achieve strict glycemic control, and early deliveries were associated with improved fetal outcome, leading to new clinical recommendations (Pederson 1977; Pedersen and Brandstrup 1956; White 1949). As a result of such recommendations and several advances in diagnosis and treatment in recent decades (i.e., advances in technology to monitor maternal glucose level more frequently, new forms of insulin and practical methods for administering insulin, and improvements in obstetric and neonatal care and obstetric anesthesia) in recent years, many women with diabetes have been able to achieve perinatal outcomes comparable to those of women without diabetes (Babbe 2008). Nonetheless, recent trends suggest that preexisting diabetes in pregnancy is becoming an important public health challenge. First, although most early studies of pregnancies complicated by diabetes reported findings mainly related to type 1 diabetes (Evers et al. 2004; Jensen et al. 2004; Penney et al. 2003; Platt et al. 2002; Vaarasmaki et al. 2000), recent reports suggest that around the world there is an increasing proportion of pregnancies complicated by type 2 diabetes (Bell et al. 2008; CEMACH 2005; Cheung et al. 2005; Dunne 2005; Lawrence et al. 2008). Second, many pregnancies among women with preexisting diabetes are unplanned (CEMACH 2005; Holing et al. 1998), and achieving sufficient glycemic control to prevent maternal and fetal complications among such pregnancies remains a major challenge (CEMACH 2005). Third, an increasing prevalence of obesity among younger age groups is likely to lead to an increasing prevalence of diabetes among women of childbearing age and an increasing prevalence of pregnancies complicated by pregestational diabetes.

Gestational Diabetes

The clinical detection of GDM is accomplished in different ways within and between countries. In general clinical detection involves screening for glucose intolerance among pregnant women not already known to have diabetes using one or more of the following procedures: (1) clinical risk assessment; (2) glucose tolerance screening; and (3) formal glucose tolerance testing. Current diagnostic criteria assign a diagnosis of GDM to women with glucose levels in the upper ~5%–10% of the population distribution (Buchanan et al. 2007). Within this group of women the distribution of hyperglycemia levels can vary from levels that would be consistent with those seen in diabetes outside of pregnancy to levels that are asymptomatic but associated with some increased risk for fetal and offspring complications. To maintain proper glucose control during pregnancy, pancreatic β cells of the mother must increase insulin secretion enough to counteract the corresponding decrease in tissue sensitivity to insulin. However pregnant women who develop GDM are unable to increase insulin production to compensate for their increased resistance to insulin. Although the causes of this pancreatic β cell dysfunction in GDM have not been fully defined, the rapid resolution of insulin resistance after delivery suggests a major role of placental hormones among some women. The fact that a majority of women with GDM eventually develop type 2 diabetes within 10 years after pregnancy suggests a chronic underlying β cell dysfunction present before and after pregnancy (Barbour et al. 2007; Buchanan et al. 2007).

This predisposition to type 2 diabetes raises concerns about potential increases in prevalence of GDM around the world. In the United States the proportion of pregnancies complicated by GDM has been increasing (Ferrara 2007). For instance in 1988 of 100 pregnancies complicated by diabetes, 88 were affected by GDM and 12 by preexisting diabetes (Engelgau et al. 1995); more recently (1995–2005), of 100 pregnancies complicated by diabetes, 85 were affected by GDM and 15 by preexisting diabetes (Lawrence et al. 2008). Published prevalence data from developing countries are scant. Recent studies suggest that GDM is becoming a more prevalent condition in developing countries, possibly due to an increasing prevalence of obesity in the population (Ma and Chan 2009; Mahtab and Habib 2009). However, determining the extent to which variations in GDM prevalence over time and across populations reflects variations in testing, diagnostic criteria, and demographics of the population versus changes in modifiable risk factors such as obesity is made difficult by the lack of population-based prevalence data on GDM.

■ Burden

Prevalence

Preexisting Diabetes

Until recently, published reports on the prevalence of pregnancies complicated by preexisting diabetes had been relatively nonexistent. However, increasing trends in the prevalence of obesity and GDM among reproductive-age women in the United States (Dabelea et al. 2005; Ferrara 2007; Ferrara et al. 2004; Flegal et al. 2002; Kim et al. 2007) recently prompted an evaluation of the prevalence of preexisting diabetes among pregnant women (Lawrence et al. 2008). Based on analyses of clinical databases from Kaiser Permanente hospitals in southern California and birth certificate information, Lawrence and colleagues (Lawrence et al. 2008) found an increase in the prevalence of pregnancies complicated by preexisting diabetes from 0.81 per 100 in 1999 to 1.82 per 100 in 2005, a pattern that was evident across various race/ethnic groups (see Fig. 10.1). The prevalence of preexisting diabetes among pregnancies was higher among non-white than among white women, with the highest prevalence noted among blacks followed by Hispanics and Asian/

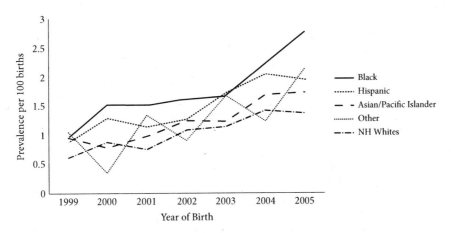

FIGURE 10.1. Trends in age-adjusted prevalence of preexisting diabetes among pregnant women, Kaiser Permanente Southern California, 1999–2005, by race/ethnicity. (Source: Lawrence et al. 2008.)

Pacific Islanders. The increasing trend in prevalence of preexisting diabetes among pregnant women was also evident across all age groups examined, 13–19, 20–24, 25–30, 30–34, 35–39, and ≥40 years. Given the increasing trends in the prevalence of obesity in the population, it is going to be important to collect population-based surveillance data on preexisting diabetes that can facilitate assessments of the evolving public health aspects of preexisting diabetes in pregnancy, temporal trends, and variations in prevalence of preexisting diabetes in pregnancy across population subgroups (e.g., age groups, ethnicity, socioeconomic status, and geographic regions), and ongoing evaluations of the effectiveness of multidisciplinary teams in reaching high–risk populations.

Gestational Diabetes

Studies from different populations from industrialized countries have reported increasing trends in the annual age-adjusted prevalence of GDM in recent years (see Table 10.1). The South Australia study reported a statistically significant increasing trend in the age-adjusted prevalence of GDM among deliveries to non-Aboriginal Australians ($n = 225,168$) and a suggestion of an increasing trend in age-adjusted prevalence of GDM in the smaller sample of pregnancies among Aboriginal Australians ($n = 4843$) (Ishak and Petocz 2003). The Northern California Kaiser Permanente Study reported a statistically significant increase in the age-adjusted prevalence of GDM among all pregnant women from 4.9% to 7.1% (Ferrara et al. 2004). The Colorado Kaiser Permanente Study reported statistically significant increases in the prevalence of GDM in each of the four race/ethnicity groups studied (Dabelea et al. 2005). The study based on the National Hospital Discharge Survey showed that the prevalence of GDM in the United States increased dramatically between 1989 and 2004 among whites as well as among blacks (Getahun et al. 2008).

TABLE 10.1 *Studies of Trends in Age-Adjusted Prevalence of Gestational Diabetes Mellitus (GDM), 1988–2005*

Location	Study Period	Criteria for GDM Definition	Change in Prevalence	p-Value[*]
South Australia (Ishak and Petocz 2003)	1988–1999	Australasian Diabetes in Pregnancy Society (Ishak and Petocz 2003) and World Health Organization (1985)	1.8% to 3.1% in non-Aboriginal	<0.0001[†]
			5.2% to 5.8% in Aboriginal	NS
Northern California Kaiser Permanente (Ferrara et al. 2004)	1991–2000	2000 American Diabetes Association or diagnosis (Ferrara, Kahn et al. 2004)	4.9% to 7.3% overall	
			7.2% to 9.7% for Asians	
			7.2% to 8.3% for Hispanics	
			4.1% to 6.4% for African Americans	
			3.9% to 5.7% for whites	
Colorado Kaiser Permanente (Dabelea et al. 2005)	1994–2002	National Diabetes Data Group (1979)	2.1% to 4.1% overall	<0.001
			7.9% to 6.8% for Asians	<0.001
			2.8% to 5.4% for Hispanics	<0.001
			3.8% to 5.5% for African Americans	<0.001
			1.7% to 3.1% for non-Hispanic whites	0.002

Study	Period	Source/Method	Result	Significance*
United States (Getahun et al. 2008)	1989–2004	International Classification of Diseases, Ninth Revision, Clinical Modification code 648.8, National Hospital Discharge Survey	2.0% to 3.6% for whites, percentage change of 80% (95% confidence interval 79%–82%)	
			1.5% to 4.1% for blacks, percentage change of 172% (95% confidence interval 166%–178%)	
Southern California Kaiser Permanente (Lawrence et al. 2008)	1999–2005	American Diabetes Association (2004; 2007)	7.4% to 7.5% overall	NS†
			10.2% to 10.3% for Asian/Pacific Islanders	NS
			8.6% to 8.6% for Hispanics	NS
			6.1% to 8.5% for other races	NS
			6.0% to 5.2% for blacks	NS
			5.1% to 4.9% for non-Hispanic whites	NS

*Test for trend.

†Not significant.

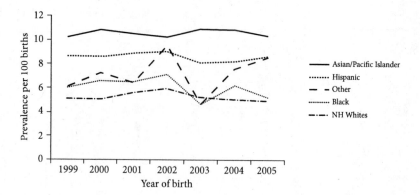

FIGURE 10.2. Trends in age-adjusted prevalence of gestational diabetes mellitus among pregnant women, Kaiser Permanente Southern California, 1999–2005, by race/ethnicity. (Source: Lawrence et al. 2008.)

The only study that did not observe an increase in age-adjusted prevalence of GDM in any of the race/ethnicity groups studied was the Southern California Kaiser Permanente Study (Lawrence et al. 2008) (see Fig. 10.2). However, this study reported higher levels of age-adjusted prevalence of GDM for the various race/ethnicity groups examined compared to previous studies. Whether the prevalence levels observed in the Southern California study represent the levels at which the prevalence of GDM is going to plateau in this population is unclear. Although published data on trends in prevalence of GDM are limited for populations from countries that are becoming more industrialized, recent reports suggest that GDM is not only one of the more common complications of pregnancy in such countries but also a significant public health burden. For example a recent community-based study in Tamilnadu state, India, using WHO criteria (1985) reported a prevalence of GDM of 13.9%, with the rate of GDM being twice as high among women with a prepregnancy body mass index (BMI) greater than 25 and 25 years of age and older (Seshiah et al. 2009).

In recent decades, the age at onset of diabetes has been shifting to younger age groups, with type 2 diabetes becoming more prevalent among children and adolescents (Matyka 2008). These trends and similar trends in the prevalence of obesity in childhood and adolescence suggest that in future years there will be an increasing number of women of childbearing age with preexisting and gestational diabetes. Accordingly, further studies are needed on trends in prevalence of pregnancies complicated by preexisting and gestational diabetes in different populations around the world. Such studies are likely to provide a better understanding of the magnitude of the public health burden of diabetes in pregnancy globally, the variation in prevalence among population subgroups, and a better insight into the underlying reasons for variations in prevalence that might be amenable to intervention.

Complications

Because women with diabetes or gestational diabetes are at increased risk for pregnancy and delivery complications, and gestational diabetes is associated with an increased risk for future diabetes in affected mothers (Kjos and Buchanan 1999), an assessment of the burden of diabetes in pregnancy needs to consider also the scope of maternal and offspring complications.

Preexisting Diabetes

Maternal complications. Women with preexisting diabetes have an increased risk for a wide range of complications, including hypoglycemia, ketoacidosis, thyroid disorders, cardiovascular disease, coronary heart disease, cardiovascular autonomic neuropathy, heart failure, ischemic stroke, peripheral arteriosclerotic vascular disease, hypertension, dyslipidemia, nephropathy, retinopathy, and peripheral neuropathy (Kitzmiller and American Diabetes Association 2008). During pregnancy, women with preexisting diabetes are also at risk for pregnancy–induced hypertension, preeclampsia, worsening of chronic complications, and maternal mortality (Langer and Langer 2006) (see Table 10.2). There is limited published information on the frequency of these complications during pregnancy, on whether pregnancy modifies the risk of such complications, and on the magnitude of the attributable risk for such complications associated with pregnancy. However available literature on some complications (i.e., retinopathy, nephropathy, gestational hypertension, and preeclampsia) provides some insights on the impact of diabetes in pregnancy on maternal complications. Pregnancy is an independent risk factor for the acceleration of retinopathy, but other pregnancy-related factors can in turn aggravate the acceleration of retinopathy (DCCT 2000; Verier-Mine et al. 2005). These factors include hyperglycemia at the start of pregnancy, rapid normalization of blood glucose, hypertension, duration of diabetes, and state of the retina. The prevalence of diabetic nephropathy (defined as total protein excretion of >300–500 mg/day) among diabetic pregnant women is estimated as 5%–6% in type 1 diabetes, compared with 1%–4% in type 2 diabetes (Kitzmiller and American Diabetes Association 2008).

Recent studies indicating that with excellent control of glucose, blood pressure, lipids, and weight, pregnancy may not constitute a risk factor for long-term progression of diabetic microvascular complications (DCCT 2000; Pettitt et al. 2005; Verier-Mine et al. 2005) offer some promise for potential prevention interventions. However, translation of such research results to pregnant women with preexisting diabetes is likely to remain a challenge, particularly among women with severe complications of diabetes and among women who present late for antenatal care and/or who are noncompliant in their management of diabetes during pregnancy. To gain a better understanding of the current prevalence of maternal complications

TABLE 10.2 *Potential Maternal and Offspring Complications from Diabetes in Pregnancy by Type of Diabetes*

	Potential Complication	Preexisting Diabetes	Gestational Diabetes
Maternal	Hypoglycemia, ketoacidosis	X	
	Pregnancy-induced hypertension	X	
	Preeclampsia	X	
	Pyelonephritis, other infections	X	
	Dyslipidemia	X	X
	Worsening of chronic complications: coronary heart disease, retinopathy, nephropathy, lower extremity arterial disease	X	
	Preterm labor	X	
	Cesarean section	X	X
	Impaired glucose tolerance postdelivery	X	X
Offspring	Birth defects	X	
	Intrauterine growth restriction	X	
	Preterm birth	X	X
	Large for gestational age, macrosomia	X	X
	Birth trauma	X	X
	Asphyxia	X	
	Respiratory distress syndrome	X	
	Hypoglycemia	X	X
	Hypocalcemia	X	
	Hypomagnesemia	X	
	Increased red blood cells and hyperviscosity	X	
	Hyperbilirubinemia	X	
	Stillbirths	X	X
	Perinatal mortality	X	
	Obesity in childhood and adolescence	X	X
	Diabetes in childhood and adolescence	X	X

X = potential complication.

from diabetes in pregnancy and of trends over time in relation to the implementation of prevention interventions, more efforts are needed to monitor the occurrence of maternal complications of diabetes in pregnancy. A surveillance system of such complications would represent a first step in addressing an important knowledge gap and in identifying possible health disparities and barriers for timely access to preconception and prenatal care.

Offspring complications. Preexisting diabetes has been associated with a wide range of perinatal complications (Langer et al. 2005), including: preterm delivery, small for gestational age, large for gestational age, birth defects, stillbirths, shoulder dystocia, perinatal mortality, jaundice, hypoglycemia, polycythemia, respiratory distress syndrome, and need for neonatal intensive care (see Table 10.2). Although many of these perinatal complications have decreased in frequency over the past few decades, several of them continue to occur with greater frequency among offspring of women with preexisting diabetes than in the general population (see Table 10.3). This excess risk of perinatal complications associated with maternal preexisting diabetes is particularly true for preterm delivery, intrauterine growth retardation, large for gestational age, birth defects, stillbirths, and perinatal mortality (i.e., the number of stillbirths and neonatal deaths per 100 total births [live births and stillbirths]).

Maternal preexisting diabetes is associated with an increased risk for a wide range of birth defects, with the most common being defects of the cardiovascular, central nervous and musculoskeletal systems, and for an increased risk of multiple defects (Correa et al. 2008). Although the pathophysiology of perinatal complications in diabetic pregnancies is unclear, poor glycemic control is regarded as an important risk factor. It is estimated that poor glycemic control accounts for 50%–75% of stillbirths in these pregnancies. For perinatal deaths and birth defects among diabetic pregnancies, the risk of these outcomes has been shown to be related to the mean blood glucose level (Karlsson and Kjellmer 1972; Schaefer-Graf et al. 2000). For birth defects, preconception care (Dunne et al. 2003; Ray et al. 2001), particularly good glycemic control (Dunne et al. 2003), has been associated with a reduction in risk of birth defects to levels comparable to those in the general population. Prematurity (spontaneous and due to indicated preterm delivery) is one of the principal causes of neonatal mortality in diabetic pregnancies (Melamed et al. 2008). Preeclampsia, which is more common in diabetic pregnancies, is one of the indications for induced preterm delivery. The combination of preterm delivery and delayed lung development in infants of diabetic mothers results in an increased susceptibility for respiratory distress of the newborn, which is associated with an increased risk of neonatal mortality. The risk of perinatal asphyxia, another important risk factor for neonatal death, is increased among infants of diabetic mothers. Fetal macrosomia, which is more common among infants of overweight and diabetic mothers, is associated with shoulder dystocia, birth trauma, and perinatal asphyxia. Neonatal hypoglycemia, which occurs within a few hours of birth and

TABLE 10.3 *Rates, Rate Ratios and Attributable Risks for Maternal and Perinatal Complications Associated with Diabetes in Pregnancy, by Type of Diabetes, 1986–2003*

Type of Diabetes	Reference	Years	Population	Complication	Rate in Diabetic Group	Rate in General Population/ Reference Group	Estimate of Relative Risk (RR/OR)	Attributable Risk*
Preexisting	Sheffield et al. (2002)	1991–2000	Dallas, Texas	Birth defects	6.1%	1.5%	4.4	77%
	Penney et al. (2003)	1998–1999	Scotland	Birth defects	6%	2.8%	2	50%
				Stillbirths	1.8%	0.5%	3.6	72%
				Perinatal mortality	2.8%	0.8%	3.5	71%
	Evers et al. (2004)	1999–2000	Netherlands	Pre-eclampsia	12.7%	1.05%	12.1	92%
				Maternal mortality	0.6%	0.01%	60	98%
				Preterm delivery	32%	7.1%	4.5	78%
				Birth defects	8.8%	2.6%	3.4	71%
				Macrosomia	45.1%	10.0%	4.5	78%
				Perinatal mortality	2.8%	0.8%	3.5	71%

Sharpe et al. (2005)	1986–2000	South Australia	Birth defects	10.1%	5.1%	2.0	50%
CEMACH (2005)	2002–2003	England, Wales, and Northern Ireland	Elective or emergency cesarean section	42.7%	11%	3.9	74%
			Birth defects	4.2%	2.1%	2.0	50%
			Spontaneous preterm delivery	9.4%	4.7%	2.0	50%
			Macrosomia	21%	11%	1.9	47%
			Stillbirths	2.7%	0.6%	4.7	79%
			Perinatal death	3.2%	0.8%	3.8	74%
			Neonatal death	0.9%	0.4%	2.6	62%
Macintosh et al. (2006)	2002–2003	UK	Stillbirths	2.7%	0.6%	4.7	78%
			Perinatal mortality	3.2%	0.8%	3.8	74%
Yang et al. (2006)	1988–2002	Nova Scotia, Canada	Pregnancy-induced hypertension	27.5%	9.1%	3.0	67%

(continued)

TABLE 10.3 (continued)

Type of Diabetes	Reference	Years	Population	Complication	Rate in Diabetic Group	Rate in General Population/ Reference Group	Estimate of Relative Risk (RR/OR)	Attributable Risk*
				Birth defects	9.1%	3.1%	3.0	67%
				Preterm birth	27.7%	5.2%	5.3	81%
				Small for gestational age	5%	10.0%	0.5	
				Large for gestational age	45.2%	12.6%	3.6	72%
				Stillbirths	0.97%	0.4%	2.4	58%
Gestational	Sheffield et al. (2002)	1991–2000	Dallas, Texas	Birth defects	Normal fasting, 1.2%	1.5%	0.8	
					Elevated fasting, 4.8%		3.4	71%
	Sharpe et al. (2005)	1986–2000	South Australia	Birth defects	6.0%	5.1%	1.19	16%
	Langer et al. (2005)	1990–1999	San Antonio, Texas	Large for gestational age	29%	11%	3.28	70%
				Hypoglycemia	18%	2%	10.4	90%
				Stillbirths	0.54%	0.2%	1.91	48%

*Unadjusted attributable risk among women with risk factor = (RR − 1)/RR.

is more common among infants of diabetic mothers, can also result in neonatal mortality if not detected and treated appropriately. Offspring of diabetic mothers are also noted to be at increased risk for impaired neurobehavioral development (Petersen et al. 1988; Rizzo et al. 1991; Sells et al. 1994). One offspring complication of increasing public health concern is the increased risk for diabetes in childhood and adolescence among infants of diabetic mothers (Pettitt et al. 1988; Dabelea et al. 2000a, 2000b). This excess risk reflects the fetal programming effects of the intrauterine diabetic environment in the transmission of diabetes susceptibility across generations among female offspring of diabetic mothers (Chan et al. 2009; Freinkel 1980; Yajnik 2009). These observations suggest the need for more dedicated and vigorous efforts to improve the early-life environment, as such primary prevention efforts could potentially prove to be more cost-effective for preventing some cases of preexisting diabetes than efforts to control unhealthy lifestyle factors later in life.

Gestational Diabetes

Maternal complications. Although the range of potential maternal and offspring complications is smaller for pregnancies complicated by GDM than for pregnancies complicated by preexisting diabetes (see Table 10.2), women with GDM have an increased risk for spontaneous preterm labor, induced labor and caesarean delivery to prevent fetal complications. After delivery women with a history of GDM have an increased risk of developing GDM in subsequent pregnancies. During the first decade after the index pregnancy, over 50% of women with GDM go on to develop diabetes outside of pregnancy (Kim et al. 2002). A recent systematic review and meta-analysis of 20 published studies of women with a history of GDM and follow-up from 1 to 28 years after delivery (Bellamy et al. 2009) estimates that, compared with women with normoglycemic pregnancies, women with GDM have a 7-fold risk (relative risk = 7.43, 95% confidence interval 4.79–1.51) of developing diabetes outside of pregnancy.

Offspring complications. Gestational diabetes has been associated with an increased risk for fetal and perinatal complications, including birth defects, stillbirths, large for gestational age, birth trauma, infant respiratory distress syndrome, cardiomyopathy, neonatal hypoglycemia and hypocalcemia, polycythemia, and hyperviscosity (Reece et al. 2009) (see Table 10.2). Recent published data on the risks of these complications from population-based studies around the globe are limited. However, recent studies from Texas (Sheffield et al. 2002) and South Australia (Sharpe et al. 2005) estimate the attributable risk for birth defects among pregnancies complicated by GDM to range from 16% to 71% (see Table 10.3). For stillbirths, large for gestational age, and neonatal hypoglycemia, the Texas study provides estimates of attributable risks among pregnancies complicated by GDM of 48%, 70%, and 90%, respectively. Most of these complications are thought to be related to maternal increased glucose levels and other associated metabolic fuels (i.e., plasma lipids, and amino acids, but not insulin). These metabolites can cross the placenta and result in exposure of the fetus to higher concentrations of fuels and growth factors than normal, resulting in increased birth weight and neonatal body fat among infants of mothers with GDM (Catalano et al. 2003). An evaluation of the neonatal body composition and anthropometrics in appropriate for gestational age (AGA) infants of women with GDM and normal glucose tolerance showed that the AGA infants of women with GDM had a significant increase in fat mass, percentage body mass, and skinfold measures, without a significant increase in body weight (Catalano et al. 2009). This observation suggests that birth weight alone may not be a sensitive enough measure of the effects of GDM on fetal growth.

Infants of GDM mothers are also at increased risk for obesity and glucose intolerance/type 2 diabetes in childhood and young adulthood (Clausen 2008; Dabelea et al. 2000a, 2000b; Sebire 2001; Vohr 2008; Yogev and Visser 2009). Among Pima Indians, a group of Native Americans residing in Arizona and known to have high rates of pregnancies complicated by GDM, the cumulative risk of type 2 diabetes at 24 years of age among offspring of mothers with GDM in the third trimester was 30% compared with a cumulative incidence of 19% among offspring of mothers with glucose tolerance in the upper normal range and 8% among offspring of mothers with glucose tolerance in the low normal range (Franks et al. 2006).

■ Modifiable Risk Factors

Pregnancies Complicated by Preexisting Diabetes

Risk factors for the development of type 2 diabetes that have become important drivers of diabetes in pregnancy because of their increasing prevalence include adiposity, weight gain and duration of overweight status, impaired glucose tolerance/ fasting glucose, and history of gestational diabetes (Balkau et al. 2008; Bellamy et al. 2009; Ferrara 2007; Langer 2006; Retnakaran et al. 2008; Vohr and Boney 2008), in addition to ethnicity (Langer 2006; Lawrence et al. 2008). A recent systematic review and meta-analysis of studies on the contribution of previous history of GDM on risk of type 2 diabetes (Bellamy et al. 2009) showed that there was a 7.4-fold risk of type 2 diabetes associated with history of GDM (rate in exposed = 0.125, rate in the unexposed = 0.0114), giving an attributable risk among women with a history of GDM of 91% ({[0.125 − 0.114]/0.125} × 100). Thus, about 91% of the cases of type 2 diabetes occurring among women with GDM could be prevented with the prevention of GDM. Despite the growing importance of upstream risk factors for type 2 diabetes, there are remarkably few published reports of population-based studies of evaluations of recent trends in prevalence of these factors among women of childbearing age and of their respective attributable or etiologic fractions as main and joint effects across population groups. Such studies are needed to better understand the drivers behind the increasing prevalence of pregnancies complicated by preexisting diabetes.

Studies of the management of pregnancies complicated by preexisting diabetes that adhere to established clinical recommendations (Babbe 2008; Kitzmiller and American Diabetes Association 2008) and of perinatal outcomes in relation to preconception care (CEMACH 2005; Kitzmiller and American Diabetes Association 2008; Kitzmiller et al. 1996) have demonstrated the effectiveness of these downstream interventions in the control and prevention of maternal and fetal complications associated with diabetes in pregnancy. By corollary, it can be inferred that modifiable risk factors for maternal and offspring complications from diabetes in pregnancy today can be related to lack of access to and/or lack of compliance with an adequate glycemic management plan before and during pregnancy. These factors include: unplanned pregnancy/lack of pregnancy counseling, lack of prepregnancy glycemic testing, lack of an adequate diabetes management plan, noncompliance with a prescribed glycemic management plan, and undiagnosed type 2 diabetes.

Of public health concern is that these factors appear to continue to be prevalent in developed regions of the world such as Europe, where the 1989 St. Vincent's Declaration set a clear target of achieving pregnancy outcomes in women with diabetes equivalent to those of the general maternity population within 5 years (CEMACH 2005). With this in mind, it is particularly disturbing to find that a 2002 survey of women with preexisting diabetes in England, Wales, and Northern Ireland reports that several of these factors continue to occur before, during, and after pregnancy. In particular this report (CEMACH 2005) noted, among other findings, that: (1) babies of women with preexisting diabetes continued to have a 3.8-fold increased risk of perinatal mortality compared with babies of mothers in the general population of England, Wales, and Northern Ireland; (2) women with diabetes were poorly prepared for pregnancy as evidenced by the fact that only 35% had received preconception counseling; (3) 37% had a preconception glycemic control measurement; (4) 39% had taken folic acid supplements before conception; (5) only 38% of those with HbA1c measurements had documentation of a HbA1c below 7%; and (6) babies of mothers with diabetes had a twofold increased risk of macrosomia compared with babies born to mothers in the general reference population. The extent to which lack of access to quality of preconception care prevails in other regions of the world is unclear as published literature or reliable surveillance data are scant.

Pregnancies Complicated by Gestational Diabetes

Several nonmodifiable and modifiable risk factors have been identified for GDM. Nonmodifiable risk factors for GDM include older maternal age; non-white race or ethnicity; history of unexplained fetal demise; a suspect glucose intolerance test or delivery of a macrosomic infant; history of GDM; high parity, family history of type 2 diabetes or gestational diabetes in a first-degree relative; polycystic ovarian syndrome; and low stature combined with reduced leg length (Bellamy et al. 2009;

Ben-Haroush et al. 2004; Dabelea et al. 2005; Reece et al. 2009; Solomon et al. 1997). The main potentially modifiable risk factors for GDM identified thus far are prepregnancy overweight status and obesity (Chu et al. 2007; Torloni et al. 2009). A recent systematic review of 70 observational studies related to prepregnancy BMI and diagnosis of GDM (Bottalico 2007) estimates that, compared with women who are of normal weight prepregnancy, women who are overweight prepregnancy have two times the odds of developing GDM, obese women have three times the odds, and morbidly obese women have greater than five times the odds of developing GDM (odds ratios and 95% confidence intervals are 1.97 [1.77–2.1], 3.01 [2.34–3.87] and 5.55 [4.27–7.21], respectively). Data from the Nurses' Health Study provide estimates of GDM of 10.5% among women with prepregnancy obesity (body mass index ≥30 kg/m^2) and 4.6% in the reference population (Solomon et al. 1997), which translates into a relative risk of 2.3 and an unadjusted attributable risk among women with obesity of 56.2% (attributable risk among those with obesity = [rate of GDM among women with obesity – rate of GDM among women in reference group]/rate of GDM among women with obesity). With the increase in overweight and obesity, especially among women of child-bearing age prepregnancy (Chu et al. 2009; Kim et al. 2007), it can be expected that GDM will continue to be a public health burden in the near future. Although other potentially modifiable risk factors for GDM such as sedentary lifestyle, diet, and weight gain during pregnancy are being examined, evidence on their independent or joint effects with overweight and obesity on the prevalence of GDM and on the race/ethnic variation in GDM prevalence is limited at this time. There is a need for further research to identify other potentially modifiable risk factors that may aid in the identification, implementation, and evaluation of effective and acceptable prevention interventions.

■ Prevention Interventions and Public Health Translational Research Issues

Preexisting Diabetes

Existing interventions for pregnancies complicated by preexisting diabetes can be classified into two broad groups: (1) upstream interventions aimed at the prevention of type 1 or type 2 diabetes among women of childbearing age; and (2) downstream interventions aimed at the prevention of complications from diabetes in pregnancy.

Upstream Interventions

Modifiable risk factors for preexisting diabetes among pregnant women or women of childbearing age are essentially those modifiable risk factors for type 2 diabetes, namely: history of GDM, obesity, weight gain, and impaired glucose tolerance/

hyperglycemia (Langer 2006). A number of interventions have been proposed to prevent GDM in some high risk populations with the hope of reducing the risk of type 2 diabetes (Liu et al. 2008; Oostdam et al. 2009). These are described in the next section on the prevention of GDM. How successful such interventions will be likely remains to be determined.

Downstream Interventions

Multidisciplinary programs developed for the management of pregnancies complicated by preexisting diabetes have been shown to be efficacious in reducing the risk of maternal, fetal, and neonatal complications associated with diabetes. Models of care with a responsible patient at the center of the management team have had the best success. The book *Management of Preexisting Diabetes and Pregnancy* (Kitzmiller and American Diabetes Association. 2008) describes models of care with an informed and responsible patient at the center of the management team and the roles of the different clinicians in multidisciplinary diabetes and pregnancy programs. These models of care are based on nonrandomized interventions among nonpregnant diabetic women or among nondiabetic pregnant women, and on observational studies of women with preexisting diabetes, before and during pregnancy. Some of the key principles of such models of care include: (1) education of women with diabetes and childbearing potential about the need for good glucose control before pregnancy as well as active participation in effective family planning; (2) whenever possible, organization of multidiscipline patient-centered team care for women with preexisting diabetes in preparation for pregnancy; (3) evaluation of women with diabetes who are contemplating pregnancy, and, if indicated, initiation of treatment for any medical complication from diabetes; (4) evaluation of medication use before conception, since drugs commonly used to treat diabetes and its complications may be contraindicated or not recommended; (5) continuation of multidisciplinary patient-centered team care throughout pregnancy and postpartum; (6) implementation of and adherence to a regular follow-up visit schedule for adjustments of the treatment plan related to the stage of pregnancy, glycemic, and blood pressure control, weight gain and individual patient needs; and (7) education of pregnant diabetic women about the strong benefits of long-term cardiovascular disease risk factor reduction, breast feeding, and effective family planning with good glycemic control before the next pregnancy.

Recently, the American Diabetes Association published a summary of evidence and consensus recommendations for diagnostic and therapeutic actions for favorable maternal and perinatal outcomes in pregnancies complicated by diabetes (Kitzmiller and American Diabetes Association 2008). Similar recommendations have been published by professional groups in other parts of the world (CEMACH 2005). However, continued reports of population-based studies of excess rates of birth defects and perinatal morbidity and mortality among pregnancies complicated by preexisting diabetes (see Table 10.3), low levels of preconception counseling for diabetic women (Kim et al. 2007), and variable levels of postpartum screening for diabetes (Almario et al. 2008; Ferrara et al. 2009) indicate that such multidisciplinary programs and recommendations vary widely in coverage, effectiveness of implementation, or both. The extent of variations in coverage of populations at risk by such programs or in implementation of recommendations, delineation of the main drivers of such variations, and descriptions of potential enablers of access to quality preconception and prenatal care across population groups are not well known as the literature on these issues remains somewhat limited. Concerted efforts are needed to improve public health surveillance and research that can describe more fully and systematically variations in access to quality preconception care and improved glycemic control throughout pregnancy among women with preexisting diabetes, identify possible determinants of such variations across populations and population subgroups, and contribute to the development of a public health framework for translational research for diabetes in pregnancy.

Gestational Diabetes

Lifestyle

Several studies, including the Diabetes Prevention Program (DPP), show that lifestyle interventions are effective for preventing type 2 diabetes or normalizing blood glucose levels in nonpregnant women at risk for the disease (Ceysens et al. 2006; Hayes and Kriska 2008; Knowler et al. 2002). However, the ability to prevent GDM with dietary and/or physical activity interventions is not as clear. Translating findings from the DPP and other studies on the prevention of type 2 diabetes in at–risk groups to women at risk of GDM has been more difficult. A handful of trials are currently being conducted around the world to see the effects of altering lifestyle in preventing progression to or onset of GDM. These include trials in the Netherlands (Oostdam et al. 2009) and the United States (Chasan-Taber et al. 2009). Other observational studies report a reduction in the risk of GDM in women who engage in physical activity during pregnancy (Dempsey et al. 2004a, 2004b; Oken et al. 2006). Data from a survey study, the National Maternal and Infant Health Study (Liu et al. 2008), show a decreased risk of GDM among women who were nonactive prepregnancy but adopted physical activity during pregnancy when compared with women who remained inactive during pregnancy. Those women who became active had 57% lower adjusted odds of developing gestational diabetes compared with those who remained inactive (odds ratio = 0.43, 95% confidence interval: 0.20–0.93). Similarly, risk of GDM is reduced among Hispanic women who engage in more household/caregiving activities or in sports and exercise activities midpregnancy (Chasan-Taber et al. 2008). However, studies show that fewer women are physically active in pregnancy than before pregnancy, and more than one–third of women are sedentary in pregnancy (Evenson et al. 2004), with only 13%–20% meeting physical activity guidelines (Gollenberg et al. 2008; Zhang and Savitz 1996). Any translational research that is conducted for the prevention of GDM must consider these findings.

Specific dietary factors have been researched for their role in the development of first-time and recurrent GDM, although, as with physical activity, results are difficult to interpret. Increased dietary fat intake has been implied as an independent risk factor for both hyperglycemia in pregnancy (Bo et al. 2001) and recurrent GDM (Moses et al. 1997). Glucose intolerance has also been associated specifically with decreased polyunsaturated fat and increased saturated fat intakes (Wang et al. 2000). Among the Nurses' Health Study cohort, consumption of red and processed meat in particular is associated with increased risk of GDM (Zhang et al. 2006). This and other associations of dietary intakes and GDM risk, however, have not been shown in other studies (Gonzalez-Clemente et al. 2007; Radesky et al. 2008). In a recent Cochrane review, the authors conclude that more research trials with larger samples and longer follow-up times are needed to determine the role of diet in the prevention of both first-onset and recurrent GDM (Tieu et al. 2008).

Preconception Care

Since one modifiable risk factor for GDM is prepregnancy overweight or obesity status, preconception care should focus on activities to maintain a healthy weight. These can involve physical activity and dietary modifications. Several studies support that increased physical activity levels prepregnancy are protective of GDM during pregnancy. In Seattle and Tacoma, Washington (Dempsey et al. 2004b), women who reported engaging in any recreational physical activity in the year prior to pregnancy had a 66% reduction in the risk of developing GDM compared with women who engaged in no recreational physical activity (relative risk = 0.34, 95% confidence interval: 0.17, 0.70). Results were only slightly attenuated after adjustment for maternal age, race, parity, and prepregnancy BMI, although they remained significant. Particularly among high-risk race and ethnic groups within which GDM disparities exist, the importance of a healthy weight when entering pregnancy in the prevention of GDM should be stressed. However, there is also need for structured interventional studies in women prepregnancy to highlight effective strategies a woman can take preconception for the prevention of GDM.

Prediabetes: The Hyperglycemia and Adverse Pregnancy Outcomes Study

Another challenge for the prevention of diabetes and pregnancy complications associated with diabetes is the fact that, during pregnancy, prediabetes or advanced hyperglycemia—without resulting in a diagnosis of GDM—is also associated with adverse maternal and fetal outcomes. The recent multicenter Hyperglycemia and Adverse Pregnancy Outcomes (HAPO) Study, involving over 23,000 pregnant women, shows the effects of differing levels of hyperglycemia on birth outcomes. Results from this influential study show that various degrees of maternal glucose intolerance—measured from fasting, 1-hour, and 2-hour plasma glucose obtained from a 75-g oral glucose tolerance test—less severe than in overt GDM are associated with adverse pregnancy outcomes, including birth weight greater than the 90th percentile and umbilical cord–blood serum C-peptide level above the 90th percentile (fetal hyperinsulinemia) (Metzger et al. 2008). Findings show that these outcomes, as well as incidence of cesarean delivery and incidence of neonatal hypoglycemic episodes, all increase in direct proportion to increasing maternal glucose levels. These results were consistent after adjustment for confounding factors including maternal age, prepregnancy BMI, and blood pressure.

A purpose of this study was to translate findings into meaningful, outcome-based clinical practices for diagnostic criteria of GDM; however, the controversy over diagnostic criteria and strategies for detection and management of GDM and hyperglycemia during pregnancy continues. The findings of the HAPO study, as well as those of others (Langer 2006), underscore the fact that with respect to adverse maternal and fetal effects from hyperglycemia in pregnancy, the threshold levels below which no adverse effects could manifest may vary by type of health outcome and could well be below those considered diagnostic of diabetes or GDM.

■ Future Developments

Diabetes in pregnancy is very complex in its biology, acute maternal and fetal effects, and long-term maternal and offspring consequences. Recent increasing trends in prevalence of diabetes in pregnancy and risk factors for diabetes, as well as younger age at onset, and concerns about undiagnosed and inadequate treatment of diabetes during pregnancy indicate that diabetes in pregnancy is also a complex public health problem with costly consequences for present and future generations of affected individuals as well as society. Although a scientific base for primary and secondary prevention of diabetes in pregnancy has been developed or is being developed, continued reports of increasing trends in prevalence of diabetes in pregnancy as well as ongoing reports of the long-term maternal and known and newly learned functional effects in offspring of diabetic mothers suggest that currently available prevention interventions have had limited uptake or effectiveness in their target populations. Prevention and control of diabetes in pregnancy and its adverse maternal, fetal, and offspring effects are likely to require first the development of a translation framework that addresses the challenges associated with the management of undiagnosed or inadequately treated diabetes among women of childbearing age. Such a framework probably should include as its core components (1) promotion of a life-cycle approach as well as a lifestyle approach to prevention of diabetes; (2) empowerment of patients through education and access to quality health services; (3) availability of multidisciplinary teams of well-trained health promotion and health care providers; (4) organizational systems committed to achieving prevention and control objectives through total quality management by providing ongoing population-based surveillance to identify possible health disparities, quality of care assessments to identify inhibiting and enabling factors, and feedback and training; and (5) allocation of resources to prevention initiatives commensurate with estimates of direct and indirect costs of the acute and long-term effects of diabetes in pregnancy.

There is a need for more research aimed at (1) identifying barriers and enabling factors among women with diabetes or at risk for diabetes to take appropriate actions to improve their pregnancy outcomes through preconception preparation; (2) developing, implementing, and evaluating effective partnerships of women with diabetes with multidisciplinary teams of health professionals; and (3) implementing innovative organizational systems that conduct surveillance of risk factors and outcomes for diabetes in pregnancy, quality of care research, translate research findings into prototypes for prevention initiatives of risk factors and outcomes of diabetes in pregnancy among high-risk population groups, and inform deliberations on the development of more effective prevention policies and interventions. The need for concerted efforts to bring about improved preconception and prenatal health and health care for women with diabetes is a priority.

■ References

Almario CV, et al. (2008). Obstetricians seldom provide postpartum diabetes screening for women with gestational diabetes. *Am J Obstet Gynecol* **198** (5), 528 e1–5.

American Diabetes Association (2004). Gestational diabetes mellitus. *Diabetes Care* **27** (Suppl 1), S88–90.

American Diabetes Association (2007). Diagnosis and classification of diabetes mellitus. *Diabetes Care* **30** (Suppl. 1), S42–7.

Babbe SG (2008). Foreword. In Kitzmiller JL et al., eds. *Managing Preexisting Diabetes and Pregnancy: Technical Reviews and Consensus Recommendations for Care*, pp xiii–xiv. Alexandria, VA: American Diabetes Association.

Balkau B, et al. (2008). Predicting diabetes: clinical, biological, and genetic approaches: data from the Epidemiological Study on the Insulin Resistance Syndrome (DESIR). *Diabetes Care* **31**(10), 2056–61.

Barbour LA, et al. (2007). Cellular mechanisms for insulin resistance in normal pregnancy and gestational diabetes. *Diabetes Care* **30** (Suppl 2), S112–9.

Bell R et al. (2008). Trends in prevalence and outcomes of pregnancy in women with pre-existing type I and type II diabetes. *Bjog* **115**(4), 445–52.

Bellamy L et al. (2009). Type 2 diabetes mellitus after gestational diabetes: a systematic review and meta-analysis. *Lancet* **373**(9677), 1773–9.

Ben-Haroush A et al. (2004). Epidemiology of gestational diabetes mellitus and its association with Type 2 diabetes. *Diabetic Medicine* **21**(2), 103–13.

Bo S et al. (2001). Dietary fat and gestational hyperglycaemia. *Diabetologia* **44**(8), 972–8.

Bottalico JN (2007). Recurrent gestational diabetes: risk factors, diagnosis, management, and implications. *Seminars in Perinatology* **31**(3), 176–84.

Buchanan TA et al. (2007). What is gestational diabetes? *Diabetes Care* **30** (Suppl. 2), S105–11.

Catalano PM et al. (2003). Gestational diabetes and insulin resistance: role in short- and long-term implications for mother and fetus. *Journal of Nutrition* **133** (5 Suppl. 2), 1674S–83S.

Catalano PM et al. (2009). Fetuses of obese mothers develop insulin resistance in utero. *Diabetes Care* **32**(6), 1076–80.

CEMACH (2005). *Confidential Enquiry into Maternal and Child Health: Pregnancy in Women with Type 1 and Type 2 Diabetes in 2002–03, England, Wales, and Northern Ireland*, pp 1–76. London, CEMACH.

Ceysens G et al. (2006). Exercise for diabetic pregnant women. *Cochrane Database of Systematic Reviews* **3**, CD004225.

Chan JC et al. (2009). Diabetes in Asia: epidemiology, risk factors, and pathophysiology. *JAMA* **301**(20), 2129–40.

Chasan-Taber L et al. (2009). A randomized controlled trial of prenatal physical activity to prevent gestational diabetes: design and methods. *Journal of Women's Health (Larchmont)* **18**(6), 851–9.

Chasan-Taber L et al. (2008). Physical activity and gestational diabetes mellitus among Hispanic women. *Journal of Women's Health (Larchmont)* **17**(6), 999–1008.

Cheung NW et al. (2005). Type 2 diabetes in pregnancy: a wolf in sheep's clothing. *Australia and New Zealand Journal of Obstetrics and Gynaecology* **45**(6), 479–83.

Chu SY et al. (2007). Maternal obesity and risk of gestational diabetes mellitus. *Diabetes Care* **30**(8), 2070–6.

Chu SY et al. (2009). Prepregnancy obesity prevalence in the United States, 2004–2005. *Maternal and Child Health Journal* **13**(5), 614–20.

Correa A et al. (2008). Diabetes mellitus and birth defects. *American Journal of Obstetrics and Gynecology* **199**(3), 237 e1–9.

Dabelea D et al. (2000a). Intrauterine exposure to diabetes conveys risks for type 2 diabetes and obesity: a study of discordant sibships. *Diabetes* **49**(12), 2208–11.

Dabelea D et al. (2000b). Effect of diabetes in pregnancy on offspring: follow–up research in the Pima Indians. *Journal of Maternal and Fetal Medicine* **9**(1), 83–8.

Dabelea D et al. (2005). Increasing prevalence of gestational diabetes mellitus (GDM) over time and by birth cohort: Kaiser Permanente of Colorado GDM Screening Program. *Diabetes Care* **28**(3), 579–84.

Diabetes Control and Complications Trial (DCCT) (2000). Effect of pregnancy on microvascular complications in the diabetes control and complications trial. The Diabetes Control and Complications Trial Research Group. *Diabetes Care* **23**(8), 1084–91.

Dempsey JC et al. (2004a). A case-control study of maternal recreational physical activity and risk of gestational diabetes mellitus. *Diabetes Research & Clinical Practice* **66**(2), 203–15.

Dempsey JC et al. (2004b). Prospective study of gestational diabetes mellitus risk in relation to maternal recreational physical activity before and during pregnancy. *American Journal of Epidemiology* **159**(7), 663–70.

Dunne F (2005). Type 2 diabetes and pregnancy. *Seminars in Fetal and Neonatal Medicine* **10**(4), 333–9.

Dunne F et al. (2003). Pregnancy in women with Type 2 diabetes: 12 years outcome data 1990–2002. *Diabetic Medicine* **20**(9), 734–8.

Engelgau MM et al. (1995). The epidemiology of diabetes and pregnancy in the U.S., 1988. *Diabetes Care* **18**(7), 1029–33.

Evenson KR et al. (2004). Leisure-time physical activity among pregnant women in the US. *Paediatric and Perinatal Epidemiology* **18**(6), 400–7.

Evers IM et al. (2004). Risk of complications of pregnancy in women with type 1 diabetes: nationwide prospective study in the Netherlands. *British Medical Journal* **328**(7445), 915.

Ferrara A (2007). Increasing prevalence of gestational diabetes mellitus: a public health perspective. *Diabetes Care* **30** (Suppl. 2), S141–6.

Ferrara A et al. (2004). An increase in the incidence of gestational diabetes mellitus: Northern California, 1991–2000. *Obstetrics and Gynecology* **103**(3), 526–33.

Ferrara A et al. (2009). Trends in postpartum diabetes screening and subsequent diabetes and impaired fasting glucose among women with histories of gestational diabetes mellitus: A report from the Translating Research Into Action for Diabetes (TRIAD) Study. *Diabetes Care* **32**(2), 269–74.

Flegal KM et al. (2002). Prevalence and trends in obesity among US adults, 1999–2000. *JAMA* **288**(14), 1723–7.

Franks PW et al. (2006). Gestational glucose tolerance and risk of type 2 diabetes in young Pima Indian offspring. *Diabetes* **55**(2), 460–5.

Freinkel N (1980). Banting Lecture 1980. Of pregnancy and progeny. *Diabetes* **29**(12), 1023–35.

Getahun D et al. (2008). Gestational diabetes in the United States: temporal trends 1989 through 2004. *American Journal of Obstetrics and Gynecology* **198**(5), 525 e1–5.

Gollenberg A et al. (2008). Dietary behaviors, physical activity, and cigarette smoking among pregnant Puerto Rican women. *American Journal of Clinical Nutrition* **87**(6), 1844–51.

Gonzalez–Clemente JM et al. (2007). Increased cholesterol intake in women with gestational diabetes mellitus. *Diabetes and Metabolism* **33**(1), 25–9.

Hayes C, Kriska A (2008). Role of physical activity in diabetes management and prevention. *Journal of the American Dietetic Association* **108**(4 Suppl 1), S19–23.

Holing EV et al. (1998). Why don't women with diabetes plan their pregnancies? *Diabetes Care* **21**(6), 889–95.

Ishak M, Petocz P (2003). Gestational diabetes among Aboriginal Australians: prevalence, time trend, and comparisons with non-Aboriginal Australians. *Ethnicity & Disease* **13**(1), 55–60.

Jensen DM et al. (2004). Outcomes in type 1 diabetic pregnancies: a nationwide, population-based study. *Diabetes Care* **27**(12), 2819–23.

Karlsson K, Kjellmer I (1972). The outcome of diabetic pregnancies in relation to the mother's blood sugar level. *American Journal of Obstetrics and Gynecology* **112**(2), 213–20.

Kim C et al. (2002). Gestational diabetes and the incidence of type 2 diabetes: a systematic review. *Diabetes Care* **25**(10), 1862–8.

Kim C et al. (2007). Preventive counseling among women with histories of gestational diabetes mellitus. *Diabetes Care* **30**(10), 2489–95.

Kim SY et al. (2007). Trends in pre-pregnancy obesity in nine states, 1993–2003. *Obesity (Silver Spring)* **15**(4), 986–93.

Kitzmiller J et al. (1996). Pre-conception care of diabetes, congenital malformations, and spontaneous abortions. *Diabetes Care* **19**(5), 514–41.

Kitzmiller JL, American Diabetes Association (2008). *Managing Preexisting Diabetes and Pregnancy: Technical Reviews and Consensus Recommendations for Care.* Alexandria, VA: American Diabetes Association.

Kjos SL, Buchanan TA (1999). Gestational diabetes mellitus. *New England Journal of Medicine* **341**(23), 1749–56.

Knowler WC et al. (2002). Reduction in the incidence of type 2 diabetes with lifestyle intervention or metformin. *New England Journal of Medicine* **346**(6), 393–403.

Lain KY, Catalano PM (2007). Metabolic changes in pregnancy. *Clinical Obstetrics and Gynecology* **50**(4), 938–48.

Langer O (2006). *The Diabetes in Pregnancy Dilemma: Leading Change with Proven Solutions.* Lanham, MD: University Press of America.

Langer O, Langer N (2006). *Diabetes Mellitus: From Antiquity to the 21st Century. The Diabetes in Pregnancy Dilemma,* pp 3–9. Lanham, MD: University Press of America.

Langer O et al. (2005). Gestational diabetes: the consequences of not treating. *American Journal of Obstetrics and Gynecology* **192**(4), 989–97.

Lawrence JM et al. (2008). Trends in the prevalence of preexisting diabetes and gestational diabetes mellitus among a racially/ethnically diverse population of pregnant women, 1999–2005. *Diabetes Care* **31**, 899–904.

Liu J et al. (2008). Does physical activity during pregnancy reduce the risk of gestational diabetes among previously inactive women? *Birth* **35**(3), 188–95.

Ma RC, Chan JC (2009). Pregnancy and diabetes scenario around the world: China. *International Journal of Gynaecology and Obstetrics* **104** (Suppl. 1), S42–5.

Macintosh MC et al. (2006). Perinatal mortality and congenital anomalies in babies of women with type 1 or type 2 diabetes in England, Wales, and Northern Ireland: population based study. *British Medical Journal* **333**(7560), 177.

Mahtab H, Habib SH (2009). Social and economic consequences of diabetes in women from low-income countries: a case study from Bangladesh. *International Journal of Gynaecology and Obstetrics* **104** (Suppl. 1), S14–6.

Matyka KA (2008). Type 2 diabetes in childhood: epidemiological and clinical aspects. *British Medical Bulletin* **86**, 59–75.

Melamed N et al. (2008). Spontaneous and indicated preterm delivery in pregestational diabetes mellitus: etiology and risk factors. *Archives of Gynecology and Obstetrics* **278**(2), 129–34.

Metzger BE et al. (2008). Hyperglycemia and adverse pregnancy outcomes. *New England Journal of Medicine* **358**(19), 1991–2002.

Moses RG et al. (1997). The recurrence of gestational diabetes: could dietary differences in fat intake be an explanation? *Diabetes Care* **20**(11), 1647–50.

National Diabetes Data Group (1979). Classification and diagnosis of diabetes mellitus and other categories of glucose intolerance. *Diabetes* **28**(12), 1039–57.

Oken E et al. (2006). Associations of physical activity and inactivity before and during pregnancy with glucose tolerance. Obstetrics & Gynecology **108**(5), 1200–7.

Oostdam N et al. (2009). Design of FitFor2 study: the effects of an exercise program on insulin sensitivity and plasma glucose levels in pregnant women at high risk for gestational diabetes. *BMC Pregnancy and Childbirth* **9**, 1.

Papaspyros NS (1952). *The History of Diabetes Mellitus*. Stuttgart: Thieme.

Pedersen J (1977). *The Pregnant Diabetic and Her Newborn*. Baltimore: Williams & Wilkins.

Pedersen J, Brandstrup E (1956). Fœtal mortality in pregnant diabetics; strict control of diabetes with conservative obstetric management. Lancet **267**(6923), 607–10.

Penney GC et al. (2003). Outcomes of pregnancies in women with type 1 diabetes in Scotland: a national population-based study. *Bjog* **110**(3), 315–8.

Petersen MB et al. (1988). Early growth delay in diabetic pregnancy: relation to psychomotor development at age 4. *British Medical Journal (Clinical Research Edition)* **296**(6622), 598–600.

Pettitt DJ et al. (1988). Congenital susceptibility to NIDDM. Role of intrauterine environment. *Diabetes* **37**(5), 622–8.

Pettitt DJ et al. (2005). Decreasing the risk of diabetic retinopathy in a study of case management: the California Medi-Cal Type 2 Diabetes Study. *Diabetes Care* **28**(12), 2819–22.

Platt MJ et al. (2002). St Vincent's Declaration 10 years on: outcomes of diabetic pregnancies. *Diabetic Medicine* **19**(3), 216–20.

Radesky JS et al. (2008). Diet during early pregnancy and development of gestational diabetes. *Paediatric and Perinatal Epidemiology* **22**(1), 47–59.

Ray JG et al. (2001). Preconception care and the risk of congenital anomalies in the offspring of women with diabetes mellitus: a meta-analysis. *Quarterly Journal of Medicine* **94**(8), 435–44.

Reece EA et al. (2009). Gestational diabetes: the need for a common ground. *Lancet* **373**(9677), 1789–97.

Retnakaran R et al. (2008). Glucose intolerance in pregnancy and future risk of pre-diabetes or diabetes. *Diabetes Care* **31**(10), 2026–31.

Rizzo T et al. (1991). Correlations between antepartum maternal metabolism and child intelligence. *New England Journal of Medicine* **325**(13), 911–6.

Schaefer-Graf UM et al. (2000). Patterns of congenital anomalies and relationship to initial maternal fasting glucose levels in pregnancies complicated by type 2 and gestational diabetes. *American Journal of Obstetrics and Gynecology* **182**(2), 313–20.

Sells CJ et al. (1994). Long-term developmental follow-up of infants of diabetic mothers. *Journal of Pediatrics* **125**(1), S9–17.

Seshiah V et al. (2009). Pregnancy and diabetes scenario around the world: India. *International Journal of Gynaecology and Obstetrics* **104** (Suppl. 1), S35–8.

Sharpe PB et al. (2005). Maternal diabetes and congenital anomalies in South Australia 1986–2000: a population-based cohort study. *Birth Defects Research Part A Clinical and Molecular Teratology* **73**(9), 605–11.

Sheffield JS et al. (2002). Maternal diabetes mellitus and infant malformations. *Obstetrics and Gynecology* **100** (5 Part 1), 925–30.

Skyler JS et al. (2009). Intensive glycemic control and the prevention of cardiovascular events: implications of the ACCORD, ADVANCE, and VA diabetes trials: a position statement of the American Diabetes Association and a scientific statement of the American College of Cardiology Foundation and the American Heart Association. *Diabetes Care* **32** (1), 187–92.

Solomon CG et al. (1997). A prospective study of pregravid determinants of gestational diabetes mellitus. *JAMA* **278**(13), 1078–83.

Tieu J et al. (2008). Dietary advice in pregnancy for preventing gestational diabetes mellitus. *Cochrane Database of Systematic Reviews* **2**, CD006674.

Torloni MR et al. (2009). Prepregnancy BMI and the risk of gestational diabetes: a systematic review of the literature with meta-analysis. *Obesity Reviews* **10** (2), 194–203.

Vaarasmaki M et al. (2000). Outpatient management does not impair outcome of pregnancy in women with type 1 diabetes. *Diabetes Research and Clinical Practice* **47** (2), 111–7.

Verier-Mine O et al. (2005). Is pregnancy a risk factor for microvascular complications? The EURODIAB Prospective Complications Study. *Diabetic Medicine* **22** (11), 1503–9.

Vohr BR, Boney CM (2008). Gestational diabetes: the forerunner for the development of maternal and childhood obesity and metabolic syndrome? *Journal of Maternal-Fetal and Neonatal Medicine* **21** (3), 149–57.

Wang Y et al. (2000). Dietary variables and glucose tolerance in pregnancy. *Diabetes Care* **23** (4), 460–4.

White P (1949). Pregnancy complicating diabetes. *American Journal of Medicine* **7** (5), 609–16.

World Health Organization (1985). Diabetes mellitus. Report of a WHO Study Group. *World Health Organization Technical Report Series* **727**, 1–113.

Yajnik CS (2009). Nutrient-mediated teratogenesis and fuel-mediated teratogenesis: two pathways of intrauterine programming of diabetes. *International Journal of Gynaecology and Obstetrics* **104** (Suppl 1), S27–31.

Yang J et al. (2006). Fetal and neonatal outcomes of diabetic pregnancies. *Obstetrics and Gynecology* **108** (3 Part 1), 644–50.

Zhang C et al. (2006). A prospective study of dietary patterns, meat intake and the risk of gestational diabetes mellitus. *Diabetologia* **49** (11), 2604–13.

Zhang J, Savitz DA (1996). Exercise during pregnancy among US women. *Annals of Epidemiology* **6** (1), 53–9.

11. DIABETES AND DISABILITY, COGNITIVE DECLINE, AND AGING-RELATED OUTCOMES

Stefano Volpato and Cinzia Maraldi

■ Main Public Health Messages

- The prevalence of diabetes increases with age and is expected to increase further in older persons worldwide in the next decades.
- In older patients, diabetes synergistically interacts with multiple aged-related pathophysiological modifications, thereby increasing the incidence of numerous geriatric syndromes, including disability, falls, and dementia.
- Lifestyle modification, including exercise and moderate weight loss combined with a healthy diet, is the best intervention to prevent diabetes and its complications in older people.
- There is a pressing need for randomized clinical trials specifically designed for older patients with diabetes. These trials must include important geriatric syndromes as main outcomes.
- Models of care that integrate traditional diabetes care and multidimensional assessment should be developed, tested, and implemented.

■ Introduction

Diabetes mellitus is one of the most prevalent chronic diseases in Western countries. Its prevalence rises steeply with age, and, as a result of the ongoing demographic transition and aging of the overall population, in Western countries older people account for more than one-third of the adult population with diabetes. As a consequence, the clinical picture of type 2 diabetes in older adults in these countries is evolving profoundly. In the past few years epidemiologic and clinical studies have consistently associated diabetes with numerous clinical outcomes that are typical of the oldest population, outcomes that are referred to as geriatric syndromes. These conditions, of which physical and cognitive impairment, falls, and depression are among the most common, are increasingly affecting the older diabetic population and already represent a looming sword of Damocles for patients and health care systems in term of quality of life and health care costs. This chapter summarizes the most compelling evidence for the relationship between diabetes and these emerging late-life complications and discusses potential avenues for secondary and tertiary prevention.

■ Epidemiology

Diabetes in Older Persons

Diabetes is one of the most common chronic diseases among older persons. For community-dwelling people in the United States, its prevalence is routinely estimated in the National Health Interview Survey (NHIS), in which a representative subsample of households is selected every year. Based on these data, in 2005 diabetes had been diagnosed in 17% of Americans aged 65 years or older (Pleis and Lethbridge-Çejku 2006). Of all people with diagnosed diabetes in the United States in that year, almost 40% were 65 or older (5.9 million people), of whom 2.5 million were 75 or older. The rate of diagnosed diabetes rises with age, and in 2005 it peaked at 19.1% in the 65–74 age group (Pleis and Lethbridge-Çejku 2006). Diabetes ranks with cardiovascular disease and cancer as a major cause of morbidity in persons aged 65 years or older, although arthritis and hypertension are even more common. Its prevalence is even more impressive in older people living in nursing homes (who comprise 4% of older Americans). Based on different surveys that used the Minimum Data Set records, the estimated prevalence of diabetes in the nursing home population was 18.1% between 1992 and 1996 and 26% in 2006 (Travis et al. 2004).

In addition to the high rates of diagnosed diabetes in the United States, many older people meet fasting blood glucose criteria for the disease (≥126 mg/dL) but have not yet been diagnosed. According to the National Health and Nutrition Examination Survey (NHANES) for the period of 1999–2002, 6.0% of the U.S. population aged 65 years and older had undiagnosed diabetes. When estimated rates of diagnosed and undiagnosed diabetes are considered together, one sees that more than 22% (or one in every four to five people) of the older population has diabetes (Cowie et al. 2006).

These extremely high prevalence rates reflect in part the increasing rate of new cases in this age group. In 2005, the incidence of diagnosed diabetes was highest among adults aged 65–79 years (13.1 per 1000) (http://www.cdc.gov/diabetes/statistics/incidence/fig3.htm), a rate that was 17% higher than in 1995 (11.2%) (see Fig. 11.1) and more than twice that of 1990 (6.0%).

The current high prevalence of diabetes and its recognition as a major public threat notwithstanding, recent projections suggest that the future burden of diabetes will be even more dramatic. According to the Census Bureau's population projection, the number of Americans aged 75 years or older with diabetes will

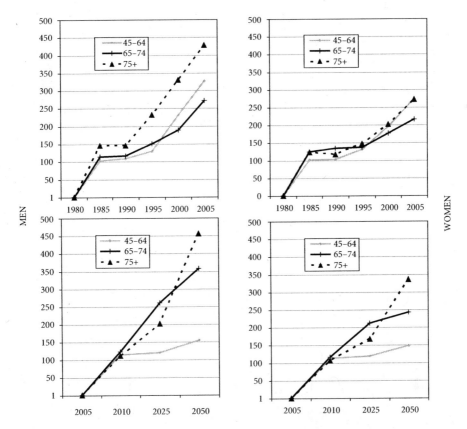

FIGURE 11.1. Observed (1980–2005) and estimated (2005–2050) number of diabetes cases as a percentage of the 1980 and 2005 number, by sex and age group for selected years (United States of America). (Source: Centers for Disease Control and Prevention. National diabetes fact sheet: general information and national estimates on diabetes in the United States, 2005. Atlanta, GA: U.S. Department of Health and Human Services, Centers for Disease Control and Prevention, 2005 and U.S. Bureau of Census.)

quadruple from 2005 to 2050, when the total number of patients with diabetes in that age group will approximate 9 million.

Diabetes as a Risk Factor for Physical Disability in Older Persons

Several epidemiologic studies conducted in the United States and other countries have found diabetes to be among the major chronic conditions associated with disability in different domains of physical function. These studies are summarized in Table 11.1.

For example, among the over 6000 participants examined at the sixth annual follow-up in the Established Populations for Epidemiologic Studies in the Elderly (EPESE), prevalent diabetes (based on self-reports) was associated with twice the probability of disability in activities of daily living (ADL) and mobility tasks, including walking one-fourth of a mile. Very similar results have been obtained using data

TABLE 11.1 *Selected Epidemiologic Studies Estimating Prevalence and Odds of Disability for Selected Domains of Function According to Diabetes Status and Sex*

| | | | | | Domains of Physical Function | | | | | | | |
| | | | | | ADL | | Walking ¼ Mile | | Climbing Stairs | | |
Study	Sex	Age, years	Diabetes	n	%	Odds Ratio (95% CI)	%	Odds Ratio (95% CI)	%	Odds Ratio (95% CI)	Adjustment Variables
EPESE* (1993)	Men	70–103	No	1,815	15.4	1	26.7	1	14.7	1	Age, race, BMI, education, comorbidity
			Yes	385	26.8	2.0 (1.4–2.7)	38.6	1.6 (1.2–2.1)	21.7	1.4 (0.9–1.9)	
	Women	70–103	No	3,420	20.6	1	43.6	1	22.8	1	
			Yes	648	30.1	1.7 (1.4–2.2)	58.9	1.7 (1.4–2.1)	34.4	1.7 (1.4–2.2)	
Framingham (Guccione et al. 1994)	Men/ women	≥60	No	1648	—	—	17.0	1	5.3	1	Age, sex, comorbidity
			Yes	110	—	—	29.8	1.7 (1.1–2.7)	13.8	2.9 (1.5–5.8)	
PAQUID (Bourdel-Marchasson et al. 1997)	Men/ women	≥65	No	2,555	13.2	1	19.3	1	25	1	Unadjusted
			Yes	237	16.5	1.4 (0.9–1.9)	30	1.8 (1.3–2.5)	36.2	1.7 (1.3–2.3)	

Study	Sex	Age	Obese	N							Adjustment
NHANES (Gregg et al. 2000)	Women	≥60	No	2,891	—	—	30.3	1	45.9	1	Age, race, education, BMI
			Yes	584	—	—	51.2	2.1 (1.5–2.9)	30.0	1.7 (1.5–2.9)	
	Men	≥60	No	2,667	—	—	21.2	1	27.8	1	Age, race, education, BMI
			Yes	446	—	—	32.8	1.9 (1.3–2.6)	18.6	1.6 (1.1–2.4)	
WHAS (Maty et al. 2004)	Women	≥65	No	483	14.4	1	35.4	1	22.4	1	Unadjusted
			Yes	3,087	27.3	2.2 (1.8–2.8)	51.8	1.9 (1.6–2.4)	38.5	2.2 (1.8–2.6)	
ILSA (Maggi et al. 2004)	Women	65–85	No	2,237	33.0	1	NA	—	23.7	1	Unadjusted
			Yes	349	49.1	1.7 (1.2–2.2)	NA	—	33.3	1.5 (1.02–2.2)	

ADL, activities of daily living; CI, confidence interval; BMI, body mass index; EPESE, Established Population for Epidemiologic Studies of the Elderly; PAQUID, Personnes Agées Quid study; NHANES, National Health and Nutrition Examination Survey; WHAS, Women's Health and Aging Study; ILSA, Italian Longitudinal Study of Aging.

¹Personal unpublished data.

from the Third NHANES (NHANES III) (Gregg et al. 2000) and from epidemiologic studies conducted in Europe. In NHANES III, also based on self-reports, 51%
of women with diabetes had some degree of difficulty in walking one-fourth of a
mile, versus 30% of women without diabetes. As for other chronic complications of
diabetes, the adjusted likelihood of having physical disability increases with longer
duration of the disease in both men and women (Gregg et al. 2000).

Evidence for a disabling effect of diabetes is further supported by a study of
nondisabled older individuals in which persons with diabetes were more likely
than their counterparts without diabetes to perform poorly on time-based performance tests using the lower extremities. Furthermore this study found that diabetic
patients with poor glycemic control (hemoglobin A1C >7%) had a 50% greater risk
of functional limitation than patients with optimal metabolic control (de Rekeneire
et al. 2003). Globally taken, these results suggest that independent of the background prevalence of diabetes and disability in the studied population, diabetes
is associated with a 50%–100% excess risk of disability in both men and women.
The cross-sectional relationship between diabetes and disability includes a broad
range of physical and functional domains, although the strength of the association
is particularly evident for mobility and other activities related to lower-extremity
function.

Fewer studies have investigated the longitudinal association between diabetes
and disability. However the prospective studies in which onset of new disability was
evaluated as a function of diabetes status in persons free of disability at baseline
show a fairly consistent pattern of associations supporting the existence of a causal
relationship. At least four properly designed studies have reported an increased incidence of functional limitation or lower-extremity disability in older patients with
diabetes. For example, in the EPESE study, self-reported diabetes at baseline predicted a 10%–60% increased risk of loss of lower-extremity mobility over the 4-year
follow-up, independent of demographic characteristics and prevalent chronic conditions (Guralnik et al. 1993). A more recent longitudinal study from the Hispanic
EPESE (Al Snih et al. 2005) found that older Mexican Americans with diabetes had
increased risks for ADL and mobility disability ranging from 50%–100% over a
7-year follow-up.

Elsewhere, the Study of Osteoporotic Fractures enrolled over 8344 older women,
of whom 527 had prevalent diabetes at baseline. Over the 8-year follow-up average
yearly incidence of any disability was 9.8% for women with diabetes and 4.7% for
women without diabetes. In this study the most common disability outcomes were
inability to perform heavy housework (8.5% versus 4.0%) and being unable to walk
one-fourth of a mile (4.3% versus 1.9%) (Gregg et al. 2002). The public health implication of the effect of diabetes on the disablement process of older people is rein-
forced by the population-attributable fraction for diabetes. Combining incidence
data from the Study of Osteoporotic Fractures with the overall prevalence of diabetes estimated in the 1988–1994 NHANES, we find the unadjusted population attributable fraction for diabetes was 17% for any disability, 19.3% for inability to walk

one-fourth of a mile, and 17.6% for heavy housework, suggesting that almost one out of five cases of disability was due to the disabling effect of diabetes. In this study statistical adjustment for potential confounders or mediators only partially attenuated the strength of the association between diabetes and disability, suggesting a direct disabling effect of diabetes. In the Women's Health and Aging Study, a 3-year prospective study of older women with functional impairment or mild disability, women with diabetes were at greater risk for further decline in objective measures of lower-extremity function and for transition to severe mobility and ADL disability than women without diabetes (Volpato et al. 2003). These results suggest that the disabling effect of diabetes on physical function is still present and clinically significant, even in the subgroup of frail, physically impaired, and oldest women.

■ The Pathway from Diabetes to Physical Disability

The biological mechanisms explaining the association between diabetes and physical disability in older adults have not been completely elucidated, but at the population level the association is certainly multifactorial. Identification of the causal factors linking diabetes to disability is of great importance for implementing effective strategies for secondary and tertiary prevention. Several diseases and impairments, including cardiovascular diseases, peripheral neuropathy, obesity, and visual deficits, are more prevalent in patients with diabetes and may explain the greater burden of disability associated with the disease. Figure 11.2 depicts a putative pathway, constructed on the model proposed by Nagi, summarizing the multiple mechanisms that can lead to disability in a person with diabetes.

The roles of several comorbidities associated with diabetes have been evaluated in different studies, but results have varied according to the studied populations

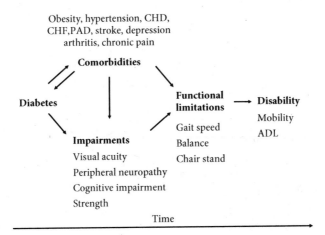

FIGURE 11.2. Theoretical model of the pathway from diabetes to disability. CHD, coronary heart disease; CHF, congestive heart failure; PAD, peripheral arterial disease

and the studies' designs. In NHANES III coronary heart disease and obesity were the most important mediators among women, accounting for more than 50% of the excess risk for disability observed in people with diabetes. Among men, on the other hand, coronary heart disease and stroke were the most important explanatory factors, explaining 25% and 21% of the excess disability risk, respectively. In the Study of Osteoporotic Fractures (Gregg et al. 2002), age, coronary heart disease, arthritis, physical inactivity, body mass index (BMI), and visual impairment were key predictors of incident disability among diabetic women who were free of disability at baseline. In the Women's Health and Aging Study, which had standardized, objective information on lower-extremity diseases, peripheral nerve dysfunction, peripheral arterial disease, and depression were the main mediators of physical disability, accounting for 20%–30% (depending on the type of physical outcome considered) of the excess risk of disability associated with diabetes (Volpato et al. 2002). In each of these studies, however, a significant excess risk of disability associated with diabetes remained, even after controlling for diabetes-related complications. For example in the Women's Health and Aging Study, even after adjustment for all covariates, there was a 40% remnant of the association between diabetes and walking disability. Globally taken, these results suggest either that diabetes has a direct intrinsic effect on physical performance and in turn on onset of disability or that other unmeasured or undiscovered diabetes-related complications influence the risk for disability.

Sarcopenia, a term that describes decreased skeletal muscle mass and strength, is common in the geriatric population and is a powerful risk factor for ADL and mobility disability. Although older patients with type 2 diabetes, because of their increased overall body mass, often have adequate muscle mass, recent reports from the Health, Aging, and Body Composition (Health ABC) Study (Park et al. 2006) found that such patients have poorer muscle quality at baseline and a steeper decline in leg strength over time than older adults without diabetes. Interestingly, about 50% of the observed decline in strength was not accounted for by a greater loss of lower-extremity muscle mass, suggesting that in older adults diabetes is associated with decline in muscle quality independent of potential loss of muscle mass (Park 2007).

Diabetes is associated with increased levels of several inflammatory markers that in turn are powerful risk factors for physical disability in older adults. Yet, only one study has formally investigated the hypothesis that systemic inflammation might mediate the association between diabetes and disability. This study, however, demonstrated that the increased risk of future limitation in mobility observed in older adults with diabetes is independent of baseline levels of C-reactive protein and interleukin-6. Despite this result this hypothesis might deserve further research in the next future. Understanding the mechanism underlying the decline in muscle strength and quality in people with diabetes might open important therapeutic options.

None of the studies mentioned above evaluated the role of chronic pain as a potential mediator of the association between diabetes and disability, and yet chronic pain is an important problem in older persons with diabetes. Indeed, one recent survey (based on self-reports) found that almost 55% of patients aged 60 and older with diabetes and older had chronic pain (Krein et al. 2005). There are several potential sources of pain in older patients with diabetes and often two or more painful conditions coexist, including peripheral neuropathies, foot ulcers, peripheral arterial disease, arthritis, and other sources of musculoskeletal pain. Regardless of the underlying conditions that cause pain, the presence of persistent pain, and particularly back and lower-extremity pain, might have an effect on multiple steps of the disabling process. Moreover, this direct disabling effect of pain might interact with other diabetes-related mechanisms, greatly enhancing the risk for functional limitation or disability (Leveille and Volpato 2007).

In the Health ABC Study, diabetes and obesity were more common among those with the most severe back pain than in those without back pain, and persons with the most severe back pain had the lowest scores on mobility performance tests and self-reported functioning, suggesting that coexisting pain might, at least in part, explain the association between diabetes and functional decline (Weiner et al. 2003).

In summary, a variety of conditions might contribute to the onset of disability in older adults with diabetes (see Table 11.2). Although at the individual level one single complication may fully account for the presence of disability, at the population level multiple conditions need to be considered simultaneously. Most of the conditions identified as potential risk factors for disability among patients with diabetes are amenable to intervention and should represent the targets for preventive strategies aimed at reducing the diabetes-associated burden of disability.

TABLE 11.2   *Putative Risk Factors for Disability in Older Adults with Diabetes*

Nonmodifiable	Potentially Modifiable
• Age • Duration of diabetes • Genetic background	• Obesity • Glycemic control • Peripheral arterial diseases • Peripheral neuropathies • Visual impairment • Congestive heart failure • Stroke • Cognitive impairment • Depressive symptoms • Arthritis • Widespread and lower-extremity pain • Poor muscle quality • Low-grade systemic inflammation

Cognitive Decline and Dementia

Cognitive impairment and diabetes, both among the most pressing public health problems facing the older population, share a number of features, including high prevalence after age 65 years (and increasing prevalence with added years), an important impact on the patient's and caregiver's quality of life, and substantial health care costs. Analysis of observational studies on cognitive impairment in patients with diabetes or impaired glucose tolerance supports the association between diabetes and moderate cognitive impairment (Pasquier et al. 2006). Although most studies are cross-sectional analyses or case-control studies affected by methodological issues, at least five large and well-designed population-based longitudinal studies found a significant association between diabetes or hyperglycemia at baseline and the risk of incident cognitive impairment (Biessels et al. 2006). The association was observed for both global cognitive decline and specific domains, including memory and executive functions. The role of diabetes as a risk factor for cognitive impairment was independent of the effect of associated cardiovascular comorbidities like hypertension, dyslipidemia, and obesity, but important interactions were found among diabetes, blood pressure levels, and the Apo E (apolipoprotein E) genotype.

Further support for the hypothesis of a causal biological link between diabetes and late-life cognitive disorders comes from epidemiologic studies that investigated the risk of incident dementia as a function of diabetes. The incidence of any type of dementia was increased in people with diabetes in most of the studies reporting this outcome, with an excess risk ranging from 50%–100% in comparisons with people without diabetes. The Rotterdam study, in examining incident dementia, estimated a population attributable risk as high as 8.8% for diabetes (Ott et al. 1999). Most studies provided separate figures for Alzheimer disease and vascular dementia. Although the strength of the association was more impressive for the vascular subtype (range of excess risk: 100%–200%), a fairly consistent pattern was found also for the Alzheimer form. In one population-based cohort study of older Japanese-American men, including 216 subjects who underwent autopsy, the association between diabetes and risk of a clinical diagnosis of Alzheimer disease was corroborated by the finding of a greater number of neurofibrillary tangles and neuritic plaques in men with diabetes than in those without diabetes (Peila, Rodriguez, and Launer 2002).

Diabetes mellitus, being a complex metabolic disorder, is a powerful atherogenic risk factor closely associated with other risk factors for cognitive impairment in the general population, including hypertension, dyslipidemia, and chronic cerebrovascular disease. These risk factors, together with demographic and socioeconomic influences, diabetes complications, and genetic factors, are likely to act as important modulators of the association between diabetes and dementia. Most of the studies showing an excess risk of cognitive impairment and dementia in older people with diabetes have statistically accounted for the effect of potential confounders and of preexisting vascular disease, thereby supporting the hypothesis that diabetes may have a direct and causal relationship with cognitive decline (see Table 11.3). Furthermore, some papers have suggested that the effect of diabetes may be synergistically enhanced by the presence of other risk factors (hypertension) (Xu et al. 2004) or by genetic predisposition (Apo E genotype) (Peila, Rodriguez, and Launer 2002). Conversely, the potential mediating effects of diabetes complications and diabetes-related comorbidities on the relationship with cognitive decline have not been fully analyzed. Therefore, there is scant information on the roles of diabetes duration, glycemic control, type of therapy, level of insulin resistance or sensitivity, and microvascular complications. For example, some studies indicate that the risk of dementia is highest in those who are treated with insulin, but whether this is related to a longer duration of diabetes, higher severity of the disease, higher rates of hypoglycemic events, or a direct effect of insulin itself, is still unknown. From this point of view, high-quality studies specifically designed to investigate the effects of diabetes and its related complications on the risk of dementia would provide valuable information.

Overall, the results of epidemiologic studies strongly indicate that the risks of both Alzheimer disease and vascular dementia are increased in patients with diabetes, although the controversies and problems of clinical diagnostic criteria for dementia types should be considered.

There are many biological mechanisms that could explain an association between diabetes and dementia. For example, there is mounting evidence that the brain of older people affected by dementia is commonly characterized by a mixture of pathologies related to both Alzheimer and vascular disease. Diabetes may facilitate the clinical onset of any type of dementia through its associations with stroke and other cerebrovascular disease, causing vascular dementia or accelerating cognitive decline and thereby "unmasking" Alzheimer disease at an earlier stage. Furthermore, vascular reactivity may be adversely affected by metabolic abnormalities and advanced glycosylation end products, resulting in perfusion abnormalities. The increased risk of Alzheimer disease may also be mediated by the exacerbation of β-amyloid neurotoxicity by advanced glycosylation end products identified in the matrix of neurofibrillary tangles and amyloid plaques. In addition, hyperinsulinemia, a common metabolic abnormality in type 2 diabetes, has been identified as a risk factor for accelerated cognitive decline and dementia. Part of this association is likely to be mediated through vascular disease because insulin is an independent risk factor for vascular disease, but insulin might also have direct effects on the brain. Finally, chronic hypoglycemia might also have an important role, particularly among the oldest patients.

Depression

Depression, a key geriatric syndrome associated with diabetes, strongly affects the quality of life of older adults, and several studies have reported an increased prevalence of clinically significant depressive symptoms among subjects with diabetes.

TABLE 11.3   *Major Population-Based Longitudinal Studies Estimating Incidence and Relative Risk of Dementia According to Diabetes Status*

| | | | | | | Dementia Type | | | | | | | |
| | | | | | | All | | Alzheimer | | Vascular | | |
Study	Sex	Age (Years)	Follow-up (Years)	Diabetes	n	%	Relative Risk (95% CI)	%	Relative Risk (95% CI)	%	Relative Risk (95% CI)	Adjustment for
HISAYAMA (Yoshitake et al. 1995)	Men/women	≥65	7.0	No	758	—	—	—	1	—	1	Age, race, education,
				Yes	70	—	—	—	2.2 (1.0–4.9)	—	2.8 (1.6–3.0)	
CAMBRIDGE (Brayne et al. 1998)	Women	≥75	2.4	No	351	20.0	1	13.0	1	—	—	Age, sex
				Yes	25	8.8	2.6 (0.9–7.8)	8.8	1.4 (1.1–17.0)	—	—	
ROTTERDAM (Ott et al. 1999)	Men/women	≥55	2.1	No	5678	1.6	1	—	1	—	1	Age, sex
				Yes	692	4.9	1.9 (1.3–2.8)	—	1.9 (1.2–3.1)	—	2.0 (0.7–5.6)	
WHICAP (Luchsinger et al. 2001)	Men/women	≥65	4.3	No	1007	—	—	12.1	1	2.1	1†	Demographic and vascular risk factors
				Yes	255	—	—	13.7	1.3 (0.8–1.9)	5.9	3.4 (1.7–6.9)	

Study	Sex	Age			N							Adjustment
HAAS (Peila et al. 2002)	Men	≥65	2.9	No	1674	4.5	1	2.2	1	1.0	1	Demographic and vascular risk factors
				Yes	900	5.9	1.5 (1.0–2.2)	3.5	1.8 (1.1–2.9)	1.9	2.3 (1.1–5.0)	
CSHA (MacKnight et al. 2004)	Men/women	≥65	5	No	5071	NA	1	NA	1	NA	1	Demographic and vascular risk factors
				Yes	503	NA	1.3 (0.9–1.8)	NA	1.3 (0.8–2.0)	NA	1.6 (1.1–2.3)	
KUNGSHOLMEN (Xu et al. 2004)	Men/women	≥75	4.7	No	1187	6.1*	1	4.7*	1	0.9*	1	Demographic and vascular risk factors
				Yes	114	8.9*	1.5 (1.0–2.1)	6.1*	1.3 (0.9–2.1)	2.2*	2.6 (1.2–6.1)	

CI, confidence interval; WHICAP, Washington Heights and Inwood Columbia Aging Project; HAAS, Honolulu-Asia Aging Study; CSHA, Canadian Study of Health and Aging.
*Incidence rates per 100 person-years.
†Stroke-associated dementia.

A meta-analysis of studies on the association between diabetes and depression reported that subjects with diabetes had twice the likelihood of depression as those without diabetes (Anderson et al. 2001). In addition, prospective studies of subjects with diabetes have suggested that their course of depression is often unfavorable, and persistent depression is common. However, the causal mechanisms and the temporal sequence of the diabetes–depression association have not been clearly delineated. Evidence from prospective studies suggests that depression may increase the risk of the onset of diabetes (Knol et al. 2006). On the other hand, diabetes is among the most psychologically and behaviorally demanding chronic illnesses, and vascular brain damage is yet another of the many burdens to which diabetes patients are more susceptible, considerations suggesting that the temporal sequence may well be diabetes and then depression. Moreover, neuroendocrine abnormalities associated with diabetes, including altered activity of the hypothalamic-pituitary-adrenocortical axis with a higher level of plasma cortisol, may be involved in the pathophysiology of mood disorders. From this point of view, it is interesting that a recent prospective study among older adults found diabetes to be associated with an increased risk of developing significant depressive symptoms, with the risk being higher for patients with poor metabolic control (Maraldi et al. 2007).

Depressive disorders significantly decrease quality of life and have important socioeconomic consequences as well. The presence of depressive symptoms is significantly associated with higher levels of hemoglobin A1C, a well-established predictor of diabetes complications, and depression increases the risk of mortality among persons with diabetes (Zhang et al. 2005). Reduction in quality of life and adverse effects on functional ability caused by depression set up the possibility of a synergic effect of diabetes and depression on functional outcomes. Depressive symptoms may lead to poor adherence to treatment and undesirable lifestyle behaviors, such as inappropriate diet, inactivity, and continued use of tobacco. Altogether these effects may lead to increasing complications and severity of the diabetes, which in turn may further aggravate depressive symptoms, leading to a downward spiral in the patient's health status. From the public health perspective, one sees the worsening of medical outcomes, along with the increased use of health care resources associated with depressed mood, leading to higher health care costs.

In conclusion, depression, either as a risk factor or as a consequence of diabetes, affects progression of the disease, compliance with treatment, performance status, and quality of life. From this point of view, an essential component of a complete clinical approach and high-quality care for the patient with diabetes should include appropriate screening for the early detection and effective treatment of depressive symptoms.

Urinary Incontinence

The high prevalence among older people of age-related changes in the lower urinary tract, functional and cognitive impairment, and associated comorbidities hinders a straightforward understanding of the independent pathophysiological role of diabetes in bladder dysfunction. Current understanding of this condition sees it as a progressive problem encompassing a broad spectrum of lower urinary tract symptoms that include urinary urgency, frequency, nocturia, and both urge and stress incontinence. Although bladder cystopathy, a condition defined as reduced bladder sensation, poor contractility, and increased post-void residual, most likely represents end-stage bladder failure and is relatively uncommon, urinary incontinence is a classic and common geriatric syndrome with multiple risk factors, including physical limitations, visual and hearing decline, cognitive and affective impairment, and other predisposing factors. In older persons, therefore, diabetes and diabetes-related comorbidity can lead to urinary incontinence in multiple ways.

The epidemiologic studies published so far, although their designs and findings are to an important degree heterogeneous, demonstrate that in women diabetes is clearly associated with the likelihood of urinary incontinence or lower urinary tract symptoms, with the degree of excess risk ranging from 30%–100% (Smith 2006). The association with diabetes is stronger for more severe urinary incontinence and tends to increase as a function of the severity of diabetes when measured as longer duration of the disease (>5 years) or need for insulin treatment. Two studies provided the proportion of cases of urinary incontinence attributable to diabetes: in the Study of Osteoporotic Fractures (Brown et al. 1996), diabetes accounted for 4% of prevalent cases of daily incontinence, whereas longitudinal analysis of the Nurses' Health Study (Lifford et al. 2005) found that up to 17% of weekly incontinence could be attributable to diabetes and up to 50% when severe cases were considered.

In men, lower urinary tract symptoms are common, age-related complaints that are often attributed to benign prostatic hyperplasia. However, among men with diabetes, similar symptoms may also result from bladder dysfunction due to denervation and poor contractility of the detrusor muscle. Common problems of older men with diabetes include symptoms of urgency, frequency, and nocturia that may occur from an overactive detrusor muscle resulting from prostatic hyperplasia but also from microvascular complications of diabetes. The effects of diabetes on lower urinary tract symptoms and benign prostatic hyperplasia have been less investigated than have the effects of prostatic hypertrophy on urinary symptoms, and results are still controversial. Recent evidence suggests that lower urinary tract symptoms may occur more frequently among men with diabetes, with an estimated 25% to nearly 100% increased risk of lower urinary tract symptoms in men with diabetes. On the other hand, no convincing evidence supports the role of diabetes as an independent risk factor for benign prostatic hyperplasia, but among men with this condition, diabetes seems to enhance the onset of lower urinary tract symptoms.

Falls and Fractures

Older people with diabetes are particularly vulnerable to falls and related complications, and several epidemiologic studies have demonstrated that diabetes is associated with an increased risk of falls over time. The relationship between diabetes and falls has been studied predominantly in women but has been reported also in men. The excess risk of falls related to diabetes has been demonstrated across the whole spectrum of functional status, including well-functioning persons, those who are disabled, and nursing home residents. The presence of peripheral neuropathy; prevalent stroke or cardiovascular disease; orthostatic hypotension; poor lower-extremity performance, including problems with balance; insulin therapy; obesity; and widespread musculoskeletal pain are important predictors of the likelihood of falling (Volpato et al. 2005). Most of these are common diabetes-related complications that may be prevented or postponed by optimal glycemic control. Nevertheless, in older people, intensive glycemic control is associated with increased risk of severe hypoglycemia that in turn is a risk factor for falls, fractures, and mortality. Indeed, a recent analysis of the Health ABC Study reported that among older diabetic patients intensive glycemic control (A1C $\leq$6%) achieved with insulin therapy was associated with an adjusted odds ratio (OR) of 4.1 (95% confidence interval [CI] 1.2–13.5) for risk of falling (Schwartz et al. 2008).

Of note, diabetes increases not only the risk of falls but also the risk of fracture. In the Health ABC Study, diabetes was associated with a 64% (95% CI 7–151%) increased risk of nontraumatic fracture that was independent of the hip bone's mineral density and other risk factors for fracture. Patients with type 2 diabetes are usually characterized by elevated bone mineral density, and this apparent paradox of higher bone density but increased risk of fracture might be explained by a combination of more frequent falls and poorer bone quality (Strotmeyer et al. 2005).

Frailty

Frailty, which is defined as a syndrome of decreased reserve and less resistance to stressors, can precede the onset of multiple poor health outcomes. Operational definitions of frailty vary widely according to the conceptual framework: some authors consider frailty in a broad sense that encompasses physical, social, cognitive, and psychological dimensions plus comorbidity, whereas others define the syndrome more restrictively, mainly on the basis of performance parameters such as gait speed, grip strength, and physical activity. Regardless of the definition used, frailty has high predictive value for adverse outcomes, such as disability, hospitalization, admission to a nursing home, and mortality. Only two studies have formally investigated the association between diabetes and the frailty syndrome in older people. In the Cardiovascular Health Study, the unadjusted prevalence of frailty was 23.5% in older people with diabetes and 11.3% in those without the disease (OR 2.4; 95% CI 1.8–3.2), with a population attributable fraction for diabetes of 14% (Fried et al. 2001). Among the older disabled women enrolled in the Women's Health and Aging Study, after adjustment for demographic characteristics, BMI, and major chronic diseases, diabetes was associated with an OR of 3.9 for risk of frailty (95% CI

1.5–10.3) (Blaum et al. 2005). These results strongly suggest that diabetes interacts with many aspects of the aging process, accelerating the loss of functional reserve and the functions of multiple physiologic systems and in turn reducing the likelihood of successful aging.

Quality of Diabetes Care in the Older, Frail Patient

For older patients the goals of diabetes care need to be individually tailored on the basis of a careful evaluation of benefits and potential risks associated with a specific diagnostic and/or therapeutic intervention. Clinical picture, functional status, and life expectancy are highly variable in the older population, making the benefit-risk ratio of any intervention less predictable than in the middle-aged adult population; providers caring for older adults with diabetes must take this heterogeneity into account when planning the goals of treatment.

The American Geriatric Society guidelines (California Healthcare Foundation/American Geriatrics Society 2003) distinguish between older patients who are relatively healthy and functioning well and those older patients who are frail and /or have significant physical impairment, comorbidity, and limited life expectancy. The first group is encouraged to achieve the same level of goals as those indicated for the general population. Conversely, the second and more vulnerable group is believed to have an unfavorable risk-benefit ratio for both intensive glucose and blood pressure control. In the case of intensive glucose control, frail patients are thought to be less likely to benefit from optimal metabolic control but at the same time to be at higher risk for hypoglycemia and adverse drug reactions. Consequently, the American Geriatric Society panel, in agreement with the American Diabetes Association (American Diabetes Association 2008), recommends a less strict A1C target such as 8% for frail, older patients. Similarly, older frail patients with diabetes are at high risk for orthostatic hypotension and falls, and for them a less intensive systolic blood pressure target of 140 mm Hg has been established. Treatment of other cardiovascular risk factors should be planned and implemented on the basis of time frame of benefit, the patient's characteristics, and considerations about polypharmacy. Lipid-lowering medications and antithrombotic therapy should be offered to patients with a life expectancy at least equal to the time frame of primary and secondary prevention trials. With regard to diagnostic assessment and screening for the complications of diabetes, particular attention should be paid to complications that can develop over a short time and to problems that would impair functional status. In this perspective, older patients with diabetes, besides receiving usual diabetes care, should benefit from multidimensional geriatric assessment, which is a systematic evaluation of multiple domains of health and functions that has been demonstrated effective in the prevention of multiple geriatric syndromes. Even so, this instrument has not been specifically tested in the older population with diabetes.

■ Prevention of Diabetes and Its Aging-Related Complications

The best way to prevent the diabetes-related complications is to prevent or postpone the onset of the disease. There is now substantial evidence that type 2 diabetes can be prevented or delayed. Individuals at high risk of developing diabetes include those with impaired fasting glucose or impaired glucose tolerance, those who are overweight, and those with a family history of the disease. Randomized clinical trials have shown that the onset of diabetes can be efficiently postponed in high-risk people. Prevention strategies include intensive lifestyle modification (weight loss and regular physical exercise) and pharmacological agents (metformin, acarbose, orlistat, or rosiglitazone) (Hussain et al. 2007). Unfortunately none of the randomized trials was specifically designed for older people. Nevertheless, a post hoc analysis of the Diabetes Prevention Program analyzed the effect of lifestyle intervention and metformin in the subgroup of persons aged 60–85 (The Diabetes Prevention Program Research Group 2006). The incidence of diabetes did not differ by age in the placebo group, but there were significant age differences in the responses to the two types of intervention. Although lifestyle intervention was effective in all age groups, diabetes incidence rates fell with increasing age (6.3 versus 4.9 versus 3.3 cases per 100 person-years in the 25- to 44-, 45- to 59-, and 60- to 85-year age groups, respectively; p for trend <0.007). In contrast in the metformin group, diabetes incidence was directly correlated with age (6.7 versus 7.7 versus 9.3 cases per 100 person-years in the three age groups; p for trend = 0.07) and consequently lifestyle intervention became significantly more effective than metformin with increasing age ($p = 0.005$). Based on this and other studies the American Diabetes Association strongly recommends lifestyle modification and weight reduction and does not recommend the use of metformin to prevent diabetes in older people.

In middle-aged patients the prevention and management of diabetes complications are based on intensive glucose control and optimal treatment of associated comorbidities, including hypertension and lipid abnormalities. In older persons there are few long-term studies demonstrating the benefits of intensive glycemic, blood pressure, and lipids control, and no studies have formally investigated the influence of glycemic control on the risk of disability, cognitive decline, falls, or frailty. One study reported an increased incidence of depressive symptoms in diabetes patients with poor glycemic control, but a causal relationship was not demonstrated.

Public health messages should encourage behavioral changes to achieve a healthy lifestyle, and health care professionals and the managers of health care systems should follow suit. Primary and secondary prevention policies that focus on lifestyle modification, specifically modest weight loss and increased physical activity, are very likely to have additional health benefits. Indeed, in older people, regular physical activity has been related not only to amelioration of cardiovascular risk profile and metabolic controls but also to lower risk of physical and cognitive decline.

■ Areas of Uncertainty and Controversy and Future Research and Developments

A considerable amount of high-quality research has been conducted on the cross-sectional and longitudinal associations between diabetes and several geriatric syndromes. Although not yet demonstrated by experimental data, the available data strongly support a causal relationship between diabetes and these important age-related complications. Long duration of the disease and severity of the metabolic impairment, either expressed as a need for insulin therapy or an elevated A1C, are also associated with a greater likelihood of most aging-related complications, but the biological mechanisms are partially unknown. In older persons traditional microvascular and macrovascular complications explain only in part the excess risk of geriatric syndromes like disability and dementia. From this point of view, the benefits of intensive glycemic control and optimal treatment of hyperglycemia and associated comorbidities have not been specifically investigated in older persons. This issue assumes particular importance in frail, older patients because of their increased risk of side effects and adverse drug reactions. Further research is necessary to understand the effect of optimal diabetes care on the onset and progression of aging-related diabetes complications. Future clinical trials need to enroll an adequate number of older patients and to include disability, cognitive decline, falls, and other geriatric syndromes as major end points. An example of this type of study is the Action to Control Cardiovascular Risk in Diabetes–Memory in Diabetes (ACCORD-MIND) study, an ongoing randomized clinical trial sponsored by the National Heart, Lung, and Blood Institute with support from the National Institute on Aging (Williamson et al. 2007). The trial is using 2977 patients aged 55 years or older to test whether there is a difference in the rate of cognitive decline and structural brain change between patients whose diabetes is treated with standard-care guidelines and those treated with intensive-care guidelines.

A pressing need in geriatric diabetes care is to develop, validate, and implement effective interventions that hit the multifaceted nature of this disabling disease. These strategies should include a model of diabetes care for older people built on the recognition that the traditional metabolic model would address only in part the complex multi-domain needs of older patients with diabetes. A modern and probably more effective model should integrate traditional areas of assessment and care with elements related to functional evaluation (focus on both cognitive and physical performance), risk of hypoglycemia or adverse drug reactions, and rehabilitation.

■ References

Al Snih S et al. (2005). Diabetes mellitus and incidence of lower body disability among older Mexican Americans. *The Journals of Gerontology. Series A, Biological Sciences and Medical Sciences* **60**, 1152–6.

American Diabetes Association (2008). Standards of medical care in diabetes—2008. *Diabetes Care* **31**, S12–54.

Anderson RJ et al. (2001). The prevalence of comorbid depression in adults with diabetes. *Diabetes Care* **24**, 1069–78.

Biessels GJ et al. (2006). Risk of dementia in diabetes mellitus: a systematic review. *Lancet Neurology* **5**, 64–74.

Blaum CS et al. (2005). The association between obesity and the frailty syndrome in older women: the women's health and aging studies. *Journal of the American Geriatrics Society* **53**, 927–34.

Bourdel-Marchasson I et al. (1997). Prevalence of diabetes and effect on quality of life in older French living in the community: the PAQUID Epidemiological Survey. *Journal of the American Geriatrics Society* **45**, 295–301.

Boyle JP et al. (2001). Projection of diabetes burden through 2050: impact of changing demography and disease prevalence in the U.S. *Diabetes Care* **24**, 1936–40.

Brayne C et al. (1998). Vascular risks and incident dementia: results from a cohort study of the very old. *Dementia and Geriatric Cognitive Disorders* **9**, 175–80.

Brown JS et al. (1996). Urinary incontinence in older women: who is at risk? Study of osteoporotic fractures research group. *Obstetrics and Gynecology* **87**, 715–21.

Brown JS et al. (2005). Urologic complications of diabetes. *Diabetes Care* **28**, 177–85.

California Healthcare Foundation/American Geriatrics Society Panel in Improving Care for Elders with Diabetes (2003). Guidelines for improving the care of the older person with diabetes mellitus. *Journal of the American Geriatrics Society* **51**, 265–80.

Cowie CC et al. (2006). Prevalence of diabetes and impaired fasting glucose in adults in the U.S. Population: National Health and Nutrition Examination Survey 1999–2002. *Diabetes Care* **29**, 1263–8.

de Rekeneire N (2003). Diabetes is associated with subclinical functional limitation in nondisabled older individuals: the Health, Aging, and Body Composition study. *Diabetes Care* **26**, 3257–63.

DiMatteo MR, Lepper HS, Croghan TW (2000). Depression is a risk factor for noncompliance with medical treatment: meta-analysis of the effects of anxiety and depression on patient adherence. *Archives of Internal Medicine* **160**, 2101–7.

Fried LP et al. (2001). Frailty in older adults: evidence for a phenotype. *The Journals of Gerontology. Series A, Biological Sciences and Medical Sciences* **56**, M146–57.

Gregg EW et al. (2000). Diabetes and physical disability among older U.S. adults. *Diabetes Care* **23**, 1272–7.

Gregg EW et al. (2002). Diabetes and incidence of functional disability in older women. *Diabetes Care* **25**, 61–7.

Guccione AA et al. (1994). The effects of specific medical conditions on the functional limitations of elders in the Framingham study. *American Journal of Public Health* **84**, 351–8.

Guralnik JM et al. (1993). Maintaining mobility in late life. I. Demographic characteristics and chronic conditions. *American Journal of Epidemiology* **137**, 845–57.

Hussain A et al. (2007). Prevention of type 2 diabetes: a review. *Diabetes Research and Clinical Practice* **76**, 317–26.

Knol MJ et al. (2006). Depression as a risk factor for the onset of type 2 diabetes. A meta-analysis. *Diabetologia* **49**, 837–45.

Krein SL et al. (2005). The effect of chronic pain on diabetes patients' self-management. *Diabetes Care* **28**, 65–70.

Lifford KL et al. (2005). Type 2 diabetes mellitus and risk of developing urinary incontinence. *Journal of the American Geriatrics Society* **53**, 1851–7.

Leveille SG, Volpato S (2007). Chronic pain and disability in diabetes. In: Munshi MN, Lipsitz LA, eds. *Geriatric Diabetes,* pp 127–42. New York: Informa Healthcare.

Luchsinger JA et al. (2001). Diabetes mellitus and risk of Alzheimer's disease and dementia with stroke in a multiethnic cohort. *American Journal of Epidemiology* **154**, 635–41.

MacKnight C et al. (2002). Diabetes mellitus and the risk of dementia, Alzheimer's disease and vascular cognitive impairment in the Canadian Study of Health and Aging. *Dementia and Geriatric Cognitive Disorders* **14**, 77–83.

Maggi S et al. (2004). Physical disability among older Italians with diabetes. The ILSA study. *Diabetologia* **47**, 1957–62.

Maraldi C et al. (2007). Diabetes mellitus, glycemic control, and incident depressive symptoms among 70- to 79-year-old persons: the health, aging, and body composition study. *Archives of Internal Medicine* **167**, 1137–44.

Maty SC et al. (2004). Patterns of disability related to diabetes mellitus in older women. *The Journals of Gerontology. Series A, Biological Sciences and Medical Sciences* **59**, 148–53.

Ott A et al. (1999). Diabetes mellitus and the risk of dementia: the Rotterdam Study. *Neurology* **53**, 1937–42.

Park et al. (2006). Decreased muscle strength and quality in older adults with type 2 diabetes: the health, aging, and body composition study. *Diabetes* **55**, 1813–8.

Park et al. (2007). Accelerated loss of skeletal muscle strength in older adults with type 2 diabetes: the health, aging, and body composition study. *Diabetes Care* **30**, 1507–12.

Pasquier F et al. (2006). Diabetes mellitus and dementia. *Diabetes & Metabolism* **32**, 403–14.

Peila R, Rodriguez BL, Launer LJ (2002). Type 2 diabetes, APOE gene, and the risk for dementia and related pathologies: the Honolulu-Asia Aging Study. *Diabetes* **51**, 1256–62.

Pleis JR, Lethbridge-Çejku M (2006). Summary health statistics for U.S. adults: National Health Interview Survey, 2005. *Vital and Health Statistics, Series 10* (232), 1–153.

Schwartz AV et al. (2008). Diabetes-related complications, glycemic control, and falls in older adults. *Diabetes Care* **31**, 391–6.

Smith DB (2006). Urinary incontinence and diabetes: a review. *Journal of Wound, Ostomy, and Continence Nursing* **33**, 619–23.

Strotmeyer ES et al. (2005). Nontraumatic fracture risk with diabetes mellitus and impaired fasting glucose in older white and black adults: the health, aging, and body composition study. *Archives of Internal Medicine* **165**, 1612–7.

The Diabetes Prevention Program Research Group (2006). The influence of age on the effects of lifestyle modification and metformin in prevention of diabetes. *The Journals of Gerontology. Series A, Medical Sciences* **61**, 1075-81.

Travis SS et al. (2004). Analyses of nursing home residents with diabetes at admission. *Journal of the American Medical Directors Association* **5**, 320–32.

Volpato S et al. (2002). Comorbidities and impairments explaining the association between diabetes and lower extremity disability: the women's health and aging study. *Diabetes Care* **25**, 678–83.

Volpato S et al. (2003). Progression of lower extremity disability in older women with diabetes: the Women's Health and Aging Study. *Diabetes Care* **26**, 70–5.

Volpato S et al. (2005). Risk factors for falls in older disabled women with diabetes: the women's health and aging study. *The Journals of Gerontology. Series A, Medical Sciences* **60**, 1539–45.

Weiner DK et al. (2003). How does low back pain impact physical function in independent, well-functioning older adults? Evidence from the health ABC cohort and implications for the future. *Pain Medicine* **4**, 311–20.

Williamson JD et al. (2007). The action to control cardiovascular risk in diabetes memory in diabetes study (accord-mind): Rationale, design, and methods. *American Journal of Cardiology* **99**, 112i–22i.

Xu WL et al. (2004). Diabetes mellitus and risk of dementia in the Kungsholmen project: a 6-year follow-up study. *Neurology* **63**, 1181–6.

Yoshitake T et al. (1995). Incidence and risk factors of vascular dementia and alzheimer's disease in a defined elderly Japanese population: the Hisayama study. *Neurology* **45**, 1161–8.

Zhang X et al. (2005). Depressive symptoms and mortality among persons with and without diabetes. *American Journal of Epidemiology* **161**, 652–60.

12. The Associations of Diabetes with Digestive, Oral, and Liver Disease, and Autonomic Neuropathy

Jeanne M. Clark, Christopher H. Gibbons, and Indra Mustapha

■ Main Public Health Messages

- Diabetes increases both incidence and mortality rates for gallstone disease and several gastrointestinal cancers.
- Reductions in the incidence and complications of common gastrointestinal conditions through prevention and increased screening could improve the health of people with diabetes and decrease costs.
- A bidirectional relationship exists between diabetes and periodontal disease, and both can be detected in their early stages by a collaborative approach between dentists and physicians.
- Public health policies aimed at preventing diabetes and periodontal disease will reduce associated morbidity, mortality, and heath care costs.
- Diabetes resulting from liver disease and the hepatic complications of diabetes are generally underappreciated in clinical practice and public health.
- Public health strategies to reduce liver disease and diabetes could have mutually beneficial effects.
- Autonomic neuropathy is common in both type 1 and type 2 diabetes and is associated with significant increases in morbidity and mortality.
- Diabetic autonomic neuropathy is generally underappreciated by general practitioners, and new guidelines are necessary to promote education about this common complication of diabetes and appropriate testing for its presence.

■ Diabetes and Digestive Diseases

Digestive diseases, which are very common in the United States as well as around the world, impose enormous economic costs. Many of the most common and costly digestive conditions are associated with diabetes mellitus. In this section we review the associations between diabetes and several digestive diseases, including gastro-intestinal cancers; the associations of liver disease with diabetes are covered separately later in this chapter.

Epidemiology

Gallbladder Disease

On the basis of ultrasound data from the Third National Health and Nutrition Examination Survey (NHANES III), the latest population-based data for the United States, 20.5 million people were found to have gallbladder disease, including 8% of adult men and 17% of adult women (Everhart et al. 1999). Gallstones are commonly asymptomatic, but 30%–50% of affected individuals will develop symptoms. In 2005 the rate of cholecystectomy was 13.5 per 10,000 population—making it the most common gastrointestinal operation if endoscopies are excluded (DeFrances et al. 2007). Thus it is not surprising that gallbladder disease is also the second most expensive digestive disease, with an estimated $6.0 billion in direct and indirect costs in 1998 (Sandler et al. 2002). Although data from case-control studies are mixed, data from NHANES III showed that people with diabetes have more than 50% greater odds of gallbladder disease after controlling for age, body mass index (BMI), and race/ethnicity, with the risk slightly higher in women (odds ratio [OR] 1.63, 95% confidence interval [CI] 1.12–2.36) than in men (OR 1.54, 95% CI 1.03–2.30) (Everhart et al. 1999).

Celiac Disease

Celiac disease, a chronic, autoimmune disorder affecting the small intestines, is induced by exposure to gluten proteins found in wheat, barley, and rye. Active celiac disease may cause malabsorption, abdominal pain, weight loss or failure to thrive, osteopenia, and gastrointestinal lymphomas. The majority of cases may actually be subclinical or silent. The incidence of celiac disease is much higher in children and adults with type 1 diabetes (4.1%, range 0–16%) than in the general population (range 0.3%–0.5%) (Freemark et al. 2003; Rewers et al. 2004). Some data suggest that celiac disease may predispose to type 1 diabetes, but such a connection remains unproven.

Digestive Disease Cancers

As shown in a large prospective study from Japan, diabetes increases the risk of several digestive disease cancers (see Table 12.1), including colon, pancreatic, and

TABLE 12.1 *Incidence and Mortality Rates for Digestive Disease Cancers in Men and Women with and without Diabetes*

Cancer Site	Incidence Rate (per 100,000)			Mortality Rate (per 100,000)		
	People with DM*	People w/o DM*	Adjusted HR* (95% CI)	People with DM†	People w/o DM†	Adjusted RR† (95% CI)
Men						
Esophagus‡	60	34	1.40 (0.84–2.32)	18	15	1.20 (0.94–1.53)
Stomach	288	194	1.23 (0.98–1.54)	19	17	0.99 (0.77–1.27)
Colon	152	97	1.36 (1.00–1.85)	67	53	1.20 (1.06–1.37)
Rectum	50	50	0.80 (0.47–1.36)	9	9	1.07 (0.75–1.51)
Liver	172	57	2.24 (1.64–3.04)	28	11	2.19 (1.76–2.72)
Bile duct	33	17	1.63 (0.84–3.17)	NA	NA	NA
Gallbladder	NA	NA	NA	5	3	1.46 (0.92–2.30)
Pancreas	53	22	1.85 (1.07–3.20)	68	45	1.48 (1.27–1.73)
Women						
Stomach	123	63	1.61 (1.02–2.54)	10	7	1.25 (0.90–1.73)
Colon	62	54	0.83 (0.42–1.61)	50	37	1.24 (1.07–1.43)
Rectum	49	27	1.65 (0.80–3.39)	5	5	0.90 (0.57–1.42)
Liver	62	20	1.94 (1.00–3.73)	8	5	1.37 (0.94–2.00)

(continued)

TABLE 12.1 (continued)

Cancer Site	Incidence Rate (per 100,000)			Mortality Rate (per 100,000)		
	People with DM*	People w/o DM*	Adjusted HR* (95% CI)	People with DM†	People w/o DM†	Adjusted RR† (95% CI)
Bile duct	12	16	0.55 (0.13–2.24)	NA	NA	NA
Gallbladder	NA	NA	NA	5	4	1.19 (0.77–1.83)
Pancreas	31	16	1.33 (0.53–3.31)	47	31	1.44 (1.21–1.72)

DM, diabetes mellitus; HR, hazard ratio; RR, relative risk; CI, confidence interval; NA, not available.

*Inoue et al. (2006). Japan Public Health Center-Based Prospective Study. Adjustments made for age, study site, cardiovascular disease, coronary heart disease, smoking, alcohol, body mass index, physical activity, intake of green vegetables, and coffee intake.

†Coughlin et al. (2004). U.S.-based Cancer Prevention II Study. Adjustments made for age, race, education, body mass index, smoking, alcohol, physical activity, intake of red meat, citrus fruit and juice intake, vegetable intake, and family history of that cancer.

‡Data on esophageal cancer available only for men.

liver cancer in men and stomach and liver cancer in women (Inoue et al. 2006). In this study each increased risk remained after adjustment for risk factors and after removal of cases occurring within the first 5 years of the study. Studies of single cancers have yielded similar results. For example, a large meta-analysis found an association between diabetes and pancreatic cancer (Huxley et al. 2005).

People with diabetes also appear to have increased rates of *mortality* from digestive disease cancers. In men with diabetes there is an increased risk of mortality from colon cancer (adjusted relative risk [ARR] 1.20, 95% CI 1.06–1.33) and pancreatic cancer (ARR 1.48, 95% CI 1.27–1.73). Women with diabetes have a similarly increased risk of mortality from colon and pancreatic cancer (Coughlin et al. 2004).

Studies such as these often have several important limitations, however, particularly the presence of confounders such as smoking, obesity, and other lifestyle risk factors that can be associated with both diabetes and cancer. Fortunately, most recent studies have attempted to control for these factors. Reverse causality is also a concern in studies of pancreatic cancer and diabetes, but excluding cases within the first few years of a study reduces this possibility. Additionally, increased cancer mortality may not be due solely to increased incidence, as delayed diagnosis and less effective treatment may be contributing factors. Finally, many studies do not distinguish between type 1 and type 2 diabetes, and studies confined to type 1 often lack sufficient cases to be conclusive.

These concerns notwithstanding, there is biological plausibility for the idea that diabetes may increase the risk of certain cancers. In type 2 diabetes, for example, increased levels of insulin and insulin-like growth factors can stimulate cell proliferation. Furthermore, beyond its apparent relationships with gastrointestinal cancers, diabetes is associated with increased incidence and mortality of some other cancers, including kidney and breast (Coughlin et al. 2004; Inoue et al. 2006).

Public Health Preventive and Interventional Strategies

Gallbladder disease

Even though gallstones are very common, their exact pathophysiology is not well understood. Gallstones can develop when there is a change in bile composition that permits precipitation of cholesterol or other liquids into crystals that eventually form stones; such stones can also result from impaired contractility of the gallbladder. There is no proven way to prevent the formation of gallstones, but eating regular meals and maintaining a normal body weight are often recommended.

Fortunately, most individuals with gallstones remain asymptomatic and develop no complications. Thus, for the general population, expectant management is the standard of care, with therapy only for symptomatic disease. In people with both diabetes and gallstones, prophylactic cholecystectomy was previously recommended because of a fear that such persons were at higher risk for complications, but more recent evidence suggests that the complication rate in people with diabetes is not higher.

Celiac Disease

Several antibody assays are available to screen for celiac disease, but an intestinal biopsy is recommended for diagnosis and to assess disease activity. Currently, screening is recommended for patients with type 1 diabetes who develop symptoms of celiac disease (American Diabetes Association 2008), but screening has been proposed for all patients with type 1 diabetes because celiac disease (1) may lead to hypoglycemia, growth failure, osteopenia, anemia, subfertility, hepatocellular dysfunction, and possibly small bowel lymphoma; (2) is not always recognized and diagnosed in clinical practice; and (3) can be treated with a gluten-free diet, which can ameliorate and even reverse the complications (Freemark et al. 2003). The advocacy of screening all type 1 patients remains controversial, however, because the data on the risks and efficacy of treatment in subclinical disease are weaker, the diagnosis requires an invasive test, and the treatment is onerous.

Digestive Disease Cancers

Although the incidence of colorectal cancer and mortality from this disease are increased in people with diabetes, currently there are no recommendations that call for a different pattern of colorectal screening for those who have diabetes. Several measures to prevent the formation of colonic polyps and subsequent cancer in the general population have been studied, but a detailed review is beyond the scope of this chapter. In brief although chronic therapy with nonsteroidal anti-inflammatory drugs (NSAIDs) may reduce polyps and cancer, such a regimen is not routinely recommended because of the adverse side effects (Rostom et al. 2007). Furthermore, this preventive therapy has not been extensively studied in people with diabetes.

At present no screening tests are recommended for other digestive disease cancers in either the general population or in people with diabetes. Of course if diabetes leads to an increased risk of several gastrointestinal cancers, then prevention of diabetes (which has been accomplished in persons at risk for type 2 disease) should reduce these risks and prevent excess cancer mortality. At this time, however, there is no evidence to support the hypothesis that prevention of diabetes actually reduces the risk of certain kinds of gastrointestinal cancer.

Implications for Health Policy

If screening for celiac disease or more frequent screening for colon cancer among persons with diabetes is proven effective, screening recommendations might change and related morbidity and mortality might decline. At the same time more widespread efforts to prevent diabetes in the population could reduce the prevalence and costs of associated digestive diseases. Finally, determining the etiology of the observed increases in cancer mortality could have important policy implications. For instance if the increased mortality is linked to suboptimal screening, policies to enhance cancer screening might be beneficial. If, however, the standard cancer treatments are less effective or more toxic in people with diabetes, further research and drug development would be indicated.

Areas of Uncertainty

It is unclear whether having celiac disease predisposes someone to type 1 diabetes and whether the person's risk is affected by the duration of exposure to gluten. In terms of gastrointestinal cancer and associated mortality, although there is good evidence that diabetes increases these risks, the exact degree to which these relationships are independent of obesity and the explanations for the increase in mortality are less certain. Finally, there are little data on whether control of diabetes affects the development of these digestive diseases or associated mortality rates.

■   Diabetes and Periodontal Disease

Periodontitis, which is the loss of the fibrous periodontal ligament attachment around teeth, occurs primarily in response to oral pathogenic bacteria and can lead to tooth loss if not treated successfully. Periodontal pathogens, such as *Porphyromonas gingivalis*, infect sites around teeth and initiate a systemic host immune response. Periodontitis can manifest as bleeding gingiva, halitosis, periodontal abscesses, loose teeth, and pain. Periodontal inflammation is closely associated with systemic diseases such as diabetes, cardiovascular disease, rheumatoid arthritis, and obesity (Moore et al. 2003).

Epidemiology

Diabetes and Periodontal Disease

Diabetes doubles the odds of periodontal disease in the U.S. population after adjustment for age and income (OR 2.06, 95% CI 1.06–4.01) (Hyman et al. 2003). Although the prevalence of periodontitis has changed little over the last 30 years (13%–15% of the U.S. population), severe forms are more common in individuals with diabetes (who have a prevalence of 30%–45%) (Taylor 2001). Because studies earlier than 2000 often combined people with type 1 and type 2 diabetes when periodontal status was assessed, separating that data is now difficult. The pathogenic bacteria involved, however, are notably similar in the two types.

Several factors may contribute to the development of periodontal disease in persons with diabetes. Advanced glycation end products appear to play a role by inducing secretion of inflammatory mediators such as interleukin-1, tumor necrosis factor-α, and prostaglandin-E_2. The loss of a tooth's attachment has been attributed to this inflammatory response, which can be precipitated by both hyperglycemia and periodontal bacteria. Additionally, thickening of basement membranes by glycosylation may cause vascular changes that affect the diffusion of oxygen or antibodies to sites of inflammation. Finally, a family history of diabetes is associated with a localized decrease in chemotaxis of polymorphonuclear leukocytes, suggesting a genetic basis for periodontal inflammation (Mealey 1999).

Diabetes and Xerostomia

Diminished salivary flow, or xerostomia, has been reported in some studies of people with diabetes, but other studies have not confirmed these findings. The protective effects of saliva are diminished in xerostomic patients, and accumulation of plaque is generally heavier and more frequent. This buildup of plaque is comprised mostly of microbiota that predispose individuals to dental caries and periodontal disease. The pathogenesis of xerostomia may involve both the basement membrane changes of parotid ducts in those with diabetes and the consequences of diabetes medications (Mealey 1999).

Diabetes, Periodontitis, and Cardiovascular Disease and Mortality

Both periodontitis and diabetes are independent risk factors for mortality from coronary heart disease and stroke. Early cardiovascular disease, as measured by thickening of the carotid intima media, has been observed in subjects exposed to periodontal pathogens in cross-sectional studies (see Fig. 12.1) (Mustapha et al. 2007). Chronic hyperglycemia is also associated with increased odds for thickening of the carotid intima media in people with diabetes (OR 2.62, 95% CI 1.36–5.06).

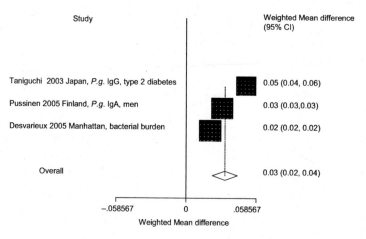

FIGURE 12.1. Forest plot of studies using carotid intima-media thickness (CIMT) as a continuous outcome, measured by ultrasound (exposure: periodontal disease). Author, year of publication, location, systemic marker, and population restriction as described. Combined effect by random effects model estimated a significant average mean increase of CIMT of 0.03 (95% CI 0.02–0.04). P.g. = *Porphyromonas gingivalis*. (From Mustapha et al. 2007.)

The close relationship among periodontitis, diabetes, and cardiovascular disease likely reflects some interrelated pathways. The association between diabetes and periodontal disease is thought to be bidirectional, and both periodontal disease and diabetes have been shown to independently increase the risk of cardiovascular disease (Janket et al. 2005). Furthermore among people with diabetes, those who have advanced periodontal disease are 3.2 times as likely to die from ischemic heart disease or diabetic nephropathy as are those without advanced periodontal disease (Saremi et al. 2005).

Public Health Strategies and Interventions

Treating periodontal disease may improve diabetes control and prevent cardiovascular morbidity and mortality. Even so, a meta-analysis found that nonsurgical periodontal therapies, such as scaling and root planing, systemic antibiotic therapy, and antibiotic placement around affected teeth, resulted in only a nonsignificant 0.7% decrease in hemoglobin A1C (95% CI –2.3% to +0.9%) (Janket et al. 2005). Recommended oral hygiene practices, such as brushing and flossing and regular dental visits, can prevent periodontitis and lower blood glucose levels (Mealey 1999). The effect of surgical periodontal intervention, commonly indicated for more severe periodontitis, on diabetes control has not been reported. Finally, there is no evidence to recommend periodontal treatment for the prevention of cardiovascular disease.

People with well-controlled diabetes have been found to benefit from periodontal therapy as much as do healthy controls (Taylor 2001). Medication to control diabetes may also improve or prevent periodontal disease by reducing inflammation. For instance, thiazolidinediones have been shown to decrease serum C-reactive protein levels, which are elevated during active periodontal disease (Qayyum et al. 2006). Uncontrolled diabetes, in contrast, may increase the risk of periodontitis (Taylor 2001).

As the prevalence of diabetes increases, dentists will likely see an increasing number of patients with diagnosed or undiagnosed diabetes. The American Dental Association now recommends that dental offices be equipped with glucometers. Educating patients about the importance of preventing and treating periodontal disease and diabetes is the role of both physicians and dentists (Ship 2003).

Recommendations for Health Policy

Research

Studies of the pathogenesis and complications of diabetes should include experts in both medicine and dentistry because inflammation from the oral cavity has known systemic effects. To allow comparison across studies, however, there needs to be a consensus on how to classify periodontal disease (Hyman et al. 2003). The assessment of inflammatory mediators, periodontal pathogens, and antibody

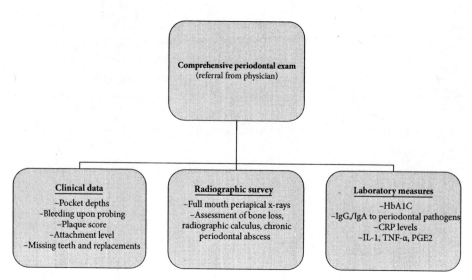

FIGURE 12.2. Data collection relevant to assessing relationship between periodontal disease and diabetes

titers to periodontal pathogens, in addition to clinical and radiographic examinations, should be considered (see Fig. 12.2). These data will help define the biological mechanisms and provide direction for future interventions. An efficient method for linking medical and dental charts for data abstraction would enhance tracking of the use, type, and duration of interventions for diabetes and periodontal disease.

Screening

Although the American Diabetes Association does not include formal recommendations about dental care in its clinical practice guidelines, the American Dental Association recommends more frequent dental visits and more intensive treatment of oral inflammation in patients with diabetes. These guidelines also suggest regular communication between physicians and dentists on the issue of glycemic control (Ship 2003). The cost-effectiveness and outcomes of screening programs for periodontal disease among populations with prediabetes can be reliably assessed only if providers routinely refer at-risk individuals to dental professionals.

Insurance coverage for dental care should be mandated for people with diabetes because this population has more to gain from the prevention and treatment of early periodontal disease (Moore et al. 2003). The health of the public will be served by public policies that focus on the prevention and control of periodontitis, diabetes, and, where possible, cardiovascular disease. Because the prognosis for periodontal disease is best if the problem is treated at its earliest stages, programs aimed at patient education and health promotion may limit the burden of sequelae associated with diabetes and periodontal disease.

Areas of Uncertainty

Although a bidirectional pathway between periodontal disease and diabetes has been proposed, the preponderance of evidence is in one direction, that diabetes increases the risk of periodontal disease. Only animal studies have isolated a bidirectional relationship that confirms the independent contribution of periodontitis and diabetes to each other. However, the biological mechanisms are poorly understood, and human models of low-dose chronic endotoxemia, which mimic the inflammation produced in response to periodontitis, are not available to perform mechanistic studies.

Large-scale studies of the association between diabetes and periodontitis are mainly cross-sectional and thus temporality can not be ascertained. Cohort studies have not routinely included dental exams, or they have included them at only one time point. Confounders, such as obesity and diet, have typically not been addressed, and their omission weakens existing studies. Unfortunately, because periodontitis, diabetes, and cardiovascular disease are chronic diseases, observational studies to address temporality and quantify the contribution of each disease would be lengthy, costly, and burdened by the potential for residual confounding. The effect of periodontal diseases on insulin resistance has not been extensively explored. Studying gingivitis, the earliest form of periodontal inflammation, may yield the most sensitive ascertainment of the effect of subtle changes of oral health on diabetes.

The effect of missing teeth on prediabetes and diabetes (through changes in dietary intake) has not been extensively studied. The effect of the ill-fitting dental prostheses sometimes used to replace missing teeth needs further evaluation. Accounting for confounding from obesity and traditional risk factors, such as smoking, socioeconomic status, and age, may change the previously reported risk estimates of diseases. Finally, the relationships among multiple diseases (diabetes, periodontitis, cardiovascular disease, obesity) are complex and not likely to be understood by a single study, regardless of its design. Synthesis of existing and future studies will be helpful in elucidating these relationships and should provide the direction for public health policies aimed at reducing the burden of these disorders on the general public.

■ Diabetes and Liver Disease

The liver plays an important role in normal glucose metabolism, including processing glucose absorbed from the gut, storing it as glycogen or metabolizing it into amino acids or fatty acids, and generating glucose de novo. The liver also metabolizes insulin, and this organ appears to have the potential to adversely affect both peripheral insulin resistance and β-cell function through undefined mechanisms, perhaps through systemic inflammation and/or portal hypertension. Given many of these functions, it is not surprising that a liver diseased from any cause could have deleterious effects on the metabolism of glucose and insulin. Furthermore, it is easy to see how impaired homeostasis of glucose and insulin could also affect the liver. However, despite the strong association between diabetes and disorders of the liver, both diabetes resulting from liver disease and the hepatic complications of diabetes are generally underappreciated in both clinical practice and public health.

Epidemiology

In 2004 in the United States chronic liver disease and cirrhosis (considered together) were the 12th-leading cause of death overall and the 7th-leading cause in individuals aged 25–64 years. The majority of these deaths were classified as *unrelated* to alcohol. Notably, cirrhosis of the liver is implicated in 80% of cases of hepatocellular carcinoma.

People with diabetes have significantly higher mortality rates for liver disease (twice or 2.5 times as high) and hepatocellular carcinoma (two to four times as high) than the general population. Furthermore, among people with known liver disease, the presence of diabetes is associated with an OR in excess of 4 for hepatocellular carcinoma and above 10 when diabetes is combined with heavy alcohol consumption. Finally, diabetes appears to increase the risk of postoperative complications and decrease survival in people with hepatocellular carcinoma (Harrison 2006).

There are several reasons for the increased rates of mortality from liver disease in people with diabetes. First, diabetes may directly lead to liver disease in the form of nonalcoholic fatty liver disease (NAFLD). NAFLD includes a spectrum of disease from simple steatosis, to hepatic inflammation and necrosis known as nonalcoholic steatohepatitis, to fibrosis and cirrhosis. The histopathology of NAFLD is indistinguishable from alcoholic liver disease, but the former occurs in the absence of significant alcohol intake. Because insulin resistance appears to be key to its pathogenesis, and because it coexists with other conditions such as central adiposity, hypertriglyceridemia, and low-HDL (high-density lipoprotein) cholesterol, NAFLD has also been called part of the metabolic syndrome. In population-based studies, type 2 diabetes is associated with an OR of approximately 1.5 to 3 for NAFLD as well as increased odds of significant hepatic fibrosis (Clark 2006).

In addition to causing liver disease, diabetes is associated with a poorer prognosis among those who have liver diseases, including hepatocellular carcinoma and chronic hepatitis C. Finally, people who undergo liver transplantation have lower survival if they have diabetes, as discussed below (Moscatiello et al. 2007).

Diabetes and liver disease are also associated because cirrhosis that is secondary to any liver disease can cause diabetes. In fact, up to 80% of people with cirrhosis from any cause will develop insulin resistance, and 20%–63% will develop diabetes, sometimes called hepatogenous diabetes. Furthermore, the incidence of type 2 diabetes is three times higher in patients with chronic hepatitis C infection, a disease frequently characterized by microvesicular steatosis, than in the general population. In addition, the risk of impaired glucose metabolism begins in the early stages of the hepatitis C infection, well before cirrhosis is present (Mehta et al. 2003). Last, there is growing evidence that NAFLD may precede type 2 diabetes in some cases (Hanley et al. 2004), but most of these studies have lacked rigorous ascertainment of either diabetes or liver disease.

Liver disease and diabetes also occur together in people undergoing liver transplantation. Indeed, approximately 16% of patients undergoing liver transplantation have preexisting type 1 or type 2 diabetes. As reported earlier in this chapter, those with preexisting diabetes have significantly poorer overall (67% vs. 75%) and graft (61% vs. 67%) survival than those without diabetes. In general people with type 1 diabetes fare worse than those with type 2. Furthermore, whereas transplantation cures two-thirds of cases of hepatogenous diabetes, one-third of those with preoperative hepatogenous diabetes have enough β-cell failure to prevent a cure. Finally, diabetes occurs de novo after liver transplantation in 15%–31% of cases, rates similar to those for other organ transplantations (Harrison 2006; Moscatiello et al. 2007). Risk factors for posttransplant diabetes include the typical risk factors for type 2 diabetes, the type of liver disease (e.g., alcohol related, hepatitis C, and NAFLD), and the immunosuppressive regimens, with the highest rates occurring with use of corticosteroids and tacrolimus.

Finally diabetes and liver disease are linked not only pathophysiologically but also through medications used to treat both conditions. As noted earlier in this chapter, medications used after liver transplantation can induce diabetes or worsen glycemic control in those with preexisting diabetes. Many medications used to treat diabetes, including biguanides, thiazolidinediones, and sulfonylureas, can cause elevated liver enzymes, acute hepatitis, and rarely, acute liver failure. Lastly, acute liver failure from idiosyncratic reaction to any medication appears to be about two-thirds higher in people with diabetes than in the general population: 2.3 versus 1.4 cases per 10,000 person-years (Moscatiello et al. 2007).

Public Health Preventive and Intervention Strategies

Preventing disease is preferable to treating disease when the costs and benefits of prevention outweigh the risks of treatment. Although relevant studies are lacking, it seems likely that preventing diabetes would prevent or reduce many of the downstream hepatic consequences detailed earlier in this chapter, including preventing NAFLD and improving the effectiveness of treatment and survival rates for hepatitis C infection and liver transplantation. Lifestyle modifications that are effective in preventing diabetes, such as physical activity and caloric restriction to produce weight loss, are already recommended for treatment of NAFLD despite limited data. Furthermore because obesity is also a risk factor for the progression of liver disease as well as less effective treatment in both hepatitis C and alcoholic liver disease, adopting a lifestyle that promotes weight loss or weight maintenance could also be beneficial. Finally, several medications that have been shown to prevent or delay the onset of diabetes, including metformin and thiazolidinediones, have been shown to be effective treatments for NAFLD in pilot studies. Thus in people at risk for both diabetes and NAFLD, use of some treatments might impart a dual benefit. Such predictions are preliminary, however, and await the results of ongoing studies of insulin sensitizers to treat NAFLD.

Similarly, strategies to prevent chronic liver disease, cirrhosis, and the subsequent need for liver transplantation are likely to reduce the prevalence of type 2 diabetes. As noted earlier in this chapter, treatments recommended for and being studied in NAFLD are already known to prevent diabetes. Additionally, effective use of vaccinations as well as other public health strategies to prevent infection with viral hepatitis, as well as preventive lifestyle strategies for alcoholic and nonalcoholic liver disease, could reduce the incidence of diabetes associated with cirrhosis. The logic of this approach notwithstanding, data on the effectiveness of successful treatment of liver disease for preventing diabetes are lacking.

Implications for Health Policy

Both diabetes and chronic liver disease are common and costly conditions in the United States. The overlap between these conditions is substantial, stemming from both the physiological overlap and the consequences of treatment. Although this interplay can make treating each condition more difficult, its potential benefits should not be ignored. Rather, the intersection could be leveraged to improve the health of the affected populations by pooling resources to enact prudent screening, preventive, and treatment strategies. With greater understanding, clinical practice guidelines could then include recommendations about screening for diabetes in chronic liver disease and for chronic liver disease in diabetes. Public health information campaigns could also begin to highlight the overlap between these conditions.

Areas of Uncertainty

Because the relationships between certain liver diseases, such as NAFLD and advanced hepatitis C infection, and diabetes have been demonstrated in both directions, causality remains uncertain. Similarly because many studies are cross-sectional rather than prospective, it remains unclear whether preexisting diabetes causes more progressive liver disease or develops from the advanced liver disease. Assuming causal relationships exist, the exact pathogenesis in many cases remains unknown. Hypothesized pathways include altered portal blood flow, systemic inflammation and oxidative stress, the balance of adipokines and cytokines, and altered growth hormone and insulin-like growth factor-1 (IGF-1) homeostasis. Finally, as noted earlier in this chapter, proof that treatment strategies for one condition will improve the other is lacking (Picardi et al. 2006).

Future Developments

More research is needed to tease out how diabetes and chronic liver diseases are related. In particular, given the substantial overlap, accurately and prospectively monitoring the presence and development of diabetes in studies of patients with liver disease, and vice versa, seems prudent. Once the relationships are clarified, the roles of screening, preventive strategies, and treatment can be elucidated. Such advances could lead to the development of new medications, new application of existing medications, and broader recommendations for lifestyle and behavioral therapies. Finally, for patients with end-stage liver disease who require transplantation, new treatments with lower risks of diabetes are needed.

■ Diabetes and Autonomic Neuropathy

Diabetes affects the peripheral nervous system through a variety of mechanisms and may result in large-fiber, small-fiber, or autonomic neuropathies. Injury to nerve fibers may occasionally be isolated to one specific nerve subtype, but it more frequently presents as a compilation of sensory, motor, and autonomic neuropathies. Clinically significant peripheral neuropathy is common in both type 1 and type 2 diabetes, with prevalence rates of 66% and 59%, respectively (Dyck et al. 1993).

Although a common complication of diabetes, autonomic neuropathy is comparatively underrecognized and frequently overlooked. The autonomic nervous system innervates the cardiovascular, gastrointestinal, genitourinary, sudomotor (sweat glands), and pupillomotor systems. The characteristics and epidemiology of these disorders are described below.

Epidemiology

Epidemiologic data on diabetic autonomic neuropathy are inconsistent, and prevalence rates range from 7% to 90% in patients with type 1 diabetes and from 18% to 54% in type 2 (Vinik et al. 2007). Gastroparesis, for example, is seen in 35%–50% of patients with diabetes and is likely underrecognized. This wide variability likely reflects different study designs and the particular organ systems of interest. Large cohort studies frequently follow patients for one condition (e.g., cardiovascular disease) and report the prevalence of autonomic dysfunction only *in that particular organ system*.

Unfortunately, studies of the frequency of diabetic autonomic neuropathy across all organ systems also lead to widely disparate results. Variability in the populations and selection bias explain some of these differences. Additional confounders include inconsistent definitions of diabetic autonomic neuropathy, variability in measurement tools, grouping of type 1 and type 2 diabetes, and disagreement in interpretation of the results (Vinik et al. 2007). Despite these differences, important information has been obtained.

Diabetic autonomic neuropathy presents across multiple organ systems with a wide variety of symptoms. Similarly, the strength of the epidemiologic evidence varies widely. The prevalence of autonomic neuropathy and a listing of its common clinical findings are detailed in Table 12.2.

The association between diabetic autonomic neuropathy and mortality risk (all causes) has been well described. Diabetic cardiac autonomic neuropathy (for both type 1 and type 2 diabetes) was associated with an OR of about 5 for 5-year mortality and a relative risk (RR) of death of 2.14 (95% CI 1.83–2.51) in 15 pooled studies of 2900 patients (Vinik et al. 2007). The pooled risk for development of silent myocardial ischemia was 1.96 (95% CI 1.53–2.51).

Autonomic neuropathy has also been identified as an independent risk factor for the development of foot ulceration and a reduction in wound-healing capacity (RR 1.36, 95% CI 1.17–1.58) (Boyko et al. 1999). Autonomic neuropathy also appears to be associated with reduced bone mineral density, resulting in an increased risk of Charcot joint.

Public Health Preventive and Intervention Strategies

The Diabetes Control and Complications Trial (DCCT) clearly determined that tight glucose control reduces the risk of diabetic autonomic neuropathy and slows its progression in people with type 1 diabetes (The Diabetes Control and Complications Trial 1998). These findings are consistent with those for microvascular complications of diabetes, such as retinopathy and nephropathy. Preventing diabetic autonomic neuropathy is especially important because there is no treatment for most of its clinical features. Although many trials to repair nerve damage or to return nerve function have been heralded with great enthusiasm, to date, not one has been successful in humans. These lackluster results have left aggressive glucose control as the only recourse.

Implications for Health Policy

Consensus Panels for Identification of Autonomic Neuropathy

Two consensus meetings on diabetic neuropathy were held jointly by the American Diabetes Association and the American Academy of Neurology in 1988 and 1992. These meetings raised awareness of diabetic autonomic neuropathies, and suggestions were made for the standardization of testing of the autonomic nervous system in clinical trials. However the consensus panels focused almost exclusively on cardiac autonomic neuropathy, with little discussion of other affected systems. Since the last consensus statement a number of scientific advances have been made in the

TABLE 12.2 Organ Systems Affected by and Clinical Manifestations of Autonomic Neuropathy

Organ System	Clinical Manifestations	Epidemiology	Evidence
Cardiovascular	Tachycardia; painless myocardial infarction; orthostatic hypotension; impaired cardiac function.	7%–80% of patients with diabetes have some form of cardiac autonomic neuropathy; those with severe cardiac neuropathy have five times the risk of mortality (absolute mortality rates of 27%–53% over 5 years in that group).	Strong: Multiple well-designed studies clearly documenting risks and the natural history of the process.
Gastrointestinal	Esophageal dysmotility; gastroparesis; diarrhea; constipation.	35%–50% of patients with DM have some gastroparesis with testing. Diarrhea and/or constipation reported in 15%–42% of diabetic subjects.	Weak: Many assessments through questionnaires, few objective measurements. Confounding variables not well controlled (medications, comorbidities).
Urogenital	Neurogenic bladder; erectile dysfunction; retrograde ejaculation.	43%–87% of patients with type 1 DM have physiologic evidence of bladder dysfunction. 35%–75% of men with diabetes report erectile dysfunction.	Moderate: Many studies documenting abnormalities of function and reported symptoms; confounding variables limit interpretation.
Sudomotor (sweat glands)	Anhidrosis, central compensatory hyperhidrosis.	51% of patients with type 1 DM and 62% of patients with type 2 DM had some sudomotor abnormalities on testing.	Weak: Several studies documenting abnormalities of sudomotor function in patients with known diabetic neuropathy, little information about the prevalence and natural history in a large diabetic population.
Pupillary	Small nonreactive pupils.	23%–59% of patients with diabetes, depending on disease duration.	Weak: Studies clearly documenting frequency of findings but not ruling out other potential causes of papillary abnormalities.

DM, diabetes mellitus.

evaluation and treatment of noncardiac autonomic neuropathy (Low 2003). A recent statement by the American Diabetes Association provides a more comprehensive review of peripheral and autonomic neuropathies by outlining testing guidelines and suggesting treatment strategies (Boulton et al. 2005).

Screening Tools for Use in Large Populations

The consensus meetings on diabetic neuropathy identified three screening tests for identifying diabetic cardiovascular autonomic neuropathy in large populations: the response of the heart rate (1) to deep breathing, (2) to standing, and (3) to a Valsalva maneuver. The expert panels also recommended two tests for identification of blood pressure control: the response of the blood pressure (1) to standing (or tilting) and (2) to handgrip exercise. They also determined that there was inadequate evidence for routine testing of sudomotor, gastrointestinal, genitourinary, or pupillomotor autonomic function (Vinik et al. 2007). The consensus meetings established screening guidelines for autonomic neuropathy to standardize testing in clinical trials, but they did not make recommendations regarding screening of the general population with diabetes.

Economic Issues and Implications

Due to uncertain estimates of the prevalence of diabetic autonomic neuropathy, data on the related health care costs to society are limited. Furthermore, the economic burdens are reported according to organ system, and no studies have attempted to combine these reports. Diabetic cardiac autonomic neuropathy has the most substantive epidemiologic data, suggesting that mortality rates are five times as high as in the general population, with a corresponding increase in medical costs. These consequences do not account for comorbid cardiac, renal, or other disease. Clearly additional study is required to understand the health care costs and perspectives.

Areas of Uncertainty

Despite the evidence that tight glucose control can prevent diabetic autonomic neuropathy, the long-term impact of such control on overall morbidity and mortality in large populations is unclear. An ongoing clinical trial of people with type 1 diabetes, the Epidemiology of Diabetes Interventions and Complications study (EDIC), may provide answers to these questions. However the EDIC study is also focused on cardiovascular autonomic neuropathy; further study is essential to understand the true risks, epidemiology, and health care costs of noncardiac autonomic neuropathies.

Future Developments

Aggressive public health initiatives to combat the growing epidemics of obesity and diabetes are the only way to truly reduce the burden of diabetic autonomic neuropathy. Even so the early identification and aggressive treatment of patients with diabetes or impaired glucose tolerance are likely to have major impacts on at-risk individuals. Multiple novel therapeutic agents to treat diabetic *sensorimotor* neuropathy are in development, but not one has shown efficacy in humans to date. This is an area of intense interest for both patients and industry, and it may play a major role in future treatments and economic costs. However, the effect these agents might have on *autonomic* neuropathy needs investigation.

■ References

American Diabetes Association (2008). Executive summary: standards of medical care in diabetes—2008. *Diabetes Care* **31** (Suppl. 1), S5–11.

Boulton AJ et al. (2005). Diabetic neuropathies: a statement by the American Diabetes Association. *Diabetes Care* **28**, 956–62.

Boyko EJ et al. (1999). A prospective study of risk factors for diabetic foot ulcer. The Seattle Diabetic Foot Study. *Diabetes Care* **22**, 1036-42.

Clark JM (2006). The epidemiology of nonalcoholic fatty liver disease in adults. *Journal of Clinical Gastroenterology* **40** (Suppl. 1), S5–10.

Coughlin SS et al. (2004). Diabetes mellitus as a predictor of cancer mortality in a large cohort of US adults. *American Journal of Epidemiology* **159**, 1160–7.

DeFrances CJ, Hall MJ (2007). 2005 National Hospital Discharge Survey. *Advance Data* **385**, 1–19.

Diabetes Control and Complications Trial Research Group (1998). The effect of intensive diabetes therapy on measures of autonomic nervous system function in the Diabetes Control and Complications Trial (DCCT). *Diabetologia* **41**, 416–23.

Dyck PJ et al. (1993). The prevalence by staged severity of various types of diabetic neuropathy, retinopathy, and nephropathy in a population-based cohort: the Rochester Diabetic Neuropathy Study. *Neurology* **43**, 817–24.

Everhart JE et al. Prevalence and ethnic differences in gallbladder disease in the United States. *Gastroenterology* **117**, 632–9.

Freemark M, Levitsky LL (2003). Screening for celiac disease in children with type 1 diabetes: two views of the controversy. *Diabetes Care* **26**, 1932–9.

Hanley AJ et al. (2004). Elevations in markers of liver injury and risk of type 2 diabetes: the insulin resistance atherosclerosis study. *Diabetes* **53**, 2623–32.

Harrison SA et al. (2006). Liver disease in patients with diabetes mellitus. *Journal of Clinical Gastroenterology* **40**, 68–76.

Huxley RA et al. (2005). Type-II diabetes and pancreatic cancer: a meta-analysis of 36 studies. *British Journal of Cancer* **92**, 2076–83.

Hyman JJ, Reid BC (2003). Epidemiologic risk factors for periodontal attachment loss among adults in the United States. *Journal of Clinical Periodontology* **30**, 230–7.

Inoue MM et al. (2006). Diabetes mellitus and the risk of cancer: results from a large-scale population-based cohort study in Japan. *Archives of Internal Medicine* **166**, 1871–7.

Janket SJ et al. (2005). Does periodontal treatment improve glycemic control in diabetic patients? A meta-analysis of intervention studies. *Journal of Dental Research* **84**, 1154–9.

Low PA (2003). Testing the autonomic nervous system. *Seminars in Neurology* **23**, 407–21.

Mealey B (1999). Diabetes and periodontal diseases. *Journal of Periodontology* **70**, 935–49.

Mehta SH et al. (2003). Hepatitis C virus infection and incident type 2 diabetes. *Hepatology* **38**, 50–6.

Moore PA, Zgibor JC, Dasanayake AP (2003). Diabetes: a growing epidemic of all ages. *Journal of the American Dental Association* **134** (Special No.), 11S–15S.

Moscatiello SR, Manini R, Marchesini G (2007). Diabetes and liver disease: an ominous association. *Nutrition, Metabolism, and Cardiovascular Diseases* **17**, 63–70.

Mustapha IZ et al. (2007). Markers of systemic bacterial exposure in periodontal disease and cardiovascular disease risk: a systematic review and meta-analysis. *Journal of Periodontology* **78**, 2289–302.

Picardi A et al. (2006). Diabetes in chronic liver disease: from old concepts to new evidence. *Diabetes/Metabolism Research and Reviews.* **22**, 274–83.

Qayyum R, Adomaityte J (2006). Meta-analysis of the effect of thiazolidinediones on serum C-reactive protein levels. *American Journal of Cardiology* **97**, 655–8.

Rewers M et al. (2004). Celiac disease associated with type 1 diabetes mellitus. *Endocrinology and Metabolism Clinics of North America* **33**, 197–214, xi.

Rostom A et al. (2007). Nonsteroidal anti-inflammatory drugs and cyclooxygenase-2 inhibitors for primary prevention of colorectal cancer: a systematic review prepared for the U.S. Preventive Services Task Force. *Annals of Internal Medicine* **146**, 376–89.

Sandler RS et al. (2002). The burden of selected digestive diseases in the United States. *Gastroenterology* **122**, 1500–11.

Saremi A et al. (2005). Periodontal disease and mortality in type 2 diabetes. *Diabetes Care* **28**, 27–32.

Ship JA (2003). Diabetes and oral health: an overview. *Journal of the American Dental Association* **134** (Special Number), 4S–10S.

Taylor GW (2001). Bidirectional interrelationships between diabetes and periodontal diseases: an epidemiologic perspective. *Annals of Periodontology* **6**, 99–112.

Vinik AI, Ziegler D (2007). Diabetic cardiovascular autonomic neuropathy. *Circulation* **115**, 387–97.

13. Diabetes and Mortality

Sharon H. Saydah and Mark S. Eberhardt

■ Main Public Health Messages

- In the population with diabetes, the risk of dying from this disease has decreased.
- Improvements in diabetes care specifically and in health care overall have contributed to the decrease in risk of dying from diabetes.
- In the U.S. population, the age-adjusted death rate from diabetes (calculated using diabetes as an underlying cause of death) has declined slightly in recent years. Even so, diabetes remains a leading cause of death, and the age-adjusted diabetes-related death rate (based on any mention of diabetes on the death certificate) has not declined.
- The absence of a decline in diabetes-related mortality in the U.S. population is due to increased incidence and prevalence of the disease.
- Current estimates of diabetes-related deaths may underestimate diabetes-related mortality because of underreporting of diabetes on death certificates.
- Disparities in diabetes mortality exist by sex, race/ethnicity, and socioeconomic status.

■ Introduction

Diabetes mortality has been and continues to be a topic of keen interest. Since 1999 the age-adjusted diabetes-related death rate (based on any mention of diabetes on the death certificate) has remained stable for the U.S. population (National Center for Health Statistics 2008; Office of Disease Prevention and Health Promotion, U.S. Department of Health and Human Services 2006). In contrast, the estimated rate of diabetes-related deaths among people with diabetes has decreased (National Center for Health Statistics 2008; Office of Disease Prevention and Health Promotion, U.S. Department of Health and Human Services 2006). In this group recent reports have documented improvements in both diabetes mortality and survival

The views and interpretations presented in this chapter are those of the authors and do not necessarily represent the official position of the Centers for Disease Control and Prevention.

(Gregg et al. 2007; Office of Disease Prevention and Health Promotion, U.S. Department of Health and Human Services 2006). Nevertheless, important challenges remain, such as disparities in diabetes mortality by race/ethnicity and other variables and the lack of decline in diabetes-related U.S. death rates despite continued declines in all-cause death rates (DiLiberti and Lorenz 2001; Kung et al. 2008; National Center for Health Statistics 2008; Office of Disease Prevention and Health Promotion, U.S. Department of Health and Human Services 2006). In 2007 the U.S. Congress introduced legislation to improve the collection of diabetes mortality data (HR 3373: Catalyst to Better Diabetes Care Act of 2007, Congressional Record— House 2007), demonstrating Congress's continued interest in this matter.

This chapter summarizes the changes in diabetes mortality for the entire population and among persons with diabetes. It examines sociodemographic differences in deaths from diabetes and the contribution of diabetes to other causes of death. Factors that are related to mortality, especially modifiable factors, are discussed. Measurement issues, such as factors associated with diabetes when diabetes is listed as the underlying rather than a related cause of death on death certificates, are also discussed.

■ Background and Historical Perspective

Diabetes was recorded on death certificates in the United States as early as 1860 (Billings 1896). As early as 1907 researchers using mortality statistics concluded that diabetes would be a growing problem in the United States and that health behaviors might be important contributors to diabetes. The 1907 federal Mortality Statistics report (Mortality Statistics 1909) stated,

> The total number of deaths from diabetes for the year 1907 in the registration area of the United States was 5801, an increase of 470 over the number reported for 1906 (5331). The death rate rose from 13 per 100,000 of population for each of the years 1905 and 1906 to 13.9 per 100,000 for the year 1907. This rate is low, as compared with the rates of tuberculosis, cancer, and other important diseases, but the mortality from diabetes is of increasing significance.... Up to the present time public health administration has concerned itself chiefly with the acute infectious diseases, such as smallpox, diphtheria, and scarlet fever.... In a few years to come—a quarter or a half century is a short period in the life of a nation—the public health authorities will be equally insistent on the prevention of such diseases as diabetes, organic heart disease, cirrhosis of the liver, and other organic diseases which may originate in improper modes of living.

Figure 13.1 presents trends in the number of deaths for diabetes, in crude and age-adjusted death rates for diabetes as an underlying cause of death, and in all-cause mortality. The observed diabetes mortality pattern has been influenced by numerous factors, including changes in mortality reporting, in diabetes classification, in health care, and in population demographics. In 1900, less than 1% of death certificates in the reporting states specified diabetes as the underlying cause

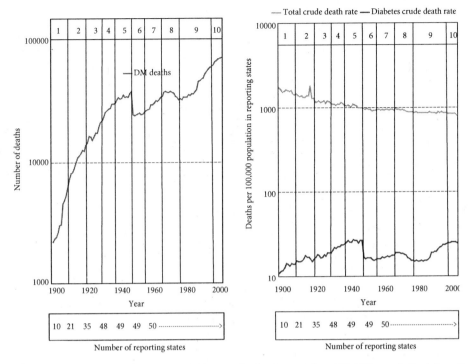

FIGURE 13.1. Number of diabetes deaths, crude death rates (per 100,000 population) for all deaths and diabetes deaths (as noted for underlying cause on death certificates using ICD 1-10) from reporting states and number of reporting states in the United States, 1900–2004

of death; by 2005 this share had increased to 3.1% (Centers for Disease Control and Prevention 2000; Kung et al. 2008).

Over the course of the last century there have been 10 revisions to the International Classification of Diseases (ICD), which is used to code causes of death (Centers for Disease Control and Prevention 2007). These changes have had observable impacts on the diabetes mortality pattern.

Improvements in diabetes management have had a demonstrable impact on diabetes mortality. All-cause death rates among children aged 5 to 14 years experienced a steady decrease from 1900 to 1940; in contrast, diabetes death rates in this age group increased 15% from 1900 to 1921. However, from 1922 (the year after insulin was discovered) until 1940, this age-specific death rate decreased 64%, surpassing the all-cause decrease of 52% for the period (National Center for Health Statistics 1947).

■ Epidemiology of Diabetes Mortality

Trends in Diabetes Mortality

Trends in diabetes mortality can be examined (1) for the U.S. population using vital statistics or (2) for people with diabetes using prospective cohort studies or other data sources. Vital statistics data collected on death certificates are used to examine diabetes mortality in the general population, which allows the examination of trends in diabetes mortality versus other causes of death. Mortality trends reflect both trends in the incidence and prevalence of diabetes in the general population and case fatality rates among people with diagnosed diabetes.

Trends in diabetes mortality are based on either underlying cause of death or all reported causes of death recorded on death certificates (diabetes-related mortality). Underlying cause of death is defined as "the disease or injury that initiated the train of events leading directly to death" (Kung et al. 2008). Cause of death in national mortality statistics is attributed to one underlying condition based on information listed on the death certificate and using the international rules for selecting underlying cause of death from the conditions listed on the death certificate. Diabetes-related mortality or diabetes as a "multiple" cause of death refers to deaths with any report of diabetes on the death certificate as an underlying or as an associated cause of death. Statistics on diabetes-related mortality complement information on the underlying cause of death. Among persons aged 65 years or older, diabetes is more than twice as likely to be listed as a related cause of death than as the underlying cause of death (Gorina and Lentzer 2008). Examining diabetes deaths based on vital statistics using multiple causes of death provides information on diabetes as an important contributor to mortality, and it is also useful for examining both crude and age-adjusted death rates. The crude death rate measures overall mortality burden and is used to rank causes of death. Age adjustment eliminates differences between rates that result from differences in age composition and is used to compare rates at two or more time points or between population subgroups. Issues in measuring diabetes mortality from death certificates are discussed later in this chapter.

Based on U.S. vital statistics for underlying cause of death, the age-adjusted death rate from diabetes increased by 38% from 1980 to 2000 and then declined by almost 2% from 2000 to 2005 (National Center for Health Statistics 2007). In contrast there was an overall decrease in all-cause mortality of 23% from 1980 to 2005 (National Center for Health Statistics 2007). The increase in diabetes mortality from 1980 to 2000 (based on underlying cause of death) was probably due to a combination of factors, including an increased prevalence of diabetes and an increased propensity for physicians, who certify the cause of death, to report diabetes on the death certificate. One factor leading to the increased prevalence of diabetes is the increased incidence of this disease, which in turn is secondary to the increasing prevalence of two major risk factors (i.e., obesity and sedentary lifestyle). Factors leading to changes in reporting of diabetes on the death certificate may include changes to the certificate's format, improvements in awareness among patients and providers that the diagnosis of diabetes is present, and changes in the understanding of the relationship of diabetes to other disease processes.

To prospectively examine mortality among people with diagnosed diabetes, one must be able to identify a group of persons with diabetes and determine their subsequent mortality. Various data sources have been used to do this, including national health surveys linked to vital statistics (Gregg et al. 2007), population-based prospective cohort studies with follow-up for mortality status (Lotufo et al. 2001), and diabetes registries (Pambianco et al. 2006). In addition mortality data from vital records in combination with denominator estimates of diabetes prevalence can be used to estimate trends in death rates among people with diagnosed diabetes (Healthy People 2010 Progression Review: Focus Area 5: Diabetes 2006; Office of Disease Prevention and Health Promotion, U.S.Department of Health and Human Services 2006).

Follow-up of people with type 1 diabetes indicates that their mortality rates were lower if their diabetes was diagnosed in the 1960s or later than if they were diagnosed prior to 1960 (Pambianco et al. 2006). Similarly, diabetes mortality among persons with *either* type 1 or type 2 diabetes has been lower among persons diagnosed since 1960 than among persons diagnosed before 1960 (Pambianco et al. 2006). Trends in diabetes mortality vary by sex and race/ethnicity; for example, the improvement in mortality experience among people with diabetes has been more pronounced among men than among women. Follow-up of national samples of adults with diabetes found that all-cause mortality rates among men with diabetes decreased 43% between 1971–1986 and 1988–2000 but did not decrease among women in the same time period (Gregg et al. 2007).

Mortality from heart disease, which is the leading cause of death among people with or without diabetes, has declined since 1971 in the United States. This trend has been observed in persons with and without diabetes. However, heart disease mortality has not decreased as much in persons with diabetes as in those without the disorder (Gregg et al. 2007; Gu et al. 1999). Similar trends are seen among persons with diabetes in Canada (Booth et al. 2006).

Overall Patterns of Diabetes Mortality

Deaths from Diabetes

Death rates from diabetes increase with age. In the United States in 2005, among adults aged 45 to 54 years the death rate (per 100,000 population) from diabetes was 13; this increased to 37 at 55 to 64 years, 87 at 65 to 74 years, 177 at 75 to 84 years, and 312 at 85 years or older (Kung et al. 2008).

Mortality risk from diabetes also differs by sex and race and ethnicity. In 2005, vital records indicate that males were about 30% more likely to die from diabetes than females based on age-adjusted underlying cause-of-death rates. Non-Hispanic whites and Asians and Pacific Islanders have lower age-adjusted death rates from diabetes than non-Hispanic blacks, Hispanics, and American Indians/Alaska Natives (National Center for Health Statistics 2007; Kung et al. 2008). In the general U.S. population in 2005, non-Hispanic blacks were 2.2 times as likely to die from diabetes based on age-adjusted underlying cause of death as non-Hispanic whites, and

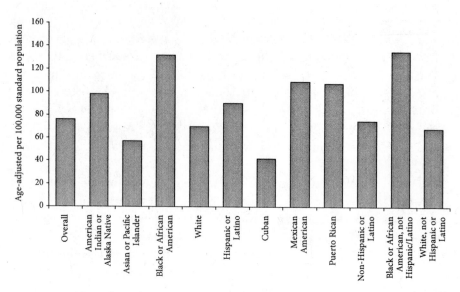

FIGURE 13.2. Age-adjusted mortality for diabetes overall and by race and ethnicity, United States 2004

Hispanics were 1.6 times as likely to die from diabetes as non-Hispanic whites (Kung et al. 2008). An excess of diabetes death rates among blacks versus whites is also present in children and teens (Centers for Disease Control and Prevention 2007).

Based on U.S. death certificates for underlying cause of death, the age-adjusted death rate from diabetes for American Indians or Alaska Natives was almost twice that for non-Hispanic whites in 2005 (National Center for Health Statistics 2007). However other research suggests that death rates for American Indians or Alaska Natives are underestimates because these two populations are underreported in the space for race on the death certificate (Stern 1998; Rosenberg et al. 1999). Figure 13.2 compares the age-adjusted diabetes-related death rates based on multiple causes of death by race/ethnicity in the United States in 2005.

Diabetes-related death rates also differ by education level. Among persons aged 25 to 64 years in 2005 (using data from 22 states), age-adjusted diabetes-related death rates were higher among those with less than a high school education (64 per 100,000) than they were among high school graduates (41 per 100,000), and they were far lower among those with at least some college (17 per 100,000) (National Center for Health Statistics 2008).

Mortality Experience of People with Diabetes Compared with the General Population

Overall, people with diabetes have twice the risk of death borne by the general population (Huxley et al. 2006; Lotufo et al. 2001; Mulnier et al. 2006; Nilsson et al. 1998). At age 50, life expectancy is approximately 7 to 8 years shorter for someone with diabetes than for a person without the disease (by 7 years for men and 8 years for women) (Franco et al. 2007; Gu et al. 1999; Narayan et al. 2003). The relative risk of death among people with diabetes compared with the population without the disease is highest at the youngest ages and decreases with increasing age. However, the risk of mortality attributable to diabetes does not decrease with age. The burden of death attributable to diabetes can be measured by the population-attributable risk, which is the percentage of deaths in the population that are associated with diabetes and could potentially be postponed by eliminating the disease. To determine the mortality attributable to diabetes, the population-attributable risk can be calculated based on the prevalence of diabetes and the relative risk of death among people with diabetes compared with people without diabetes. Because of the increasing prevalence of diabetes in the older ages, the percentage of deaths attributable to diabetes increased with age from 3.1% for adults aged 30–49 years to 4.9% for persons aged 50–64 years and then to 6.9% for those aged 65–74 years (Saydah et al. 2002) in a U.S. nationally representative study conducted from 1974 to 1992.

Diabetes is often cited as "eliminating or reducing" the female protective advantage for risk of cardiovascular disease (Barrett-Connor and Wingard 1983; Barrett-Connor et al. 1991), and this appears to be true for cardiovascular disease mortality among people with diabetes (Barrett-Connor and Wingard 1983; Barrett-Connor et al. 1991), where the relative risk of death in among people with diabetes from heart disease was 2.5 for men and 3.4 for women. In the general population, life expectancy at birth was 5.2 years longer for females than for males in 2005 (Minino et al. 2007).

However, the relative risk of death among females with diabetes using females without diabetes as the referent ranges from 2.1 to 3.7, whereas the relative risk of death among males with diabetes (versus males without diabetes) ranges from 1.7 to 2.2 (Huxley et al. 2006; Mulnier et al. 2006; Nilsson et al. 1998).

Lower education levels are associated with increased mortality in the general population and among people with diabetes. The patterns of mortality by education level are similar among people with and without diabetes, with lower attained education level associated with an increased risk of death (Chaturvedi et al. 1998).

Major Causes of Death among People with Diabetes

Vascular diseases, both macrovascular and microvascular, are the leading complications of diabetes and one of the leading underlying causes of death among people with diabetes. Cardiovascular disease, which includes both macrovascular and microvascular disease, accounted for over 40% of combined deaths among people with type 1 or type 2 diabetes in 1978 to 1988 (Portuese and Orchard 1995; Geiss et al. 1995; Morrish et al. 2001). Deaths from renal disease, a microvascular disease, are also common. Other common causes of death among people with diabetes include acute metabolic events, pneumonia and influenza, and malignant neoplasms (Portuese and Orchard 1995; Geiss et al. 1995; Morrish et al. 2001). Causes of death are similar by gender among persons with diabetes, although women are more likely to die from renal disease than are men.

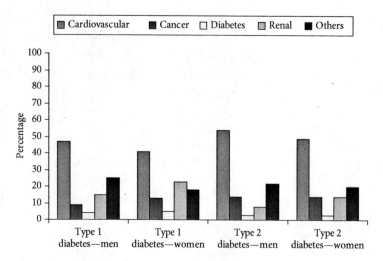

FIGURE 13.3. Major causes of death among people with diabetes. (Adapted from Morrish et al. 2001.)

Patterns for type 1 and type 2 diabetes differ slightly. Figure 13.3 illustrates the major causes of death (assigned by a committee of physicians as part of the World Health Organization [WHO] Multinational Study of Vascular Disease in Diabetes from 10 internal study centers) among people with diabetes by gender and diabetes type. Renal disease accounted for 21% of the deaths for people with type 1 diabetes versus 11% of the deaths for people with type 2 (Morrish et al. 2001). Deaths from cardiovascular disease accounted for 52% of deaths among people with type 2 and 44% of deaths for type 1. All other causes of death accounted for 20%–25% of all deaths for both type 1 and type 2.

Risk Factors for Mortality among People with Diabetes

Numerous factors are associated with an increased risk of death among people with diabetes, including age, gender, race/ethnicity, education, diabetes duration, insulin use, smoking, microvascular and macrovascular disease, and comorbid depression.

Many risk factors that are associated with increased mortality in the general population also predict increased mortality among people with diabetes. For example cohort studies of people with diabetes report excess mortality among older adults, males, and some racial/ethnic subpopulations (including African Americans and American Indians) (Gregg et al. 2007; Gu et al. 1999; Lee et al. 1998). In addition lower-attained levels of education are associated with higher mortality among adults with diabetes (Nilsson et al. 1998; Wilder 2003). Finally, smoking has consistently been associated with increased risk of mortality among people with diabetes (Geiss et al. 1995; Portuese and Orchard 1995). As would be expected a longer duration of diabetes is associated with increased risk of mortality after adjusting for age (Brun et al. 2000; Mulnier et al. 2006).

Use of insulin for treatment of diabetes, which may be a marker for disease severity, is associated with increased risk of mortality (Kronmal et al. 2006). Elevated cholesterol levels and high blood pressure are also associated with increased risk of mortality among people with diabetes (Geiss et al. 1995; Portuese and Orchard 1995; Stevens and Holman 2004; Vaccaro et al. 1998), as are microvascular and macrovascular diseases. A prospective cohort study of patients with type 2 diabetes found that elevated glucose levels and hypertension increased the risk of death from all causes and from cardiovascular disease (Bruno et al. 1999; Mulnier et al. 2006). Comorbid depression among adults with diabetes is common, with a prevalence ranging from 11% to 15% (Anderson RJ et al. 2001), and is associated with increased mortality. Among a large cohort of patients with type 2 diabetes enrolled in a health maintenance organization, both minor and major depression increased the risk of death by 43%–46% after adjustment for other potential confounders (Katon et al. 2005).

Among people without a clinical diagnosis of diabetes, undiagnosed diabetes or hyperglycemia, such as prediabetes or impaired fasting glucose, has been associated with increased mortality. Studies have consistently found undiagnosed diabetes to be associated with increased risk of mortality (DECODE Study Group 1999; de Vegt et al. 1999; Saydah et al. 2001). Many studies have also found that levels of glucose that are elevated but not enough for a diagnosis of diabetes, such as impaired fasting glucose, are associated with increased mortality (DECODE Study Group 1999; de Vegt et al. 1999; Saydah et al. 2001). Part of this increased risk may be explained by a conversion to actual diabetes among persons with impaired fasting glucose (Rijkelijkhuizen et al. 2007). Regardless, whether the relationship of glycemia and mortality follows a threshold effect or is continuous is debated (Balkau et al. 1999; Gerstein 1999). A meta-analysis of prospective cohort studies found a threshold effect at 100 mg/dl between fasting glucose and cardiovascular disease mortality, but a linear relationship was found between 2-hour glucose values from an oral glucose tolerance test and this kind of mortality (Levitan et al. 2004).

■ Public Health Preventive or Intervention Strategies

Public health strategies to decrease diabetes mortality have a dual focus on (1) reducing the burden of diabetes-related complications through research, health promotion efforts, and public education, and on (2) reducing the risk of developing diabetes. Numerous epidemiologic studies and clinical trials have demonstrated the benefit of improved diabetes care in terms of lowering diabetes-related complications and subsequent mortality (Nathan et al. 2005; Schrier et al. 2007; Vijan and Hayward 2004). Much of this success involves improved glycemic, blood pressure, and lipid control (Fuller et al. 2001; Miettinen et al. 1996). More details about these prevention efforts are discussed later in this chapter under "Diabetes Control Programs and Policy." Health promotion efforts include expanded Medicare coverage for diabetes screening (Medicare Preventive Services: Diabetes Screening 2008), assessments of the quality of diabetes care by the Agency for Health Care Research and Quality (AHRQ 2008), and conducting surveillance activities to inform health policy officials of progress toward achieving national diabetes mortality objectives set forth in *Healthy People 2010* (Healthy People 2010 Progression Review: Focus Area 5: Diabetes 2006). Improved public education regarding diabetes and its risk factors is accomplished through many private and public efforts, such as the National Diabetes Education Program (National Institutes of Health 2007), which has a campaign to reduce the risk factors for heart disease, as noted earlier the leading cause of death among people with diabetes.

■ Implications for Health Policy

Research on mortality provides guidance for primary, secondary, and tertiary prevention efforts for diabetes. People with impaired glucose tolerance have a 40% increased risk for mortality even if they do not develop clinically defined diabetes (DECODE Study Group 1999; Qiao et al. 2003). These results, in combination with evidence from clinical trials (UK Prospective Diabetes Study [UKPDS] Group 1998), laid the groundwork for current clinical guidelines for persons with prediabetes (American Diabetes Association 2008). Findings reported in 2000 suggested that each decrease in systolic blood pressure of 10 mm Hg was associated with an average 15% reduction in diabetes-related death rates (Adler et al. 2000). These results contributed to a consensus among diabetes and hypertension experts that the recommended level of blood pressure for people with diabetes should be lowered (American Diabetes Association 2003; National Heart, Lung and Blood Institute, National Institutes of Health 2004).

Others have used mortality data to develop standards of medical care for hospitalized patients with hyperglycemia (American College of Endocrinology Position Statement on Inpatient Diabetes and Metabolic Control 2004). To reduce premature mortality, free access to some pharmacologic therapies is being explored for persons with diabetes (Gavin 2006; Rosen et al. 2005). This effort was guided by recent research combining data on mortality with economic research that showed the cost-effectiveness of pharmacologic therapies (Rosen et al. 2005). In addition to improving the standards of care for people with diabetes, research on mortality has led to actions to reduce the burden of diabetes. With the knowledge that diabetes was a leading cause of death, in 1974 the U.S. Congress directed federal officials to establish state-based diabetes control programs (National Diabetes Mellitus Research and Education Act, 1974). In 1977 five programs began with federal assistance (State-Based Diabetes Prevention & Control Programs 2007). The current system of diabetes control and prevention programs, which includes all states, U.S. territories, and island jurisdictions (State-Based Diabetes Prevention & Control Programs 2007), arose in response to several concerns, among them the increased burden of diabetes, interest in improving the quality of health care, and reducing mortality. Information on diabetes mortality was important in the passage of state laws to improve health insurance coverage for people with diabetes (National Conference of State Legislatures 2007). In addition, researchers have presented findings that demonstrate racial/ethnic disparities in diabetes mortality (Fiscella 2003; Statehealthfacts.org 2007). Recognition of these disparities lends support to decisions made by the National Diabetes Education Program to offer health education efforts that target particular races or ethnicities (National Institutes of Health 2007).

Since 1990 national health objectives have included goals to reduce diabetes mortality, and progress has indeed been made in reducing the age-adjusted diabetes-related death rate among persons with diabetes. The 2010 objective, established in 2000, was to reduce diabetes-related deaths per 1000 persons with diabetes from 8.8 in 1999 to 7.8. By 2001, this goal had already been achieved, and in 2005 the death rate was 6.9 per 1000 (Healthy People 2010 Progression Review: Focus Area 5: Diabetes 2006; National Center for Health Statistics 2008; Office of Disease Prevention and Health Promotion, U.S. Department of Health and Human Services 2006). And yet, despite improvements in health practices for people with diabetes (Saaddine et al. 2006), little progress has been made toward the 2010 objective to reduce the age-adjusted death rate for diabetes-related deaths among the *total* U.S. population to 46 per 100,000. The estimates (per 100,000 U.S. population) for both the baseline year (1999) and for 2005 were 77 (National Center for Health Statistics 2008). This stable rate is due, in part, to the increasing proportion of the population with diabetes (Cowie et al. 2006).

■ Areas of Uncertainty or Controversy

In estimating diabetes mortality a variety of errors can be made. One such error is to assume that all deaths among people with diabetes can be attributed solely to diabetes (Saydah et al. 2002). This assumption, which often is made in cohort studies comparing mortality of people with and without diabetes, may lead to an overestimation of deaths due to diabetes (Andresen et al. 1993; Centers for Disease Control [CDC] 1991; Saydah et al. 2002). An alternative method in determining the mortality attributable to diabetes is to calculate the population attributable risk, as described earlier in this chapter.

Another concern is underreporting of diabetes on death certificates. Several studies have calculated the sensitivity of diabetes reporting on death certificates among persons known to have diabetes and who died from diabetes-related causes. These studies found that the sensitivity of death certificates for listing diabetes as one of the causes of death ranged from 32% to 68%, with a median of 43.6% (Saydah et al. 2004). The sensitivity dropped from 29% to 7% (median 12.7%) when underlying cause of death rather than any listed cause was used (Saydah et al. 2004). One recent study found that diabetes is more likely to be reported on death certificates in the context of cardiovascular disease (Cheng et al. 2008). A few states, such as North Dakota and New Jersey, have attempted to address this issue by including a single check box on the state death certificate for the physician to indicate if the decedent had diabetes. Kentucky has two check box questions to indicate diabetes; the first question asks whether the decedent had diabetes and the second whether the diabetes was an underlying or contributing cause of death. A recent analysis of death certificates from Kentucky showed that the use of a second check box may have contributed to a slight increase in diabetes listed as the underlying cause of death but an overall decrease in diabetes listed as a cause of death (Heron and Anderson 2006).

Diabetes death rates can also be influenced by other changes in the death certificate. Between 1988 and 1989 there was an unexpected 14% increase in diabetes death rates in the United States; rather than a sudden rise in deaths from diabetes, this was thought to result from changes in reporting diabetes on death certificates (Hoyert et al. 2000; National Center for Health Statistics 1992). Specifically, it was proposed that this increase was due to changes by physicians in their documentation of diabetes on the death certificate. The changes in the death certificate included instructions and examples of proper cause-of-death certification, of which diabetes was one of the examples. Periodic revisions of the ICD also have affected estimates of diabetes mortality. The change from the 9th to the 10th Revision of the ICD, which was implemented in the United States in 1999, resulted in minimal changes in the diabetes death rates (Anderson RN et al. 2001), but the change between ICD-5 and ICD-6 resulted in a drop in diabetes deaths as observed in Figure 13.1.

The recording of diabetes on death certificates varies by country. In general countries follow a two-part format as recommended by WHO. Part I lists diseases or injuries that caused the death, while Part II lists other significant conditions. For example, physicians in the United States are less likely to report diabetes in Part I of the death certificate (19%) than are physicians in Sweden (46%) or Taiwan (56%) (Lu et al. 2006). Given the differences in completing death certificates by country, international comparisons of diabetes mortality based on death certificates should be interpreted carefully.

There are numerous reasons why diabetes may not be reported on a death certificate. For example, if a person with diabetes died from an accident or injury, diabetes may not be included on the death certificate (Heron M, personal communication 2007; Lu et al. 2006; Murray et al. 2008). Or, the certifying physician may not know the person had diabetes; this may especially be true if the person died in the emergency room. Physicians may also be less likely to report diabetes on a death certificate if the person's diabetes is considered to be under control, because the physician may not consider diabetes to be a contributing cause of death in that situation (Heron M, personal communication 2007; Lu et al. 2006; Murray et al. 2008).

■ Developments over the Next 5 to 10 Years

The prevalence of diabetes in the United States is likely to continue to increase in the next 5 to 10 years (Narayan et al. 2006). The exact impact of this continued increase on future diabetes death rates is unknown. In general mortality has decreased among people with diabetes. More generally trends are likely to differ between population-based and patient-based diabetes death rates. The increased prevalence of diabetes may result in an increase in diabetes-related death rates in the United States. On the other hand, continued improvements in diabetes care may increase life expectancy among people with diabetes and thereby lower the death rate in this group. In the general population continued efforts to diagnose and treat diabetes may improve overall mortality from this disease.

■ References

Adler AI et al. (2000). Association of systolic blood pressure with macrovascular and microvascular complications of type 2 diabetes (UKPDS 36): prospective observational study. *British Medical Journal* **321**, 412–9.

Agency for Healthcare Research and Quality (2008). Available at www.ahrq.gov. Accessed April 21, 2008.

American College of Endocrinology (2004). Position Statement on Inpatient Diabetes and Metabolic Control *Endocrine Practice* **10** (1), 77–82.

American Diabetes Association. (2003) Treatment of hypertension in adults with diabetes. *Diabetes Care* **26**, S80–2.

American Diabetes Association. (2008). Standards of Medical Care in Diabetes–2008. *Diabetes Care* **30** (S1), S41.

Anderson RJ et al. (2001). The prevalence of comorbid depression in adults with diabetes: a meta-analysis. *Diabetes Care* **24**, 1069–78.

Anderson RN et al. (2001) Comparability of cause of death between ICD-9 and ICD-10: preliminary estimates. *National Vital Statistics Report* **49** (2), 1–32.

Andresen EM et al (1993). Underreporting of diabetes on death certificates, King County, Washington. *American Journal of Public Health* **83**, 1021–4.

Balkau B et al. (1999) Is there a glycemic threshold for mortality risk? *Diabetes Care* **22**, 696–9.

Barrett-Connor E, Wingard DL. (1983). Sex differential in ischemic heart disease mortality in diabetics: a prospective population-based study. *American Journal of Epidemiology* **118**, 489–96.

Barrett-Connor EL et al. (1991). Why is diabetes mellitus a stronger risk factor for fatal ischemic heart disease in women than in men? The Rancho Bernardo Study. *JAMA* **265**, 627–31.

Billings JS (1896). Report on Vital and Social Statistics at the 11th Census, 1890, Part I Analysis and Rate Tables. Available at http://www.cdc.gov/nchs/data/vsushistorical/vsush_1890_1.pdf. Accessed August 1, 2007.

Booth GL et al. (2006). Recent trends in cardiovascular complications among men and women with and without diabetes. *Diabetes Care* **29**, 32–7.

Brun E et al. (2000). Diabetes duration and cause-specific mortality in the Verona Diabetes Study. *Diabetes Care* **23**, 1119–23.

Bruno G et al. (1999) Impact of glycaemic control, hypertension and insulin treatment on general and cause-specific mortality: an Italian population-based cohort of type II (non-insulin-dependent) diabetes mellitus. *Diabetologia* **42**, 297–301.

Centers for Disease Control (CDC) (1991). Sensitivity of death certificate data for monitoring diabetes mortality—Diabetic Eye Disease Follow-up Study, 1985–1990. *MMWR Morbidity and Mortality Weekly Report* **40**, 739–41.

Centers for Disease Control and Prevention (CDC) (2007). Racial disparities in diabetes mortality among persons aged 1–19 years, United States 1979–2004. *MMWR Morbidity and Mortality Weekly Report* **56** (45), 1184–7.

Centers for Disease Control and Prevention National Center for Health Statistics (2000). Leading Causes of Death, 1900–1998. Available at http://www.cdc.gov/nchs/data/dvs/lead1900_98.pdf. Accessed September 5, 2007.

Centers for Disease Control and Prevention National Center for Health Statistics. (2007) International Classification of Diseases, Tenth Revision. Centers for Disease Control and Prevention, National Center for Health Statistics. Available at www.cdc.gov/nchs/about/major/dvs/icd10des.htm. Accessed August 31, 2007.

Chaturvedi N et al. (1998). Socioeconomic gradient in morbidity and mortality in people with diabetes: cohort study findings from the Whitehall Study and the WHO Multinational Study of Vascular Disease in Diabetes. *British Medical Journal* **316**, 100–5.

Cheng WS et al. (2008). Sensitivity and specificity of death certificates for diabetes. *Diabetes Care* **31**, 279–84.

Cowie CC et al. (2006). Prevalence of diabetes and impaired fasting glucose in adults in the U.S. population: National Health and Nutrition Examination Survey 1999–2002. Diabetes Care **29**, 1263–8.

DECODE Study Group (1999). Glucose tolerance and mortality: comparison of WHO and American Diabetes Association diagnostic criteria. The DECODE study group. European Diabetes Epidemiology Group. Diabetes Epidemiology: Collaborative Analysis Of Diagnostic Criteria in Europe. *Lancet* **354**, 617–21.

de Vegt F et al. (1999). Hyperglycaemia is associated with all-cause and cardiovascular mortality in the Hoorn population: the Hoorn Study. *Diabetologia* **42**, 926–31.

DiLiberti JH, Lorenz RA (2001). Long-term trends in childhood diabetes mortality: 1968–1998. *Diabetes Care* **24**, 1348–52.

Fiscella K (2003). Assessing Health Care Quality for Minority and Other Disparity Populations. U.S. Department of Health and Human Services, Agency for Healthcare Research and Quality; Report AHRQ Publication No. 03-0047-EF. Available at http://www.ahrq.gov/qual/qdisprep.pdf. Accessed April 16, 2010.

Franco OH et al. (2007). Associations of diabetes mellitus with total life expectancy and life expectancy with and without cardiovascular disease. *Archives of Internal Medicine* **167**, 1145–51.

Fuller JH et al. (2001) Risk factors for cardiovascular mortality and morbidity: the WHO Multinational Study of Vascular Disease in Diabetes. *Diabetologia* **44** (Suppl. 2), S54–64.

Gavin K (2006). University unveils plan to encourage use of medications to control diabetes. University of Michigan News Service . 5-2-2006. (Accessed 8-17-2007) Available at http://www.umich.edu/~urecord/0506/Apr24_06/00.shtml Accessed August 17, 2007.

Geiss L et al. (1995) Mortality in Non-Insulin Dependent Diabetes. In Harris MI et al., eds. *Diabetes in America*. 2nd ed., pp 233–55. National Institutes of Health, National Institute of Diabetes and Digestive and Kidney Diseases, NIH Publication No. 95-1468, Bethesda, MD

Gerstein HC. (1999) Is glucose a continuous risk factor for cardiovascular mortality? *Diabetes Care* **22**, 659–60.

Gorina Y, Lentzer H. (2008). Multiple causes of death in old age. Aging Trends. Report No. 9 Hyattsville, MD: National Center for Health Statistics (accessed September 29, 2008) Available at http://www.cdc.gov/nchs/data/ahcd/agingtrends/09causes. htm. Accessed April 16, 2010

Gregg EW et al. (2007). Mortality trends in men and women with diabetes, 1971 to 2000. *Annals of Internal Medicine* **147**, 149–55.

Gu K et al. (1999). Diabetes and decline in heart disease mortality in US adults. *JAMA* **281**, 1291–7.

Healthy People 2010 Progression Review: Focus Area 5: Diabetes (2006). U.S. Department of Health and Human Services. Available at http://www.cdc.gov/ nchs/about/otheract/hpdata2010/focusareas/fa05-diabetes2.htm. Accessed August 17, 2007.

Heron M, Anderson RN (2006). Diabetes reporting on death certificates in Kentucky, 2002–2003. 2006 National Center for Health Statistics Data Users Conference. Available at: http://www.cdc.gov/nchs/ppt/duc2006/heron_8.ppt. Accessed September 29, 2008.

Hoyert DL et al. (2000). Effect of changes in death certificate format on cause-specific mortality trends, United States, 1979–92. In Death certification and mortality statistics: An international perspective. Report 64. Office for National Statistics; London.

HR 3373: Catalyst to Better Diabetes Care Act of 2007, Congressional Record—House (2007). August 3, 2007. Available at http://www.govtrack.us/congress/bill. xpd?bill=h110-3373. Accessed April 16, 2010.

Huxley R et al. (2006) Excess risk of fatal coronary heart disease associated with diabetes in men and women: meta-analysis of 37 prospective cohort studies. *British Medical Journal* **332**, 73–8.

Katon WJ et al. (2005) The association of comorbid depression with mortality in patients with type 2 diabetes. *Diabetes Care* **28**, 2668–72.

Kronmal RA, et al. (2006). Mortality in pharmacologically treated older adults with diabetes: the Cardiovascular Health Study, 1989–2001. *PLoS Medicine* **3** (10), e400.

Kung HC et al. (2008) Deaths: final data for 2005. *National Vital Statistics Report* **56** (10), 1–120.

Lee ET et al. (1998) All-cause mortality and cardiovascular disease mortality in three American Indian populations, aged 45–74 years, 1984–1988. The Strong Heart Study. *American Journal of Epidemiology* **147**, 995–1008.

Levitan EB et al. (2004). Is nondiabetic hyperglycemia a risk factor for cardiovascular disease? A meta-analysis of prospective studies. *Archives of Internal Medicine* **164**, 2147–55.

Lotufo PA et al. (2001) Diabetes and all-cause and coronary heart disease mortality among US male physicians. *Archives of Internal Medicine* **161**, 242–7.

Lu TH et al. (2006) Certifying diabetes-related cause-of-death: a comparison of inappropriate certification statements in Sweden, Taiwan and the USA. *Diabetologia* **49**, 2878–81.

Medicare Preventive Services: Diabetes Screening, Supplies and Self-Management Training (2008). Available at http://www.medicare.gov/Health/Diabetes.asp. Accessed April 20, 2008.

Miettinen H et al (1996). Retinopathy predicts coronary heart disease events in NIDDM patients. *Diabetes Care* **19**, 1445–8.

Minino AM et al. (2007). Deaths: final data for 2004. *National Vital Statistics Report* **55** (19), 1–120.

Morrish NJ et al. (2001). Mortality and causes of death in the WHO Multinational Study of Vascular Disease in Diabetes. *Diabetologia* **44** (Suppl. 2), S14–21.

Mortality Statistics (1909). Mortality Statistics 1907. Eighth Annual Report. Available at http://www.cdc.gov/nchs/data/vsushistorical/mortstatsh_1907.pdf. Accessed April 16, 2010.

Mulnier HE et al. (2006). Mortality in people with type 2 diabetes in the UK. *Diabetic Medicine* **23**, 516–21.

Murray CJ et al. (2008). Improving the comparability of diabetes mortality statistics in the U.S. and Mexico. *Diabetes Care* **31**, 451–8.

Narayan KM et al. (2003). Lifetime risk for diabetes mellitus in the United States. *JAMA* **290**, 1884–90.

Narayan KM et al. (2006). Impact of recent increase in incidence on future diabetes burden: U.S., 2005–2050. *Diabetes Care* **29**, 2114–6.

Nathan DM et al. (2005) Intensive diabetes treatment and cardiovascular disease in patients with type 1 diabetes. *New England Journal of Medicine* **353**, 2643–53.

National Center for Health Statistics (1947). Vital Statistics in the United States, 1900–1940. Table 14. Available at http://www.cdc.gov/nchs/data/vsus/vsrates1900_40.pdf. Accessed August 1, 2007.

National Center for Health Statistics (1992). Advance Report of Final Mortality Statistics, 1989. Monthly Vital Statistics National Center for Health Statistics; Vol. 40, No. 8, Suppl. 2. p 1–52. Available at http://www.cdc.gov/nchs/data/mvsr/supp/mv40_08s2.pdf. Accessed April 16, 2010.

National Center for Health Statistics (2007). Health, United States, 2007 with Chartbook on Trends in Health of Americans. Available at http://www.cdc.gov/nchs/hus.htm. Accessed August 1, 2008.

National Center for Health Statistics. (2008). DATA2010. Available at http://wonder. cdc.gov/data2010. Accessed July 14, 2008.

National Conference of State Legislatures (2007). State Laws Mandating Diabetes Health Coverage. National Conference of State Legislatures. Available at http://www.ncsl.org/programs/health/diabetes.htm. Accessed August 17, 2007.

National Diabetes Mellitus Research and Education Act (1974). § Public Law 93-354.

National Heart, Lung, and Blood Institute, National Institutes of Health, National High Blood Pressure Education Program (2004). The Seventh Report of the Joint National Committee on Prevention, Detection, Evaluation, and Treatment of High Blood Pressure. Bethesda, MD: U.S. Department of Health and Human Services, National Institutes of Health, Publication No. 04-5230.

National Institute of Health National Institute for Diabetes and Digestive and Kidney Diseases (2007). National Diabetes Education Program. Available at http://ndep. nih.gov/. Accessed September 29, 2008.

Nilsson PM et al. (1998). Low educational status is a risk factor for mortality among diabetic people. *Diabetic Medicine* **15**, 213–9.

Office of Disease Prevention and Health Promotion, U.S. Department of Health and Human Services (2006). Summary Report, Healthy People 2010 Progress Review, Diabetes. Available at http://www.healthypeople.gov/data/2010prog/ focus05/2006Focus5.pdf. Accessed August 17, 2007.

Pambianco G et al. (2006). The 30-year natural history of type 1 diabetes complications: the Pittsburgh Epidemiology of Diabetes Complications Study experience. *Diabetes* **55**, 1463–9.

Portuese E, Orchard T (1995). Mortality in insulin-dependent diabetes. In Harris MI et al., eds. *Diabetes in America*, 2nd ed., pp 221–32. Bethesda, MD: National Institutes of Health, National Institute of Diabetes and Digestive and Kidney Diseases, NIH Publication No. 95-1468.

Qiao Q et al. (2003). Predictive properties of impaired glucose tolerance for cardiovascular risk are not explained by the development of overt diabetes during follow-up. *Diabetes Care* **26**, 2910–4.

Rijkelijkhuizen JM et al. (2007). High risk of cardiovascular mortality in individuals with impaired fasting glucose is explained by conversion to diabetes: the Hoorn study. *Diabetes Care* **30**, 332–6.

Rosen AB et al. (2005). Cost-effectiveness of full medicare coverage of angiotensin-converting enzyme inhibitors for beneficiaries with diabetes. *Annals of Internal Medicine* **143**, 89–99.

Rosenberg HM et al. (1999). Quality of death rates by race and Hispanic origin: a summary of current research, 1999. *Vital and Health Statistics Series* **2** (128), 1–13.

Saaddine JB, et al. (2006). Improvements in diabetes processes of care and intermediate outcomes: United States, 1988–2002. *Annals of Internal Medicine* **144**, 465–74.

Saydah SH et al. (2001). Subclinical states of glucose intolerance and risk of death in the U.S. *Diabetes Care* **24**, 447–53.

Saydah SH et al. (2002). Age and the burden of death attributable to diabetes in the United States. *American Journal of Epidemiology* **156**, 714–9.

Saydah SH et al. (2004). Review of the performance of methods to identify diabetes cases among vital statistics, administrative, and survey data. *Annals of Epidemiology* **14**, 507–16.

Schrier RW et al (2007). Appropriate blood pressure control in hypertensive and normotensive type 2 diabetes mellitus: a summary of the ABCD trial. *Nature Clinical Practice Nephrology* **3**, 428–38.

State-Based Diabetes Prevention & Control Programs. Centers for Disease Control and Prevention, Division of Diabetes Translation (2007). Available at http://www.cdc.gov/diabetes/states/index.htm. Accessed September 5, 2007.

Statehealthfacts.org (2007). *Key Health and Healthcare Indicators by Race/ethnicity and State.* The Henry J. Kaiser Family Foundation . Available at http://www.kff.org/minorityhealth/upload/7633.pdf. Accessed August 17, 2007.

Stern MP (1998). Invited commentary: cardiovascular mortality in American Indians: paradox explained? *American Journal of Epidemiology* **147**, 1009–10.

Stevens RJ, Holman R (2004). Comparative study of prognostic value for coronary disease risk between the U.K. Prospective diabetes study and Framingham models: response to Protopsaltis et al. *Diabetes Care* **27**, 1843–4.

UK Prospective Diabetes Study (UKPDS) Group (1998). Intensive blood-glucose control with sulphonylureas or insulin compared with conventional treatment and risk of complications in patients with type 2 diabetes (UKPDS 33). UK Prospective Diabetes Study (UKPDS) Group. *Lancet* **352**, 837–53.

Vaccaro O et al. (1998) Sixteen-year coronary mortality in black and white men with diabetes screened for the Multiple Risk Factor Intervention Trial (MRFIT). *International Journal of Epidemiology* **27**, 636–41.

Vijan S, Hayward RA (2004). Pharmacologic lipid-lowering therapy in type 2 diabetes mellitus: background paper for the American College of Physicians. *Annals of Internal Medicine* **140**, 650–8.

Wilder RP (2003). Education and mortality in type 2 diabetes. *Diabetes Care* **26**, 1650.

14. Impact of Ethnic and Socioeconomic Factors on Diabetes-Related Health and Management

Arleen F. Brown, Andrew J. Karter, and Dean Schillinger

■ Main Public Health Messages

- Many people with diabetes experience well-documented, often interrelated, social disparities in access to care, quality of care, and rates of complications.
- Research suggests that many social disparities are attenuated among insured patients with diabetes, particularly those in managed care.
- Many of the explanatory factors for the social disparities are modifiable, but only a modest number of patient, health care provider, health care system, and community-level interventions have been found to improve care and outcomes for socially disadvantaged persons with diabetes.
- More research is needed to understand the principal drivers of disparities, to refine our understanding of critical components of successful interventions, and to generate evidence-based policy to improve outcomes for socially disadvantaged persons with diabetes.

■ Introduction

Type 2 diabetes disproportionately affects socially disadvantaged populations, including racial and ethnic minority groups and low-income and less-educated persons (Barker 1999; Barker, Gardner, and Power 1982; Burke et al. 1999; Pincus, Callahan, and Burkhauser 1987; Robbins et al. 2000; Winkleby et al. 1999). The evidence-based therapies available for managing diabetes and for preventing or treating its complications are underused in these groups (Brown et al. 2003; Cowie and Eberhardt 1995; Karter et al. 2000). It is less clear how much these social disparities in the use of therapies are associated with differences in access to care versus underutilization of offered or available care. Social disadvantage may affect diabetes outcomes through a variety of pathways, including access to care, the quality of care received, functional limitations, burden of morbidity, psychosocial characteristics, and neighborhood or community factors (Brown et al. 2004). Because of the high prevalence of diabetes among socially disadvantaged persons, interventions to reduce racial/ethnic and social disparities in health overall may have a profound impact on the morbidity and mortality associated with diabetes. In this chapter we focus on social disparities in diabetes-related care and health, with special attention paid to mediators of the association between (1) racial/ethnic and socioeconomic factors and (2) diabetes outcomes and management. We also discuss evidence on interventions at the individual, provider, health care system, and community levels that have the potential to reduce disparities in diabetes. Finally, we highlight gaps in our understanding of social disparities and how they affect health for persons with diabetes.

■ Background/Historical Perspective

The elimination of ethnic differences in the incidence and prevalence of diabetes and its complications by the year 2010 is a central component of the "Healthy People 2010" initiative (http://www.health.gov/healthypeople). There has been considerable debate, however, as to the definition of race and ethnicity and the appropriate analytic approach to studying racial and ethnic disparities in health outcomes (Bhopal 1997; Kaufman, Cooper, and McGee 1997; Morgenstern 1997; Moy 1989). We refer to Williams's definition of ethnicity: "a complex multidimensional construct reflecting the confluence of biological factors and geographical origins, culture, economic, political and legal factors, as well as racism" (Williams 1997). The concepts of "race" and "ethnicity," despite their somewhat inconsistent usage, have public health value in light of the historic and current disparities in health and the importance to rigorously monitor our progress toward eliminating ethnic health disparities even if we do not yet fully grasp their causes (Karter 2003a, 2003b).

Disentangling race/ethnicity from socioeconomic status (SES) is difficult because vulnerabilities often co-occur. In this chapter, we focus on race/ethnicity and education as two key social determinants of health in diabetes. Researchers often favor using educational attainment as the measure of SES because it is generally stable by the end of early adulthood (e.g., after the age of 25) and remains so over the life course. It is also rarely influenced by diabetes health status, because diabetes-related complications typically occur later in the life course. Moreover because education is a strong predictor of subsequent income, income may be considered as a mediator (on the causal pathway) between education and health outcomes.

■ Epidemiology

Race/Ethnicity, Socioeconomic Status, and Diabetes Outcomes

Much of the morbidity and mortality attributed to diabetes is due to chronic complications of the disease (e.g., heart attacks, stroke, end-stage renal disease [ESRD], amputation) rather than acute complications (e.g., diabetic ketoacidosis, hypogly-cemia). Most of the annual U.S. health care expenditures for diabetic care are also attributable to complications, primarily for the management of macrovascular complications (Caro, Ward, and O'Brien 2002; Huse et al. 1989). Generally, find-ings suggest an excess in microvascular complications (Hamman et al. 1991), such as ESRD (Brancati et al. 1992; Cowie 1993; Klag et al. 1997; Stephens et al. 1990) and nontraumatic, lower-extremity amputations (LEA) (Bild et al. 1989; Gujral et al. 1993; Lavery et al. 1996; Lee et al. 1993), among minority populations, with whites having higher rates of cardiovascular disease. In population-based studies, ethnic minorities with diabetes have significantly higher rates of diabetes-related complications than non-Hispanic white patients (henceforth, whites). African Americans have two to four times the rate of renal disease, blindness, amputa-tions, and amputation-related mortality experienced by whites (Carter, Pugh, and Monterrosa 1996; Emanuele 2005; Lanting et al. 2005). Similarly, Latinos have higher rates of renal disease and retinopathy than whites (Carter, Pugh, and Monterrosa 1996; Harris et al. 1998; Lanting et al. 2005; Lavery et al. 1997). Diabetes mortality rates (per 100,000) in California in 1998 were 98 for African Americans and 60 for Latinos, versus 38 for whites (California MediCal Type 2 Diabetes Study 2004). Diabetes-related mortality is 4.3 times as high in American Indians/Alaskan Natives as in whites (Governing Council of the APHA 1999).

Racial/ethnic differences are evident even in populations with uniform health coverage, but they are attenuated relative to findings from population-based samples. A study of over 60,000 patients from Kaiser Permanente found inconsistent patterns of ethnic differences in macrovascular and microvascular complications (Karter et al. 2002). Relative to whites, adjusted incidence rates for myocardial infarction were 26%, 32%, and 34% lower in Latinos, Asians, and African Americans, respec-tively. For stroke they were 18% and 24% lower in Latinos and Asians; for conges-tive heart failure, 32% and 36% lower in Latinos and Asians; for LEA, 64% lower in Asians (p <0.01 for all comparisons); whereas for ESRD they were 41%, 44%, and 112% higher in Latinos, Asians, and African Americans, respectively. There were no differences between African Americans and whites for stroke, congestive heart failure, or LEA, nor were there Latino-white differences for LEA. In the Translating Research Into Action for Diabetes (TRIAD) study, a multicenter study of diabetes care in managed care, Latinos had significantly lower rates of all-cause mortality than other ethnic groups (McEwen et al. 2007).

In summary, in population-based studies, racial/ethnic minorities with dia-betes have higher rates of microvascular complications and higher mortality than whites; in insured populations, minority patients also have higher rates of some microvascular complications, but their rates of macrovascular complication and death appear to be lower. These observations suggest that socioeconomic factors contribute to some racial/ethnic diabetes disparities but that improved access to care can attenuate the relationship between race/ethnicity and diabetes-related complications.

Educational Differences in Diabetes-Related Health Outcomes

Social disadvantage as measured by education, individual or household income, employment, occupation, or living in an underprivileged area has been associated with poorer physical and emotional health (Chaturvedi et al. 1998; Olivera, Duhalde, and Galiardino 1991; Robinson et al. 1990; Robinson, Stevens, and Protopapa 1993; Ware et al. 1996), all-cause mortality, and higher rates of fatal and nonfatal cardio-vascular disease in general populations (Cabrera et al. 2001; Chaturvedi et al. 1998; Dorman et al. 1985; Matsushima et al. 1996; Nielsson, Johansson, and Sundqvist 1998; Robinson, Lloyd, and Stevens 1998; Ware et al. 1996). Several European studies have demonstrated an educational gradient in diabetes outcomes, including prolif-erative retinopathy and prevalent heart disease (Marmot et al. 1998). In the United States, in contrast, fewer associations between education and diabetes complications have been observed, although a lower level of education has been associated with higher mortality (Lynch and Kaplan 2000; Wei et al. 1996). There is some evidence of an inverse relationship between education and diabetes mortality, microvascular complications, and macrovascular complications.

■ Explanatory Factors

Spectrum of Modifiable Explanatory Factors

In our efforts to understand, and potentially reduce, social disparities in health it is of primary interest to identify potentially modifiable explanatory factors that link social factors (e.g., race, ethnicity, or education) with differing rates of diabetes-related complications. Potential explanatory factors (mediators) either (1) differen-tially affect the risk of complications or (2) have similar impact but are distributed differently across social groups. Identifying mediators with substantially differing effect size or prevalence across social groups would facilitate targeted interventions attempting to reduce existing disparities. These mediators can operate at the patient, provider, health care system, or neighborhood level.

Patient-Level Mediators

Control of Intermediate Risk Factors

Compared with whites, African Americans, Latinos, Asians/Pacific Islanders, and Native Americans have poorer glycemic control, and many minority subgroups also have poorer control of blood pressure and low-density lipoprotein (LDL) choles-terol, even in populations with uniform access to care (Kirk et al. 2006). Lower SES has been associated with worse glycemic control in type 2 diabetes in some U.S. studies (Haan, Kaplan, and Camacho 1987), although other research has not shown this association (Haffner et al. 1989; Harris 2001). Educational gradients have been consistently observed for proteinuria, total cholesterol, and triglycerides, all potent risk factors for diabetic complications (Marmot et al. 1998).

Health Behaviors

Social disparities in health behaviors and self-care behaviors are thought to be a main reason for disparities in health among adults with diabetes (Evefrson et al. 2002). A complex range of self-care behaviors are required to manage diabetes, among them self-monitoring of blood glucose (SMBG), periodic examination of the feet, dietary restrictions, regular exercise, adherence to and management of multiple medications and dosing schedules, and maintaining glycemic control during intercurrent illness. Although no studies have simultaneously addressed all the health behaviors required to control blood sugar, lipids, and blood pressure as well as associated chronic conditions among persons with diabetes, recent studies have shed light on the social disparities in diabetes-related health behaviors.

Among adults with diabetes, low income, less education, and living in a poverty area have been associated with higher rates of smoking (Caddick et al. 1994; Connolly and Kesson 1996; Cubbin, Hadden, and Winkleby 2001), lower rates of SMBG (Beckles et al. 1998; Harris, Cowie, and Howie 1993; Karter et al. 2000), less vigorous exercise (Chaturvedi et al. 1998; Cubbin, Hadden, and Winkleby 2001), poorer adherence to medications (Heisler et al. 2007), and underuse of recommended preventive health screening (Brechner et al. 1993; Karter et al. 2007; Witkin and Klein 1984). Recent data from TRIAD indicate that approximately half of poorly educated, young adults with diabetes in that study smoked, magnifying the health risk associated with early-onset diabetes (Karter et al. 2008).

An analysis of Health and Retirement Study (Heisler et al. 2007) data suggested that one of the dominant mediators of the association between minority status and poorer glycemic control was poorer adherence to medication among African Americans and Latinos. Other researchers have not found this association between race/ethnicity and adherence (Adams et al. 2008). The lack of consistent findings suggests that more work is needed to understand the causal pathways underlying social disparities in intermediate health outcomes.

Access to Care

Evidence from multiple studies indicates that inadequate access to care (e.g., due to lack of health insurance) may be an important contributor to the current state of social disparities in diabetes outcomes. People with only a primary or secondary education have more contacts with their general practitioner and dieticians but fewer visits with specialists (e.g., endocrinologists) or diabetes nurses, and they undergo fewer assessments of their body weight and receive fewer influenza vaccinations. However, the educational gradient in complications does not appear to be mediated by disparities in health service utilization. The persistence of some disparities even in managed care settings (Schneider, Zaslavsky, and Epstein 2002) and in countries with universal health insurance (Chaturvedi et al. 1998; Larsson, Lager, and Nilsson 1999; Muhlhauser et al. 1998; Roper et al. 2001; Van der Meer and Mackenbach 1999) suggests that neither access to care nor having insurance is sufficient to improve diabetes outcomes.

Insurance

For persons with diabetes, access to health insurance is also important for the receipt of high-quality care (Beckles et al. 1998; Burge, Lucero Rassam, and Schade 2000; Piette 2000). Although cross-sectional studies have estimated that, overall, approximately 93% of patients with diabetes have some form of health insurance (Harris 1999; Harris, Cowie, and Eastman 1994), both the 1989 National Health Interview Survey and the Third National Health and Nutrition Examination Survey (NHANES III, 1988–94) indicated that a much greater proportion of minorities with diabetes lacked insurance (Harris 1999; Harris, Cowie, and Eastman 1994). Uninsured adults with diabetes receive fewer recommended processes of care, including dilated eye examinations, foot examinations, and other preventive health care services, than insured persons (Beckles et al. 1998). Uninsured diabetic adults also have poorer intermediate and longer-term outcomes, such as poorer glycemic control (Gregg et al. 2001), and they have almost seven times the odds of having diabetic eye disease as their insured counterparts (Baker et al. 1998). Finally, lack of insurance has been shown to predict higher rates of microvascular complications in Latinos with diabetes (Pugh et al. 1992).

Quality of Care

Race and ethnicity (Brown et al. 2005; Harris 1999; Heisler et al. 2003; Schneider, Zaslavsky, and Epstein 2002), income (Kelly et al. 1993, 1994), and education (Beckles et al. 1998; Chin, Zhang, and Merrell 1998) have all been associated with gradients in processes of care. In one national study minorities were less likely to have a lipid test and a dilated ophthalmologic examination than were whites (Thackeray, Merrill, and Neiger 2004). Another study found that ethnic disparities in quality and access to care can be substantially reduced, if not eliminated, within health care organizations that provide uniform care to large populations (Brown et al. 2005). Still, although there have been exceptions, reports from diverse settings indicate that the quality of diabetes care for socially disadvantaged persons is inferior to that of more affluent persons (Beckles et al. 1998; Kirk et al. 2005; Peters et al. 1996).

Financial Barriers

Financial incentives in health care systems may disproportionately disadvantage socially vulnerable adults with diabetes. For example poorer patients in Kaiser were more likely to have a steep, negative association between the costs of glucometer strips and the use of those strips than were wealthier patients (Karter et al. 2000).

Although intuitive, this pattern of increasing price sensitivity among the poor has not been observed consistently in other cross-sectional (Karter et al. 2003) or longitudinal studies (Karter et al. 2007) in similar settings.

Language Barriers

In a study of a managed care population, patients with type 2 diabetes who reported difficulty with English monitored their blood sugars less frequently than persons with no language barriers (Karter et al. 2000). Spanish-speaking Latinos are less likely than those who speak English to have a regular source of care, and they receive less screening, report lower rates of use of preventive services (Fiscella et al. 2002; Hu and Covell 1986; Schur and Albers 1996), and are less satisfied with their health care (Morales et al. 1999) than either whites or English-speaking Latinos. We expand on the contributions of language discordance in the section on mediators at the provider level.

Mental Health

Persons with diabetes have twice the odds of depression as people in the general population (Anderson et al. 2001; Egede, Zheng, and Simpson 2002), and adults with diabetes who have relatively less education have significantly higher rates of depression (Tellez-Zenteno and Cardiel 2002). In diabetic adults, depression may adversely influence self-management behaviors, glycemic control, communication with providers, and mortality (Ciechanowski, Katon, and Russo 2000; Katon et al. 2005; Lustman et al. 2000; Swenson et al. 2008). In addition self-reported data indicate that adults with depression have more primary care and emergency department visits and more hospitalizations, and their total costs of care are four times as high as those of diabetic adults who are not depressed (Ciechanowski, Katon, and Russo 2000; Egede, Zheng, and Simpson 2002). Although a recent randomized trial suggests that successful treatment of depression may not be associated with better self-care or glycemic control, it may reduce overall costs of care (Katon et al. 2008; Lin et al. 2006).

Social Support and Competing Demands for Time

Evidence is strong for a relationship between having supportive social ties and better physical and mental health (Glasgow et al. 2000) and, conversely, between social isolation and greater morbidity and mortality (Berkman and Syme 1979). In the aggregate, among persons with diabetes, higher levels of social support have been associated with better self-management, including adherence to recommended diet and exercise regimens, better glycemic control (Ford, Tilley, and McDonald 1998), and less vulnerability to social stressors (Griffith, Field, and Lustman 1990). Social support may be particularly important for minority or low-income patients with diabetes. For example African Americans with diabetes rely more heavily on informal social networks to meet their disease management needs (Ford, Tilley, and McDonald 1998), and poorer persons are more likely to be socially isolated and to have fewer supportive social ties (Oakley and Rajan 1991).

Although empiric data are sparse on how social support influences health outcomes for persons with diabetes, better self-management skills and improved access (through the health-seeking behaviors of the persons themselves or their social network) and quality (because of better communication with physicians) likely play a role.

On the other hand social ties may result in detrimental effects, as in the case of obligations that result in financial expenditures, demands on time, and criticism from social contacts (Finch et al. 1989; Rook 1984; Schuster, Kessler, and Aseltine 1990). In addition the health care needs of persons who are caregivers for disabled elders can compete with the physical and emotional needs of their dependents, and these caregivers often fail to obtain adequate health care for themselves (Zarit, Reever, and Bach-Peterson 1980). These effects are likely accentuated among the poor and African Americans and possibly other ethnic minorities, among whom the caregiver role is common (Batts et al. 2001).

Stress

Stress associated with social deprivation and ethnic isolation undoubtedly has physical consequences, explaining some portion of the linkage between low SES and poor health (Adler and Newman 2002; Epel et al. 1999). Inadequate blood glucose control has been closely linked to stress in studies of type 1 and type 2 diabetes (Kramer et al. 2000), and stress management can result in modest but sustained reductions in glycemic control independent of any changes in health behaviors such as diet or exercise (Surwit et al. 2002). Allostatic load, which is the cumulative biologic burden associated with the body's adaptation to chronic stress, may be a particularly important mechanism through which low SES affects health outcomes for persons with diabetes (Seeman et al. 2001).

Provider-Level Mediators

Patient–Provider Communication

Effective communication between patients and providers (Greenfield et al. 1988; Kaplan, Greenfield, and Ware 1989) and shared decision making (Berger and Muhlhauser 1999; Golin et al. 2002; Olivarius et al. 2001) positively influence health behaviors and the process and outcomes of care for persons with diabetes. Patients' ratings of providers' general and diabetes-specific communication are associated with self-care for diabetes (Heisler et al. 2002; Piette et al. 2003). Unfortunately, a growing body of research shows that communication is more likely to be suboptimal for socially vulnerable patients. Physicians are more likely to adopt a more directive (less participatory) approach with less-educated patients, who are then less likely to have their expectations met (Fiscella et al. 2002).

Language Barriers and Health Literacy

Language barriers appear to influence diabetes self-care behaviors and outcomes, and a provider's ability to successfully communicate with patients may counter the effects of inadequate English proficiency and poor comprehension of verbal instructions (Fernandez et al. 2004). Persons with diabetes who have low functional health literacy (health literacy is "the ability to read and comprehend prescription bottles, appointment slips, and the other essential health-related materials required to successfully function as a patient") (Ad Hoc Committee on Health Literacy 1999) are less likely to know the symptoms of hypoglycemia (Williams et al. 1998). Limited functional health literacy has also been associated with difficulty in understanding physicians' explanations and with impaired shared decision making in patients with type 2 diabetes (Schillinger et al. 2004), and it appears to be an important mediating factor linking limited education to health outcomes such as inadequate glycemic control and retinopathy (Schillinger et al. 2002, 2006). In encounters with patients who have limited health literacy, physicians often use unclarified jargon that can interfere with their patients' comprehension of recommendations for care (Castro et al. 2007). New research suggests, however, that closing the communication loop between the provider and diabetic patient by using the "teach-back" technique, in which patients, before leaving the office, repeat in their own words what the provider has told them, can increase patients' understanding of the medical information conveyed despite their low literacy (Schillinger et al. 2003).

Discrimination and Trust in Health Care Providers

The bias of providers against low-SES or minority patients, even when unintentional or subtle, and stereotypes about the behaviors or health of socially disadvantaged patients may influence the provider's willingness or ability to provide counseling on healthy behaviors and disease management, reinforce the tendency of patients of low SES not to engage in these behaviors, and lead to differential treatment of minority patients (Smedley, Stith, and Nelson 2002; van Ryn and Burke 2000). This bias can also influence patient health via the impact of internalized racism (Krieger, Sidney, and Coakley 1998; Tull and Chambers 2001). In one study, 8% of minority patients reported discrimination by their doctors or the office staff due to their race, education, or income (Piette, Bibbins-Domingo, and Schillinger 2006). Patients who reported racial discrimination in health care settings were more likely to report other types of discrimination (i.e., due to sex, language, income, or education) and reported worse health and glycemic control.

The provision of culturally competent care has been associated with better rapport, trust, and exchange of information (Fernandez et al. 2004), but it may be hindered by physicians' preconceptions about socially disadvantaged patients' behavioral risks, intelligence, and likelihood of adherence to treatment (van Ryn and Burke 2000). These attitudes not only interfere with provision of care but may also reduce a patient's confidence and self-efficacy, further undermining treatment, behavior, and adherence (Sherbourne et al. 1992). Patients' and providers' attitudes may influence each other reciprocally; if patients convey mistrust, demonstrate poor adherence, and refuse treatment, providers are likely to become less engaged in the treatment process and less clinically aggressive (Smedley, Stith, and Nelson 2002).

Characteristics of the Health Care System

Among the specific features of health care organizations that can improve diabetes outcomes are targeting either the practices of health care providers or the organization of diabetes care, identifying persons with diabetes and tracking their care via registries, educating patients, providing participatory care, and offering training in empowerment (Norris, Engelgau, and Narayan 2001; Norris et al. 2002). It is not known whether the impact of these interventions varies by race/ethnicity or SES.

Although health care organizations can promote access (for example, by reducing financial barriers to care), various characteristics of these health systems also have the potential to negatively affect access, process, and health behaviors and to worsen health outcomes. Management of specialty referrals through a gatekeeper, for example, may lead to more appropriate referral patterns (Martin et al. 1989; Moore, Martin, and Richardson 1983), but restrictions on referrals to specialists that are differentially applied to poorer or less-educated persons may adversely influence health. In addition health care organizations may promote intensive diabetes management, but a recent analysis of data from the TRIAD study found little evidence that obtaining care in health care systems with more intensive diabetes management (e.g., through referral systems, diabetes registries, or provider feedback) reduced social disparities in quality of care, suggesting that the reduction of many disparities requires more tailored approaches (Duru et al. 2006).

Because persons of low SES may be clustered in certain health care systems (Schneider, Zaslavsky, and Epstein 2002) or within a few facilities associated with a health care network, the gradient of SES and health may be explained by the kinds of systems in which less-affluent persons receive their care.

Some financial and organizational arrangements may pose greater obstacles for persons of lower SES. Patient co-payments have been most closely studied, and low-income persons may be particularly sensitive to even modest changes in cost sharing, as they spend a higher proportion of their income on out-of-pocket expenses than do higher-income enrollees (Karter et al. 2003). The associations are complex, however. In a recent study, although patients did not increase utilization of SMBG test strips when fees were removed, they reduced utilization when a small fee was reintroduced (Karter et al. 2007).

Financial incentives for physicians may affect diabetes outcomes, and these effects may be more pronounced for low-SES patients. For example, more-educated patients and those who do not face language barriers may be more effective at negotiating with clinicians or health plans to get their needs met in the face of potential disincentives to provide care (Schillinger et al. 2002), and wealthier patients have a greater ability to purchase alternate health care.

Neighborhood Characteristics

Characteristics of communities or neighborhoods, such as the availability and accessibility of health services, the built environment, prevailing attitudes toward health, and levels of stress and social support, may influence general health outcomes (Connolly et al. 2000; Diez-Roux 1998; Pickett and Pearl 2001). Poor persons, particularly those with a chronic condition like diabetes, are more likely to experience multiple dimensions of neighborhood disadvantage, among them poorer-quality foods, high crime rates, and poor-quality housing and schools, and management of a chronic disease may be much more difficult in low-SES areas (Brown, Ang, and Pebley 2007).

Several community-level characteristics are thought to contribute to disparities in diabetes management. Adults with diabetes who report more neighborhood problems have higher rates of smoking and worse blood pressure control (Gary et al. 2008). Price disincentives to eating healthy food are greater in poor than in wealthier neighborhoods (Sooman, Macintyre, and Anderson 1993), and low-income communities have fewer supermarkets than more affluent neighborhoods (Morland, Diez Roux, and Wing 2006; Morland, Wing, and Diez Roux 2002). Moreover, access to foods recommended for adults with diabetes, e.g., fresh fruits and vegetables, whole grains, diet sodas, and low-fat milk, is limited in low-income and predominantly minority areas (Horowitz et al. 2004; Zenk et al. 2006). Ease of access to parks and recreational facilities and the safety of the neighborhood may influence the ability or willingness of persons with diabetes to engage in regular exercise, another important strategy in diabetes management. Transportation may be an underappreciated element in managing diabetes, as lack of transportation is an important barrier to receiving appropriate health services (Rittner and Kirk 1995) and may influence other environmental factors, such as access to food, health care, and social networks (Bostock 2001).

■ Public Health Preventive or Intervention Strategies

Several comprehensive reviews have assessed the effectiveness of interventions to improve diabetes care at the patient, provider, health care system, and community levels (Armour et al. 2005; Norris, Engelgau, and Narayan 2001; Norris et al. 2002a, 2002b, 2002c). These studies suggest that education and support for self-management, family interventions, disease management, case management, and use of community health workers can improve diabetes outcomes. Relatively little work, however, has addressed whether these interventions reduce racial/ethnic or socioeconomic disparities in health among adults with diabetes.

There is some evidence that more intensive health care interventions may benefit those with poor education more than those who are better educated in terms of improving adherence and self-management and thus in reducing disparities (Goldman and Smith 2002). A relatively small number of controlled trials have been identified that measured the effectiveness of interventions to improve diabetes care among socially disadvantaged groups, some of which were included in recent systematic reviews (Glazier et al. 2006; Peek, Cargill, and Huang 2007). Features of interventions are described below.

Features of Successful Interventions

Successful interventions to improve diabetes outcomes among vulnerable populations tend to occur in community settings, address the social context, and occur at multiple levels (Eakin et al. 2002). Features of successful interventions include cultural tailoring of the intervention, use of community educators or laypeople as leaders, one-on-one interventions with individualized assessment, use of treatment algorithms by lay health providers, use of feedback to participants about their diabetes control, and high-intensity programs (more than 10 contacts) delivered over a long duration ($\geq$6 months) (Glazier et al. 2006). In contrast, methods such as traditional didactic teaching and interventions focused on diabetes knowledge were less likely to be effective in improving care for socially disadvantaged groups. A more recent review that assessed the effectiveness of diabetes interventions to improve health outcomes or reduce diabetes-related disparities among racial/ethnic minorities (Peek, Cargill, and Huang 2007) found that hemoglobin A1C values were reduced by 0.36% more among persons exposed to the intervention than in control participants. The next sections review the rationale for and evidence of effective interventions at the patient, provider, health care system, and community levels to improve diabetes care for socially disadvantaged adults with diabetes.

Interventions at the Patient Level

Several interventions have been directed at disadvantaged patients (Eakin et al. 2002; Glazier et al. 2006; Peek, Cargill, and Huang 2007), with most targeting low-income patients and focusing on increasing their knowledge, skills, attitudes, and behaviors. Many of the successful interventions have been tailored to the language, cultural context, or literacy levels of the populations studied. Interventions to improve effective patient–provider communication may also improve diabetes outcomes among vulnerable groups. Additionally, improving social support may be the mechanism through which many of the patient-level interventions improve diabetes-related behaviors and outcomes.

Interventions at the Clinician Level

Only a few interventions to reduce diabetes disparities have focused on clinicians (Eakin et al. 2002; Glazier et al. 2006; Peek, Cargill, and Huang 2007). In urban areas where clinicians were serving low-SES patients, strategies such as giving reminder cards to patients and the provider's receipt of A1C results at the time of the clinic visit were associated with better outcomes. However it not clear how much these findings would differ from those observed in nonvulnerable populations.

Interventions at the Health Care System Level

Among the small number of controlled trials that have studied the influence of the health care system on health disparities, all were delivered by a licensed health care professional, several tailored the intervention to the language and/or literacy level of the patients, but just a few tailored the intervention to cultural characteristics of the patients (Eakin et al. 2002; Glazier et al. 2006; Peek, Cargill, and Huang 2007). A recent study that tested the effects of a multilingual intervention providing proactive automated telephone care management within a safety net health system demonstrated higher degrees of participation among those with limited health literacy and limited English proficiency, resulting in robust improvements in health behaviors and functional status (Schillinger et al. 2007) and improved safety, relative to usual care (Sarkar et al. 2008). Little work directly addresses how reducing organizational barriers to care, such as eliminating or reducing copayments or improving access to needed specialty care, affects diabetes disparities.

Interventions at the Community Level

There are only limited data on the influence of community-based interventions on the self-management of chronic conditions and virtually no data from randomized trials (Gilmer, Philis-Tsimikas, and Walker 2005; U.S. Department of Housing and Urban Development 2003). Given the strong association between contextual factors and health, more intervention studies are needed.

■ Conclusions

We have summarized some of the key disparities in diabetes care and outcomes by race/ethnicity or SES, discussed the evidence on the main mediators for the observed differences, and reviewed strategies for reducing these disparities. There are many unanswered questions related to both our understanding of the causes and consequences of disparities and the relative effectiveness of strategies to reduce them.

Limitations in Extant Literature on Social Disparities

Most of the research on social disparities in care has been based on utilization records, but these data do not allow us to distinguish between "offered" and "accepted" care. Thus researchers have not been able to tease apart the factors associated with (1) poor access to care, versus (2) underutilization of offered or available care, versus (3) community-level determinants of self-management behavior. Most studies to date have published racial-/ethnic-specific incidence rates for single diabetes-related complications and have compared the largest racial/ethnic groups, that is, non-Latino whites, Latinos, and African Americans. Few studies have had sufficient samples to concurrently examine rates of multiple complications in smaller ethnic groups such as Filipinos, Pacific Islanders, South Asians, and Native Americans. Education and income are not available in many studies despite being important determinants of health. Moreover education and income are confounded by factors like nativity (the value of a high school education often differs among foreign-born), age (college education is less common among the elderly), employment status (retiree incomes are generally substantially lower than the incomes of wage earners), and geographic region (income varies substantially across the country).

Evidence on patterns of discrimination is quite limited, as is research on the extent to which providers' perceptions may modify the willingness to prescribe therapies that require greater levels of health literacy or numeracy (e.g., insulin pump). Little is known regarding the extent to which dysfunctional patient–provider relationships result in clinical inertia among providers, poor patient adherence, and adverse clinical outcomes in diabetes. Even less is known as to whether these hypothesized associations between patient–provider communication and health care differ by patients' social status and ethnicity. Finally, the scope and quality of practice-based research to either improve diabetes care for vulnerable populations or reduce disparities in diabetes care are still very limited relative to the extent of the problem.

Limitations in Our Understanding of Strategies to Reduce Disparities

A better understanding is needed as to whether targeting just clinically at-risk individuals or socially vulnerable groups, or not targeting any group but instead using an intervention for the general population, would have more of an impact on reducing social disparities in diabetes-related health.

Several mechanisms through which disparities may affect diabetes outcomes deserve additional attention. It remains unclear whether all groups have benefited from recent improvements in strategies for managing diabetes, or whether socioeconomic differences and health literacy/language barriers have continued to contribute to racial/ethnic disparities (Frohlich and Potvin 2008). Also unclear is whether extant health disparities are attributable to racial/ethnic differences in the prevalence and/or the effect size of modifiable risk factors (e.g., hypertension). More work is needed to evaluate racial/ethnic differences in quality of care (going beyond simple screening tests), the diffusion of innovations, adherence to treatment, health behaviors, and patient–provider relationships. For example mental health may be an important mediator of the relationship between social disadvantage and poorer diabetes outcomes, and yet few interventions to address this question have been conducted that focused on racial/ethnic minority groups or low-income persons. At the provider and health care system levels research is needed on interventions that have the potential to reduce health disparities. These might include improvement of providers' communication skills to accommodate inadequate health literacy, selective reduction of co-payments to address financial barriers, provision of translation services for those with limited English proficiency, the offering of training in cultural sensitivity, application of lay health worker models that have been shown to be effective, and implementation of tailored communication technologies. At the neighborhood level there is a need for rigorous studies of interventions that target the built environment, promote access to nutritious foods and other health-related resources, or identify ways to build sustainable support for diabetes management in community settings. Finally, more work is needed on how to integrate and coordinate care across levels to improve health and health care for socially disadvantaged persons with diabetes.

■ References

Ad Hoc Committee on Health Literacy for the Council on Scientific Affairs AMA (1999). Health literacy: report of the Council on Scientific Affairs. *JAMA* **281**, 552–7.

Adams AS et al. (2008). Medication adherence and racial differences in A1C control. *Diabetes Care* **31**, 916–21.

Adler NE, Newman K (2002). Socioeconomic disparities in health: pathways and policies. *Health Affairs (Millwood)* **21**, 60–76.

Anderson R et al. (2001). The prevalence of comorbid depression in adults with diabetes. *Diabetes Care* **24**, 1069–78.

Armour T et al. (2005). The effectiveness of family interventions in people with diabetes mellitus: a systematic review. *Diabetic Medicine* **22**, 1295–305.

Baker R et al. (1998). Demographic and clinical characteristics of patients with diabetes presenting to an urban public hospital ophthalmology clinic. *Ophthalmology* **105**, 1373–9.

Barker D (1999). The fetal origins of type 2 diabetes mellitus. *Annals of Internal Medicine* **130**, 321–3.

Barker D, Gardner MJ, Power C (1982). Incidence of diabetes amongst people aged 18–50 years in nine British towns: a collaborative study. *Diabetologia* **22**, 421–5.

Batts M et al. (2001). Patient priorities and needs for diabetes care among urban African American adults. *Diabetes Educator* **27**, 405–12.

Beckles G et al. (1998). Population-based assessment of the level of care among adults with diabetes in the U.S. *Diabetes Care* **21**, 1432–8.

Berger M, Muhlhauser I (1999). Diabetes care and patient-oriented outcomes. *JAMA* **281**, 1676–8.

Berkman L, Syme SL (1979). Social networks, host resistance, and mortality: a nine-year follow-up study of Alameda County residents. *American Journal of Epidemiology* **109**, 186–204.

Bhopal R (1997). Is research into ethnicity and health racist, unsound, or important science? *British Medical Journal* **314**, 1751–6.

Bild D et al. (1989). Lower-extremity amputation in people with diabetes. Epidemiology and prevention. . *Diabetes Care* **12**, 24–31.

Bostock L (2001). Pathways of disadvantage? Walking as a mode of transport among low-income mothers. *Health & Social Care in the Community* **9**, 11–8.

Brancati F et al. (1992). The excess incidence of diabetic end-stage renal disease among blacks. A population-based study of potential explanatory factors. *JAMA* **268**, 3079–84.

Brechner R et al. (1993). Ophthalmic examination among adults with diagnosed diabetes mellitus. *JAMA* **270**, 1714–8.

Brown A et al. (2003). Income-related differences in the use of evidence-based therapies in older persons with diabetes mellitus in for-profit managed care. *Journal of the American Geriatric Society* **51**, 665–70.

Brown A et al. (2004). Socioeconomic position and health for persons with diabetes: a conceptual framework and review of the literature. *Epidemiologic Reviews* **26**, 63–77.

Brown A et al. (2005). Race, ethnicity, socioeconomic position, and quality of care for adults with diabetes enrolled in managed care: the Translating Research Into Action for Diabetes (TRIAD) study. *Diabetes Care* **28**, 2864–70.

Brown A, Ang A, Pebley AR (2007). The relationship between the neighborhood socioeconomic environment and self-rated health for adults with chronic conditions. *American Journal of Public Health* **97**, 926–32.

Burge M, Lucero Rassam AG, Schade DS (2000). What are the barriers to medical care for patients with newly diagnosed diabetes mellitus? *Diabetes, Obesity & Metabolism* **2**, 351–4.

Burke J et al. (1999). Rapid rise in the incidence of type 2 diabetes from 1987 to 1996: results from the San Antonio Heart Study. *Archives of Internal Medicine* **159**, 1450–6.

Cabrera C et al. (2001). Socioeconomic status and mortality in Swedish women: opposing trends for cardiovascular disease and cancer. *Epidemiology* **12**, 532–6.

Caddick S et al. (1994). Hospital admissions and social deprivation of patients with diabetes mellitus. *Diabetic Medicine* **11**, 981–3.

Caro J, Ward AJ, O'Brien JA (2002). Lifetime costs of complications resulting from type 2 diabetes in the U.S. *Diabetes Care* **25**, 476–81.

Carter J, Pugh JA, Monterrosa A (1996). Non-insulin-dependent diabetes mellitus in minorities in the United States. *Annals of Internal Medicine* **125**, 221–2.

Castro CM et al. (2007). Babel babble: physicians' use of unclarified medical jargon with patients. *American Journal of Health Behavior* **31** (Suppl. 1), S85–95.

Chaturvedi N et al. (1998). Socioeconomic gradient in morbidity and mortality in people with diabetes: cohort study findings from the Whitehall Study and the WHO Multinational Study of Vascular Disease in Diabetes. *British Medical Journal* **316**, 100–5.

Chaturvedi N, Stephenson JM, Fuller JH (1996). The relationship between socioeconomic status and diabetes control and complications in the EURODIAB IDDM Complications Study. *Diabetes Care* **19**, 423–30.

Chin M, Zhang JX, Merrell K (1998). Diabetes in the African-American Medicare population. Morbidity, quality of care, and resource utilization. *Diabetes Care* **21**, 1090–5.

Ciechanowski P, Katon WJ, Russo JE (2000). Depression and diabetes: impact of depressive symptoms on adherence, function, and costs. *Archives of Internal Medicine* **160**, 3278–85.

Connolly V et al. (2000). Diabetes prevalence and socioeconomic status: a population based study showing increased prevalence of type 2 diabetes mellitus in deprived areas. *Journal of Epidemiology and Community Health* **54**, 173–7.

Connolly V, Kesson CM (1996). Socio-economic status and membership of the British Diabetic Association in Scotland. *Diabetic Medicine* **13**, 898–901.

Cowie C (1993). Diabetic renal disease: racial and ethnic differences from an epidemiologic perspective. *Transplant Proceedings* **25**, 2426–30.

Cowie C, Eberhardt MS (1995). Sociodemographic characteristics of persons with diabetes. In: Harris MI et al., eds. *Diabetes in America*, 2nd ed., pp 85–116. Bethesda, MD: National Institutes of Health.

Cubbin C, Hadden WC, Winkleby MA (2001). Neighborhood context and cardiovascular disease risk factors: the contribution of material deprivation. *Ethnicity & Disease* **11**, 687–700.

Diez-Roux A (1998). Bringing context back into epidemiology: variables and fallacies in multilevel analysis. *American Journal of Public Health* **88**, 216–22.

Dorman J et al. (1985). The Pittsburgh Insulin-Dependant Diabetes Mellitus (IDDM) Morbidity and Mortality Study: case-control analyses of risk factors for mortality. *Diabetes Care* **8** (Suppl. 1), 54–60.

Duru O et al. (2006). The association between clinical care strategies and the attenuation of racial/ethnic disparities in diabetes care: the Translating Research Into Action for Diabetes (TRIAD) Study. *Medical Care* **44**, 1121–8.

Eakin E et al. (2002). Reaching those most in need: a review of diabetes self-management interventions in disadvantaged populations. *Diabetes/Metabolism Research and Reviews* **18**, 26–35.

Egede L, Zheng D, Simpson K (2002). Comorbid depression is associated with increased health care use and expenditures in individuals with diabetes. *Diabetes Care* **25**, 464–70.

Emanuele N et al. (2005). Ethnicity, race, and baseline retinopathy correlates in the veterans affairs diabetes trial. *Diabetes Care* **28**, 1954–8.

Epel E et al. (1999). Social status, anabolic activity, and fat distribution. *Annals of the New York Academy of Sciences* **896**, 424–6.

Everson S et al. (2002). Epidemiologic evidence for the relation between socioeconomic status and depression, obesity, and diabetes. *Journal of Psychosomatic Research* **53**, 891–5.

Fernandez A et al. (2004). Physician language ability and cultural competence. An exploratory study of communication with Spanish-speaking patients. *Journal of General Internal Medicine* **19**, 167–74.

Finch J et al. (1989). Positive and negative social ties among older adults: measurement models and the prediction of psychological distress and well-being. *American Journal of Community Psychology* **17**, 585–605.

Fiscella K et al. (2002). Disparities in health care by race, ethnicity, and language among the uninsured. *Medical Care* **40**, 52–9.

Ford M, Tilley BC, McDonald PE (1998). Social support among African-American adults with diabetes, Part 2: a review. *Journal of the National Medical Association* **90**, 425–32.

Frohlich KL, Potvin L (2008). Transcending the known in public health practice: the inequality paradox: the population approach and vulnerable populations. *American Journal of Public Health* **98**, 216–21.

Gary TL, et al. (2008) Perception of neighborhood problems, health behaviors, and diabetes outcomes among adults with diabetes in managed care: the Translating Research Into Action for Diabetes (TRIAD) study. *Diabetes Care* **31**, 273–8.

Gilmer TP, Philis-Tsimikas A, Walker C (2005). Outcomes of Project Dulce: a culturally specific diabetes management program. *Annals of Pharmacotherapy* **39**, 817–22.

Glasgow R et al. (2000). A social-ecologic approach to assessing support for disease self-management: the Chronic Illness Resources Survey. *Journal of Behavioral Medicine* **23**, 559–83.

Glazier R et al. (2006). A systematic review of interventions to improve diabetes care in socially disadvantaged populations. *Diabetes Care* **29**, 1678–88.

Goldman D, Smith JP (2002). Can patient self-management help explain the SES health gradient? *Proceedings of the National Academy of Science U.S.A.* **99**, 10929–34.

Golin C et al. (2002). Impoverished diabetic patients whose doctors facilitate their participation in medical decision making are more satisfied with their care. *Journal of General Internal Medicine* **17**, 857–66.

Governing Council of the American Public Health Association (1999). Policy statements adopted. *American Journal of Public Health* **89**, 428–50.

Greenfield S et al. (1988). Patients' participation in medical care: effects on blood sugar control and quality of life in diabetes. *Journal of General Internal Medicine* **3**, 448–57.

Gregg E et al. (2001). Use of diabetes preventative care and complications risk in two African-American communities. *American Journal of Preventive Medicine* **21**, 197–202.

Griffith L, Field BJ, Lustman PJ (1990). Life stress and social support in diabetes: association with glycemic control. *International Journal of Psychiatry in Medicine* **20**, 365–70.

Gujral J et al. (1993). Ethnic differences in the incidence of lower extremity amputation secondary to diabetes mellitus. *Diabetic Medicine* **10**, 271–4.

Haan M, Kaplan GA, Camacho T. Poverty and health. Prospective evidence from the Alameda County Study. *American Journal of Epidemiology* **125**, 989–98.

Haffner S et al. (1989). Effects of socioeconomic status on hyperglycemia and retinopathy levels in Mexican Americans with NIDDM. *Diabetes Care* **12**, 128–34.

Hamman R et al. (1991). Microvascular complications of NIDDM in Hispanics and non- Hispanic whites. San Luis Valley Diabetes Study. *Diabetes Care* **14**, 655–64.

Harris M (1999). Racial and ethnic differences in health insurance coverage for adults with diabetes. *Diabetes Care* **22**, 1679–82.

Harris M (2001). Racial and ethnic differences in health care access and health outcomes for adults with type 2 diabetes. *Diabetes Care* **24**, 454–9.

Harris M, Cowie CC, Eastman R (1994). Health-insurance coverage for adults with diabetes in the U.S. population *Diabetes Care* **17**, 585–91.

Harris M, Cowie CC, Howie LJ (1993). Self-monitoring of blood glucose by adults with diabetes in the United States population. *Diabetes Care* **16**, 1116–23.

Harris MI et al. (1998). Is the risk of diabetic retinopathy greater in non-Hispanic blacks and Mexican Americans than in non-Hispanic whites with type 2 diabetes? A U.S. population study. *Diabetes Care* **21**, 1230–5.

Heisler M et al. (2002). The relative importance of physician communication, participatory decision making, and patient understanding in diabetes self-management. *Journal of General Internal Medicine* **17**, 243–52.

Heisler M et al. (2003). Racial disparities in diabetes care processes, outcomes, and treatment intensity. *Medical Care* **41**, 1221–32.

Heisler M et al. (2007). Mechanisms for racial and ethnic disparities in glycemic control in middle-aged and older Americans in the health and retirement study. *Archives of Internal Medicine* **167**, 1853–60.

Horowitz C et al. (2004). Barriers to buying healthy foods for people with diabetes: evidence of environmental disparities. *American Journal of Public Health* **94**, 1549–54.

Hu DJ, Covell RM (1986). Health care usage by Hispanic outpatients as function of primary language. *Western Journal of Medicine* **144**, 490–3.

Huse D et al. (1989). The economic costs of non-insulin-dependent diabetes mellitus. *JAMA* **262**, 2708–13.

Kaplan S, Greenfield S, Ware JE (1989). Assessing the effects of physician-patient interactions on the outcomes of chronic disease. *Medical Care* **27** (3 Suppl.), S110–S127.

Karter A (2003a). Commentary: race, genetics and disease—in search of a middle ground. *International Journal of Epidemiology* **32**, 26–28.

Karter A (2003b). Race and ethnicity: vital constructs for diabetes research. *Diabetes Care* **7**, 2189–93.

Karter A et al. (2000). Self-monitoring of blood glucose: language and financial barriers in a managed care population with diabetes. *Diabetes Care* **23**, 477–83.

Karter A et al. (2002). Ethnic disparities in diabetic complications in an insured population. *JAMA* **287**, 2519–27.

Karter A et al. (2003). Out-of-pocket costs and diabetes preventive services: the Translating Research Into Action for Diabetes (TRIAD) study. *Diabetes Care* **26**, 2294–9.

Karter A et al. (2007a). Effect of cost-sharing changes on self-monitoring of blood glucose. *American Journal of Managed Care* **13**, 408–6.

Karter AJ et al. (2007b). Educational disparities in health behaviors among patients with diabetes: the Translating Research Into Action for Diabetes (TRIAD) Study. *BMC Public Health* **7**, 308.

Karter AJ et al. (2008). Educational disparities in rates of smoking among diabetic adults: the Translating Research Into Action for Diabetes Study. *American Journal of Public Health* **98**, 365–70.

Katon W et al. (2005). The association of comorbid depression with mortality in patients with type 2 diabetes. *Diabetes Care* **28**, 2668–72.

Katon WJ et al. (2008). Long-term effects on medical costs of improving depression outcomes in patients with depression and diabetes. *Diabetes Care* **31**, 1155–9.

Kaufman J, Cooper RS, McGee DL (1997). Socioeconomic status and health in blacks and whites: the problem of residual confounding and the resiliency of race. *Epidemiology* **8**, 621–8.

Kelly W et al. (1993). Influence of social deprivation on illness in diabetic patients. *British Medical Journal* **307**, 1115–6.

Kelly W et al. (1994). Geographical mapping of diabetic patients from the deprived inner city shows less insulin therapy and more hyperglycemia. *Diabetic Medicine* **11**, 344–8.

Kirk JK et al. (2005). Ethnic disparities: control of glycemia, blood pressure, and LDL cholesterol among US adults with type 2 diabetes. *Annals of Pharmacotherapy* **39**, 1489–501.

Kirk JK et al. (2006). Disparities in HbA1c levels between African-American and non-Hispanic white adults with diabetes: a meta-analysis. *Diabetes Care* **29**, 2130–6.

Klag M et al. (1997). End-stage renal disease in African-American and white men. 16-year MRFIT findings. *JAMA* **277**, 1293–8.

Kramer J et al. (2000). Stress and metabolic control in diabetes mellitus: methodologic issues and an illustrative analysis. *Annals of Behavioral Medicine* **22**, 17–28.

Krieger N, Sidney S, Coakley E (1998). Racial discrimination and skin color in the CARDIA study: implications for public health research. Coronary Artery Risk Development in Young Adults. *American Journal of Public Health* **88**, 1308–13.

Lanting L et al. (2005). Ethnic differences in mortality, end-stage complications, and quality of care among diabetic patients *Diabetes Care* **28**, 2280–88.

Larsson D, Lager I, Nilsson PM (1999). Socio-economic characteristics and quality of life in diabetes mellitus relation to metabolic control. *Scandinavian Journal of Public Health* **27**, 101–5.

Lavery L et al. (1996). Variation in the incidence and proportion of diabetes-related amputations in minorities. *Diabetes Care* **19**, 48–52.

Lavery L et al. (1997). Mortality following lower extremity amputation in minorities with diabetes mellitus. *Diabetes Research and Clinical Practice* **37**, 41–47.

Lee J et al. (1993). Lower-extremity amputation. Incidence, risk factors, and mortality in the Oklahoma Indian Diabetes Study. *Diabetes* **42**, 876–82.

Lin E et al. (2006). Effects of enhanced depression treatment on diabetes self-care. *Annals of Family Medicine* **4**, 46–53.

Lustman P et al. (2000). Depression and poor glycemic control: a meta-analytic review of the literature. *Diabetes Care* **23**, 934–42.

Lynch J, Kaplan GA (2000). Socioeconomic factors **337**, 13–35.

Marmot M et al. (1998). Contribution of psychosocial factors to socioeconomic differences in health. *Milbank Quarterly* **76**, 403–48.

Martin D et al. (1989). Effect of a gatekeeper plan on health services use and charges: a randomized trial. *American Journal of Public Health* **79**, 1628–32.

Matsushima M et al. (1996). Socioeconomic and behavioural risk factors for mortality of individuals with IDDM in Japan: a population-based case-control study. Diabetes Epidemiology Research International (DERI) US-Japan Mortality Study. *Diabetologia* **39**, 710–6.

McEwen LN et al. (2007). Risk factors for mortality among patients with diabetes: the Translating Research Into Action for Diabetes (TRIAD) Study. *Diabetes Care* **30**, 1736–41.

Moore S, Martin DP, Richardson WC (1983). Does the primary-care gatekeeper control the costs of health care? Lessons from the SAFECO experience. *New England Journal of Medicine* **309**, 1400–2.

Morales L et al. (1999). Are Latinos less satisfied with communication by health care providers? *Journal of General Internal Medicine* **14**, 409–17.

Morgenstern H (1997). Defining and explaining race effects. *Epidemiology* **8**, 609–611.

Morland K, Diez Roux AV, Wing S (2006). Supermarkets, other food stores, and obesity: the atherosclerosis risk in communities study. *American Journal of Preventive Medicine* **30**, 333–9.

Morland K, Wing S, Diez Roux A (2002). The contextual effect of the local food environment on residents' diets: the atherosclerosis risk in communities study. *American Journal of Public Health* **92**, 1761–7.

Moy CS et al. (1989). Heritage research: the next generation of migrant studies. *American Journal of Epidemiology* **130**, 819–20.

Muhlhauser I et al. (1998). Social status and the quality of care for adult people with type 1 (insulin-dependent) diabetes mellitus—a population-based study. *Diabetologia* **41**, 1139–50.

Nielsson P, Johansson S-E, Sundqvist J (1998). Diabetes mortality and social class in Sweden—influence of age and gender. *Diabetic Medicine* **15**, 213–9.

Norris S et al. (2002a). Self-management education for adults with type 2 diabetes: a meta-analysis of the effect on glycemic control. *Diabetes Care* **25**, 1159–71.

Norris S et al. (2002b). Increasing diabetes self-management education in community settings. A systematic review. *American Journal of Preventive Medicine* **22** (4 Suppl.), 39–66.

Norris S et al. (2002c). The effectiveness of disease and case management for people with diabetes. A systematic review. *American Journal of Preventive Medicine* **22** (4 Suppl.), 15–38.

Norris S, Engelgau MM, Narayan KM (2001). Effectiveness of self-management training in type 2 diabetes: a systematic review of randomized controlled trials. *Diabetes Care* **24**, 561–87.

Oakley A, Rajan L (1991). Social class and social support: the same or different? *Sociology* **25**, 31–59.

Olivarius N et al. (2001). Randomised controlled trial of structured personal care of type 2 diabetes mellitus. *British Medical Journal* **323**, 970–5.

Olivera E, Duhalde EP, Galiardino JJ (1991). Costs of temporary and permanent disability induced by diabetes. *Diabetes Care* **14**, 593–6.

Peek ME, Cargill A, Huang ES (2007). Diabetes health disparities: a systematic review of health care interventions. *Medical Care Research and Review* **64** (5 Suppl.), 101S–56S.

Peters A et al. (1996). Quality of outpatient care provided to diabetic patients. A health maintenance organization experience. *Diabetes Care* **19**, 601–6.

Pickett K, Pearl M (2001). Multilevel analyses of neighbourhood socioeconomic context and health outcomes: a critical review. *Journal of Epidemiology and Community Health* **55**, 111–22.

Piette J (2000). Perceived access problems among patients with diabetes in two public systems of care. *Journal of General Internal Medicine* **15**, 797–804.

Piette JD et al. (2003). Dimensions of patient-provider communication and diabetes self-care in an ethnically diverse population. *Journal of General Internal Medicine* **18**, 624–33.

Piette JD, Bibbins-Domingo K, Schillinger D (2006). Health care discrimination, processes of care, and diabetes patients' health status. *Patient Education and Counseling* **60**, 41–8.

Piette JD et al. (2006). Use of telephone care in a cardiovascular disease management programme for type 2 diabetes patients in Santiago, Chile. *Chronic Illness* **2**, 87–96.

Pincus T, Callahan LF, Burkhauser RV (1987). Most chronic diseases are reported more frequently by individuals with fewer than 12 years of formal education in the age 18–64 United States population. *Journal of Chronic Disease* **40**, 865–74.

Pugh J et al. (1992). The influence of outpatient insurance coverage on the microvascular complications of non-insulin-dependent diabetes in Mexican Americans. *Journal of Diabetes and Its Complications* **6**, 236–41.

Rittner B, Kirk AB (1995). Health care and public transportation use by poor and frail elderly people. *Social Work* **40**, 365–73.

Robbins J et al. (2000). Excess type 2 diabetes in African-American women and men aged 40–74 and socioeconomic status: evidence from the Third National Health and Nutrition Examination Survey. *Journal of Epidemiology and Community Health* 54, 839–845.

Robinson N et al. (1990). Employment problems and diabetes. *Diabetic Medicine* 7, 16–22.

Robinson N, Lloyd CE, Stevens LK (1998). Social deprivation and mortality in adults with diabetes mellitus. *Diabetic Medicine* **15**, 205–12.

Robinson N, Stevens LK, Protopapa LE (1993). Education and employment for young people. *Diabetic Medicine* **10**, 983–9.

Rook K (1984). The negative side of social interaction: impact on psychological well-being. *Journal of Personality and Social Psychology* **46**, 1097–108.

Roper N et al. (2001). Excess mortality in a population with diabetes and the impact of material deprivation: longitudinal, population based study. *British Medical Journal* **322**, 1375–6.

Sarkar U et al. (2008). Preferences for self-management support: findings from a survey of diabetes patients in safety-net health systems. *Patient Education and Counseling* **70**, 102–10.

Schillinger D et al. (2002). Association of health literacy with diabetes outcomes. *JAMA* **288**, 475–82.

Schillinger D et al. (2003). Closing the loop: physician communication with diabetic patients who have low health literacy. *Archives of Internal Medicine* **163**, 83–90.

Schillinger D et al. (2004). Functional health literacy and the quality of physician-patient communication among diabetes patients. *Patient Education and Counseling* **52**, 315–23.

Schillinger D et al. (2006). Does literacy mediate the relationship between education and health outcomes? A study of a low-income population with diabetes. *Public Health Reports* **121**, 245–54.

Schillinger D et al. (2007). Seeing in 3-D: examining the reach of diabetes self-management support strategies in a public health care system. *Health Education and Behavior*

Schneider E, Zaslavsky AM, Epstein AM (2002). Racial disparities in the quality of care for enrollees in Medicare managed care. *JAMA* **287**, 1288–94.

Schur C, Albers LA (1996). Language, sociodemographics, and health care use of Hispanic adults *Journal of Health Care for the Poor and Underserved* **7**, 140–58.

Schuster T, Kessler RC, Aseltine RH Jr (1990). Supportive interactions, negative interactions, and depressed mood. *American Journal of Community Psychology* **18**, 423–438.

Seeman TE et al. (2001). Allostatic load as a marker of cumulative biological risk: MacArthur studies of successful aging. *Proceedings of the National Academy of Sciences U.S.A.* **98**, 4770–5.

Sherbourne C et al. (1992). Antecedents of adherence to medical recommendations: results from the Medical Outcomes Study. *Journal of Behavioral Medicine* **15**, 447–68.

Smedley B, Stith AY, Nelson AR (2002). *Unequal Treatment: Confronting Racial and Ethnic Disparities in Health Care*. Washington, DC: National Academy Press.

Sooman A, Macintyre S, Anderson A (1993). Scotland's health—a more difficult challenge for some? The price and availability of healthy foods in socially contrasting localities in the west of Scotland. *Health Bulletin (Edinburgh)* **51**, 276–84.

Stephens G et al. (1990). Racial differences in the incidence of end-stage renal disease in types I and II diabetes mellitus. *American Journal of Kidney Disease* **15**, 562–7.

Surwit R et al. (2002). Stress management improves long-term glycemic control in type 2 diabetes. *Diabetes Care* **25**, 30–4.

Swenson SL et al. (2008). The influence of depressive symptoms on clinician-patient communication among patients with type 2 diabetes. *Medical Care* **46**, 257–65.

Tellez-Zenteno J, Cardiel MH (2002). Risk factors associated with depression in patients with type 2 diabetes mellitus. *Archives of Medical Research* **33**, 53–60.

Thackeray R, Merrill RM, Neiger BL (2004). Disparities in diabetes management practice between racial and ethnic groups in the United States. *Diabetes Educator* **30**, 665–75.

The California Medi-Cal Type 2 Diabetes Study (2004). Closing the gap: effect of diabetes case management on glycemic control among low-income ethnic minority populations: the California Medi-Cal type 2 diabetes study. *Diabetes Care* **27**, 95–103.

Tull ES, Chambers EC (2001). Internalized racism is associated with glucose intolerance among Black Americans in the U.S. Virgin Islands. *Diabetes Care* **24**, 1498.

U.S. Department of Housing and Urban Development Office of Policy Development and Research (2003). Moving to opportunity interim impacts evaluation: final report. Available at http://www.abtassociates.com/reports/2003302754569_71451.pdf.

Van der Meer J, Mackenbach JP (1999). The care and course of diabetes: differences according to level of education. *Health Policy* **46**, 127–41.

van Ryn M, Burke J (2000). The effect of patient race and socio-economic status on physicians' perceptions of patients. *Social Science & Medicine* **50**, 813–28.

Ware JJ et al. (1996). Differences in 4-year health outcomes for elderly and poor, clinically ill patients treated in HMO and fee-for-service systems. Results from the Medical Outcomes Study. *JAMA* **276**, 1039–47.

Wei M et al. (1996). Migration status, socioeconomic status, and mortality rates in Mexican Americans and non-Hispanic whites: the San Antonio Heart Study. *Annals of Epidemiology* **6**, 307–13.

Williams D (1997). Race and health: basic questions, emerging directions. *Annals of Epidemiology* **7**, 322–33.

Williams M et al. (1998). Relationship of functional health literacy to patients' knowledge of their chronic disease. A study of patients with hypertension and diabetes. *Archives of Internal Medicine* **158**, 166–72.

Winkleby M et al. (1999) Pathways by which SES and ethnicity influence cardiovascular disease risk factors. *Annals of the New York Academy of Sciences* **896**, 191–209.

Witkin S, Klein R (1984). Ophthalmologic care for persons with diabetes. *JAMA* **251**, 2534–37.

Zarit S, Reever KE, Bach-Peterson J (1980). Relatives of the impaired elderly: correlates of feelings of burden. *Gerontologist* **20**, 649–55.

Zenk S et al. (2006). Fruit and vegetable access differs by community racial composition and socioeconomic position in Detroit, Michigan. *Ethnicity & Disease* **16**, 275–80.

SECTION 3
PREVENTION OF DIABETES
AND ITS COMPLICATIONS

15. Prevention of Type 2 Diabetes
Accomplishments and Challenges

William C. Knowler, Mary Hoskin, Jeffrey M. Curtis,
Robert G. Nelson, and Robert L. Hanson

■ Main Public Health Messages

- People at high risk of developing type 2 diabetes can often be identified with simple clinical tests.
- Many of the risk factors—such as obesity, physical inactivity, and subdiagnostic elevations in glycemia—that predict which of these people are most likely to develop diabetes are potentially modifiable.
- Randomized clinical trials reported in the last two decades confirm that treatment of diabetes risk factors in high-risk persons can reduce the development of new cases of diabetes.
- Genetic data have so far had limited use in predicting the risk of type 2 diabetes or in guiding preventive interventions, but early studies in this field suggest that progress will be made in this area.
- None of the tested interventions are fully successful at preventing diabetes, indicating that more effective interventions are needed.

■ Why Should Type 2 Diabetes Be Preventable?

Type 2 diabetes results from a combination of genetic and environmental factors. The genetic basis for susceptibility remains elusive and appears to involve many different genes, each with small effects on diabetes susceptibility (Hanson, Nelson, and Knowler chapter 28, this volume). Due to the small sizes of these effects and our limited ability to target susceptibility mechanisms with drug or behavioral interventions, knowledge of genetic determinants has so far had little impact on the prevention of type 2 diabetes. Nevertheless type 2 diabetes has been proposed as a preventable disease because (1) at least some of its risk factors, such as obesity and physical activity, are potentially modifiable; (2) it is relatively easy to identify people at high risk of developing the disease; and (3) the often prolonged periods of abnormal glucose regulation that precede diabetes might be controllable with drugs or behavioral interventions (Knowler et al. 1995). The major factors that have been targeted for behavioral interventions are obesity and physical inactivity (Knowler et al. 1995). Obesity, itself, is a complex condition resulting from poorly understood genetic factors and environmental influences including availability of food, demands for physical activity, and social influences on eating and exercise behavior. In some situations the development of obesity is also influenced by transgenerational effects, such as exposure to diabetes in utero, that defy simple genetic or environmental explanations (Dabelea et al. 2000; Pettitt et al. 1988).

■ Randomized Clinical Trials in Preventing Type 2 Diabetes

Although early attempts at preventing type 2 diabetes were disappointing, the past two decades have brought much new evidence from randomized clinical trials about the prevention of type 2 diabetes mellitus, as recently reviewed in detail by Crandall et al. (2008) and summarized here. Early clinical trials in the United Kingdom and Sweden examined effects of drugs then commonly used to treat diabetes, tolbutamide and phenformin, in persons identified at high risk of type 2 diabetes by virtue of having impaired glucose tolerance (Jarrett et al. 1979; Keen et al. 1982; Sartor et al. 1980). Preventive effects, if any, of these three clinical trials were modest, but importantly, the studies were very small compared with those performed later, resulting in very wide confidence intervals of effects (Crandall et al. 2008; Knowler et al. 1995). Accordingly, these studies were inconclusive. The next major clinical trials were not reported until the late 1990s and 2000s.

Major clinical trials reported since 1997 showed that, in high-risk persons, diabetes could be prevented or delayed by several different means, including drug treatment or lifestyle interventions focused on diet, exercise, and weight loss (reviewed by Crandall et al. 2008). Drugs used to treat type 2 diabetes, such as metformin (DPP Research Group 2002; Ramachandran et al. 2006), acarbose (Chiasson et al. 2002), troglitazone (Buchanan et al. 2002; DPP Research Group 2005a), and rosiglitazone (DREAM Trial Investigators 2006), were also effective in preventing or limiting the rise in glycemia in nondiabetic persons to levels diagnostic of diabetes.

The results of these pharmacologic intervention trials are perhaps not surprising, given that these drugs control hyperglycemia in diabetes. Some have argued, however, that it is inappropriate to consider their use in nondiabetic persons as "preventing" diabetes rather than simply "treating" hyperglycemia at levels below those diagnostic of diabetes. This semantic argument of treatment or prevention is actually of little clinical importance; the important question is whether such treatment or prevention leads to real improvements in health, as discussed below.

Lifestyle or behavioral interventions designed to induce weight loss, improve diet, or increase habitual physical activity are also effective. The Da Qing, China, clinical trial compared approaches involving changes in diet, exercise, or both.

There was little difference in these three approaches, each of which was modestly effective in reducing the incidence of diabetes (Pan et al. 1997). The Finnish Diabetes Prevention Study tested a behavioral intervention that included the following goals: weight reduction of ≥5%, dietary fat intake of <30% of energy, saturated fat intake <10% of energy, fiber intake of ≥15 g per 1000 kcal, and moderate exercise for ≥30 minutes per day. This intensive intervention group was compared with a control group receiving limited health advice. The behavioral intervention reduced the diabetes incidence rate by 58% over 3 years (Tuomilehto et al. 2001), with a somewhat smaller reduction in a period following cessation of the active intervention (Lindström et al. 2006). The U.S. Diabetes Prevention Program tested both metformin and a lifestyle intervention with goals of ≥7% weight loss, initially through dietary fat reduction to <30% of calories, and moderate physical activity for ≥150 minutes per week. There was a greater reduction in the incidence rate of diabetes by the lifestyle intervention (58% rate reduction) than by metformin (31% rate reduction), both compared with placebo (DPP Research Group 2002). In the Indian Diabetes Prevention Program, by contrast, a behavioral weight-loss intervention, metformin, and a combination of the two led to similar reductions in diabetes incidence (Ramachandran et al. 2006). Unfortunately no other clinical trials of comparable scope to these have compared lifestyle with pharmacologic approaches in participants meeting similar criteria. Thus there are limited data comparing pharmacological with lifestyle approaches and even fewer comparing different drugs with each other or with drug-lifestyle combinations. Bariatric surgery for weight loss, although not subjected to randomized clinical trials, may have some value in preventing diabetes in extremely obese persons, as reviewed elsewhere (Crandall et al. 2008).

■ Remaining Gaps in Our Knowledge

Despite this dramatic progress resulting from randomized clinical trials, major gaps in our knowledge persist, and a number of questions remain unanswered.

Why have the "successful" interventions been only partially successful? Both the clinical trials reporting the greatest benefit of lifestyle interventions (DPP Research Group 2002; Tuomilehto et al. 2001) achieved a 58% reduction in the annual incidence rate of diabetes in high-risk adults. Although these results were very encouraging, prevention was not complete. Even among those receiving the lifestyle interventions, 19% developed diabetes after 6 years in the Finnish Diabetes Prevention Study (Tuomilehto et al. 2001), and 21% developed diabetes after 4 years in the U.S. Diabetes Prevention Program (DPP Research Group 2002) (approximate numbers estimated from the published figures). Among the lifestyle intervention groups of these two clinical trials, the reduction of diabetes incidence was directly related to the participants' success in meeting goals in the Finnish Diabetes Prevention Study (Tuomilehto et al. 2001) or in losing weight in the U.S. Diabetes Prevention Program (DPP Research Group 2006). In the three lifestyle intervention groups in the Da Qing clinical trial, the 6-year cumulative incidence of diabetes ranged from 44% to 47% (Pan et al. 1997). The results of these three clinical trials suggest that diabetes incidence rates could be reduced even further if better methods were available for inducing diet and exercise behavior change. The extent to which such behavioral interventions can be improved and the degree of prevention attainable, however, are not known. Similarly we do not known how much risk reduction could have been achieved in the drug studies had adherence to the study drugs been complete; nor do we know the extent to which imperfect adherence was due to unacceptable side effects or inadequate understanding and motivation on the part of the participants.

Can different approaches to intervention be more successful? Many other types of interventions should be considered. Just as the optimal dietary approach to treating type 2 diabetes is quite controversial (Nield et al. 2009), the optimal dietary approach to preventing type 2 diabetes has not been evaluated. For example although low-carbohydrate, high-fat diets can be effective for weight loss and thus might be effective in preventing diabetes, they have not, to our knowledge, been evaluated in diabetes prevention clinical trials, nor have programs of vigorous aerobic or resistance exercise or their combination. There has been little study of combinations of two or more drugs or of a drug with a lifestyle intervention.

Should preventive interventions be offered to different types of people than those enrolled in clinical trials so far? Eligibility for diabetes prevention clinical trials thus far has required some level of abnormal plasma glucose, usually following an oral glucose load and sometimes also requiring elevated fasting glucose. If intervention programs were not restricted to people with such characteristics, many more could be offered interventions, but their average incidence of diabetes would be lower. Therefore, formal evaluation of benefit in randomized clinical trials would require much larger or longer trials than have been performed so far, making it unlikely that such trials will be performed.

Persons might be selected for diabetes prevention efforts based on their genotypes at genes conferring susceptibility to diabetes. Although research in this area is in its infancy, the Diabetes Prevention Program addressed this question in adults who were selected for the clinical trial based on high-risk characteristics assessed independently of genotype. Those subsequently found to have high-risk genotypes at two susceptibility genes, *TCF7L2* (Florez et al. 2006) and *ENPP1* (Moore et al. 2009), appeared to derive greater benefit from the lifestyle intervention that those with lower-risk genotypes, suggesting the possibility of using genetic factors to recruit those with the greatest potential to benefit from prevention interventions. Such an approach, however, would risk inappropriately excluding people with the lower-risk genotypes. In the Diabetes Prevention Program people with the lower-risk genotypes for these two genes were in the majority and comprised the largest number of incident cases of diabetes, and the intervention further reduced their incidence of diabetes (Florez et al. 2006; Moore et al. 2009).

Should preventive interventions be started earlier in life? Genetic suscepti-bility to type 2 diabetes begins at conception. Intrauterine hyperglycemia and conditions at birth and infancy are powerful predictors of risk of type 2 diabe-tes later in life (Dabelea et al. 2000; Franks et al. 2006; Pettitt et al. 1988, 1997) Optimally, the prevention of diabetes would target the potentially modifiable factors operating early in life, such as hyperglycemia in pregnancy and lack of breast feeding of infants. Such programs, however, will be extremely difficult to evaluate because of the long time frame from conception to the typical onset of type 2 diabetes.

To what extent should prevention be focused on individuals or on societies as a whole? The increasing incidence rates of obesity and type 2 diabetes in the United States and many other parts of the world are due in part to increased availability of food, including food of high caloric density, and to the decreased demands for phys-ical activity. Therefore, it may be much more effective to target these risk factors by group or societal interventions in addition to individual approaches. Such interven-tions extend beyond usual medical activities, as they involve economic and physical attributes of our living environments, and thus they will be difficult to implement and evaluate.

Would resources be better allocated to early detection and treatment of dia-betes rather than prevention? This is a major question regarding competition for health care resources for type 2 diabetes. Several, but not all, economic analyses of costs and benefits of diabetes prevention indicate good value for the resources spent, although not cost savings (Crandall et al. 2008; DPP Research Group 2005b; Eddy, Schlessinger, and Kahn 2005; Engelgau 2005). The ultimate answer to this question depends on whether diabetes prevention, as currently defined by the clinical trials reviewed here, will have health benefits beyond controlling hyperglycemia and other risk factors. That is, will detection and treatment of hyperglycemia at a point earlier than what is now defined as diabetes ultimately lead to less microvascular and macrovascular disease and early mortality than will a policy of detection and intensive treatment only when current diabetes diagnostic criteria are met? Ideally, this question would be answered by a ran-domized clinical trial of diabetes "prevention" compared with early detection and treatment of diabetes as currently defined. Such a trial, the design of which would need to account for different enrollment criteria causing different "lead times" and which might require many years of follow-up, has not been initiated as far as we know.

What are the implications for diabetes diagnostic criteria? If it is ultimately decided that degrees of hyperglycemia that we now label as impaired glucose regu-lation (impaired fasting glucose or impaired glucose tolerance) (Expert Committee 1997) warrant intensive efforts toward detection and intervention, then they may be treated essentially as disease states. In such a situation, the diagnostic categories of normal, impaired glucose regulation, and diabetes might be abandoned in favor of dealing with hyperglycemia as a continuum.

■ **Acknowledgment**

This work was supported, in part, by the Intramural Research Program of the National Institute of Diabetes and Digestive and Kidney Diseases.

■ **References**

Buchanan TA et al. (2002). Preservation of pancreatic beta-cell function and prevention of type 2 diabetes by pharmacological treatment of insulin resistance in high-risk Hispanic women. *Diabetes* **51**, 2796–2803.

Chiasson JL et al. (2002). Acarbose for prevention of type 2 diabetes mellitus: the STOP-NIDDM randomized trial. *Lancet* **359**, 2072–7.

Crandall JP et al. (2008). The prevention of type 2 diabetes. *Nature Clinical Practice: Endocrinology and Metabolism* **4**, 382–93.

Dabelea D et al. (2000). Intrauterine exposure to diabetes conveys risks for type 2 diabetes and obesity: a study of discordant sibships. *Diabetes* **49**, 2208–11.

Diabetes Prevention Program Research Group (2002). Reduction in the incidence of type 2 diabetes with lifestyle intervention or metformin. *New England Journal of Medicine* **346**, 393–403.

Diabetes Prevention Program Research Group (2005a). Prevention of type 2 diabetes with troglitazone in the Diabetes Prevention Program. *Diabetes* **54**, 1150–6.

Diabetes Prevention Program Research Group (2005b). The cost-effectiveness of lifestyle modification or metformin in preventing type 2 diabetes in adults with impaired glucose tolerance. *Annals of Internal Medicine* **142**, 323–32.

Diabetes Prevention Program Research Group, prepared by Hamman RF et al. (2006). Effect of weight loss with lifestyle intervention on risk of diabetes. *Diabetes Care* **29**, 2102–7.

DREAM (Diabetes Reduction Assessment with ramipril and rosiglitazone medication) Trial Investigators (2006). Effect of rosiglitazone on the frequency of diabetes in patients with impaired glucose tolerance or impaired fasting glucose: a randomized controlled trial. *Lancet* **368**, 1096–1105.

Eddy DM, Schlessinger L, Kahn R (2005). Clinical outcomes and cost-effectiveness of strategies for managing people at high risk for diabetes. *Annals of Internal Medicine* **143**, 251–64.

Engelgau MM (2005). Trying to predict the future for people with diabetes: a tough but important task. *Annals of Internal Medicine* **143**, 301–2.

Expert Committee on the Diagnosis and Classification of Diabetes Mellitus (1997). Report of the expert committee on the diagnosis and classification of diabetes mellitus. *Diabetes Care* **20**, 1183–97.

Florez JC et al. (2006). TCF7L2 polymorphisms and progression to diabetes in the Diabetes Prevention Program. *New England Journal of Medicine* **355**, 241–50.

Franks PW et al. (2006). Gestational glucose tolerance and risk of type 2 diabetes in young Pima Indian offspring. *Diabetes* **55**, 460–5.

Jarrett RJ et al. (1979). Worsening to diabetes in men with impaired glucose tolerance ("borderline diabetes"). *Diabetologia* **16**, 25–30.

Keen H et al. (1982). The ten-year follow-up of the Bedford survey (1962–1972): glucose tolerance and diabetes. *Diabetologia* **22**, 73–8.

Knowler WC et al. (1995). Preventing non-insulin-dependent diabetes mellitus. *Diabetes* **44**, 483–8.

Lindström J et al. (2006). Sustained reduction in the incidence of type 2 diabetes by lifestyle intervention: follow-up of the Finnish Diabetes Prevention Study. *Lancet* **368**, 1673–9.

Moore AF et al. (2009). The association of *ENPP1* K121Q with diabetes incidence is abolished by lifestyle modification in the Diabetes Prevention Program. *Journal of Clinical Endocrinology and Metabolism* **94**, 449–55.

Nield L et al. (2009). Dietary advice for treatment of type 2 diabetes mellitus in adults (review). *The Cochrane Collaboration, The Cochrane Library* 2009, issue 1.

Pan XR et al. (1997). Effects of diet and exercise in preventing NIDDM in people with impaired glucose tolerance. The Da Qing IGT and Diabetes Study. *Diabetes Care* **20**, 537–44.

Pettitt DJ et al. (1988). Congenital susceptibility to non-insulin-dependent diabetes mellitus: role of intrauterine environment. *Diabetes* **37**, 622–8.

Pettitt DJ et al. (1997). Breastfeeding and incidence of non-insulin-dependent diabetes mellitus in Pima Indians. *Lancet* **350**, 166–8.

Ramachandran A et al. (2006). The Indian Diabetes Prevention Programme shows that lifestyle modification and metformin prevent type 2 diabetes in Asian Indian subjects with impaired glucose tolerance (IDPP-1). *Diabetologia* **49**, 289–97.

Sartor G et al. (1980). Ten-year follow-up of subjects with impaired glucose tolerance: prevention of diabetes by tolbutamide and diet regulation. *Diabetes* **29**, 41–9.

Tuomilehto J et al. (2001). Prevention of type 2 diabetes mellitus by changes in lifestyle among subjects with impaired glucose tolerance. *New England Journal of Medicine* **344**, 1343–50.

16. Implementing Programs for the Primary Prevention of Diabetes in Non-Health-Care Settings

From Evidence to Practice

Ronald T. Ackermann and David G. Marrero

■ Main Public Health Messages

- There is compelling evidence that improvements in diet and physical activity, particularly when they lead to modest weight loss, can prevent type 2 diabetes.
- Evidence is strong that structured lifestyle interventions to prevent diabetes are cost-effective when offered to overweight or obese adults with impaired glucose tolerance, but it is unclear whether policies or programs that offer less intensive lifestyle interventions to other groups are also cost-effective.
- Strategies to prevent diabetes outside of the health care setting should consider multilevel approaches that provide structured programs for high-risk adults with impaired glucose tolerance (IGT) in concert with more general, population-level initiatives to support regular physical activity and healthy eating behaviors.
- Structured lifestyle interventions to prevent diabetes outside of the health care setting could be more sustainable through health care partnerships that help to identify high-risk adults with IGT and provide one future avenue toward payment by health plan coverage mechanisms.
- Multilevel, population-based initiatives to prevent diabetes that involve institutional, community, and public policy sectors are likely to have greater impact and sustainability if they are designed using participatory approaches to community involvement and coalition building.

■ Introduction

Extensive research demonstrates the effectiveness of two broad strategies to prevent or delay the onset of type 2 diabetes in adults—pharmacologic therapy and structured lifestyle interventions (Burnet et al. 2006; Gillies et al. 2007). To date, however, high-quality preventive services have proved particularly challenging to deliver in health care settings, even when there is compelling evidence for their clinical cost-effectiveness (Bodenheimer, Wagner, and Grumbach 2002a, 2002b; Garfield et al. 2003; Grumbach and Bodenheimer 2002). Conversely, resources and policies to support modest weight loss and moderate physical activity behaviors have a stronger capacity to reach vast segments of the population when offered in non-health-care community settings. In this context, this chapter considers the current evidence base for cost-effective prevention of diabetes and explores implications and emerging research for implementing policies and programs to prevent type 2 diabetes in non-health-care settings.

■ Background/Historical Perspective

What Is Evidence-Based Diabetes Prevention?

Large, prospective observational studies have demonstrated strong associations between reduction of diabetes risk and healthier diets, regular physical activity, and modest weight loss (Colditz et al. 1995; Hu FB et al. 1999; Hu G et al. 2003; Koh-Banerjee et al. 2004; Schulze and Hu 2005; Wannamethee, Shaper, and Alberti 2000; Weinstein et al. 2004). Although this rich epidemiologic evidence strongly suggests that lifestyle changes might reduce the development of diabetes in broad populations, these studies relied largely on self-reports to indicate the development of diabetes, and participants were not systematically assessed for undiagnosed diabetes. In this context it is possible that persons with less healthy lifestyle behaviors who were experiencing weight gain were more likely to seek medical advice, undergo testing for diabetes, and receive a diagnosis. Thus these studies were limited by both potential recall bias (because of the reliance on self-reports) and incomplete ascertainment of diabetes development as an outcome. Moreover these epidemiologic studies do not provide insight into the human and financial costs required to successfully achieve and maintain modest lifestyle changes. Thus although this research supports the notion that almost any broad efforts to improve diet and physical activity behaviors might help to stem the tide of diabetes in the population, it does not help to inform policies about how to distribute limited societal resources to support successful lifestyle changes, nor does it answer whether payment for these efforts would prove cost-effective for a particular stakeholder group, such as health payers, employers, individuals at high risk for diabetes, or society as a whole.

Since the mid-1990s several large randomized trials have been implemented to overcome the limitations of past epidemiologic research and to assess the health and economic benefits of structured lifestyle programs to reduce the development of diabetes. Recent systematic reviews have summarized direct evidence from these high-quality randomized trials (Burnet et al. 2006; Gillies et al. 2007; Santaguida et al. 2005). One of the largest and most pivotal of these studies was the U.S. Diabetes Prevention Program (DPP). The DPP was a 27-site clinical trial that randomly assigned over 3200 overweight or obese adults with impaired glucose tolerance to receive intensive lifestyle modification (diet and regular physical activity), metformin, or placebo. Participants were ethnically diverse and had a mean age of 51 years and baseline body mass index (BMI) of 34 (kg/m^2). After 24 weeks in the study, half of the lifestyle intervention participants had reached the study's treatment goal of ≥7% weight reduction, and 74% had reached the goal of ≥150 minutes per week of moderate physical activity (equivalent to brisk walking). An average of about 2 years later, 38% of lifestyle participants were still at the weight goal, and 58% were maintaining the exercise goal. At this level of success, the lifestyle intervention reduced the cumulative incidence of type 2 diabetes by 58%. By contrast, study participants assigned to receive metformin had a 31% reduction in the development of type 2 diabetes.

One key theme across the DPP and other randomized prevention trials has been the use of cognitive and behavioral strategies to help individuals achieve and maintain *modest* weight reduction (5% to 7% of baseline body mass) through dietary restriction and moderate daily physical activity. These trials primarily employed dietary strategies that focused on restriction of dietary fat intake to less than 25%–30% of total kilocalories, with stricter total caloric restriction if initial attempts to achieve weight loss were unsuccessful (Burnet et al. 2006; Gillies et al. 2007). Most successful intervention programs also recommended moderate-intensity physical activity (e.g., walking) for 30 minutes a day on 5 to 7 days per week. To achieve these behavioral goals interventions typically included *structured*, one-on-one or group meetings that were held every 1 to 4 weeks for a period of 3 to 6 months in order to work individually with participants to achieve early successes and employ tailored problem-solving strategies to overcome barriers. Initial, more intensive phases of most interventions were typically followed by maintenance visits that recurred at intervals of every 1–3 months. Using these approaches, structured, ongoing lifestyle interventions were found to reduce the hazard of type 2 diabetes (i.e., new cases of diabetes per 100 person-years of treatment) across studies by 51% (Gillies et al. 2007).

When considering implications for resource allocation in efforts to implement evidence-based diabetes prevention in the real world, it is important to realize that randomized trials have focused almost exclusively on adults who are at high risk for developing diabetes by virtue of having impaired glucose tolerance (IGT) (Burnet et al. 2006; Caro et al. 2004; Gillies et al. 2007; Herman et al. 2005; Palmer et al. 2004). IGT is a clinical diagnosis, defined by an elevated plasma (blood) glucose concentration collected 2 hours after administration of a 75-g oral glucose challenge—a test that is only feasible to perform in health care settings (Screening for type 2 diabetes 2003). To date no high-quality clinical trials have demonstrated whether low-intensity community programs or broad environmental policies with the same goals for modest behavioral change can make a comparable impact in terms of diabetes prevention or will be cost-effective when offered to nonselected populations or to groups with other known indicators of diabetes risk, such as elevated BMI, a high waist-to-hip ratio, hyperinsulinemia, or impaired fasting glucose (Gillies et al. 2007).

■ Implications for Non-Health-Care Programs and Policies

Compelling research indicates that the modest weight loss achieved through dietary changes and moderate physical activities can improve health for most populations, not just high-risk subgroups that are identified in health care settings (McTigue et al. 2003). However there are simply no clinical trials that directly assess the cost-effectiveness of preventing diabetes via less structured programs or policies in non-health-care settings or in unselected populations. Clearly, however, an absence of such trials is quite different from having clinical trials that demonstrate no benefit. Furthermore, there is a wealth of research demonstrating that lower-intensity, non-health-care policies and programs can successfully support modest improvements in lifestyle behaviors (Brownson, Haire-Joshu, and Luke 2006; Guide to Community Preventive Services 2007). The real question is how these broader initiatives should fit into an integrated, population-wide strategy that seeks to modify common risk factors for developing diabetes while also offering formal programs that have proved cost-effective for preventing diabetes in high-risk persons with IGT.

The Lessons of Cost-Effectiveness Research

Even low-intensity policies and programs can be costly to implement, particularly when they are offered to large segments of the population. Moreover, many formal programs in non-health-care settings require participants to pay a fee, thereby presenting a significant barrier for many segments of the population. When resources are limited, estimates of cost-effectiveness can provide guidance about the costs and benefits of different programs and can help inform decisions about who should pay. Cost-effectiveness estimates are best if based on strong research evidence, but this may pose a problem, because we currently have little information about whether it is feasible or effective to pay for low-intensity diet and physical activity programs to prevent diabetes in unselected populations. On the other hand several studies have found that offering highly structured lifestyle intervention programs to overweight or obese adults with IGT is likely to be highly cost-effective (Caro et al. 2004; Gillies et al. 2008; Herman et al. 2006; Icks et al. 2007; Jacobs-van der Bruggen et al. 2007; Palmer et al. 2004; Ramachandran et al. 2007).

We also need to consider whether economically disadvantaged persons with diabetes risk factors will pay a fee to access structured community programs if they are not aware that they are at high risk. Perceptions of risk, personal experience, and motivation of adults at high risk for developing diabetes may play a role in the successful adoption and maintenance of modest lifestyle changes (Kim et al. 2007; Kramer et al. 2007; Walker et al. 2007). Moreover, persons who believe that they are at high risk for developing diabetes often report that they are willing to pay more to access programs to help them prevent the development of diabetes, particularly if those programs offer more intensive and structured resources that provide ongoing support for successful weight loss and adoption of physical activity (Johnson et al. 2006). Thus, whereas non-health-care policies and programs have a clear impact on health behaviors that are tightly linked to the development of type 2 diabetes, we need to also consider novel approaches for identifying those at high risk, increasing awareness about risk, and enabling broader access to programs that offer greater structure and ongoing support for modest weight loss and physical activity, even if these efforts increase the overall costs of diabetes prevention.

Implementing Diabetes Prevention in the Real World—Shared Goals, Shared Realities

Although clinical trials tell us that lifestyle changes resulting in modest weight reduction appear to be a principal mediator of successful diabetes prevention (Hamman et al. 2006), maintaining successful lifestyle changes has not proved easy or cheap. Systematic reviews of interventions designed to achieve and maintain weight loss indicate that they are more successful when they combine cognitive and behavioral strategies to improve *both* diet and physical activity behaviors and provide *ongoing, long-term* contact at least every month. Briefer interventions delivered by health care providers can help motivate patients to consider initiating new lifestyle behaviors, to direct patients to supportive lifestyle programs, and to provide follow-up to reinforce the maintenance of new behaviors. However, there is insufficient evidence that such interventions alone can result in meaningful levels of weight loss by individual patients (Behavioral counseling in primary care to promote physical activity: recommendation and rationale 2002; Eden et al. 2002; McTigue et al. 2003; Pignone et al. 2003). By contrast non-health-care settings provide greater reach to broad segments of the population and have an enhanced capacity to provide ongoing behavioral support and follow-up. Unfortunately it is not feasible in most non-health-care settings to identify persons who are at the highest risk for developing diabetes, to prescribe potentially beneficial medications for diabetes prevention, or to provide ongoing follow-up tests or treatment for persons who develop type 2 diabetes (Screening for type 2 diabetes 2003).

Partnerships that combine health care and non-health-care resources could strengthen population-wide goals for achieving successful diabetes prevention. Indeed, the major public health achievements over the past three decades to lower the burden of tobacco use should teach us that behavioral interventions to prevent diabetes on a population scale are most effective when implemented as community-wide, multi-stakeholder initiatives involving local governments, employers, health care payers and providers, public health agencies, and other community organizations (Fiore et al. 2000; Thompson, Lynn, and Shopland 1995). Although behavioral initiatives to prevent diabetes could well be more sustainable, have greater impact, and reach a larger population if they are offered outside of health care settings, such initiatives might benefit considerably from partnerships with the health care system, for two reasons: (1) these partnerships could identify persons at high risk for developing diabetes; and (2) resources that are part of the health care system could be leveraged to deliver more structured lifestyle programs that have proved cost-effective for preventing diabetes in these individuals. Lack of financing for structured programs in the community may be one factor that has prevented passive diffusion of evidence-based diabetes prevention beyond the health care system. In this context, linkages to the health care system may provide a mechanism to enable coverage of behavioral interventions by health payers (Garfield et al. 2003; Glasgow, Orleans, and Wagner 2001; Whitlock et al. 2002). Before considering partnered approaches to diabetes prevention, however, it is important to consider first how general, population-based approaches to address obesity and metabolic risk factors may serve to expand the reach, effectiveness, and sustainability of diabetes prevention in non-health-care settings.

Framework for Behavioral Resources and Policies in Non-Health-Care Settings

Contemporary health promotion involves efforts to change organizational behavior as well as the physical, social, and economic environments of communities (Theory at a Glance: A Guide for Health Promotion Practice 2005). Successful health promotion programs that seek to address health problems across this spectrum employ a range of strategies and operate on multiple levels. The ecological perspective emphasizes the interaction among factors across each of these levels and highlights people's interactions with their physical and sociocultural environments (Theory at a Glance: A Guide for Health Promotion Practice 2005; Whittemore, Melkus, and Grey 2004). In the context of non-health-care interventions to support healthy diet and physical activity behaviors that prevent the development of type 2 diabetes, the ecological framework encompasses initiatives at the institutional, community, and public policy levels, involving community-based organizations, social institutions, work sites, schools, media, government, and the built environment. The following section briefly summarizes published evidence for strategies to reduce the development of diabetes using non-health-care institutional, community, or public policy channels.

Non-Health-Care Interventions to Prevent Diabetes

A systematic review published in 2003 summarized peer-reviewed research of formal attempts to implement population-level environmental and policy interventions to directly prevent diabetes (Satterfield et al. 2003). This review identified only 16 published reports, of which just 11 presented results, and only a few used rigorous methods to evaluate effectiveness. From this review it was not possible to identify any specific approaches to population-level diabetes prevention for which there was strong evidence of effectiveness. In this context the U.S. Centers for Disease Control and Prevention (CDC) launched an aggressive initiative to evaluate strategies to implement evidence-based diabetes prevention activities in concert with the state-based Diabetes Prevention & Control Programs (DPCPs) (Murphy, Chapel, and Clark 2004). In 2005, the CDC provided funds to support DPCP efforts in California, Massachusetts, Michigan, Minnesota, and Washington. This project, known as the Diabetes Primary Prevention Initiative 4 (DPPI 4), was intended to lay the groundwork for establishing collaborative, evidence-based diabetes prevention projects for surveillance, decision-making support for policy makers, and more focused public health and health system interventions in diverse settings.

DPPI 4 funds provided support to DPCP staff to engage stakeholders (i.e., community organizations, business and employer groups, health care staff, policy makers, and consumers) to develop a conceptual framework that could serve as a template for national dissemination of effective strategies for supporting diabetes prevention resources on a population scale. Specific objectives of the DPPI 4 included efforts to (1) design interventions for adults diagnosed with prediabetes (defined as a fasting blood glucose of 100–125 mg/dL or a plasma glucose of 140–199 mg/dL 2 hours after a glucose challenge), (2) build partnerships to allow diagnosis of prediabetes to occur within the clinical setting while permitting interventions to take place in the community, (3) use the Planned Care Model for strategic planning and implementation (Bodenheimer et al. 2002a, 2002b; Glasgow et al. 2001), (4) develop appropriate systems to provide resources for persons with newly detected diabetes as a natural consequence of efforts to identify prediabetes, and (5) develop strategies that strengthen community-based ownership, partnership, and collaboration. In 2007 the U.S. Agency for Healthcare Research and Quality issued funding for a formal evaluation of DPPI 4 intervention approaches in the hope of identifying successful implementation strategies that would help to serve as a template for broader DPCP efforts to prevent diabetes. At the time of this written work, the results of this evaluation are still forthcoming.

The limited availability of direct research evidence that non-health-care policies and programs can prevent diabetes should not dissuade public health institutions from developing diabetes prevention initiatives. As a first step to demonstrating the potential of any new intervention to affect health outcomes, researchers naturally begin by developing studies of intensive strategies for selected, high-risk persons. This increases the potential for initial research to detect even a very small impact and is a reasonable approach for interventions involving drugs or structured life-style interventions that require considerable costs to develop and implement. If research is unable to demonstrate a benefit from an intensive intervention in the highest-risk individuals, it may not be justified to study less-intensive approaches or to try to determine whether it is cost-effective to expend the same resources to treat lower-risk persons. Thus it is not surprising that studies of the impact of life-style strategies for preventing diabetes among broader, nonclinical populations will emerge more slowly.

Today, we have strong evidence that intensive lifestyle interventions are cost-effective for preventing diabetes in high-risk adults with IGT. It may be some time, however, until we have research that estimates the resources needed to successfully prevent diabetes in nonclinical, non-high-risk populations. Until then we have com-pelling epidemiologic research supporting the association between lifestyle behav-iors and diabetes risk in general populations, and we have secondary analyses of diabetes prevention trials indicating that interventions to prevent diabetes are effec-tive even at low levels of lifestyle change and that achieving effectiveness does not seem to depend on the degree of baseline diabetes risk (Hamman et al. 2006). This should encourage us to consider the potential impact of non-health-care interven-tions in all populations that result in weight loss and maintenance.

We do know from extensive past research on weight loss that success requires considerable ongoing support at substantial ongoing cost (McTigue et al., 2003). With this information we could begin by assuming that modest weight loss might have the same relative impact on reducing the development of diabetes in low-risk individuals as it does in the high-risk (about a 50% reduction in new cases). We might also assume that it would cost about the same amount per person to achieve modest weight loss in both high-risk and low-risk persons. If so fewer cases of diabe-tes would be prevented by using the same resources to target low-risk populations.

This illustration allows us to consider several things about the types of non-health-care interventions to prevent diabetes that could prove to be a good socie-tal investment. First, the cost-effectiveness of interventions to encourage lifestyle changes will improve by minimizing the costs needed to implement them, provided that lower-cost strategies still result in meaningful changes in behavior and, ide-ally, modest weight loss. Second, initiatives that are designed to extend their impact beyond diabetes prevention are likely to be more sustainable because they will increase the range of beneficial effects that result from the same dollars invested. Other benefits of general policies to increase physical activity and reduce obesity include improved functional status, better quality of life, reduced pain, and a myr-iad of other positive outcomes (McTigue et al. 2003). Third, programs that ultimately reduce the underlying prevalence of diabetes risk factors could have a profound, long-range impact on diabetes prevalence for the population. Thus initiatives that help to bring about sociocultural and environmental changes that aid in reversing the current population trend of slow annual weight gain and increasing levels of physical inactivity have the potential to leverage considerable reductions in future diabetes risk for the population. Fourth, inasmuch as structured lifestyle behavioral interventions are more feasible to implement in non-health-care settings, we should consider partnered approaches that help to identify high-risk individuals who might benefit from these programs and to invite multi-stakeholder approaches to finance these costlier approaches to preventing diabetes. In this context the following section discusses evidence that non-health-care interventions can reduce body weight by improving underlying dietary and physical activity behaviors and how partnered approaches to implement high-intensity programs in non-health-care settings might be developed.

Non-Health-Care Interventions to Support Changes in Body Weight or Underlying Lifestyle Behaviors

Peer-reviewed research to support particular non-health-care policies designed specifically for diabetes prevention is limited, but recent systematic reviews have summarized the effectiveness of more general efforts to support physical activity and dietary behaviors that could help individuals to achieve and maintain weight loss (Brownson et al. 2006; Katz et al. 2005). These reviews, performed in conjunction with the development of the *Guide to Community Preventive Services*, identified several intervention areas as having strong or sufficient evidence to support their effectiveness in supporting healthy physical activity or nutrition in adults or children (see Table 16.1).

In a separate review, the Task Force on Community Preventive Services also found strong research to support multicomponent work-site interventions involving nutrition and physical activity to control overweight or obesity (Katz et al. 2005). Commonly used work-site intervention strategies included didactic education in nutrition, prescriptions for aerobic or strength-training exercise, training in behavioral techniques, providing self-directed materials, specific dietary prescriptions, incentives achieved through payroll deduction, and group or supervised exercise.

Several additional non-health-care interventions to support lifestyle behavior change showed promise in some studies but were found by the Task Force to have mixed or insufficient evidence to support a recommendation (Katz et al. 2005). These strategies included transportation policies, economic incentives for physical activity, availability of foods and beverages in schools, media campaigns, strategies to improve access to healthy ready-to-eat foods in cafeterias and restaurants, and altering food pricing or offering incentives for healthier food choices.

Transportation policy measures, including changes in standards for designing roadways, expansion of public transportation services, or subsidization of public transportation (e.g., providing transit passes) may influence the rate of physical activity and may also be beneficial to air quality and reduce traffic congestion. However, because of too few qualified studies, these intervention strategies had insufficient evidence for the Task Force to make any type of recommendation (Katz et al. 2005).

TABLE 16.1 *Non-Health-Care Interventions with Strong or Sufficient Evidence for Promoting Healthy Lifestyle Behaviors*

Strategy	Examples of Intervention Components	Sites/Populations	Effectiveness	Other Notes
Access to facilities	• Increased access to fitness centers • Building walking/biking trails • Focus on recreational activity	Diverse settings, including work sites, universities, federal agencies, and communities	Median increase in aerobic capacity 5.1% (IQR 2.8% to 9.6%) (Kahn et al. 2002)	Only one study in ethnically diverse populations
Urban planning and policy	• Zoning regulations and building codes • Improved street lighting • Infrastructure projects to increase the ease and safety of street crossing • Policies to ensure sidewalk continuity	Includes a variety of geographic scales—from a few blocks to an entire community	Median improvement in some aspect of physical activity (e.g., number of walkers or bicyclists) was 161% (Heath et al. 2006)	Few studies are available in minority populations Effect sizes were generally large, but all except 3 studies had cross-sectional designs
School-based physical education	• Adding new PE classes • Lengthening existing PE classes • Increasing physical activity during PE class	9 U.S. studies, 1 in Crete, 2 in Australia; 10 studies in elementary school students and 2 studies in high-school students	Median increase in aerobic capacity of 8.4% (IQR 3.1% to 18.9%) (Kahn et al. 2002)	Primary barrier is the lack of consistent PE policies across states and cities

Point-of-decision prompts	• Signs placed by elevators and escalators to motivate people to use nearby stairs • Messages focusing on health benefits or weight loss	Diverse settings, including shopping malls, train/bus stations, and a university library	Median increase in stair climbing of 53.9% (Kahn et al. 2002)	Some evidence of higher effectiveness in obese individuals; no studies measured impact on fitness
Nutrition labeling and information	• Point-of-purchase labeling in cafeterias, work sites, groceries • Restaurant menu labeling	Several interventions included reduced pricing and promotion	Unavailable from primary source (Matson-Koffman et al. 2005)	Labeling of ready-to-eat foods has not been evaluated

IQR, interquartile range; PE, physical education.
Source: Adapted from Brownson et al. (2006).

Several research studies included interventions designed to improve the availability of healthy foods and beverages in schools by altering food services, preparation, and choices in cafeterias and vending machines; offering promotional activities for healthy foods and beverages; enhancing the nutrition content of classroom curricula; and informing and educating parents and teachers. Although these interventions reported small but consistent improvements in students' intake of fruits and vegetables, intake of fat, and choices of healthier food options, the Task Force concluded that evidence was insufficient to support a recommendation because effect sizes at the population level were typically quite small (Katz et al. 2005).

The Task Force also believed that evidence was promising for strategies to alter food pricing or offer incentives for healthier food choices (Katz et al. 2005). However, synthesizing this research was limited because few studies used rigorous designs or common outcome measures.

Media campaigns designed to balance or enhance health messages addressing dietary change showed mixed results or were conducted in combination with other multicomponent interventions, making it difficult to separate the independent effects of media strategies (Katz et al. 2005).

Collectively research for population-level strategies to support modest weight reduction and prevent diabetes demonstrates that a positive policy environment can support behavioral change, but the magnitude of behavioral change resulting from individual policies is not likely to have a substantial, direct, and *short-term* impact on diabetes prevention. However, these programs and policies should be considered for their potential to simultaneously improve other chronic illness outcomes and to reduce the future prevalence of underlying behavioral risk factors across the general population. It is also probable that combining strategies in the context of multi-level, multistakeholder approaches is likely to amplify the overall reach and impact of individual initiatives. Finally, it is possible that a supportive policy environment could improve the success and sustainability of efforts to place structured lifestyle programs (for directly preventing diabetes in high-risk populations) in non-health-care settings.

Structured Community-Based Programs to Prevent Diabetes—Essential and a Good Investment

Because structured lifestyle interventions that provide support for modest weight loss and physical activity in persons with IGT are likely to have favorable cost-effectiveness (Caro et al. 2004; Gillies et al. 2008; Icks et al. 2007; Jacobs-van der Bruggen et al. 2007; Herman et al. 2005; Palmer et al. 2004 Ramachandran et al. 2007), community-wide initiatives to implement and sustain such programs, particularly in the context of a more supportive policy environment, might have a strong impact on the prevention of diabetes. Moreover, structured diabetes prevention programs supported by community institutions should be particularly attractive to health care payers and purchasers because they offer a potential opportunity for resource-sharing arrangements that could improve program sustainability. One recent prediction model demonstrated that financing of a structured diabetes prevention program, modeled after the highly effective lifestyle intervention of the U.S. DPP (Knowler et al. 2002), could offer a favorable business case for a health payer that covers up to half of the direct program costs, even if implementing such an intervention achieves only half of the effectiveness observed in the original DPP clinical trial (Ackermann et al. 2006). Because the DPP also found that participants in the lifestyle intervention had fewer work absences, employers may have an added incentive for helping to support these initiatives (Ackermann et al. 2006; Herman et al. 2003). Finally, adults with prediabetes who believe that their personal risk for developing diabetes is high report that they would be willing to pay as much as $89 per month for 3 years to access a formal diabetes prevention program (Johnson et al. 2006)—an amount that should meet or exceed any residual fees required to support such a program in the community (Ackermann et al. 2006).

Although research suggests that coverage for formal diabetes prevention programs is likely to present a strong business case for employers and health payers, one remaining source of uncertainty for these stakeholders is whether non-health-care institutions offering such a program can deliver a high-quality program that helps community members with prediabetes to achieve and sustain modest weight loss. There is very little published literature in this area, but the results of several ongoing studies (see Table 16.2) should help to inform policies in the near future.

Case Example of Preventing Diabetes in the Community—the YMCA Model

Since 2003 the Indiana University Diabetes Translational Research Center has collaborated with the YMCA of Greater Indianapolis to develop, demonstrate, and evaluate novel strategies to transfer the DPP lifestyle intervention into the public health sector. This collaboration has included a community-based, pilot randomized trial to evaluate the feasibility and effectiveness of delivering a group-based adaptation of the DPP lifestyle intervention in YMCA facilities (Ackermann et al. 2008). This pilot study recruited adult community residents by conducting diabetes risk screening and counseling at two Indianapolis-area YMCA facilities. Between August 2005 and May 2006 the YMCA mailed a one-page flier to 45,000 randomly selected households within 3 miles of each of these two YMCA sites. Fliers introduced the concept of prediabetes and information about how to prevent diabetes, allowed recipients to judge their own risk status by including a short checklist of major diabetes risk factors, and invited those with self-identified risk factors to attend one of several screening events held at the YMCA.

Adults who attended screening events completed the American Diabetes Association (ADA) Diabetes Risk Assessment (Herman et al. 1995), had a casual capillary blood glucose test, and were offered brief advice guided by National Diabetes Education Program (NDEP) materials (2004). Persons who were overweight or obese with an ADA risk score ≥10 and a capillary blood glucose result of 110–199 mg/dL

TABLE 16.2   *Examples of Ongoing, NIH-Funded Community-Based Diabetes Prevention Studies*

Project Title	Principal Investigator	Target Group	Community Involvement	Brief Description
Family-Based Prevention of Diabetes and Its Complications	Julie A. Marshall	Adults and children with a family member with diabetes	Unclear	Family visits and group activities to increase physical activity and fruit and vegetable consumption and to maintain healthy body weight
Translating Research into Prevention of Diabetes (TRIP Diabetes)	David C. Goff	Overweight adults with elevated fasting glucose	Community health care practices	Group-based lifestyle intervention employing professional and lay health counselors aided by videos and other tools
Prevention and Control of Diabetes in Families	Kim D. Reynolds	Adult married couples – one with diagnosed diabetes	—	Spousal behavioral intervention to improve both the prevention and control of diabetes using health educator, computer program, and mailed materials
Middle School Prevention of Type 2 Diabetes	Tom Baranowski	African American and Hispanic children	Middle schools	Multicomponent school social and environmental intervention to support healthy diet and physical activity, combined with individual problem solving and parental education and motivational interview
Reach Out Chicago Children's Diabetes Prevention Project	Deborah Burnet	Children and parent in urban minority neighborhood		Family-based behavioral intervention to decrease overweight
Web-Based Diabetes Prevention Program for the Work Site	Royer F. Cook	Working-age adults with diabetes risk	Work sites	Web-based multimedia behavioral program
Physical Activity, Obesity and Diabetes Prevention	Ross C. Brownson	Overweight rural adults	Community advisory board and promotion of walking paths and green space	Multicomponent individual, interpersonal, and community-level interventions to promote walking and control body weight

Title	Principal Investigator	Target Population	Setting	Description
Physical Activity in Youth—Preventing Type 2 Diabetes	Joanne S. Harrell	Overweight children with hyperinsulinemia	Elementary and middle schools	School-based intervention to add a prescribed physical activity program and modify access to soft drinks at school
Exercise Strategy to Prevent Pediatric Type 2 Diabetes	Daniel M. Cooper	Children at risk for diabetes	Middle schools	School-based program involving physical activity enhancement and teacher/student education
Translating the DPP into the Community: The YMCA Model	Ronald T. Ackermann	Overweight adults at high risk for diabetes	YMCAs	Group-based adaptation of the DPP lifestyle intervention delivered by centrally trained wellness instructors in YMCA facilities
Feasibility of Diabetes Prevention in Arab Americans	Linda A. Jaber	Overweight adults in Arab American community	Community centers and cultural organizations	To develop a model for involving the community in culturally tailored approaches to implement the DPP lifestyle intervention
Lawrence Latino Diabetes Prevention Project	Ira S. Ockene	Adult Latinos at high risk for developing diabetes	Federally qualified health center with community outreach	Clinical risk factor prediction model to identify Latinos at high risk for developing diabetes and use of culturally tailored lifestyle counseling to reduce risk
Partnership for a Hispanic Diabetes Prevention Program	Beti Thompson	Hispanic community	Community advisory board	Use of participatory research principles to develop a community-centered, culturally tailored approach to diabetes prevention in a Hispanic community
Primary Care–Community Partnerships to Prevent Diabetes	Ronald T. Ackermann	Overweight adults with prediabetes	YMCAs	CQI strategies to help primary care-YMCA teams implement linkages involving testing for prediabetes and delivery of a group-based lifestyle intervention by the YMCA

were considered to be at high risk for IGT (Rolka et al. 2001) and were eligible to participate in the randomized trial. Before recruitment began, one of the two YMCA sites was randomly allocated to receive formal training in how to deliver the DPP lifestyle intervention. After enrolling, participants at both sites met with a YMCA staff member to receive additional information about available lifestyle programs that might help them to prevent type 2 diabetes. Because personnel at only one of the YMCA sites were trained to deliver the DPP intervention, only participants at this site received information about how to enroll in this "active" intervention; those at the control site received information about other existing YMCA programs.

Over a 1-year period this study tested and counseled 535 adults. Of these 143 were considered to be at high risk for developing diabetes, and 131 met inclusion criteria for the study. Ninety-two provided informed consent and enrolled. At baseline, intervention and control participants were similar with respect to age, gender, and race. The 6-month follow-up visit was completed by 85% of intervention participants and 83% of controls. There were no significant between-group differences in the age, gender, or race of nonrespondents to the follow-up evaluation. At the 6-month follow-up visit, body weight had decreased by 6.0% (95% confidence interval [CI] 4.7% to 7.3%) in intervention participants and 2.0% (95% CI 0.6% to 3.3%) in control participants ($p < 0.001$ for difference between groups). In addition, participants at the intervention YMCA had greater reductions in total cholesterol (–22 mg/dL in the intervention group vs. +6 mg/dL in controls; $p < 0.001$) (Ackermann et al. 2008). These differences were sustained after 12 months.

The results of this study provide strong support for the idea that training a community partner, in this case YMCA staff, to deliver a structured lifestyle intervention to prevent diabetes can achieve short-term weight-loss results comparable to those achieved during the DPP clinical trial. Because prior analyses of DPP data suggest that this level of weight loss would translate to at least a *50% reduction* in new cases of type 2 diabetes (Hamman et al. 2006), more research is needed to determine the feasibility and effectiveness of working with the YMCA and other community partners to deliver formal lifestyle programs for preventing diabetes nationally. Moreover because it appears that broader environmental and policy interventions targeting healthy diet and physical activity may offer additional, incremental support for behavior change, it will be important to investigate whether formal community-based diabetes prevention programs are more successful and sustainable when offered in the context of community-wide initiatives that provide a backdrop of supportive resources to adopt new behaviors, achieve weight loss, and prevent relapse.

Closing the Loop—Enhancing Sustainability by Health Care–Community Collaboration

If research continues to demonstrate that formal diabetes prevention programs are effective and can be delivered with high fidelity in community settings, it will become important for community organizations to develop sustainable strategies to work with nearby health care partners to identify and enroll adults with IGT. One good example of clinic–community partnerships to prevent diabetes in the United States comes from the Health Disparities Collaboratives (HDCs) implemented by the Bureau of Primary Healthcare of the Health Resources and Services Administration (HRSA) (Health Disparities Collaboratives 2007). Beginning with an initial focus on diabetes in 1998, the HDCs were developed to transform primary health care practices to improve the health care that is provided to underserved populations and to eliminate health disparities across all regions of the United States. As of September 2006 about 800 federally qualified health centers had participated in HDCs to address a wide variety of health priorities including asthma, depression, cardiovascular disease, cancer screening/planned care, diabetes prevention, perinatal/patient safety, and oral health. HRSA works with the Institute for Healthcare Improvement to assist HDC sites in using an approach that integrates the Planned Care Model (Bodenheimer et al. 2002a, 2002b; Glasgow et al. 2001) with principles of process-driven quality improvement and collaborative learning (Improvement Methods: How to Improve 2007) to identify health priorities and to implement and sustain local health care improvement strategies.

In 2002 HRSA invited five HDC centers to initiate a pilot diabetes prevention collaborative. Participating centers designed and implemented new strategies focusing on ways to identify patients with either form of prediabetes (impaired fasting glucose [IFG] or IGT) and to offer clinical and community resources to support modest weight loss and moderate daily physical activity. This process included the development of local registries of nondiabetic patients who were believed to be at high risk for diabetes because of factors such as a family history of diabetes, history of gestational diabetes, prior random glucose > 126 mg/dL, BMI > 30, presence of hypertension, high cholesterol, or a past cardiovascular event. As of November 2003, 3167 at-risk adults had been identified by the patient registries. Of these high-risk patients 903 (29%) had completed a 2-hour, 75-g oral glucose tolerance test; 428 (47%) of these tests were diagnostic of abnormal glucose metabolism, with 273 meeting older criteria for prediabetes (either IFG with a reading of 110–125 mg/dL or IGT with 2-hour glucose of 140–199 mg/dL) and 155 (17%) meeting criteria for newly diagnosed diabetes (Ratner 2004).

Patients found to have either IFG or IGT in these five HDC centers were offered information about effective strategies to prevent or delay the development of type 2 diabetes. Brief advice at many sites was facilitated by use of NDEP materials, which describe an approach to reducing weight and increasing levels of physical activity. Several participating sites formed linkages with nearby DPCP resources to support healthy diet and physical activity to achieve modest weight loss. DPCPs and other community partners collaborated to provide feedback and ongoing support to patients with prediabetes and to help ensure that they received follow-up clinical care, including surveillance and early initiation of intensive treatment for the development of diabetes. One center reported that 49% of patients identified with prediabetes attended at least one lifestyle intervention visit to receive counseling and information about supportive resources for weight management; 46% of these patients were reported to achieve 7% or greater weight loss while participating in the intervention (Prevention of Type 2 Diabetes 2005).

All participating HDC centers also shared information about barriers and facilitators to identifying prediabetes in clinical practice and linking with community partners to provide lifestyle resources. One common finding was that success in maintaining partners hips required a truly participatory relationship between clinical and community teams. This is typically not the case in focused clinic-centered projects that involve a simple referral from a community program without follow-up or feedback from the community partner, but a participatory and synergistic relationship appears to be essential for effective and sustainable approaches to lifestyle diabetes prevention in the community (Goodman, Yoo, and Jack 2006).

Another common challenge for HDC centers was the cost and capacity of performing oral glucose tolerance tests in a high volume in busy primary care settings. Indeed, fewer than 30% of patients whose names were in high-risk prediabetes registries at HDC sites completed an oral glucose tolerance test (Ratner 2004). Given the barriers to identifying IGT, it may prove more feasible to consider simpler strategies to identifying this condition. Examples include the use of questionnaires, risk equations, or fasting glucose tests (Santaguida et al. 2005). Although a large number of adults identified as "high risk" by these simpler strategies will not actually have IGT, it is very possible that using tests that are inherently more feasible in primary care settings and more acceptable to patients could identify more patients who truly have IGT, simply because they will be completed by a much larger population. One impact of such a choice is that persons without IGT would also be given expanded access to costly lifestyle programs. Although we do not have research today to show that offering an intensive lifestyle intervention to persons without IGT is cost-effective, there are clear health benefits from participation in such programs by overweight persons with other diabetes risk factors, such as IFG, a family history of diabetes, advancing age, or higher levels of obesity. These health benefits, including improved quality of life, less risk for depression and decline in physical function, and improvements in cardiometabolic risk factors such as high blood pressure and high cholesterol (Klein et al. 2004; Maciejewski, Patrick, and Williamson 2005) have the potential to lead to cost-effectiveness, even for persons without confirmed IGT. One recent predictive modeling study suggests that there is likely to be little difference in the lifetime cost-effectiveness of screening and prevention interventions that target adults with IFG or IGT versus those that target IGT alone (Hoerger et al. 2007). However because building and maintaining linkages between community and health care partners will introduce additional costs for formal community programs, we need additional research to determine whether enrollment of broader populations identified through simpler testing procedures will prove to be more cost effective and affordable for stakeholders to implement.

Conclusion

Type 2 diabetes is common and costly but clearly preventable. The most consistently effective strategies for preventing diabetes are structured lifestyle interventions that are designed to assist patients with a clinical diagnosis of IGT to achieve and maintain weight loss and increase their levels of physical activity. Research supports the idea that community institutions may have a greater capacity than health care settings to offer such programs on a public health scale. However, most non-health-care settings lack the resources or capacity to perform metabolic tests required to identify IGT. Thus it is imperative that clinical systems learn to partner efficiently and effectively with resources in the community to offer intensive lifestyle services that reach the greatest population of persons with prediabetes. The effectiveness of such efforts may be enhanced if they are offered in the context of broad-scale, population-based resources and policies that provide general support for healthy behaviors in the areas of diet and physical activity. In this regard, multistakeholder approaches that share the costs and benefits of diabetes prevention initiatives may be necessary to ensure feasibility and sustainability in the real world. Rapidly emerging translational research in diabetes prevention should continue to provide badly needed information about the reach, effectiveness, and sustainability of health-care–community partnerships to prevent diabetes in real-world settings. This research will prove vital to informing policy decisions about the development and implementation of integrated clinical–community strategies designed to prevent diabetes on a national and international scale.

References

Ackermann RT et al. (2006). An evaluation of cost sharing to finance a diet and physical activity intervention to prevent diabetes. *Diabetes Care* **29**, 1237–41.

Ackermann RT et al. (2008). Translating the Diabetes Prevention Program into the community. The DEPLOY Pilot Study. *American Journal of Preventive Medicine* **35**, 357–63.

Behavioral counseling in primary care to promote physical activity: recommendation and rationale (2002). *Annals of Internal Medicine* **137**, 205–7.

Bodenheimer T, Wagner EH, Grumbach K (2002a). Improving primary care for patients with chronic illness. *JAMA* **288**, 1775–9.

Bodenheimer T, Wagner EH, Grumbach K (2002b). Improving primary care for patients with chronic illness: the chronic care model, Part 2. *JAMA* **288**, 1909–14.

Brownson RC, Haire-Joshu D, Luke DA (2006). Shaping the context of health: a review of environmental and policy approaches in the prevention of chronic diseases. *Annual Reviews of Public Health* **27**, 341–70.

Burnet DL et al. (2006). Preventing diabetes in the clinical setting. *Journal of General Internal Medicine* **21**, 84–93.

Caro JJ, et al. (2004). Economic evaluation of therapeutic interventions to prevent type 2 diabetes in Canada. *Diabetic Medicine* **21** (11), 1229–36.

Colditz GA et al. (1995). Weight gain as a risk factor for clinical diabetes mellitus in women. *Annals of Internal Medicine* **122** (7), 481–6.

Eden KB et al. (2002). Does counseling by clinicians improve physical activity? A summary of the evidence for the U.S. Preventive Services Task Force. *Annals of Internal Medicine* **137** (3), 208–15.

Fiore MC. et al. (2000). *Treating Tobacco Use and Dependence. Clinical Practice Guideline.* Rockville, MD: U.S. Department of Health and Human Services. Public Health Service.

Garfield SA et al. (2003). Considerations for diabetes translational research in real-world settings. *Diabetes Care* **26** (9), 2670–4.

Gillies CL et al. (2007). Pharmacological and lifestyle interventions to prevent or delay type 2 diabetes in people with impaired glucose tolerance: systematic review and meta-analysis. *British Medical Journal* **334** (7588), 299.

Gillies CL et al. (2008). Different strategies for screening and prevention of type 2 diabetes in adults: cost effectiveness analysis. *British Medical Journal* **336** (7654), 1180–5.

Glasgow RE, Orleans CT, Wagner EH (2001). Does the chronic care model serve also as a template for improving prevention? *Milbank Quarterly* **79** (4), 579–612, iv–v.

Goodman R M, Yoo S, Jack L Jr (2006). Applying comprehensive community-based approaches in diabetes prevention: rationale, principles, and models. *Journal of Public Health Management Practice* **12** (6), 545–55.

Grumbach K, Bodenheimer T (2002). A primary care home for Americans: putting the house in order. *JAMA* **288** (7), 889–93.

Guide to Community Preventive Services (2007). Available at http://www.thecommunityguide.org/. Accessed April 20, 2007.

Hamman RF et al. (2006). Effect of weight loss with lifestyle intervention on risk of diabetes. *Diabetes Care* **29** (9), 2102–7.

Health Disparities Collaboratives (2007). Available at http://www.healthdisparities.net/hdc/html/home.aspx. Accessed April 25, 2007.

Heath GW et al. (2006). The effectiveness of urban design and land use transport policies and practices to increase physical activity. A systematic review. *Journal of Physical Activity and Health,* **3** (1 Suppl.), S55–76.

Herman WH et al. (1995). A new and simple questionnaire to identify people at increased risk for undiagnosed diabetes. *Diabetes Care* **18** (3), 382–7.

Herman WH et al. (2003). Costs associated with the primary prevention of type 2 diabetes mellitus in the diabetes prevention program. *Diabetes Care* **26** (1), 36–47.

Herman WH et al. (2005). The cost-effectiveness of lifestyle modification or metformin in preventing type 2 diabetes in adults with impaired glucose tolerance. *Annals of Internal Medicine* **142** (5), 323–32.

Herman WH et al. (2006). Managing people at high risk for diabetes. *Annals of Internal Medicine* **144** (1), 66–7; author reply 67–8.

Hoerger TJ et al. (2007). Cost-effectiveness of screening for pre-diabetes among overweight and obese U.S. adults. *Diabetes Care* **30** (11), 2874–9.

Hu FB et al. (1999). Walking compared with vigorous physical activity and risk of type 2 diabetes in women: a prospective study. *JAMA* **282** (15), 1433–9.

Hu G et al. (2003). Occupational, commuting, and leisure-time physical activity in relation to risk for type 2 diabetes in middle-aged Finnish men and women. *Diabetologia* **46** (3), 322–9.

Icks A et al. (2007). Clinical and cost-effectiveness of primary prevention of Type 2 diabetes in a 'real world' routine healthcare setting: model based on the KORA Survey 2000. *Diabetic Medicine* **24** (5), 473–80.

Improvement Methods: How to Improve (2007). Available at http://www.ihi.org/IHI/ Topics/Improvement/ImprovementMethods/HowToImprove/. Accessed April 26, 2007.

Jacobs-van der Bruggen MA et al. (2007). Lifestyle interventions are cost-effective in people with different levels of diabetes risk: results from a modeling study. *Diabetes Care.* **30** (1), 128–34.

Johnson FR et al. (2006). High-risk individuals' willingness to pay for diabetes risk-reduction programs. *Diabetes Care* **29** (6), 1351–6.

Kahn EB et al. (2002). The effectiveness of interventions to increase physical activity. A systematic review. *American Journal of Preventive Medicine* **22** (4 Suppl.), 73–107.

Katz DL et al. (2005). Public health strategies for preventing and controlling overweight and obesity in school and worksite settings: a report on recommendations of the Task Force on Community Preventive Services. *MMWR Recommendation Reports* **54** (RR-10), 1–12.

Kim C et al. (2007). Risk perception for diabetes among women with histories of gestational diabetes mellitus. *Diabetes Care* **30** (9), 2281–6.

Klein S et al. (2004). Clinical implications of obesity with specific focus on cardiovascular disease: a statement for professionals from the American Heart Association Council on Nutrition, Physical Activity, and Metabolism: endorsed by the American College of Cardiology Foundation. *Circulation* **110** (18), 2952–67.

Knowler WC et al. (2002). Reduction in the incidence of type 2 diabetes with lifestyle intervention or metformin. *New England Journal of Medicine* **346** (6), 393–403.

Koh-Banerjee P et al. (2004). Changes in body weight and body fat distribution as risk factors for clinical diabetes in US men. *American Journal of Epidemiology* **159** (12), 1150–9.

Kramer MK et al. (2007). Risk Perception and Relationship to Performance in a Modified DPP Group Lifestyle Intervention for Individuals with Metabolic Syndrome. Paper presented at the 68th Scientific Session of the American Diabetes Association, Chicago, IL.

Maciejewski ML, Patrick DL, Williamson DF (2005). A structured review of randomized controlled trials of weight loss showed little improvement in health-related quality of life. *Journal of Clinical Epidemiology* **58** (6), 568–78.

Matson-Koffman DM et al. (2005). A site-specific literature review of policy and environmental interventions that promote physical activity and nutrition for cardiovascular health: what works? *American Journal of Health Promotion* **19**(3), 167–93.

McTigue KM et al. (2003). Screening and interventions for obesity in adults: summary of the evidence for the U.S. Preventive Services Task Force. *Annals of Internal Medicine* **139** (11), 933–49.

Murphy D, Chapel T, Clark C (2004). Moving diabetes care from science to practice: the evolution of the National Diabetes Prevention and Control Program. *Annals of Internal Medicine* **140** (11), 978–84.

Palmer AJ et al. (2004). Intensive lifestyle changes or metformin in patients with impaired glucose tolerance: modeling the long-term health economic implications of the diabetes prevention program in Australia, France, Germany, Switzerland, and the United Kingdom. *Clinical Therapeutics* **26** (2), 304–21.

Pignone MP et al. (2003). Counseling to promote a healthy diet in adults: a summary of the evidence for the U.S. Preventive Services Task Force. *American Journal of Preventive Medicine* **24** (1), 75–92.

Prevention of Type 2 Diabetes (2005). New Haven, CT: Hill Health Center.

Ramachandran A et al. (2007). Cost-effectiveness of the interventions in the primary prevention of diabetes among Asian Indians: within-trial results of the Indian Diabetes Prevention Programme (IDPP). *Diabetes Care* **30** (10), 2548–52.

Ratner RE (2004). Community-Based Identification of Pre-Diabetes. Efficient Screening Techniques for Implementation of Diabetes Prevention Strategies. Paper presented at the 64th Annual Scientific Session of the American Diabetes Association, Orlando, FL.

Rolka DB et al. (2001). Performance of recommended screening tests for undiagnosed diabetes and dysglycemia. *Diabetes Care* **24** (11), 1899–903.

Santaguida P et al. (2005). *Diagnosis, Prognosis, and Treatment of Impaired Glucose Tolerance and Impaired Fasting Glucose* (Evidence Report/Technology Assessment No. 128 [Prepared by the McMaster University Evidence-based Practice Center under Contract No. 290-02-0020]). Rockville, MD: Agency for Healthcare Research and Quality.

Satterfield DW et al. (2003). Community-based lifestyle interventions to prevent type 2 diabetes. *Diabetes Care* **26** (9), 2643–52.

Schulze MB, Hu FB (2005). Primary prevention of diabetes: what can be done and how much can be prevented? *Annual Review of Public Health* **26**, 445–67.

Screening for type 2 diabetes (2003). *Diabetes Care* **26** (Suppl. 1), S21–4.

Surgeon_General (2001). *The Surgeon General's Call To Action To Prevent and Decrease Overweight and Obesity.* Rockville, MD: U.S. Department of Health and Human Services, Public Health Service, Office of the Surgeon General.

Theory at a Glance: A Guide for Health Promotion Practice (2005). Baltimore, MD: U.S. Department of Health and Human Services, National Institutes of Health, National Cancer Institute.

Thompson B, Lynn WR, Shopland DR (1995). *Community-based Interventions for Smokers: The COMMITT Field Experience. Smoking and Tobacco Control*

Monograph No. 6. NIH Pub. No. 95-4028. Bethesda, MD: National Cancer Institute (NCI/NIH).

Walker EA et al. (2007). Measuring comparative risk perceptions in an urban minority population: the risk perception survey for diabetes. *Diabetes Education* **33** (1), 103–10.

Wannamethee SG, Shaper AG, Alberti KG (2000). Physical activity, metabolic factors, and the incidence of coronary heart disease and type 2 diabetes. *Archives of Internal Medicine* **160** (14), 2108–16.

Weinstein AR et al. (2004). Relationship of physical activity vs body mass index with type 2 diabetes in women. *JAMA* **292** (10), 1188–94.

Whitlock EP et al. (2002). Evaluating primary care behavioral counseling interventions: an evidence-based approach. *American Journal of Preventive Medicine* **22** (4), 267–84.

Whittemore R, Melkus GD, Grey M (2004). Applying the social ecological theory to type 2 diabetes prevention and management. *Journal of Community Health Nursing* **21** (2), 87–99.

17. EFFECTIVENESS OF INDIVIDUAL-LEVEL INTERVENTIONS TO PREVENT VASCULAR COMPLICATIONS

Amanda I. Adler

■ Main Public Health Messages

- Randomized trials to prevent or delay the complications of diabetes have focused on diabetes-specific factors—notably, high blood glucose and other modifiable risk factors.
- Trials to date confirm the effectiveness of lowering of blood glucose, blood pressure, and LDL cholesterol.
- Aggressive lowering of blood glucose in type 2 diabetes has been associated with an increased risk of death.
- Glucose insulin potassium (GIK) infusion is not associated with favorable outcomes, although attaining excellent glycemic control during an acute illness may be associated.
- Justification for the use of aspirin and fish oil for the primary prevention of cardiovascular disease in diabetes awaits ongoing trials.
- In proliferative and severe preproliferative retinopathy, laser photocoagulation prevents severe visual loss.
- Challenges for future clinical research include achieving ever-lower values of A1C in the intervention arms of trials, the need to conduct trials that require ever-larger samples, and differentiating the effects of specific drugs from glycemic-lowering in general.

■ Introduction

Diabetes mellitus markedly increases the risk of a variety of conditions that are not specific to diabetes, including coronary, cerebrovascular, and peripheral vascular disease; renal, neuropathic, and retinal disease; as well as ophthalmologic, dermatologic, hematologic, dental, osseous, hepatic, and respiratory diseases. Hyperglycemia influences blood flow, vascular permeability, and blood clotting, and many of the diseases described result directly or indirectly from vascular disturbances. Scientists have traditionally deemed these complications of diabetes either "macrovascular" or "microvascular" disease. In all probability both microvascular and macrovascular abnormalities contribute to these problems (Witt et al. 2006).

To reduce the incidence of the complications of diabetes and the progression of existing complications, researchers have tested therapies (interventions) in randomized clinical trials. Targeting modifiable risk factors for diabetic complications that occur at higher levels in individuals with diabetes, many trials attempt to improve hyperglycemia, the sine qua non of diabetes, alter biochemical pathways downstream from hyperglycemia (Brownlee 2005), or lower blood pressure. Other trials target risk factors that are not necessarily more common in individuals with diabetes (e.g., elevated low-density lipoprotein [LDL]) or use interventions that have proven effective in nondiabetic populations, such as aspirin. In general, trials employ drugs, devices, surgery, and changes in lifestyle.

This chapter covers interventional studies aimed at lowering the incidence of cardiovascular disease (CVD), nephropathy, retinopathy, blindness, lower-extremity amputation (LEA), peripheral sensory neuropathy, and autonomic neuropathy; and at prolonging life. The chapter includes, with the exception of renal disease, studies that address clinical endpoints, and it does not include surrogate measures, for example, results of coronary angiography or calculations of cardiovascular risk. This chapter emphasizes results from studies likely to have sufficient statistical power to find meaningful differences.

■ Pharmacological Interventions

Strategies to Lower Blood Glucose

Interventions proven to lower blood glucose include exercise, diet, insulin, sulfonylureas, meglitinides, biguanides, α-glucosidase inhibitors, thiazolidinediones, glucagon-like peptide 1 analogs, dipeptidyl peptidase 4 inhibitors, and drugs that promote weight loss.

Diabetes Control and Complications Trial

The Diabetes Control and Complications Trial (DCCT) showed unambiguously that lowering blood glucose in adults with type 1 diabetes and a disease duration of an average of 6.5 years lowered the risk of microvascular complications (Diabetes Control and Complications Trial Research Group 1993). Intensive therapy significantly reduced the risk for the development or worsening of retinopathy and nephropathy and the development of neuropathy. The approximate difference in glycosylated hemoglobin (A1C) between intensive and conventional groups was 2 percentage points, with the intensive group achieving an A1C of about 7%. The intensive regimen included a basal bolus regimen (long-acting insulin plus short-acting meal-time insulin) or use of an insulin pump (short-acting insulin administered continuously and extra with meals) as well as adjustment of insulin to food intake and exercise, a diet and exercise plan, and monthly visits to study personnel. Patients randomized to intensive therapy experienced three times the frequency of hypoglycemia and gained more weight.

After the trial, investigators encouraged participants in the conventional group to adopt intensive treatment. Participants are being followed in an observational study and personal physicians have resumed their care. Although A1C levels of the two groups have equalized, individuals formerly randomized to intensive therapy have experienced fewer CVD events than those randomized to conventional therapy, with an estimated risk reduction of 42% (Nathan et al. 2005). This difference, driven in large part by greater glycemic control, provides compelling evidence for the effectiveness of lowering blood glucose as a means to prevent or delay CVD in type 1 diabetes.

University Group Diabetes Program

The University Group Diabetes Program (UGDP) started in 1960 measured "the efficacy of hypoglycemic treatments in the prevention of vascular complications in type 2 diabetes" in 1027 individuals (Meinert et al. 1970). Patients were randomized to (1) fixed-dose insulin or variable-dose insulin; (2) the biguanide phenformin or placebo; or (3) the sulfonylurea tolbutamide or placebo. Because of an apparent increase in mortality from both tolbutamide and phenformin, investigators discontinued both of those arms and compared instead the placebo arms with insulin. There were fewer hospitalizations for heart disease and better blood glucose control in the groups receiving insulin, but neither the rates of CVD nor of microvascular complications differed significantly from those in the placebo groups. Ample criticism and debate followed publication of the study (Seltzer 1972; Kilor et al. 1980; Schwartz and Meinert 2004).

Veterans Affairs Cooperative Study

The Veterans Affairs Cooperative Study on Glycemic Control and Complications in Type II Diabetes was a small (153 men) study designed to assess the feasibility of using standard treatment to lower blood glucose intensively as a means to reduce cardiovascular events. In 27 months of follow-up, investigators observed a difference in A1C of approximately 2 percentage points between groups, but no difference in rates of CVD or death (Abraira et al. 1995). Given the study's modest size and duration, it did not have sufficient power to detect a true difference between these rates.

Kumamoto Study

The Kumamoto Study tested the hypothesis, in 110 Japanese insulin-treated patients with type 2 diabetes who were without significant complications at baseline, that intensive treatment of blood glucose prevents the development or worsening of diabetic complications. One group received basal insulin plus prandial insulin and the other group basal insulin only. Although designed primarily to measure microvascular complications, the study examined rates of angina pectoris, myocardial infarction (MI), stroke, intermittent claudication, gangrene, and LEA. Over 8 years, the group receiving multiple injections achieved an A1C of 7.2% versus 9.4% in the other group. Despite equivalent dosages per kg of body weight between groups, randomization to the basal plus prandial insulin regime significantly decreased the risk of retinopathy, nephropathy, and neuropathy. Based on very small numbers, the investigators reported that total cardiovascular events in the group with multiple injections were half those of the other group (0.6 vs. 1.3 events/100 patient-years) (Shichiri et al. 2000).

United Kingdom Prospective Diabetes Study

The United Kingdom Prospective Diabetes Study (UKPDS), which recruited 5102 patients newly diagnosed with type 2 diabetes, tested whether intensive blood glucose control (vs. conventional treatment) lowered the incidence of diabetic complications. Sample size was determined from a composite endpoint comprising microvascular and macrovascular disease. MI, stroke, and death from peripheral vascular disease or LEA comprised a prespecified, aggregate macrovascular endpoint (UKPDS Group 1998b). The study randomized 3867 patients to intensive therapy, defined as initial treatment with sulfonylurea or insulin, or to conventional therapy with diet. A subsidiary study among overweight patients included an alternate randomization to metformin (UKPDS Group 1998a). The UKPDS permitted the addition of therapies to maintain the goal of fasting blood glucose values of <6 mmol/L in the intensive group and <15 mmol/L in the conventional group.

Over a median follow-up of 10 years, the group randomized to intensive therapy achieved a median A1C value of 7.0%, versus 7.9% in the conventional group. The intensively treated group experienced fewer microvascular complications, but more episodes of hypoglycemia and greater weight gain. The incidence of any diabetes-related endpoint was 12% lower in the intensive-treatment group than in the conventional group (95% confidence interval [CI] 1–21%, $p = 0.029$).

Patients randomized to intensive treatment were less likely to have an MI during follow-up, with an estimated 16% reduction in relative risk (RR; 95% CI 0–29%, $p = 0.052$) (UKPDS Group 1998b). The study showed no difference in incidence of MI among the three agents employed in the intensive group (chlorpropamide, glibenclamide, insulin), nor a difference in rates of stroke between the intensive and conventional groups (UKPDS Group 1998b). Intensive therapy was not associated with rates of death. Lowering blood glucose reduced the risk of microvascular end-points by 25% (95% CI 7–40%, $p = 0.0099$).

Investigators observed a smaller difference (–0.6 percentage points) in median A1C between the metformin and conventional groups than between the sulfonylurea or insulin and conventional groups. Patients randomized to metformin experienced fewer diabetes-related complications (reduction in RR 42% [9%–63%], $p = 0.017$) than the conventional group and a 39% lower rate of MI (11%–59%) (UKPDS Group 1998a). The degree to which metformin reduced the rate of MI exceeded that expected from the relationship between A1C and the incidence of MI, suggesting that metformin exerted effects beyond those of lowering glucose alone (Stratton et al. 2000).

In the 10 years following the end of the UKPDS patients randomized to the intensive group were less likely to die or to experience an MI, even though their A1C values had become similar (Holman et al. 2008a). This suggested a benefit from previous intensive therapy, as well as a benefit that had persisted, termed a "legacy effect." However, the possibility remains that the benefit was associated with a factor, itself associated with, but not directly due to, improved glycemic control.

Proactive Study

The Proactive Study tested whether patients randomized to pioglitazone, compared with placebo, experienced fewer events, defined as any one of all-cause mortality, nonfatal MI (including silent MI), stroke, acute coronary syndrome, revascularization of coronary or lower-extremity arteries, or LEA. This study, which randomized 5238 patients with type 2 diabetes and CVD, found a nonsignificant decrease in the risk of CVD over 2½ years at the expense of weight gain and an increased risk of congestive heart failure (CHF) (Charbonnel et al. 2004; Dormandy et al. 2005).

Action to Control Cardiovascular Risk in Diabetes Study

The Action to Control Cardiovascular Risk in Diabetes Study (ACCORD) recruited 10,251 type 2 diabetic patients with CVD or a high cardiovascular risk. ACCORD tested the hypothesis that normalizing glycemia delays or prevents CVD. The study excluded patients with a body mass index (BMI; weight in kg divided by height in m²) >45 and an A1C <7.5%. Investigators randomized patients to intensive control with a target A1C of <6.0% or standard control with a target of 7.0%–7.9% (Gerstein et al. 2007). All participants randomized to intensive control started on at least two antidiabetic agents, and investigators added further therapies when the A1C exceeded 6% or when preprandial or postprandial blood glucose exceeded target levels. The prespecified primary outcome was the first occurrence of nonfatal MI or nonfatal stroke or death from a cardiovascular cause.

The study population, which had had diabetes an average of 10 years, had an average A1C of 8.3%. After 1 year, the median A1C was 6.4% in the intensive group and 7.5% in the standard group, levels that were maintained throughout the study.

Three-and-a-half years into the study, investigators stopped the study because of a higher death rate in the intensive-therapy group. The intensive-therapy group experienced higher rates of fluid retention, hypoglycemia, and weight gain but lower rates of nonfatal MI. The primary endpoint did not differ between groups. At the time of writing, investigators do not know why patients randomized to intensive therapy were more likely to die (Gerstein et al. 2008).

ACCORD is ongoing, with 4733 of the participants also randomized to either intensive blood pressure control (target systolic <120 mm Hg) or standard control (target systolic <140 mm Hg).

Action in Diabetes and Vascular Disease

Action in Diabetes and Vascular Disease: Preterax and Diamicron Modified Release Controlled Evaluation (ADVANCE) addressed control of blood glucose (and blood pressure), enrolling 11,140 participants with type 2 diabetes over age 55 who had complications or were at high risk for CVD for another reason. Investigators randomized patients to a glucose-lowering regimen with an A1C goal of ≤6.5% or to one based on standard guidelines (Chalmers et al. 2006). Modified-release gliclazide was the only sulfonylurea permitted in the intensive arm and the only sulfonylurea not allowed in the standard-control group; both groups permitted the addition of metformin, thiazolidinediones, acarbose, and insulin. The two primary endpoints were composites of macrovascular disease and of microvascular disease.

At the beginning of the 5-year study the median A1C was 7.2% in both groups; at the end the values were 6.3% and 7.0% in the intensive- and standard-control groups, respectively. Of the two primary endpoints, only the rates of microvascular disease (hazard ratio 0.86; 95% CI 0.77 to 0.97; $p = 0.01$) were lower in the intensively treated group relative to the standard group. Compared with the UKPDS, this study had a smaller difference in A1C between groups and a lower reduction in risk for microvascular complications; nonetheless, like the UKPDS, this study supported lowering of glucose in type 2 diabetes. In addition to more frequent hypoglycemia, subjects randomized to intensive therapy were hospitalized more frequently (Patel et al. 2008).

Veterans Affairs Diabetes Trials

The Veterans Affairs Diabetes Trials (VADT), which enrolled 1792 adults with type 2 diabetes and an A1C >8.5% (Kirkman et al. 2006), tested the hypothesis that improved glycemic control lowers the incidence of major CVD events. Investigators randomized subjects to "intensive" or "usual" glycemic control, aiming to achieve a difference in A1C of at least 1.5 percentage points. Therapy in both groups included thiazolidinediones, sulfonylureas, biguanides, α-glucosidase inhibitors, natiglinide, and insulin (Abraira et al. 2003). The median A1C was 8.4% in the standard-therapy group and 6.9% in the intensive-therapy group. Despite this difference, no difference in rates for either macrovascular or microvascular complications was observed (Duckworth et al. 2009). Further analyses show that intensive control initiated in the first 15 years after diagnosis of type 2 diabetes reduced the risk of cardiovascular morbidity and mortality. By contrast, initiating intensive therapy 16–20 years after diagnosis yielded no benefit, and 20 years or more after diagnosis increased the risk of CVD events (American Diabetes Association Meeting 2009).

Glucose Insulin Potassium Infusion Trials

During periods of acute illness, including MI, researchers have investigated the treatment of hospitalized patients with intravenous glucose, insulin, and potassium (GIK) in order to improve survival. This hypothesis is based on the observation that myocardium preferentially uses glucose as a source of energy during ischemia and reperfusion; insulin permits glucose and potassium uptake, and infused potassium restores blood potassium levels. GIK trials have included patients with diabetes or with stress hyperglycemia. A meta-analysis of 38 studies found no benefit for randomization to GIK for patients with MI but noted that trials that strove for euglycemia resulted in better outcomes (Pittas et al. 2006). In analyses (Diaz et al. 2007) that combined two major studies with over 11,000 patients in each of the intervention and comparison arms, no differences were observed between arms in the 30-day rate of death or in the rate of CHF. Patients with the highest levels of blood glucose had the highest mortality, regardless of allocated treatment. For patients with stroke, a study that randomized patients with hyperglycemia to GIK or no GIK found no difference in outcome, but the study may have been underpowered (Gray et al. 2007). In studies limited to patients with diabetes, Diabetes Mellitus, Insulin Glucose Infusion in Acute Myocardial Infarction (DIGAMI) showed an increased survival beyond 3 years for patients randomized to GIK versus conventional treatment (Malmberg 1997), but DIGAMI-2 did not confirm this benefit (Malmberg et al. 2005). In review, GIK administration is not itself associated with favorable outcomes, although attaining excellent glycemic control during an acute illness may be (Langley and Adams 2007).

HEART 2-D

The Hyperglycemia and Its Effect After Acute Myocardial Infarction on Cardiovascular Outcomes in Patients With Type 2 Diabetes (HEART 2-D; Milicevic et al. 2005) study randomized patients with type 2 diabetes following MI to different insulin-based regimes. This study measured time to first recurrent cardiovascular event, defined as death from CVD, an MI or stroke, hospitalization for an acute coronary syndrome, or coronary revascularization. Patients were randomized to a "postprandial" strategy with the short-acting insulin analog lispro (with the possible inclusion of bedtime NPH insulin) or to a "basal" strategy with basal (or biphasic) insulin. This study aimed for an A1C < 7.0% in both groups, but it obtained means of 7.7% and 7.8% in the prandial and basal groups respectively. The trial was stopped early because of its inability to reach objectives; no difference in primary endpoint was observed (Raz et al. 2009).

BARI 2D

The Bypass Angioplasty Revascularization Investigation in Type 2 Diabetes (BARI 2D) trial of 2368 adults asked (1) whether elective revascularization and "aggressive" medical therapy versus "aggressive" medical therapy alone lowered all-cause mortality and (2) whether an insulin-sensitizing approach (metformin, thiazolidinediones) compared with an insulin-providing approach (insulin, sulfonylureas) lowered mortality. Both groups had a target A1C of <7.0%. Participants had ischemia and angiographically documented significant coronary disease (Brooks et al. 2006). After an average follow-up of 5 years, neither mortality nor major cardiovascular event rates differed significantly between the group receiving revascularization and medical therapy and the group receiving medical therapy alone; these outcomes did not differ significantly between the insulin-sensitizing and insulin-providing medical therapy groups (BARI 2D Study Group 2009).

RECORD

The Rosiglitazone Evaluated for Cardiac Outcomes and Regulation of Glycemia in Diabetes (RECORD) study enrolled patients on metformin or sulfonylurea. If already taking a sulfonylurea, participants were randomized to add rosiglitazone or metformin or, if taking metformin, to add rosiglitazone or a sulfonylurea. The composite primary endpoint was death or hospitalization from CVD (Home et al. 2005). The study followed 4447 patients for a mean of 5.5 years. An analysis prior to the study's end precipitated by safety concerns about rosiglitazone (Nissen and Wolski 2007; Home et al. 2007) showed an increased risk of CHF associated with rosiglitazone and no difference in rates of MI. Final results confirmed a two-fold increased risk of CHF with use of rosiglitazone (Home 2009). Rosiglitazone was associated with an increased risk of fractures, mainly in women. Rosiglitazone did not increase the risk of overall cardiovascular morbidity or mortality compared to metformin or sulfonylurea. Data were inconclusive about the effect of rosiglitazone on MI.

Other Trials Under Way or Awaiting Publication

Look AHEAD

The Look AHEAD (Action for Health in Diabetes) randomized study addresses the hypothesis that weight loss will reduce the risk of CVD among 5145 adults with type 2 diabetes. Investigators encourage weight loss via intensive diet and physical activity in the intervention group and by education alone in the control group. The composite primary endpoint includes fatal and nonfatal MI, stroke, and cardiovascular deaths (Look AHEAD Protocol Review Committee 2005; Look AHEAD Research Group 2003, 2007). One-year results showed that participants who received intensive lifestyle advice were fitter and lost more weight than controls. A1C also dropped more in the intervention group than in the control group (0.6 vs. 0.1 percentage points); whether this translates into a lower incidence of CVD awaits the study's end.

ORIGIN

The ORIGIN Study compares lowering of blood glucose with basal insulin (vs. no active agent) among individuals with newly diagnosed type 2 diabetes or in those with impaired fasting and/or impaired glucose tolerance (Barr et al. 2007; DECODE Study Group 2001). The unblinded study has two co-primary composite outcomes: (1) CVD death or nonfatal MI or nonfatal stroke; and (2) outcome 1 plus revascularization or hospitalization for CHF. Investigators strive for values of fasting plasma glucose of ≤5.3 mmol/L in the group receiving insulin and for values representing "best practice" for the other group.

Other Trials

Other trials under way include the Study on the Prognosis and Effect of Anti-Diabetic Drugs on Type-2 Diabetes Mellitus with Coronary Artery Disease (SPREADDIMCAD), which is a double-blind, randomized trial of glipizide and metformin that addresses recurrent cardiovascular events. The study's forecasted completion date is 2010. Also under way is the "A Randomized Placebo Controlled Clinical Trial to Evaluate Cardiovascular Outcomes after Treatment with Sitagliptin in Patients with Type 2 Diabetes Mellitus and Inadequate Glycemic Control on Mono- or Dual Combination Oral Antihyperglycemic Therapy" (TECOS).

Interventions to Alter the Metabolism of Blood Glucose

Various investigators have tested the use of aldose reductase inhibitors to slow the metabolism of glucose to sorbitol. A systematic review concluded that for diabetic neuropathy these agents have shown no benefit (Chalk et al. 2007), and no studies of their use in CVD exist. Aldose reductase inhibitors are not currently indicated for the prevention or treatment of diabetic complications.

Hyperglycemia can increase the activity of protein kinase C (PKC) in vascular cells (Way et al. 2001). Ruboxistaurin, an inhibitor of PKC-β, has been tested for the treatment of retinopathy, nephropathy, and neuropathy, with modest promising results (PKC-DRS Study Group 2005). A decision from the Food and Drug Administration on its use in diabetic retinopathy awaits further research.

Strategies to Lower Blood Pressure

Elevated levels of arterial blood pressure have been linked strongly and independently to death, MI, CHF, and microvascular disease in persons with diabetes (Adler et al. 2000). Lowering blood pressure in patients with diabetes and hypertension lowers morbidity and mortality, but requires multiple drugs (Sigal et al. 2006). The Blood Pressure Lowering Treatment Trialists' Collaboration confirmed the effectiveness of lowering blood pressure to prevent CVD and confirmed that angiotensin-converting enzyme (ACE) inhibitors, calcium channel blockers (CCBs), and diuretics/β-blockers have similar effects on cardiovascular events (Neal et al. 2000). For diabetes, the collaborators identified 27 trials of 33,395 individuals (Turnbull et al. 2005). The Collaboration compared intensive (more) and conventional (less) lowering of blood pressure, classes of drugs against placebo, and classes of drugs against active comparators. For patients with diabetes, both ACE inhibitors and CCBs, each compared with placebo, reduced the risk for stroke, whereas CCBs, but not ACE inhibitors, lowered the risk of coronary heart disease. Class comparisons included ACE inhibitors or CCBs versus "conventional" drugs (diuretics and/or β-blockers) and ACE inhibitors versus CCBs, showing that patients randomized to CCBs fared worse than those on conventional drugs with respect to CHF. Comparing more intensive and less intensive regimens, analyses showed a benefit for stroke but not for coronary heart disease or CHF.

Patients with diabetes, compared with those without the disease, gained greater protection from angiotensin receptor blockers (ARBs) for CHF but less protection for CVD. For patients with diabetes, head-to-head comparisons provide no differences in the effects of ACE inhibitors, CCBs, or diuretics/β-blockers for any complication. The Collaboration concluded that lowering blood pressure, rather than using a specific agent, should guide clinicians (Sigal et al. 2006; Turnbull et al. 2005).

No one blood pressure target has proven to be best (Vijan 2007), yet lower targets tend to supersede higher ones. Current guidelines generally advocate treating patients with diabetes to blood pressure at or below 130/80 mm Hg (American Diabetes Association 2007; Graham et al. 2007; Smith et al. 2006), with the exception of governmental guidelines from the United Kingdom, which advocate 130/80 mm Hg or below for patients with kidney, eye, or cerebrovascular damage and 140/80 mm Hg otherwise (National Institute for Health and Clinical Excellence 2007).

Among major trials defining a target is the HOT (The Hypertension Optimal Treatment) trial, in which investigators randomized participants to target groups of diastolic blood pressure less than or equal to 90, 85, or 80 mm Hg, treating them with multiple agents. The main endpoint was a combination of CVD events. Of 18,790 patients, 8% had diabetes. In that group, the risk of a major cardiovascular event in the <90 mm Hg target group was twice (RR 2.1 [95% CI 1.2–3.4]) the risk of that in the <80 mm Hg target group (Hansson et al. 1998). This study provided further evidence for aggressive lowering of blood pressure in diabetes patients.

The SYST-EUR (Systolic Hypertension in Europe) trial investigated whether treatment of high systolic blood pressure reduced the risk of stroke in patients over age 60 (Staessen et al. 1997). Investigators added enalapril and hydrochlorothiazide as needed to nitrendipine or placebo to lower the systolic pressure to below 150 mm Hg. A post hoc analysis of 492 diabetic participants (of 4695) (Tuomilehto et al. 1999) showed greater reduction of blood pressure in the active-treatment group and a 62% risk reduction (95% CI 19% to 80%) for all cardiovascular events. In SYST-CHINA, Chinese patients with isolated systolic hypertension were treated with nitrendipine or placebo with the addition of captopril and hydrochlorothiazide. Randomization to nitrendipine among the 98 patients with diabetes was associated with a large reduction in risk (74%, $p = 0.03$) for all cardiovascular endpoints and corroborated the estimate from SYST-EUR (Brenner et al. 2001; Tuomilehto et al. 1999; Wang et al. 2000). SHEP (Systolic Hypertension in the Elderly Program) addressed whether treating elderly persons who had isolated systolic hypertension with chlorthalidone (vs. placebo) lowered the risk of fatal and nonfatal strokes (Curb et al. 1996). Five hundred and eighty-three of 4736 participants had diabetes, among whom the use of chlorthalidone was associated with a large reduction in risk (34%, 95% CI 6–54%).

The UKPDS tested whether tight control of blood pressure prevented or delayed diabetic complications in hypertensive patients with type 2 diabetes. Investigators randomized 1148 patients with hypertension to tight control of blood pressure and secondarily to a regimen based either on captopril or atenolol, and they followed patients for a median 8.4 years. The study achieved a difference in both systolic and diastolic pressures (144/82 mm Hg vs. 154/87 mm Hg). Compared with the group with less tight control, significant reductions in risk were observed for any diabetes-related endpoints (24%, 95% CI 8% to 38%), diabetes-related deaths (32%, 6% to 51%), stroke (44%), heart failure (56%), and microvascular endpoints (37%), the last largely because of a reduced risk of retinal photocoagulation (UKPDS Group 1998c). However, the benefits of previously improved blood-pressure control were not sustained during the poststudy monitoring period (Holman et al. 2008b).

The HOPE (Heart Outcomes Prevention Evaluation) study enrolled 3577 patients with diabetes over age 55 years among 9297 participants at high risk for CVD and investigated whether ramipril (vs. placebo) lowered the incidence of primary or recurrent CVD (Heart Outcomes Prevention Evaluation Study Investigators 2000). Of note, over 40% of patients did not have hypertension. The investigators terminated the study early because of a marked benefit associated with ramipril (risk reduction for CVD 25% [95% CI 12%–36%]). The risk of each component of CVD—MI, stroke, and cardiovascular death—was significantly reduced by randomization to ramipril.

ADVANCE, as described above, enrolled 11,140 patients with type 2 diabetes at high risk for CVD. Investigators randomized patients to combined perindopril (2 mg) and indapamide (0.625 mg) or to matching placebo. During follow-up (mean 4.3 years), blood pressure was reduced (vs. placebo) by an average of 5.6 mm Hg (systolic) more and 2.2 mm Hg (diastolic) more in patients assigned active treatment. The study supported the role of lowering blood pressure in diabetes insofar as treatment reduced the risk of a combined endpoint of microvascular and macrovascular disease but did not support lowering of blood glucose with the specific intention of lowering the incidence of CVD (RR reduction 8% [95% CI –4% to 19%; $p = 0.16$]) (Patel et al. 2007).

A number of studies have addressed renal outcomes, although few have provided sufficient numbers of individuals with or who developed end-stage renal disease (ESRD). In general, ACE inhibitors are considered beneficial for type 1 diabetes (Shiplak 2007). The ABCD (Appropriate Blood Pressure Control study in Diabetes) addressed whether control of diastolic blood pressure to <75 mm Hg was superior to targeting 80–89 mm Hg in hypertensive patients with type 2 diabetes. Investigators randomized patients to enalapril or nisoldipine (intensive arm) or placebo (Estacio et al. 1998). The endpoint was a change in creatinine clearance, with no difference between arms or between drugs (Schrier et al. 2002). Randomization to intensive therapy was associated with a decrease in mortality rate ($p = 0.037$) (Estacio et al. 2000) and a lower incidence of stroke ($p = 0.03$), but these were not primary outcomes.

In the DETAIL (Diabetes Exposed to Telmisartan and Enalapril) study investigators randomized participants with type 2 diabetes to either the ARB telmisartan or the ACE inhibitor enalapril. The endpoint was the change in the glomerular filtration rate; in this study telmisartan did not differ from enalapril (Barnett et al. 2004). IRMA 2 (Irbesartan Reduction of Microalbuminuria-2) was a randomized, double-blind, placebo-controlled study of irbesartan in patients with type 2 diabetes and microalbuminuria (Parving et al. 2001); participants randomized to irbesartan were less likely to experience progressive nephropathy. The IDNT (Irbesartan Diabetic Nephropathy Trial) randomized patients with type 2 diabetes and nephropathy to treatment with irbesartan, amlodipine, or placebo. The primary endpoint, which occurred less frequently in patients randomized to irbesartan, was a composite of a doubling of base-line serum creatinine concentration, development of ESRD, or death (Lewis et al. 2001), but there was no difference for a prespecified composite cardiovascular endpoint (Berl et al. 2005).

The MARVAL (Microalbuminuria Reduction With Valsartan) study randomized patients with type 2 diabetes and microalbuminuria to valsartan or amlodipine. Valsartan improved the excretion of urinary albumin (the primary endpoint) despite no differences in blood pressure between treatment groups; investigators therefore proposed that valsartan had a "blood pressure-independent antiproteinuric effect" (Viberti and Wheeldon 2002). RENAAL (Reduction of Endpoints in NIDDM with the Angiotensin II Antagonist Losartan Study) was a double-blind, placebo-controlled study in 1513 patients with type 2 diabetes and nephropathy. Randomization to the ARB losartan reduced the risk (by 16%) of the primary endpoint (doubling of plasma creatinine, ESRD, or death). As with other studies of ARBs, the investigators suggested that the benefit exceeded that expected due to lowering of blood pressure alone.

Clinicians continue to debate whether ACEs and ARBs, advocated as first-line treatment, provide benefits above lowering of blood pressure alone (Casas et al. 2005; Whelton et al. 2005; Strippoli et al. 2006). The combination of ACE inhibitors and aldosterone inhibitors holds promise (Chrysostomou et al. 2006), but may lead to hyperkalemia. Trials of renin inhibitors exist (Parving et al. 2008), but they do not as yet include ESRD or CVD endpoints. To prevent retinopathy, lowering blood pressure is strongly advocated (Mohamed et al. 2007).

Modification of Plasma Lipid Levels

Of the lipoproteins, higher concentrations of LDL, intermediate-density lipoproteins, and small forms of very low-density lipoproteins and lower concentrations of HDL (high-density lipoprotein) are atherogenic and associated with an increased incidence of CVD. Most cholesterol is carried in LDL. LDL-lowering drugs include statins, bile acid sequestrants, ezetamibe, and, to a lesser extent, fibrates and nicotinic acid. Drugs that increase HDL include fibrates and nicotinic acid. Trials have been performed of statins and fibrates for the primary prevention of CVD in diabetes.

The Heart Protection Study (HPS) randomized over 5000 individuals with diabetes (plus others without diabetes) to simvastatin or placebo. The LDL cholesterol concentration in the active-treatment group was 0.9 mmol/L lower than in the placebo group, and the incidence of CVD at the trial's end was 24% lower. Unlike previous trials of statins, the HPS showed a clear reduction in the incidence of stroke as well as of CVD in the elderly. The benefit occurred regardless of risk of CVD and LDL level, confirming that simvastatin lowered risk in individuals with normal or even low levels of LDL (Collins et al. 2003). The study showed no difference in benefit between types of diabetes, but it was not powered to do so.

The Collaborative Atorvastatin Diabetes Study (CARDS) also tested lowering of LDL and included adults with type 2 diabetes who were otherwise at high risk for CVD. Because the study excluded patients with known CVD and those with high levels of LDL, none of the participants had an indication, per clinical practice at the time, for therapy with a statin. Patients who received active treatment with atorvastatin had levels of LDL 1.2 mmol/L lower than those on placebo and experienced a 37% reduction in major cardiovascular events, including a 48% reduction in the incidence of stroke. As in the HPS, the treatment effect did not differ by cholesterol level at study entry (Colhoun et al. 2004).

Both HPS and CARDS showed a reduction in risk proportionate to the lowering of LDL. Stronger statins have been shown to lower risk of CVD more than weaker ones, but controversy exists (Shepherd et al. 2006). Although statins may have pleiotropic properties (Yamagishi et al. 2007), these properties are unlikely to account for but a small proportion of the observed reduction in risk (Baigent et al. 2005). HPS and CARDS countered the notion of an appropriate target for LDL in diabetes, and yet, current guidelines continue to advocate targets (Buse et al. 2007). These studies support the shift in clinical practice from treating individual risk factors (e.g., cholesterol levels) to lowering overall risk (Jackson 2000). In addition treating with statins represents cost-effective spending for health (Mihaylova et al. 2006; Raikou et al. 2007).

With regard to raising concentrations of HDL as a means to lower the incidence of CVD, the Fenofibrate Intervention and Event Lowering in Diabetes (FIELD) study randomized 9795 patients with type 2 diabetes, with or without heart disease, to fenofibrate or placebo. The primary outcome was death due to coronary heart disease or a nonfatal MI. Although total cholesterol, LDL, and triglycerides changed proportionately more for LDL (absolute value −0.17 mmol/L) than did HDL, randomization to fenofibrate was not associated with a lower rate of coronary events. That patients randomized to placebo were more likely to receive statins outside of the trial which may have minimized a benefit of fenofibrate (Keech et al. 2005). The study generated the possibility that use of fenofibrate lowers the risk of retinopathy, a hypothesis embedded in the ongoing ACCORD Eye Study (Chew et al. 2007). ACCORD also tests the effect of fenofibrate (vs. placebo) on cardiovascular outcomes in patients treated with statins (Ginsberg et al. 2007).

An ongoing study is HPS2-THRIVE (Treatment of HDL to Reduce the Incidence of Vascular Events). By design, investigators will include 7000 patients with diabetes as a subset of the 20,000 participants. The placebo-controlled trial tests whether niacin plus laropiprant, a prostaglandin D receptor antagonist designed to minimize niacin-induced flushing, reduces the incidence of CVD.

To date, the evidence for the prevention and delay of CVD in diabetes with respect to modifying lipids is limited to the statins.

Antiplatelet Agents

Professional medical organizations advocate aspirin therapy in individuals with diabetes at high risk of CVD (Buse et al. 2007; International Diabetes Federation Clinical Guidelines Task Force 2002). Yet, researchers question the evidence and note the possibility of aspirin resistance (Nicolucci et al. 2007). Ongoing trials testing the use of aspirin in diabetes to lower the incidence of CVD include ASCEND (A Study of Cardiovascular Events in Diabetes), POPADAD (Prevention of Progression of Asymptomatic Diabetic Arterial Disease), ACCEPT-D (Aspirin and Simvastatin Combination for Cardiovascular Events Prevention Trial in Diabetes) (De Berardis et al. 2007), and J-PAD (Japanese Primary Prevention of Atherosclerosis With Aspirin for Diabetes) (Morimoto et al. 2007).

Clopidogrel and dipyridamole also inhibit platelet function, but studies of these agents that include sufficient numbers of patients with diabetes do not exist. Application of positive trial findings (Yusuf et al. 2001) has led to the recommendation of clopidogrel in combination with low-dose aspirin for 12 months following acute coronary syndrome (National Institute for Clinical Excellence 2004), a recommendation that also applies to patients with diabetes. Clopidrogrel and aspirin are not recommended for primary prevention of CVD (Wang et al. 2007).

Antiplatelet agents have been tested in the prevention of diabetic retinopathy. The Early Treatment Diabetic Retinopathy Study (ETDRS) (Chew et al. 1995; ETDRS Research Group 1991) showed no beneficial effect of aspirin, but neither did it show an increase in hemorrhage. Guidelines tailored for the prevention of retinopathy do not currently include aspirin, clopidogrel, or dipyrimadole (Mohamed et al. 2007).

Lowering of Homocysteine Concentrations

Meta-analyses of observational studies have shown a modest association between plasma homocysteine and CVD (Danesh and Lewington 1998; Homocysteine Studies Collaboration 1998). However, as all randomized trials in nondiabetic participants have been negative, experts do not recommend supplementation with folic acid and vitamin B_{12} (Baigent and Clarke 2007). The Study of the Effectiveness of Additional Reductions in Cholesterol and Homocysteine (SEARCH) trial (Bowman et al. 2007) with 12,064 patients (many with diabetes) found no effect of supplementation and awaits publication.

Supplementation with Fish Oil

Several studies that included individuals with diabetes have found an inverse association between the consumption of fish or fish oils and the risk of coronary heart disease and sudden cardiac death (Hu et al. 2003). Fish oils reduce the concentrations of plasma triglyceride in hypertriglyceridemic individuals, one of the putative mechanisms for their effectiveness. To date no trials restricted to people with diabetes have been completed, but two major placebo-controlled trials of fish oils for primary prevention, ASCEND and ORIGIN (discussed previously with relation to insulin treatment), will provide answers. Current reviews do not advocate treatment with fish oil (Patel 2006).

Weight Reduction Using Medications

Randomized trials have shown that orlistat and sibutramine can achieve modest weight loss in individuals with diabetes (Norris et al. 2005). The ongoing SCOUT (Sibutramine Cardiovascular Outcome Trial) study addresses the effectiveness of sibutramine use (vs. placebo) to prevent CVD in patients with type 2 diabetes (Torp-Pedersen et al. 2007). Rimonabant, a cannabinoid receptor antagonist previously licensed in Europe, reduces weight as well as glycemia in patients with diabetes (Scheen et al. 2006). The ongoing CRESCENDO study's primary objective is to show whether rimonabant reduces the risk of MI, stroke, or death from an MI or stroke in diabetic patients with abdominal obesity.

Antioxidants

Antioxidant molecules prevent the production of free radicals, which damage cells via oxidative stress. Of relevance to CVD, oxidized LDL accelerates atherosclerosis (Chait and Heinecke 1994). Common antioxidants include vitamins C and E and other components of food. In an effort to reduce CVD, a number of major trials in diabetes, including HPS and HOPE (discussed earlier in this chapter), have randomized large numbers of people to antioxidants, but with no apparent benefit.

Intraocular Corticosteroids

Injecting corticosteroids into the vitreous has been tested as a treatment for diffuse diabetic macular edema that is unresponsive to laser treatment. Currently, this treatment is recommended with caution because of the risk of cataracts and increased intraocular pressure (Mohamed et al. 2007).

Use of Antibiotics

Administration of antibiotics for infected foot ulcers remains the standard of care, but the preferred agent and the mode of administration (oral, intravenous, topical) are less clear (Cavanagh et al. 2005). Intravenous therapy does not appear more effective, with the possible exception of cases of severe infection (Cavanagh et al. 2005; Lipsky 2007; Nelson et al. 2006). Largely because studies have been small, there is no strong evidence for any particular antibiotic for preventing LEA, eradicating infection, or healing ulcers (Nelson et al. 2006).

Bisphosphonates

Bisphosphonates, which are used to arrest bone loss, have been studied in Charcot arthropathy (Smith et al. 2007). Reviewers note greater reduction in disease activity, pain, and discomfort for intervention subjects compared with controls, but there is no firm evidence for the prevention of subsequent ulceration.

Growth Factors

Subcutaneous granulocyte colony-stimulating factor (G-CSF) has been used to treat foot ulceration in diabetes, but too few trials exist to judge effectiveness (Nelson et al. 2006). Platelet-derived growth factor-B (PDGF-B) has been approved for use in diabetic ulcers, and at least one trial testing the delivery of a gene for PDGF-B has been performed. Vascular endothelial growth factor (VEGF) is an angiogenic and vascular permeability factor implicated in the pathogenesis of diabetic retinopathy. Currently licensed for the treatment of age-related macular degeneration, anti-VEGF drugs include pegaptanib and ranibizumab. Authorities have licensed bevacizumab for the treatment of bowel cancer; this drug has ocular effects similar to those of ranibizumab. The possibility of albuminuria and hypertension as side effects with these drugs (Zhu et al. 2007) highlights the importance of long-term trials.

■ Surgical and Other Nonpharmacological Interventions

Retinopathy

In proliferative and severe preproliferative retinopathy, laser photocoagulation prevents severe visual loss (Mohamed et al. 2007). A systematic review is under way for subthreshold (at the level of the retinal pigment epithelium) laser treatment for diabetic maculopathy (Cochrane Eyes and Vision Group 2006), but this treatment may not be beneficial without clinically significant macular edema (Mendrinos et al. 2007). Also under review is oral calcium dobesilate for retinopathy. Surgical vitrectomy for severe vitreous hemorrhage and significant retinopathy has been assigned an intermediate level of evidence (Mohamed et al. 2007), and a systematic review is currently under way for the indication of diabetic macular edema (Cochrane Eyes and Vision Group 2006).

Debridement

Debridement, the removal of dead or infected tissue to enhance the survival of healthy tissue, is a mainstay of practice for diabetic foot ulcers. Debridement may be surgical, physical, or chemical (with absorbing substances), or it may involve maggots. The use of hydrogels appears promising, but evidence is lacking (Smith 2002). A randomized trial of treatment with maggots is ongoing (Raynor et al. 2004).

Hyperbaric Oxygen Therapy

Hyperbaric oxygen therapy has been reviewed as a possible modality for treating ulcerated, chronically infected diabetic feet. This therapy appears to reduce the risk of major amputation, but the evidence is not sufficient to justify its routine use (Kranke et al. 2004; Hunt 2007). Moreover, the limited availability of pressurized chambers constrains its application.

Offloading

Taking weight off the foot (offloading) prevents individuals from putting pressure on a diabetic foot ulcer. Bed rest, crutches, wheelchairs, and walkers alone are not considered effective because patients are unlikely to accept them. However, plaster casting, whether removable or not, is considered vital to the healing of complicated ulcers (Cavanagh et al. 2005).

Revascularization

Revascularization for coronary disease includes angioplasty (opening narrowed or blocked coronary arteries with a catheter), stenting (using a tube or scaffold to keep open a coronary artery), and coronary arterial bypass grafting [CABG] (creating vascular routes around narrowed or blocked arteries). Balloon angioplasty compresses plaque, laser angioplasty vaporizes plaque, and coronary atherectomy cuts away plaque. Stenting may include bare-metal stents or drug-eluting stents impregnated with drugs to prevent arterial restenosis. Angioplasty and stenting comprise percutaneous intervention (PCI).

The Bypass Angioplasty Revascularization Investigation (BARI) study (BARI Investigators 2000) randomized patients with coronary heart disease to either CABG or bare-metal stents. In patients with diabetes survival was better for those who underwent CABG (Kapur et al. 2005). BARI-2D, an ongoing study in diabetes discussed earlier in this chapter, compares revascularization with medical intervention. Systematic reviews of revascularization do not distinguish between participants with and without diabetes. With respect to prevention of stroke there are no diabetes-specific recommendations for carotid revascularization. Rather, care is guided by estimated surgical risk, life expectancy, degree of carotid stenosis, and whether a patient is to undergo simultaneous CABG (Biller et al. 1998). Revascularization for peripheral vascular disease, and to augment healing of ulcers, is frequently undertaken despite scanty evidence (Cavanagh et al. 2005).

Bariatric Surgery

The Swedish Obesity Study tested the potential benefits and drawbacks of bariatric surgery in 4047 obese individuals with an average BMI of about 40. Because ethics committees were unlikely to have approved a randomized design, the study employed a matched observational cohort design. Bariatric surgery was associated with a 27% reduction in the risk of death in the presence and absence of diabetes (Sjostrom et al. 2007). No randomized trial exists of bariatric surgery among patients with diabetes in terms of CVD outcomes.

Lifestyle

Diet and Exercise

Adherence to dietary restrictions is one of the most effective means to reduce blood glucose, but it is difficult to sustain. However there is no evidence from trials that improved diet or exercise reduces the risk of diabetic complications or prolongs the life of patients with diabetes (Nield et al. 2007). Dieting to lower cholesterol levels is modestly effective (Tang et al. 1998). The observational follow-on study to the Diabetes Prevention Program (Diabetes Prevention Program Research Group 2002), the Diabetes Prevention Program Outcomes Study, will determine whether patients formerly randomized to intensive diet and exercise develop fewer diabetic complications.

Smoking Cessation

No trial of smoking cessation to reduce CVD in diabetes exists, but there is little debate that observational studies alone justify the promotion of smoking cessation in clinical and public health practice (Critchley and Capewell 2003; Weiss 1996).

■ Other Interventions

To prevent diabetic foot complications, numerous other therapies exist, but without sufficient evidence with which to recommend them. For foot ulcers, these include pressure-relieving interventions (Spencer 2000), the use of silver-containing dressings, and topical drugs (Bergin and Wraight 2006). Studies of palliative irradiation and magnetic fields in the treatment of Charcot joints yielded insufficient evidence to advocate treatment (Smith et al. 2007). A trial of limb salvage and ulcer healing using traditional Chinese herbs as an adjuvant therapy exists (Liu et al. 2006). Shock-wave treatment is currently being tested for diabetic foot ulcers, as are negative-pressure dressings and bioengineered skin equivalents (Cavanagh et al. 2005), which are deemed "likely to be beneficial" (Hunt 2007). One trial, using intravenous saline as a control, is testing the effect of autologous bone marrow cells on the growth of lower extremity collateral arteries with a primary outcome of avoiding major amputation or improving critical limb ischemia.

The merit of educating patients to prevent diabetic foot ulceration has been reviewed, but the studies' poor methodological quality prevented reviewers from advocating education (Valk et al. 2005). Regular professional surveillance for foot problems in the clinic, however, can decrease risk of amputation (Litzelman et al. 1993).

■ Combined Interventions

The STENO-2 investigators tested a "targeted, intensified, multifactorial intervention" of modifiable risk factors for diabetic complications against Danish community-standard, guideline-driven care. To decrease the occurrence of death due to CVD, MI, or stroke; of revascularization; and of LEA; the intervention targeted hyperglycemia, hypertension, dyslipidemia, microalbuminuria, and CVD. Intensive therapy was associated with a halving of the risk of CVD events over 8 years (Gaede et al. 1999). After an additional 5 years of observation, mortality, too, was reduced approximately 50% among those previously randomized to the intervention (Gaede et al. 1999; Gaede et al. 2008).

■ Implications for Health Policy

This review shows that individuals with diabetes and their providers of care can reduce the occurrence of diabetic complications by lowering glucose, blood pressure, and LDL, either alone or in combination. Nonpharmacologic interventions, chiefly those related to retinopathy and obesity, also improve outcomes. To date evidence for lowering blood glucose and blood pressure does not support the use of specific agents except possibly metformin and blockade of the angiotensin system. For LDL, statins remain the intervention of choice.

The values to which providers should direct their patients to lower plasma glucose, blood pressure, and LDL cholesterol remains unclear. Health care providers and patients with diabetes together should agree on values appropriate for that individual. For each of blood glucose, blood pressure, and LDL cholesterol epidemiologic studies show lower rates of complications with lower levels, but the increased death rates in the ACCORD study were associated with the most aggressive policy to date for lowering blood glucose. Side effects, mostly hypoglycemia and weight gain, limit treatments for lowering blood glucose. Moreover, targets have been difficult to reach, even in the clinical trial setting. Reflecting these limitations, guidelines advocate values of A1C above the nondiabetic range. Guidelines of the American Diabetes Association propose a goal in general for diabetic patients (A1C < 7%) that is less stringent than those for *individual* patients (A1C < 6%), while British guidance advocates an A1C goal of 6.5% but acknowledges that this may not be appropriate for all.

Most guidelines and physician-incentive programs continue to advocate treatment to clear targets defined by A1C, blood pressure, and lipid levels. Increasingly guidelines advocate treating above, and not below, a level of absolute risk defined by the probability that a complication will occur in a given time period. These cutoffs may be determined by analyses of cost-effectiveness, with treatment below these cutoffs representing a poor choice for health spending given limited resources.

■ Challenges and Developments over the Next 5 to 10 Years

Research in the future will define whether drugs or subgroups of patients exist with or for which glycemic control is particularly effective, or, conversely, ineffective or even deleterious. Challenges for future clinical research include achieving ever-lower values of A1C in the intervention arms of trials, the need to conduct trials that require ever-larger samples, teasing out drug-versus-glycemic-lowering effects, and recruiting to placebo-controlled trials that exist to determine the cardiovascular safety of antidiabetic agents. Measures of quality of life should accompany trials, and be performed against active comparators used in current clinical practice. Trials related to diet and physical activity will likely have benefits that extend to diseases beyond diabetes and should be designed to capture these effects. Those who synthesize clinical evidence will likely develop increasingly sophisticated methods of meta-analyses and modeling taking into account effectiveness and costs, which in turn will support the clinical guidelines that guide health care providers and individuals with diabetes.

■ References

Abraira C et al. (1995). Veterans Affairs Cooperative Study on glycemic control and complications in type II diabetes (VA CSDM). Results of the feasibility trial. Veterans Affairs Cooperative Study in Type II Diabetes. *Diabetes Care* **18**, 1113–23.

Abraira C et al. (2003). Design of the cooperative study on glycemic control and complications in diabetes mellitus type 2: Veterans Affairs Diabetes Trial. *Journal of Diabetes Complications* **17**, 314–22.

Adler A et al. (2000). Association of systolic blood pressure with macrovascular and microvascular complications of type 2 diabetes (UKPDS 36). *British Medical Journal* **321**, 412–9.

American Diabetes Association (2007). Standards of medical care in diabetes—2007. *Diabetes Care* **30** (Suppl.), S4–S411.

American Diabetes Association Meetings (2009). Presented at the Annual 2009 Scientific Meetings.

Baigent C, Clark R (2007). B vitamins for the prevention of vascular disease: insufficient evidence to justify treatment. *JAMA* **298**, 1212–4.

Baigent C et al. (2005). Efficacy and safety of cholesterol-lowering treatment: prospective meta-analysis of data from 90,056 participants in 14 randomised trials of statins. *Lancet* **366**, 1267–78.

BARI Investigators (2000). Seven-year outcome in the Bypass Angioplasty Revascularization Investigation (BARI) by treatment and diabetic status. *Journal of the American College of Cardiology* **35**, 1122–9.

BARI 2D Study Group (2009). A randomized trial of therapies for type 2 diabetes and coronary artery disease. *New England Journal of Medicine* **360** (19), 2503–15.

Barnett AH et al. (2004). Angiotensin-receptor blockade versus converting-enzyme inhibition in type 2 diabetes and nephropathy. *New England Journal of Medicine* **351**(19), 1952–61.

Barr EL et al. (2007). Risk of cardiovascular and all-cause mortality in individuals with diabetes mellitus, impaired fasting glucose, and impaired glucose tolerance: the Australian Diabetes, Obesity, and Lifestyle Study (AusDiab). *Circulation* **116** (2), 151–7.

Bergin SM, Wraight P (2006). Silver based wound dressings and topical agents for treating diabetic foot ulcers. *Cochrane Database Systematic Reviews* (1): CD005082.

Berl T et al. (2005). Impact of achieved blood pressure on cardiovascular outcomes in the Irbesartan Diabetic Nephropathy Trial. *Journal of the American Society of Nephrology* **16** (7), 2170–9.

Biller J et al. (1998). Guidelines for carotid endarterectomy: a statement for healthcare professionals from a Special Writing Group of the Stroke Council, American Heart Association. *Circulation* **97** (5), 501–9.

Bowman L et al. (2007). Study of the effectiveness of additional reductions in cholesterol and homocysteine (SEARCH): characteristics of a randomized trial among 12064 myocardial infarction survivors. *American Heart Journal* **154** (5), 815–23, 823 e1–6.

Brenner BM et al. (2001). Effects of losartan on renal and cardiovascular outcomes in patients with type 2 diabetes and nephropathy. *New England Journal of Medicine* **345**, 861–9.

Brooks MM et al. (2006). Hypotheses, design, and methods for the Bypass Angioplasty Revascularization Investigation 2 Diabetes (BARI 2D) Trial. *American Journal of Cardiology* **97** (12A), 9G–19G.

Brownlee M (2005). The pathobiology of diabetic complications: a unifying mechanism. *Diabetes* **54** (6), 1615–25.

Buse JB et al. (2007). Primary prevention of cardiovascular diseases in people with diabetes mellitus: a scientific statement from the American Heart Association and the American Diabetes Association. *Diabetes Care* **30** (1), 162–72.

Casas JP et al. (2005). Effect of inhibitors of the renin-angiotensin system and other antihypertensive drugs on renal outcomes: systematic review and meta-analysis. *Lancet* **366** (9502), 2026–33.

Cavanagh PR et al. (2005). Treatment for diabetic foot ulcers. *Lancet* **366** (9498), 1725–35.

Chait A, Heinecke JW (1994). Lipoprotein modification: cellular mechanisms. *Current Opinions in Lipidology* **5** (5), 365–70.

Chalk C et al. (2007). Aldose reductase inhibitors for the treatment of diabetic polyneuropathy. *Cochrane Database of Systematic Reviews* (4), CD004572.

Chalmers J et al. (2006). ADVANCE: breaking new ground in type 2 diabetes. *Journal of Hypertension [Suppl.]* **24** (5), S22–8.

Charbonnel B et al. (2004). The prospective pioglitazone clinical trial in macrovascular events (PROactive): can pioglitazone reduce cardiovascular events in diabetes? Study design and baseline characteristics of 5238 patients. *Diabetes Care* **27**, 1647–53.

Chew E et al. (1995). Effects of aspirin on vitreous/preretinal hemorrhage in patients with diabetes mellitus: Early Treatment Diabetic Retinopathy Study report no. 20. *Archives of Ophthalmology* **113**, 52–55.

Chew EY et al. (2007). Rationale, design, and methods of the Action to Control Cardiovascular Risk in Diabetes Eye Study (ACCORD-EYE). *American Journal of Cardiology* **99** (12A), 103i–111i.

Chrysostomou A et al. (2006). Double-blind, placebo-controlled study on the effect of the aldosterone receptor antagonist spironolactone in patients who have persistent proteinuria and are on long-term angiotensin-converting enzyme inhibitor therapy, with or without an angiotensin II receptor blocker. *Clinical Journal of the American Society of Nephrology* **1**(2), 256–62.

Cochrane Eyes and Vision Group (2006). Cochrane Eyes and Vision Group (CEVG) systematic review activity on posterior segment treatments. *Community Eye Health* **19**, 11.

Colhoun HM et al. (2004). Primary prevention of cardiovascular disease with atorvastatin in type 2 diabetes in the Collaborative Atorvastatin Diabetes Study (CARDS): multicentre randomised placebo-controlled trial. *Lancet* **364** (9435), 685–96.

Collins R et al. (2003). MRC/BHF Heart Protection Study of cholesterol-lowering with simvastatin in 5963 people with diabetes: a randomised placebo-controlled trial. *Lancet* **361** (9374), 2005–16.

Critchley JA, Capewell S (2003). Mortality risk reduction associated with smoking cessation in patients with coronary heart disease: a systematic review. *JAMA* **290** (1), 86–97.

Curb JD et al. (1996). Effect of diuretic-based antihypertensive treatment on cardiovascular disease risk in older diabetic patients with isolated systolic hypertension. Systolic Hypertension in the Elderly Program Cooperative Research Group. *JAMA* **276**, 1886–92.

Danesh J, Lewington S (1998). Plasma homocysteine and coronary heart disease: systematic review of published epidemiological studies. *Journal of Cardiovascular Risk* **5** (4), 229–32.

De Berardis G et al. (2007). Aspirin and Simvastatin Combination for Cardiovascular Events Prevention Trial in Diabetes (ACCEPT-D): design of a randomized study of the efficacy of low-dose aspirin in the prevention of cardiovascular events in subjects with diabetes mellitus treated with statins. *Trials* **8**, 21.

DECODE Study Group (2001). Glucose tolerance and cardiovascular mortality: comparison of fasting and 2-hour diagnostic criteria. *Archives of Internal Medicine* **161** (161), 397–405.

Diabetes Control and Complications Trial Research Group (1993). The effect of intensive treatment of diabetes on the development and progression of long-term complications in insulin-dependent diabetes mellitus. *New England Journal of Medicine* **329**, 977–86.

Diabetes Prevention Program Research Group (2002). Reduction in the incidence of type 2 diabetes with lifestyle intervention or metformin. *New England Journal of Medicine* **346**, 393–403.

Diaz R et al. (2007). Glucose-insulin-potassium therapy in patients with ST-segment elevation myocardial infarction. *JAMA* **298** (20), 2399–405.

Dormandy JA et al. (2005). Secondary prevention of macrovascular events in patients with type 2 diabetes in the PROactive Study (PROspective pioglitAzone Clinical Trial In macroVascular Events): a randomised controlled trial. *Lancet* **366** (9493), 1279–89.

Duckworth W et al. (2009). Glucose control and vascular complications in veterans with type 2 diabetes. *New England Journal of Medicine* **360** (2), 129–39.

Early Treatment Diabetic Retinopathy Study Research Group (1991). Effects of aspirin treatment on diabetic retinopathy: ETDRS report number 8. *Ophthalmology* **98**, 757–65.

Estacio R et al. (2000). Effect of blood pressure control on diabetic microvascular complications in patients with hypertension and type 2 diabetes. *Diabetes Care* **Suppl 2**, B54–64.

Estacio RO et al. (1998). The effect of nisoldipine as compared with enalapril on cardiovascular outcomes in patients with non-insulin-dependent diabetes and hypertension. *New England Journal of Medicine* **338**, 645–52.

Gaede P et al. (1999). Intensified multifactorial intervention in patients with type 2 diabetes mellitus and microalbuminuria: the Steno type 2 randomised study. Lancet **353**, 617–22.

Gaede P et al. (2008). Effect of a multifactorial intervention on mortality in type 2 diabetes. *New England Journal of Medicine* **358**, 580–91.

Gerstein HC et al. (2008). Effects of intensive glucose lowering in type 2 diabetes. *New England Journal of Medicine* **358**(24), 2545–59.

Gerstein HC et al. (2007). Glycemia treatment strategies in the Action to Control Cardiovascular Risk in Diabetes (ACCORD) trial. *American Journal of Cardiology* **99** (12A), 34i–43i.

Ginsberg HN et al. (2007). Evolution of the lipid trial protocol of the Action to Control Cardiovascular Risk in Diabetes (ACCORD) trial. *American Journal of Cardiology* **99** (12A), 56i–67i.

Graham I et al. (2007). European guidelines on cardiovascular disease prevention in clinical practice. *European Journal of Cardiovascular Prevention and Rehabilitation* **14** (Suppl. 2, 16), S1–113.

Gray CS et al. (2007). Glucose-potassium-insulin infusions in the management of post-stroke hyperglycaemia: the UK Glucose Insulin in Stroke Trial (GIST-UK). *Lancet Neurol* **6** (5), 397–406.

Hansson L et al. (1998). Effect of intensive blood-pressure lowering and low-dose aspirin in patients with hypertension: principal results of the Hypertension Optimal Treatment (HOT) randomised trial. *Lancet* **351**, 1755–62.

Heart Outcomes Prevention Evaluation Study Investigators (2000). Effects of ramipril on cardiovascular and microvascular outcomes in people with diabetes mellitus: results of the HOPE study and MICRO-HOPE substudy. *Lancet* **355**, 253–9.

Holman RR et al.. (2008a). Long-term follow-up after intensive glucose control in type 2 diabetes. *New England Journal of Medicine* **359**, 1577–89.

Holman RR et al. (2008b). Long-term follow-up after tight control of blood pressure in type 2 diabetes. *New England Journal of Medicine* **359**, 1565–76.

Home PD et al. (2005). Rosiglitazone Evaluated for Cardiac Outcomes and Regulation of Glycaemia in Diabetes (RECORD): study design and protocol. *Diabetologia* **48** (9), 1726–35.

Home PD et al. (2007). Rosiglitazone evaluated for cardiovascular outcomes—an interim analysis. *New England Journal of Medicine* **357** (1), 28–38.

Home PD et al. (2009). Rosiglitazone evaluated for cardiovascular outcomes in oral agent combination therapy for type 2 diabetes (RECORD): a multicentre, randomized, open-label trial. *Lancet* **373**, 2125–35.

Homocysteine Studies Collaboration (1998). Lowering blood homocysteine with folic acid based supplements: meta-analysis of randomised trials. Homocysteine Lowering Trialists' Collaboration. *British Medical Journal* **316** (7135), 894–8.

Hu FB et al. (2003). Fish and long-chain omega-3 fatty acid intake and risk of coronary heart disease and total mortality in diabetic women. *Circulation* **107** (14), 1852–7.

Hunt D (2007). Foot ulcers and amputations in diabetes. *British Medical Journal Clinical Evidence* **12**, 602.

International Diabetes Federation Clinical Guidelines Task Force (2002). Global Guideline for Type 2 Diabetes: recommendations for standard, comprehensive, and minimal care. *Diabetic Medicine* **23** (6), 579–93.
Cardiovascular risk protection. *Global guideline for type 2 diabetes*, IDF: 46–50.

Jackson R (2000). Guidelines on preventing cardiovascular disease in clinical practice. *British Medical Journal* **320** (7236), 659–61.

Kapur A et al. (2005). The Coronary Artery Revascularisation in Diabetes (CARDia) trial: background, aims, and design. *Am Heart J* **149** (1), 13–9.

Keech A et al. (2005). Effects of long-term fenofibrate therapy on cardiovascular events in 9795 people with type 2 diabetes mellitus (the FIELD study): randomised controlled trial. *Lancet* **366** (9500), 1849–61.

Kilo C et al. (1980). The Achilles heel of the University Group Diabetes Program. *JAMA* **243**, 450–7.

Kirkman MS et al. (2006). The association between metabolic control and prevalent macrovascular disease in type 2 diabetes: the VA Cooperative Study in diabetes. *Journal of Diabetes Complications* **20** (2), 75–80.

Kranke P et al. (2004). Hyperbaric oxygen therapy for chronic wounds. *Cochrane Database of Systematic Reviews* (2), CD004123.

Langley J, Adams G (2007). Insulin-based regimens decrease mortality rates in critically ill patients: a systematic review. *Diabetes Metabolism Research and Reviews* **23** (3), 184–92.

Lewis EJ et al. (2001). Renoprotective effect of the angiotensin-receptor antagonist irbesarten in patients with nephropathy due to type 2 diabetes. *New England Journal of Medicine* **345**, 851–60.

Lipsky BA (2007). Empirical therapy for diabetic foot infections: are there clinical clues to guide antibiotic selection? *Clinical Microbiology and Infection* **13** (4), 351–3.

Litzelman DK et al. (1993). Reduction of lower extremity clinical abnormalities in patients with non-insulin-dependent diabetes mellitus. *Annals of Internal Medicine* **119**, 36–41.

Liu J et al. (2006). Chinese herbal medicines for treating diabetic foot ulcers. *Cochrane Database of Systematic Reviews* (3), CD006098.

Look AHEAD Protocol Review Committee (2005). Protocol, Action for Health in Diabetes Look AHEAD Clinical Trial. Available at: https://www.lookaheadtrial.org/public/LookAHEADProtocol.pdf. Accessed December 27, 2007.

Look AHEAD Research Group (2003). Look AHEAD (Action for Health in Diabetes): design and methods for a clinical trial of weight loss for the prevention of cardiovascular disease in type 2 diabetes. *Controlled Clinical Trials* **24**, 610–28.

Look AHEAD Research Group (2007). Reduction in weight and cardiovascular disease risk factors in individuals with type 2 diabetes: one-year results of the look AHEAD trial. *Diabetes Care* **30**, 1374–83.

Malmberg K (1997). Prospective randomised study of intensive insulin treatment on long term survival after acute myocardial infarction in patients with diabetes mellitus. DIGAMI (Diabetes Mellitus, Insulin Glucose Infusion in Acute Myocardial Infarction) Study Group. *British Medical Journal* **314**, 1512–5.

Malmberg K et al. (2005). Intense metabolic control by means of insulin in patients with diabetes mellitus and acute myocardial infarction (DIGAMI 2): effects on mortality and morbidity. *European Heart Journal* **26** (7), 650–61.

Meinert C et al. (1970). A study of the effects of hypoglycemic agents on vascular complications in patients with adult-onset diabetes. *Diabetes* **19**, 789–830.

Mendrinos E et al. (2007). Diabetic Retinopathy. *British Medical Journal Clinical Evidence* **11**, 702.

Mihaylova B et al. (2006). Lifetime cost effectiveness of simvastatin in a range of risk groups and age groups derived from a randomised trial of 20,536 people. *British Medical Journal* **333** (7579), 1145.

Milicevic Z et al. (2005). Hyperglycemia and its effect after acute myocardial infarction on cardiovascular outcomes in patients with type 2 diabetes mellitus (HEART2D) Study design. *Journal of Diabetes Complications* **19** (2), 80–7.

Mohamed Q et al. (2007). Management of diabetic retinopathy: a systematic review. *JAMA* **298** (8), 902–16.

Morimoto T et al. (2007). Aspirin for primary prevention of atherosclerotic disease in Japan. *Journal of Atherosclerosis and Thrombosis* **14** (4), 159–66.

Nathan DM et al. (2005). Intensive diabetes treatment and cardiovascular disease in patients with type 1 diabetes. *New England Journal of Medicine* **353** (25), 2643–53.

National Institute for Clinical Excellence (2004). Clopidogrel in the treatment of non-ST-segment-elevation acute coronary syndrome. *Technology Appraisal 80.* London: National Institute for Clinical Excellence.

National Institute for Health and Clinical Excellence (2007). Type 2 diabetes (update): *National Clinical Guideline for the Management in Primary and Secondary Care.* London: National Institute for Health and Clinical Excellence.

Neal B et al. (2000). Effects of ACE inhibitors, calcium antagonists, and other blood-pressure-lowering drugs: results of prospectively designed overviews of randomised trials. Blood Pressure Lowering Treatment Trialists' Collaboration. *Lancet* **356** (9246), 1955–64.

Nelson EA et al. (2006). A series of systematic reviews to inform a decision analysis for sampling and treating infected diabetic foot ulcers. *Health Technology Assessment* **10** (12), iii–iv, ix–x, 1–221.

Nicolucci A et al. (2007). Aspirin and Simvastatin Combination for Cardiovascular Events Prevention Trial in Diabetes (ACCEPT-D): design of a randomized study of the efficacy of low-dose aspirin in the prevention of cardiovascular events in subjects with diabetes mellitus treated with statins. *European Heart Journal* **28** (16), 1925–7.

Nield L et al. (2007). Dietary advice for treatment of type 2 diabetes mellitus in adults. *Cochrane Database Systematic Reviews* (3), CD004097.

Nissen SE, Wolski K (2007). Effect of rosiglitazone on the risk of myocardial infarction and death from cardiovascular causes. *New England Journal of Medicine* **356** (24), 2457–71.

Norris S et al. (2005). Pharmacotherapy for weight loss in adults with type 2 diabetes mellitus. *Cochrane Database of Systematic Reviews* (3), CD004096.

Parving HH et al. (2001) Irbesartan in patients with type 2 diabetes and microalbuminuria study group. *New England Journal of Medicine* **345** (12), 870–8.

Parving HH et al. (2008). Aliskiren combined with losartan in type 2 diabetes and nephropathy. *New England Journal of Medicine* **358** (23), 2433–46.

Patel A et al. (2008). Intensive blood glucose control and vascular outcomes in patients with type 2 diabetes. *New England Journal of Medicine* **358** (24), 2560–72.

Patel A et al. (2007). Effects of a fixed combination of perindopril and indapamide on macrovascular and microvascular outcomes in patients with type 2 diabetes mellitus (the ADVANCE trial): a randomised controlled trial. *Lancet* **370** (9590), 829–40.

Patel J (2006). Dyslipidaemia in diabetes. *British Medical Journal Clinical Evidence* **2006** (12), 610.

Pittas AG et al. (2006). Insulin therapy and in-hospital mortality in critically ill patients: systematic review and meta-analysis of randomized controlled trials. *Journal of Parenteral and Enteral Nutrition* **30** (2), 164–72.

PKC-DRS Study Group (2005). The effect of ruboxistaurin on visual loss in patients with moderately severe to very severe nonproliferative diabetic retinopathy: initial results of the Protein Kinase C beta Inhibitor Diabetic Retinopathy Study (PKC-DRS) multicenter randomized clinical trial. *Diabetes* **54** (7), 2188–97.

Raikou M et al. (2007). Cost-effectiveness of primary prevention of cardiovascular disease with atorvastatin in type 2 diabetes: results from the Collaborative Atorvastatin Diabetes Study (CARDS). *Diabetologia* **50** (4), 733–40.

Raynor P et al. (2004). A new clinical trial of the effect of larval therapy. *Journal of Tissue Viability* **14** (3), 104–5.

Raz I et al. (2009). Effects of prandial versus fasting glycemia on cardiovascular outcomes in type 2 diabetes: The HEART2D trial. *Diabetes Care* **32**, 381–6.

Scheen AJ et al. (2006). Efficacy and tolerability of rimonabant in overweight or obese patients with type 2 diabetes: a randomised controlled study. *Lancet* **368** (9548), 1660–72.

Schrier R et al. (2002). Effects of aggressive blood pressure control in normotensive type 2 diabetic patients on albuminuria, retinopathy and strokes. *Kidney International* **61**, 1086–97.

Schwartz TB, Meinert CL (2004). The UGDP controversy: thirty-four years of contentious ambiguity laid to rest. *Perspectives in Biology and Medicine* **47** (4), 564–74.

Seltzer HS (1972). Avoiding the pitfalls of long-term therapeutic trials: lessons learned from the UGDP study. *Journal of Clinical Pharmacol New Drugs* **12** (10), 393–8.

Shepherd J et al. (2006). Effect of lowering LDL cholesterol substantially below currently recommended levels in patients with coronary heart disease and diabetes: the Treating to New Targets (TNT) study. *Diabetes Care* **29** (6), 1220–6.

Shichiri M et al. (2000). Long-term results of the Kumamoto Study on optimal diabetes control in type 2 diabetic patients. *Diabetes Care* **23** (Suppl. 2), B21–9.

Shiplak M (2007). Diabetic nephropathy. *British Medical Journal Clinical Evidence* **12**, 606.

Sigal R et al. (2006). Prevention of cardiovascular events in diabetes. *British Medical Journal Clinical Evidence* **2**, 601.

Sjostrom L et al. (2007). Effects of bariatric surgery on mortality in Swedish obese subjects. *New England Journal of Medicine* **357** (8), 741–52.

Smith C et al. (2007). The effectiveness of non-surgical interventions in the treatment of Charcot foot. *International Journal of Evidence-Based Healthcare* **5**, 437–49.

Smith J (2002). Debridement of diabetic foot ulcers. *Cochrane Database Systematic Reviews* (4), CD003556.

Smith SC Jr et al. (2006). AHA/ACC guidelines for secondary prevention for patients with coronary and other atherosclerotic vascular disease: 2006 update: endorsed by the National Heart, Lung, and Blood Institute. *Circulation* **113** (19), 2363–72.

Spencer S (2000). Pressure relieving interventions for preventing and treating diabetic foot ulcers. *Cochrane Database Systematic Reviews* (3), CD002302.

Staessen JA et al. (1997). Randomised double-blind comparison of placebo and active treatment for older patients with isolated systolic hypertension. The Systolic Hypertension in Europe (Syst-Eur) Trial Investigators. *Lancet* **350**, 757–64.

Stratton I et al. (2000). Association of glycaemia with macrovascular and microvascular complications of Type 2 diabetes (UKPDS 35). *British Medical Journal* **321**, 405–11.

Strippoli GF et al. (2006). Angiotensin converting enzyme inhibitors and angiotensin II receptor antagonists for preventing the progression of diabetic kidney disease. *Cochrane Database Systematic Reviews* (4), CD006257.

Tang JL et al. (1998). Systematic review of dietary intervention trials to lower blood total cholesterol in free-living subjects. *British Medical Journal* **316** (7139), 1213–20.

Torp-Pedersen C et al. (2007). Cardiovascular responses to weight management and sibutramine in high-risk subjects: an analysis from the SCOUT trial. *European Heart Journal* **28**(23), 2915–23.

Tuomilehto J et al. (1999). Effect of calcium-channel blockade in older patients with diabetes and systolic hypertension. *New England Journal of Medicine* **340**, 677–84.

Turnbull F et al. (2005). Effects of different blood pressure-lowering regimens on major cardiovascular events in individuals with and without diabetes mellitus: results of prospectively designed overviews of randomized trials. *Archives of Internal Medicine* **165** (12), 1410–9.

UKPDS Group (1998a). Effect of intensive blood-glucose control with metformin on complications in overweight patients with type 2 diabetes (UKPDS 34). *Lancet* **352**, 854–65.

UKPDS Group (1998b). Intensive blood-glucose control with sulphonylureas or insulin compared with conventional treatment and risk of complications in patients with type 2 diabetes (UKPDS 33). *Lancet* **352**, 837–53.

UKPDS Group (1998c). Tight blood pressure control and risk of macrovascular and microvascular complications in type 2 diabetes (UKPDS 38). *British Medical Journal* **317**, 703–13.

Valk GD et al. (2005). Patient education for preventing diabetic foot ulceration. *Cochrane Database Systematic Reviews* (1), CD001488.

Viberti G, Wheeldon NM (2002). Microalbuminuria reduction with valsartan in patients with type 2 diabetes mellitus: a blood pressure-independent effect. *Circulation* **106** (6), 672–8.

Vijan S (2007). Diabetes: treating hypertension. *British Medical Journal Clinical Evidence* **10**, 608.

Wang J et al. (2000). Chinese trial on isolated systolic hypertension in the elderly. Systolic Hypertension in China (Syst-China) Collaborative Group. *Archives of Internal Medicine* **160**, 211–20.

Wang TH et al. (2007). An analysis of mortality rates with dual-antiplatelet therapy in the primary prevention population of the CHARISMA trial. *European Heart Journal* **28** (18), 2200–7.

Way KJ et al. (2001). Protein kinase C and the development of diabetic vascular complications. *Diabetic Medicine* **18** (12), 945–59.

Weiss N. (1996). *Clinical Epidemiology: the Study of the Outcome of Illness*. Oxford: Oxford University Press.

Whelton PK et al. (2005). Clinical outcomes in antihypertensive treatment of type 2 diabetes, impaired fasting glucose concentration, and normoglycemia: Antihypertensive and Lipid-Lowering Treatment to Prevent Heart Attack Trial (ALLHAT). *Archives of Internal Medicine* **165** (12), 1401–9.

Witt N et al. (2006). Abnormalities of retinal microvascular structure and risk of mortality from ischemic heart disease and stroke. *Hypertension* **47** (5), 975–81.

Yamagishi S et al. (2007). A novel pleiotropic effect of atorvastatin on advanced glycation end product (AGE)-related disorders. *Medical Hypotheses* **69** (2), 338–40.

Yusuf S et al. (2001). Effects of clopidogrel in addition to aspirin in patients with acute coronary syndromes without ST-segment elevation. *New England Journal of Medicine* **345** (7), 494–502.

Zhu X et al. (2007). Risks of proteinuria and hypertension with bevacizumab, an antibody against vascular endothelial growth factor: systematic review and meta-analysis. *American Journal of Kidney Disease* **49**, 186–93.

18. QUALITY OF DIABETES CARE (CURRENT LEVELS, DISTRIBUTION, AND TRENDS) AND CHALLENGES IN MEASURING QUALITY OF CARE

Leonard M. Pogach and David C. Aron

■ Main Public Health Messages

- The Institute of Medicine defines "quality" as "the degree to which health services for individuals and populations increase the likelihood of desired health outcomes and are consistent with current professional knowledge."
- Clinical practice recommendations are based on evaluation of evidence of varying strengths: that is, randomized clinical trials, post hoc epidemiologic analyses, and expert opinion.
- Public health systems and payers/systems of care may have differing perspectives on what measures to choose based on their missions and available data sources.
- When systems or health care providers are compared or compensated, a greater strength of evidence is required than if the purpose of measurement is for quality improvement (internal use). In addition, special care must be taken to ensure that the same types of patients are compared. This may require more stringent technical specifications, for example, inclusion/exclusion criteria, risk adjustment, and/or stratification.
- In the evaluation of trends in any measurement, caution must be taken when serial cross sections are used. Trends within health care plans may reflect changes in the population, for example, in-/out-migration of sicker patients, rather than changes in quality of health care delivery.

The views expressed are solely those of the authors and do not necessarily reflect the views of the Department of Veterans Affairs.

- Although all-or-none intermediate outcome measures are currently used by both public health systems and payers/systems of care to evaluate quality, such dichotomous threshold measures have significant limitations, and thus more sophisticated measures need to be developed. These new measures should address issues of longitudinal results and continuous rather than dichotomous results.

  - Widespread implementation of the next generation of quality measures will depend on greater adoption and interoperability of electronic medical record systems.
  - The development of measures for the more humanistic aspects of care in diabetes, such as shared decision making and patient centeredness, has lagged behind the development of the more easily quantifiable aspects of diabetes care.
  - Limitations of current measures notwithstanding, there are significant deficiencies in the overall quality of care for diabetes.
  - There are significant differences in the quality of care related to gender (male/female) and ethnic background. Disparities persist even when access to care seems comparable.

■ Introduction

This chapter summarizes current definitions and approaches used in assessing the quality of diabetes care and the underlying conceptual frameworks, evidence base, and methodological issues. The chapter also summarizes both current levels and trends in the quality of diabetes care in the United States, with specific attention paid to variation and disparities by patient subgroup. Finally, we address the policy implications of quality measurement for the purpose of improving care within a health care system versus measuring quality for the purpose of public comparisons and/or payment.

■ Background/Historical Perspective

Frameworks for Assessment of Quality and Domains of Quality

The modern era of quality assessment in health care began with the work of Avedis Donabedian, who developed a framework of structure, processes, and outcomes of care based on the underlying theory that good structure increases the likelihood of good process, and good process increases the likelihood of good outcome (Donabedian 1966). This model has been adapted by many groups, including the World Health Organization (WHO), Institute of Medicine (IOM), and Organization for Economic Cooperation and Development (OECD). Structures, which are "the attributes of material resources ... human resources and ... organizational structure" (Donabedian 1966), include physical facilities and equipment, staffing and staff qualifications and training, information systems, and many other elements. For example, in diabetes these might include the existence of a diabetes clinical registry or the ratio of certified diabetes educators to patients. Processes are the actions taken by providers (and patients) in such domains as health promotion, illness prevention, and illness management. For example, the proportion of patients with diabetes whose hemoglobin A1C has been recorded in the previous 12 months is a measure of process. Sibthorpe and others have suggested that processes of care be distinguished from organizational processes, rather than being combined with them, because there are many important organizational processes worthy of identification and monitoring that do not involve direct patient care (Sibthorpe 2004). For example monitoring A1C levels in the management of diabetes, a process of care, would be facilitated by the establishment of a clinical registry, a structural variable. In terms of outcomes these run the gamut of the "5Ds"—death, disease, disability, discomfort, and dissatisfaction—each of which can be parsed in many different ways.

Diabetes lends itself to measurement of intermediate outcomes, for example, the proportion of patients with diabetes in whom the last A1C is <9% or LDL-C (low-density lipoprotein cholesterol) is <100 mg/dL or systolic blood pressure is <140 mm Hg in the previous 12 months. There are different perspectives of quality: professional, managerial (provider and purchaser), patient, and societal. Consequently different stakeholders may reasonably hold different opinions as to whether to include other domains of quality, for example, efficiency (the relationship between resource inputs, that is, costs, and intermediate or final health outcomes) and equity (is it the same for everyone?) (Institute of Medicine 1990, 2001a) . It is with this background that we examine further the IOM's approach, which cited Donabedian's conceptualization as its "unifying conceptual framework for quality measurement and assurance" (Institute of Medicine 1990).

The IOM report defined quality as "the degree to which health services for individuals and populations increase the likelihood of desired health outcomes and are consistent with current professional knowledge" (Institute of Medicine 1990). Of interest this definition includes both individuals and populations and recognizes that increasing the *likelihood* of desired health outcomes is not synonymous with *actually* increasing desired health outcomes. In a landmark 2001 publication the IOM expanded the conceptual framework for quality and measurement to include six domains: effectiveness ["providing services based on scientific knowledge to all who could benefit, and refraining from providing services to those not likely to benefit (avoiding overuse and underuse)"], equity ["providing health care of equal quality to those who may differ in personal characteristics other than their clinical condition or preferences for care"], patient safety ["avoiding injuries or harms to patients from care that is intended to help them"], patient-centered care ["establishing a partnership among practitioners, patients, and their families (when appropriate) to ensure that decisions respect patients' wants, needs, and preferences and that patients have the education and support they require to make decisions and participate in their own care"], timeliness ["obtaining needed care and minimizing unnecessary delays in getting that care"], and efficiency, that is, cost-effectiveness (Institute of Medicine 2001a, 2001b). Efficiency was noted but not included in the conceptual framework of 2001, but it was specifically addressed in a later report on pay for performance (Institute of Medicine 2006). The development and endorsement of quality of care measures for diabetes by various organizations and coalitions led to their widespread usage by payers, health care systems, and accrediting organizations and thus need to be placed in the context of evolving societal, industry, and academic perspectives on the science and purpose of measurement over the past 40 years, but primarily since the 1990s. As Donabedian noted, ". . . the definition of quality may be almost anything anyone wishes it to be, although it is, ordinarily a reflection of values and goals current in the medical care system and in the larger society of which it is part" (Donabedian 1966).

The Evolution of Measures to Assess the Quality of Diabetes Care

In 1990 the U.S. Department of Health and Human Services released *Healthy People 2000: National Health Promotion and Disease Prevention Objectives,* thereby taking the lead on public health measures specific for diabetes. One of the document's priority areas, "Diabetes and Chronic Disabling Conditions," relied upon several national data sources, including the National Health Interview Survey, the National Health and Nutrition Examination Survey (NHANES), National Hospital Discharge Survey, National Vital Statistics System—Mortality Component, and Behavioral Risk Factor Surveillance Survey (BRFSS) (Donabedian 1983; U.S. Department of Health and Human Services 2008). *Healthy People 2010*, the successor to *Healthy People 2000*, used a framework of primary, secondary, and tertiary prevention (Donabedian 1983; U.S. Department of Health and Human Services 2008). As shown in Table 18.1, *Healthy People 2010* has an emphasis on process measures, which was based not only on low rates of screening for intermediate outcomes and complications and poor control of risk factors for microvascular and macrovascular disease but also on ease of data collection (Harris 1996, 2002; Saaddine et al. 2002; Tseng et al. 2007a). Surveillance leads to earlier identification of diabetic nephropathy, neuropathy, peripheral vascular disease, and retinopathy, thus enabling interventions that can result in decreasing rates of dialysis, lower-extremity complications (ulcers and amputations), and significant visual loss. During the midcourse correction of *Healthy People 2010*, several objectives (including those for foot ulcers and gestational diabetes) had to be eliminated because of the unavailability of data.

From the early to late 1990s, a number of landmark studies such as the Diabetes Control and Complications Trial (DCCT), United Kingdom Prospective Diabetes Study (UKPDS), Scandinavian Simvastatin Survival Study (4S), West of Scotland

TABLE 18.1   *Diabetes Measures in Healthy People 2000 (and 2010)*

Goal: *Through prevention programs, reduce the disease and economic burden of diabetes, and improve the quality of life for all persons who have or are at risk for diabetes*

Number	Short Title of Objective
5-1	Diabetes education
5-2	New cases of diabetes
5-3	Overall cases of diagnosed diabetes
5-4	Diagnosis of diabetes
5-5	Diabetes deaths
5-6	Diabetes-related deaths
5-7	Cardiovascular disease deaths in persons with diabetes
5-8	Gestational diabetes*
5-9	Foot ulcers*
5-10	Lower-extremity amputations
5-11	Annual urinary microalbumin measurement
5-12	Annual glycosylated hemoglobin measurement
5-13	Annual dilated eye examinations
5-14	Annual foot examinations
5-15	Annual dental examinations
5-16	Aspirin therapy
5-17	Self-blood-glucose monitoring

*Eliminated, midcourse correction, due to lack of data source. See http://www.healthypeople.gov/data/midcourse/html/focusareas/FA05Objectives.htm.

Source: *Healthy People 2010 Diabetes*. Centers for Disease Control and Prevention, National Institutes of Health. http://www.healthypeople.gov/document/html/volume1/05diabetes.htm.

Coronary Prevention Study (WOSCOPS), Hypertension Optimal Treatment (HOT) Study, and the Renal Outcomes substudy of the Heart Outcomes Prevention Evaluation (HOPE) study (MICRO-HOPE) demonstrated that better control of glycemia, blood pressure, and LDL-C levels leads to a marked reduction in microvascular and macrovascular events and that specific medications such as statins, angiotensin-converting enzyme (ACE) inhibitors, and angiotensin receptor blockers (ARBs) decrease cardiovascular morbidity and mortality. These findings provided the basis for some process measures, for example, proportion of patients with

diabetes and hypertension taking an ACE inhibitor or ARB, and, more important, intermediate outcome measures related to levels of A1C, LDL-C, and blood
pressure.

The development of practice guidelines by a variety of organizations, both
governmental and professional, that were based on these and other studies pro-
ceeded apace (Lohr et al. 1998). However, different people can draw different
conclusions from the same evidence; not surprisingly, recommendations from different groups/agencies/professional societies/institutions differed (Hayward et al.
2005; Pogach et al. 2004). The Veterans Health Administration—Department of
Defense Guidelines, initially published in 1997, were the first to incorporate systematic reviews and provide explicit grading of evidence as well as to introduce
the concept of life expectancy and adjustment for severity of disease and complex
comorbid conditions (Pogach et al. 2004). The first comprehensive approach to
developing diabetes-specific "performance measures" was undertaken in the late
1990s by the Diabetes Quality Improvement Program (DQIP), a federal–private
sector coalition (Fleming et al. 2001). However, the ability to "translate" evidence-
based practice recommendations from guidelines was problematic due to issues of
data acquisition (frequent unavailability of data and/or the cost of collecting data)
and reliability. Indeed despite the potential of electronic medical records, abstraction of paper records remains the industry standard. Consequently the DQIP
developed a *parsimonious* set of measures that were both evidence based and easily obtainable from medical records. These included process measures for surveillance, including the performance of eye and foot examinations, monitoring for
nephropathy status, and obtaining laboratory tests (also a process measure) necessary to assess intermediate outcomes (A1C, LDL-C). The undesirable threshold
levels for intermediate outcomes were "poor" A1C ($\geq$9.5%), LDL-C ($\geq$130 mg/dL),
and blood pressure ($\geq$140/90 mm Hg). The threshold levels for these last three
measures had the strongest level of evidence in that they would be applicable for
all persons with diabetes and thus would not require risk adjustment or stratification. Furthermore if an A1C or LDL-C test was not recorded, then the measure
was considered "not met," thus avoiding intentional or unintentional selection
biases.

Finally, DQIP recommended a survey to collect smoking status and smoking cessation status. These measures were proposed by DQIP for public reporting (see Table 18.2), and eventually all were adapted or endorsed by other groups
(see Table 18.3). The National Committee for Quality Assurance—HEDIS (Health
Plan Employer Data and Information Set) incorporated those DQIP accountability
measures that could be obtained from administrative data into its Comprehensive
Care Module. This set of measures was the first nationally developed program to
include intermediate outcomes. A distinction was made between measures used
for accountability, that is, measures used externally for comparisons of different
health plans or providers and measures for improvement, that is, measures used
internally as part of quality improvement efforts (Berwick, James, and Coyne

TABLE 18.2   *DQIP 1.0 Measure Set*

- Accountability
  - From medical records or electronic data
    - HbA1c tested (annually)*
    - Poor HbA1c control (HbA1c ≥9.5%)*
    - Eye examination performed (high-risk annually, low-risk biennially)*
    - Lipid profile performed (biennially)*
    - Lipids controlled (LDL <130 mg/dL)*
    - Monitoring for diabetic nephropathy (high-risk annually, low-risk biennially)*
    - Blood pressure controlled (<140/90 mm Hg)*
    - Foot examination (annually)
  - From patient survey
    - Smoking cessation counseling (annually)
- Quality Improvement
  - From medical records or electronic data
    - Distribution of values for HbA1c (<7.0, 7.0–7.9, 8.0–8.9, 9.0–9.9, ≥10.0%, or undocumented)
    - Distribution of values for LDL cholesterol (<100, 100–129, 130–159, ≥160 mg/dL, or undocumented)
    - Distribution of values for blood pressure (<140, 141–159, 160–179, 180–209, ≥210 mm Hg systolic; <90, 90–99, 100–109, 110–119, ≥120 mm Hg diastolic, or no value documented)
  - From patient survey
    - Diabetes self-management and nutrition education
    - Interpersonal care

* Included in the NCQA Diabetes Comprehensive Care HEDIS Measures 2000.
LDL, low-density lipoprotein; HbA1c, glycosylated hemoglobin.

Source: Fleming et al. 2001.

2003). Consequently lower threshold levels of A1C (e.g., <8%, <7%), blood pressure (e.g., <130/80 mm Hg), and cholesterol (e.g., <100 mg/dL) were recommended by DQIP for internal quality improvement, with the hope that over time methodologies would be developed that would enable public reporting without biases associated with factors beyond the plans' control, such as duration and severity of disease (see Table 18.2).

TABLE 18.3 *Comparison of Quality Measures for Diabetes*

Measure/Most Recent Update	NCQA (2009)[1]	Alliance (2005)[*2]	CMS/PQRI (2010)[3]	AQA (2005)[4]	NQF Endorse (2010)[5]
HbA1C					
% with ≥ 1 HbA1C measure	☐	✓	✓	✓	✓
% with HbA1C > 9.0%	✓	✓		✓	✓
% with HbA1C < 8.0%[†]	✓				✓
% with A1C <7.0%[†]	✓				
# of HbA1C tests per patient		QI			
Distribution of HbA1C tests done		QI			
Trend of HbA1C values		QI			
Distribution of HbA1C values		QI			
Adults taking insulin with evidence of self-monitoring					✓
Lipids (mg/dL)					
% with ≥ 1 LDL measure	✓	✓	✓	✓	✓
% with LDL < 100	✓	✓	✓	✓	✓
% with LDL < 100 or on statin		QI			
% with LDL < 130		✓			✓

(continued)

TABLE 18.3 (*continued*)

Measure/Most Recent Update	NCQA (2009)[1]	Alliance (2005)*[2]	CMS/PQRI (2010)[3]	AQA (2005)[4]	NQF Endorse (2010)[5]
% with LDL < 130 or on statin		QI			
Trend of LDL values		QI			
Distribution of LDL values		QI			
% with ≥ full lipid panel		QI			
Blood pressure control					
% with BP < 140/80 mm Hg		✓	✓		✓
% with BP < 140/90 mm Hg	✓				
% with BP <130/80 mm Hg	✓	QI			
Most recent BP		✓			✓
Distribution of BP values		QI			✓
% patients on ≥ 3 meds for BP		QI			
Nephropathy					
Documentation of treatment for nephropathy OR	✓	✓			✓
% with ≥ 1 urine microalbumin OR	✓	✓	✓		✓
% w/ m'alb or on ACEI/ARB	✓	QI	✓		✓

(*continued*)

TABLE 18.3 *(continued)*

Measure/Most Recent Update	NCQA (2009)[1]	Alliance (2005)[*2]	CMS/PQRI (2010)[3]	AQA (2005)[4]	NQF Endorse (2010)[5]
Eye exam			✓		✓
% with annual or (biennial for low risk) dilated eye exam			✓	✓	✓
% with annual dilated exam	✓	✓			
% communication from ophth. to PCP			✓		
Foot exam					
% with foot examination (visual, pulse, or monofilament)	✓		✓		✓
% with ≥ neurological exam of lower extremities	QI		✓		
% who were evaluated for proper footwear and sizing			✓		
Foot care and education					✓
Tobacco use					
% smoking status ascertained	✓	✓			
% smokers offered advice to quit			✓		
% smokers offered smoking cessation	QI				

(continued)

TABLE 18.3   (*continued*)

Measure/Most Recent Update	NCQA (2009)[1]	Alliance (2005)[*2]	CMS/PQRI (2010)[3]	AQA (2005)[4]	NQF Endorse (2010)[5]
Aspirin use					
% receiving aspirin ≥ 75 mg/d		QI			
Influenza					
% received flu shot	✓	QI			

[1]National Committee for Quality Assurance. HEDIS 2009. Available at: http://www.ncqa.org/tabid/784/Default.aspx. Accessed November 2, 2008.

[2]National Quality Forum. 2006. National Voluntary Consensus Standards for Adult Diabetes Care: 2005 Update. Available at http://www.qualityforum.org/publications/reports/diabetes_update.asp. Accessed November 2, 2008.

[3]2010 PQRI Measures List. https://www.cms.gov/PQRI/Downloads/2010_PQRI_MeasuresList_111309.pdf. Accessed May 3, 2010.

[4]US Department of Health and Human Services (2006). Agency for Healthcare Research and Quality. Recommended Starter Set. The Ambulatory Care Quality Alliance. Clinical Performance Measures for Ambulatory Care. Available at: http://www.ahrq.gov/qual/aqastart.htm. Accessed November 2, 2008.

[5]http://www.qualityforum.org/Measures_List.aspx#k=diabetes&e=1&st=&sd=&s=&p=6

[*]Quality improvement (QI) measures were not designated as accountability measures because of concerns over data completeness, e.g., patients obtaining flu shots in nonmedical settings.

[†]First-year measures for 2009, will not be publicly reported.

m'alb, microalbumin; ACEI, angiotensin-converting enzyme inhibitor; ARB, angiotensin receptor blocking agent; PCP, primary care physician.

A great deal of discussion revolved around the establishment of these measures and the level of care that would be acceptable. DQIP recognized that the evidence base for defining "optimal" care for patients was problematic because even in the clinical trials that were cited, about half of subjects will be "above the mean." In addition trial values vary over time. For example in the UKPDS (1998), the average A1C over 10 years was 7.0%, but the average A1C was 7.3% in the last year of the study. Thus, choosing a single A1C value at one point in time as representing "optimal care," and not considering marginal benefit, was neither reflective of the study design nor its results. It is also worth noting that the concept of "optimal" care as a benchmark for "quality of care" is not without its critics. For example in 1983 Donabedian wrote:

> At the very least the optimal strategy balances the expected benefit and harm from technical interventions. Health care practitioners tend to specify optimal strategies based on what they consider to be best for patients, without regard to monetary cost. This is an absolutist definition of quality. Individuals may place different valuations on the outcomes, are concerned with the monetary costs to themselves, and are particularly sensitive to the attributes of the

interpersonal relationship with the practitioners. Including all of these leads to an individualized definition of the quality of care. But this specification of quality may be in conflict with a social definition of quality, which takes into account social as well as individual monetary costs, externalities, and the social distribution of quality. (Donabedian 1983)

Notwithstanding these issues the National Diabetes Quality Improvement Alliance (the successor to DQIP) lowered the level of poor A1C to 9.0%, blood pressure to 140/80 mm Hg (the same systolic pressure but a drop in the diastolic), and added a new threshold LDL-C level of 100 mg/dL while maintaining the LDL-C level of 130 mg/dL (Ahmann 2007; Sanderson and Dixon 2000). Measures of smoking cessation and of vaccination against influenza and pneumonia were not recommended for public accountability (a decision related to data issues) but were already part of the broader National Committee for Quality Assurance (NCQA)–HEDIS measures (Ahmann 2007). Because measures of aspirin use and diabetes education would require surveys, they were not implemented because of concerns of cost and response bias. In May 2006 the NCQA included measures of optimal systolic blood pressure (<130 mm Hg) and glycemic control (A1C <7%) for public reporting in 2008. Other organizations and coalitions, such as the National Quality Forum, the Physicians Consortium of the American Medical Association, and the Ambulatory Care Quality Alliance, have not included so-called optimal measures, which remain a matter of controversy (Ahmann 2007; Hayward 2007; Pogach et al. 2007a). Indeed, because of results from the ACCORD (Action to Control Cardiovascular Risk in Diabetes) study (Action to Control Cardiovascular Risk in Diabetes Study 2008), the ADVANCE (Action in Diabetes and Vascular Disease) study (ADVANCE Collaborative Group 2008), and the Veterans Affairs Diabetes Trial (Duckworth 2008), NCQA recently changed its policy by eliminating the 2008 reporting requirement for A1C of <7%. Instead, it has decided to add an indicator for A1C of <8% and refine the indicator for A1C <7% by adding exclusions for members within a specific age cohort who have certain comorbid conditions (HEDIS 2008). It is likely that the findings of the ACCORD trial (and others) for intensive blood pressure control and lipid therapy will influence and result in modification of existing measures (ACCORD Study Group, 2010a, 2010b) Although it is clear that the development and adoption of performance measurement are aspects of an evolving process that is in response to the evidence, it is also clear that the rationale by which organizations do so is neither explicit nor shared with external stakeholders (Aron and Pogach 2008).

Table 18.3 lists measures, all related to ambulatory care, that are currently endorsed or implemented by national organizations. Beyond these measures, in 2001 the Agency for Healthcare Research and Quality proposed Preventive Quality Indicators based on hospitalization rates for those conditions "for which the provision of timely and effective outpatient care prior to hospitalization" could prevent the hospitalization (Sanderson and Dixon 2000). Hospitalizations for uncontrolled diabetes, diabetic ketoacidosis, and lower-extremity amputations specifically

TABLE 18.4   *AHRQ National Healthcare Quality Report*

1.16. Adults age 40 and over with diabetes who had all three (3) recommended services—hemoglobin A1C test, retinal eye exam, and foot exam.

1.17. Adults age 40 and over with diabetes who had a hemoglobin A1C measurement at least once in past year.

1.18. Adults age 40 and over with diabetes who had a lipid profile in past 2 years.

1.19. Adults age 40 and over with diabetes who had a retinal eye examination in past year.

1.20. Adults age 40 and over with diabetes who had a foot examination in past year.

1.21. Adults with diabetes who had an influenza immunization in past year.

1.22. Adults age 40 and over with diagnosed diabetes whose hemoglobin A1C level is < 7.0% (optimal).

1.23. Adults age 40 and over with diagnosed diabetes whose total cholesterol is < 200 mg/dL.

1.24. Adults age 40 and over with diagnosed diabetes with blood pressure < 140/80 mm Hg based on average of three measurements.

1.25. Hospital admissions for uncontrolled diabetes per 100,000 population.

1.26. Hospital admissions for short-term complications of diabetes per 100,000 population.

1.27. Hospital admissions for long-term complications of diabetes per 100,000 population.

1.28. Hospital admissions for lower-extremity amputations in patients with diabetes per 1000 population.

related to diabetes were intended for surveillance purposes, primarily by communities (National Committee for Quality Assurance 2007; U.S. Department of Health and Human Services 2007a). From a public health perspective, the Agency for Healthcare Research and Quality *National Healthcare Quality Report, 2006* combines elements of HEDIS, Preventive Quality Indicators, and the *Healthy People 2010* section on public health measures for diabetes (U.S. Department of Health and Human Services 2007c). These are shown in Table 18.4. Patient-centered care is a key component of diabetes management, and the Consumer Assessment of Health Plans Survey includes many of the domains of patient-centered care (Hays et al. 1999). However, although the importance of multidisciplinary care, the need for participatory decision making, and the issue of satisfaction with care have been well studied in the literature, no current diabetes-specific surveys have been used within the performance measurement industry.

Finally, an evolving evidence base indicating that improvements in in-hospital glycemic control lead to improved mortality, especially in the intensive care setting

(Van den Bergh et al. 2001, 2006), led to inpatient guidelines for glycemic control and proposals for related measures. However, concerns over the methodologies for this approach (Goldberg et al. 2006), the strength of evidence (Weiner, Weiner, and Larson 2008), and generalization beyond surgical intensive care units, where glycemic control can be more precisely monitored, remain matters of discussion. Thus although other domains of quality are important, most quality measurement has focused on ambulatory care measures of process and/or intermediate outcomes for the purpose of measuring "quality" on a population basis or among health care systems (Geiss et al. 2005; Landon et al. 2003; National Committee for Quality Assurance 2007), while public health efforts have included surveillance for advanced complications (dialysis, blindness, amputations) and death (U.S. Department of Health and Human Services 2007b, 2008).

■ Quality of Diabetes Care in the United States: Public Health and Health Care System Perspectives

Current State and Trends

In the United States the population health of persons with diabetes is assessed within the Department of Health and Human Services by the *Healthy People 2010* initiative (the agencies responsible are the National Institute of Diabetes and Digestive and Kidney Diseases and the Centers for Disease Control and Prevention) and by the Agency for Healthcare Research and Quality's *National Healthcare Disparities Report* (U.S. Department of Health and Human Services 2005; Institute of Medicine 2002; U.S. Department of Health and Human Services 2006; U.S. Department of Health and Human Services 2000). Process and intermediate outcome measures are derived from two federally funded, nationally representative surveys: NHANES and BRFSS (CDC 2007a, 2007b). In the NHANES, which consists of nationally representative samples of the U.S. civilian, noninstitutionalized population, samples are obtained using a stratified multistage probability design with planned over-sampling of older and minority groups. Household interviews are conducted to ascertain sociodemographic characteristics and medical and family history, followed by clinical examinations conducted at a mobile examination center. In contrast BRFSS is an ongoing random-digit telephone survey of the noninstitutionalized U.S. adult population in each of the 50 states and the District of Columbia.

The most comprehensive and recent evaluation of changes in the quality of diabetes care is based on analyses of the 1988–1994 NHANES (NHANES III), NHANES 1999–2002, and the BRFSS 1995 and 2002 surveys (Saaddine et al. 2006; Table 18.5). Despite increasing recognition of the effect of diabetes on the health of the U.S. population, among most demographic groups, regardless of health care setting, there has been only modest improvement in the control of process and intermediate outcomes from the 1990s to the early 2000s. Encouragingly, during this period the percentage of individuals with A1C levels between 6% and 8% increased

TABLE 18.5 *Proportion of Persons with Diabetes 18 to 75 Years of Age Who Received Processes and Intermediate Outcomes of Care for Diabetes: National Health and Nutrition Examination Survey, 1988–1994 and 1999–2002, and Behavioral Risk Factors Surveillance System, 1995 and 2002**

Indicator	Baseline Surveys (1990s), %	Recent Surveys (2000s), %	Absolute Change (95% CI), Percentage Points
National Diabetes Quality Improvement Alliance indicators			
Hemoglobin A1C >9.0%	24.5	20.6	–3.9 (–10.4 to 2.5)
Annual lipid profile	76.3	84.6	8.3 (4.0 to 12.7)
LDL cholesterol level <3.4 mmol/L (<130 mg/dL)	42.4	64.2	21.9 (12.4 to 31.3)
Blood pressure < 140/90 mm Hg	67.6	68.0	0.4 (–6.0 to 6.7)
Absence of microalbuminuria	65.2	66.9	1.7 (–4.0 to 7.3)
Annual dilated eye examination	63.2	67.7	4.5 (0.5 to 8.5)
Annual foot examination	64.5	68.3	3.8 (–0.1 to 7.7)
Annual influenza vaccination	45.7	52.5	6.8 (2.9 to 10.7)
Aspirin therapy[†]	32.0	45.1	13.1 (5.4 to 20.7)
Smokers	20.0	19.3	–0.7 (–4.6 to 3.1)
Smokers who are trying to quit smoking	43.6	62.2	18.7 (7.6 to 29.7)
Additional indicators			
Pneumococcal vaccination	26.5	43.0	16.5 (12.7 to 20.2)
Diabetes education	NA	54.9	
Self-monitoring blood glucose level (at least once daily)	38.5	55.1	16.6 (12.7 to 20.5)
Annual dental examination	57.6	57.0	–0.6 (–6.4 to 5.3)

*LDL = low-density lipoprotein.
[†]Behavioral Risk Factors Surveillance System 1996 survey was the baseline measure used for this analysis.

Source: Reprinted from: Saaddine JB et al. (2006). Improvements in diabetes processes of care and intermediate outcomes: United States. *Annals of Internal Medicine* **144,** 465–74.

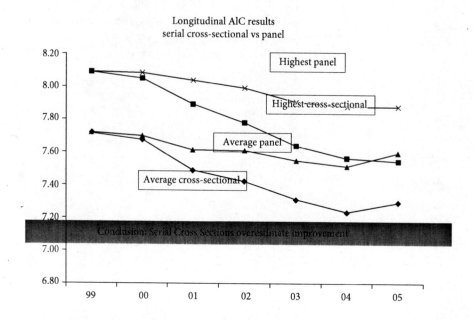

FIGURE 18.1. Comparison of trends of serial cross-sectional (within year) and longitudinal panel A1C results. A panel is comprised of continued users with longer-duration diabetes (in This panel the average duration was about 11 years), whereas the cross-sectional data include new patients as well as continued users. (From Miller and Pogach 2008.)

by about 13% to 47%, the proportion of individuals with LDL-C levels less than 3.4 mmol/L (<130 mg/dL) increased by 22% to 64%, and the frequency of aspirin use increased by 13% to 45%. However mean A1C remained unchanged, as did the percentage (about 68%) of individuals whose blood pressure was less than 140/90 mm Hg. Rates for important process measures, such as foot screening and dilated eye examinations, did not increase. Caution, however, is essential when comparing responses on cross-sectional surveys that were performed years apart, especially with an intervening change in the definition of diabetes in 1997 (which could have affected the results obtained by Saaddine and colleagues [2006]). This is illustrated in Figure 18.1, which shows the results of serial cross sections and longitudinal measures for a single cohort of patients with diabetes. Moreover changes in clinical practice could result in more patients receiving a diagnosis earlier. Because the NHANES used a sampling strategy representative of the U.S. population, we can safely extrapolate the findings to suggest that millions of Americans with diabetes are benefiting from improved glycemic and cholesterol level control, although significant deficiencies in care remain.

Improvements have also been observed within specific health care delivery systems in the private and public sectors. For example, a recent NCQA report (State of Health Care 2007) showed that from 2000 to 2009, the percentage of patients with A1C >9% dropped from 42.5% to 28.4%, from 33.4% to 29.4%, and from 54.9%

to 44.8% in commercial, Medicare, and Medicaid health care plans, respectively (National Committee for Quality Assurance 2009). Public health care systems, including the Indian Health Service, Federally Qualified Plans, and the Veterans Health Administration, as well as health maintenance organizations (HMOs) (Geiss et al. 2005; Landon et al. 2007; Wilson et al. 2005) have also reported improvements in care when benchmarked against HEDIS measures. In the case of the Veterans Health Administration cross-sectional outcomes have been demonstrated to be comparable to or in excess of commercial health care plans in direct comparisons (Kerr et al. 2004) as well as in comparisons using NCQA Quality Compass criteria (Oliver 2007).

In contrast to the large number of studies involving process or intermediate outcome measures, there are relatively few studies of longer-term outcomes. The 2006 *National Healthcare Quality Report* based on data sources noted above looked at trends in lower-extremity amputation as indicators of the quality of diabetes preventive care (U.S. Department of Health and Human Services 2007c). From 1999–2001 to 2002–2004 the overall rate of lower-extremity amputations in adults with diagnosed diabetes fell from 5.5 to 4.4 per 1000 population. By age group the declines (per 1000 people with diagnosed diabetes) were from 6.1 to 4.6 in the 45–64 group and 9.2 to 6.9 among those aged 65 or older. The *Healthy People 2010* target rate was 1.8 lower-extremity amputations per 1000 population in adults with diagnosed diabetes, however, and this has not been met, prompting a midcourse revision in the goal to 2.9 lower-extremity amputations per 1000 persons with diabetes per year (U.S. Department of Health and Human Services 2008). Moreover because denominators are population based, it is difficult to evaluate the extent to which declines in amputations result from secondary and tertiary prevention efforts versus an increase in incident diabetes over the same time period. This is a key concept to emphasize, lest an apparent decrease in rates of adverse outcomes be attributed to "improved care" when some portion of the decline is actually attributable to an increase in the denominator of persons with diabetes of more recent onset, who are unlikely to incur adverse outcomes within a 10- to 15-year period (UK Prospective Diabetes Study [UKPDS] Group 1998). This is a limitation of nonindividual-level longitudinal data that remains a methodological challenge (see below).

Disparities in Care

There are deficiencies in the quality of care for patients with diabetes generally, and these deficiencies vary by population. Ending racial/ethnic gaps in diabetes care and outcomes has been identified as a key governmental policy goal, although the definitions of disparities differ. *Healthy People 2010* states that "In pursuit of the overarching goal of eliminating health disparities, all differences among populations in measures of health and healthcare are considered evidence of disparities." In contrast, the IOM has refined and narrowed this definition to term "disparities" in health care as "differences that remain after accounting for patient's needs and preferences and the availability of health care." In the IOM's definition of quality, access to care and equity are considered to be separate domains (Institute of Medicine 2002). The *National Healthcare Disparities Report*, issued by the Agency for Healthcare Research and Quality in 2003, was the first comprehensive federal review of disparities by racial/ ethnic and socioeconomic groups (U.S. Department of Health and Human Services 2005); both stratified and multivariate analyses were included. The report found that there are multiple factors associated with poorer diabetes outcomes, including socio-economic factors, mental health conditions, access to care, and racial/ethnic/class bias, consistent with systematic reviews (Brown et al. 2004).

Given economic disparities by racial/ethnic subgroup, analyses should be per-formed both on a population basis and within systems of care in which access is comparable based upon eligibility. This requires analysis of population-based data, for example, weighted national surveys, reports from the Medicare program, and reports from comprehensive health care systems such as the Veterans Health Administration and larger HMOs.

NHANES III (1988–1994) showed some differences by race and ethnicity in health care access and utilization and in health status and outcomes for diabetic adults. However the magnitude of these differences pales in comparison with the sub-optimal health status of all three racial/ethnic groups (whites, African Americans, and Hispanics) relative to established treatment goals (Harris 1996, 2002). In the previously cited article by Saaddine and colleagues, the quality measures as defined by the National Diabetes Quality Improvement Alliance were also used to evaluate the existence of and changes in disparities in diabetes care between 1995 and 2002 based on NHANES and BRFSS (Saaddine et al. 2006) (see Table 18.6). There was some variation by demographic and clinical subgroups. For example men had sig-nificantly more improvement in the proportions receiving the flu vaccine and using aspirin than did women. Those with less than a high school education had better improvement in flu vaccination but not in aspirin use than those with more than a high school education. People who had health insurance improved in aspirin use more than those without. Although better-educated individuals with health insur-ance generally fared better, these two socioeconomic factors (education, insurance) did not consistently predict better intermediate outcomes, such as blood pressure control or LDL-C level. The proportion of people with diabetes who used insulin was also lower in the recent surveys, but this was significant only in BRFSS (i.e., not in NHANES). Overall, the analysis indicates that care remains poor overall for a substantial minority of patients: about 20% have A1C greater than 9% (with 14% having a value above 10%), 33% have uncontrolled blood pressure ($\geq$140/90 mm Hg), and 40% have poor LDL-C ($\geq$ 3.4 mmol/L [$\geq$130 mg/dL]). Fewer than 50% of patients were taking aspirin.

Differences in quality by race or ethnicity have been observed within specific health care plans. In fee-for-service Medicare in 2001, blacks were 7.6% less likely, and other races 6.4% less likely, to receive A1C tests and eye examinations than were whites (Kuo 2005). In two other studies Trivedi and coworkers reported on Medicare

TABLE 18.6 *Predictive Margins, Absolute Percentage Change, and 95% CIs According to Strata of Demographic Variables Between Baseline Surveys (National Health and Nutrition Examination Survey, 1988–1994, and Behavioral Risk Factors Surveillance System 1995) and Recent Surveys (National Health and Nutrition Examination Survey, 1999–2002, and Behavioral Risk Factors Surveillance System, 2002)**

Alliance Measures	Hemoglobin A1C >9.0%		Annual Lipid Test		LDL Cholesterol < 3.4 mmol/L (<130 mg/dL)		Blood Pressure < 140/90 mm Hg		Annual Dilated Eye Examination	
	Baseline, %	Absolute Change (95% CI) Percentage Points	Baseline, %	Absolute Change (95% CI) Percentage Points	Baseline, %	Absolute Change (95% CI) Percentage Points	Baseline, %	Absolute Change (95% CI) Percentage Points	Baseline, %	Absolute Change (95% CI) Percentage Points
Age										
18–64 y	26.9	−4.3 (−13.4 to 4.9)	74.4	8.7 (3.9 to 13.4)	43.5	21.6 (7.2 to 36.0)	73.0	1.8 (−6.4 to 10.0)	59.5	6.7 (2.1 to 11.2)
65–75 y	18.8	−5.0 (−13.3 to 3.4)	80.7	6.8 (0.5 to 13.1)	43.0	19.0 (−2.0 to 40.0)	55.8	−4.7 (−14.5 to 5.2)	67.1	6.8 (0.7 to 12.8)
Sex										
Men	23.0	−0.9 (−10.4 to 8.5)	76.5	9.7 (4.4 to 15.0)	46.3	19.7 (3.0 to 36.3)	70.7	0.8 (−7.3 to 9.0)	59.4	6.3 (1.1 to 11.6)
Women	26.1	−7.8 (−14.2 to −1.5)	75.9	6.8 (1.3 to 12.4)	39.6	22.4 (6.3 to 38.6)	65.1	−1.1 (−9.8 to 7.7)	64.0	6.9 (1.7 to 12.2)
Race or ethnicity										
Non-Hispanic white	21.2	−5.6 (−13.4 to 2.1)	78.0	7.3 (3.4 to 11.2)	49.9	24.3 (11.3 to 37.3)	70.3	−0.4 (−8.8 to 8.1)	61.4	8.3 (4.7 to 12.0)
Other	30.4	−2.3 (−10.5 to 5.9)	72.4	10.1 (1.5 to 18.7)	50.1	14.5 (−2.6 to 31.6)	63.4	0.4 (−9.3 to 10.1)	62.5	3.8 (−4.4 to 11.9)
Education										
<High school	24.7	−3.2 (−13.1 to 6.7)	77.5	3.3 (−4.3 to 10.9)	38.8	34.0 (14.6 to 53.3)	64.0	−3.3 (−14.3 to 7.7)	58.1	4.7 (−2.7 to 12.2)
>High school	24.5	−5.2 (−12.3 to 2.0)	75.8	9.8 (5.0 to 14.6)	45.2	15.6 (−10 to 32.2)	70.2	1.9 (−5.1 to 8.8)	62.9	7.3 (2.5 to 12.0)
Insulin										
Yes	34.5	−3.0 (−15.8 to 9.8)	74.6	9.4 (2.2 to 16.7)	NA‡	NA	66.7	−3.1 (15.8 to 9.6)	71.0	2.7 (−4.2 to 9.5)
No	20.7	−4.9 (−12.2 to 2.5)	77.1	7.4 (3.2 to 117)	NA	NA	68.4	1.1 (−5.8 to 7.9)	57.5	8.5 (4.2 to 12.8)
Health Insurance										
Yes	23.2	−4.7 (−11.4 to 2.1)	79.4	7.0 (3.2 to 10.8)	43.5	20.8 (8.9 to 32.6)	67.8	1.5 (−5.4 to 8.4)	65.3	5.1 (1.4 to 8.8)
No	35.4	−3.1 (−22.0 to 15.9)	55.5	16.2 (−0.4 to 32.7)	40.3	23.4 (−21.1 to 67.9)	68.1	−14.0 (−32.7 to 4.7)	37.5	18.1 (0.5 to 35.5)

(continued)

TABLE 18.6 (continued)

Alliance Measures	Flu Vaccine		Aspirin Use		Smoking Cessation		Annual Foot Examination		Negative for Microalbuminurea	
	Baseline, %	Absolute Change (95% CI) Percentage Points	Baseline, %	Absolute Change (95% CI) Percentage Points	Baseline, %	Absolute Change (95% CI) Percentage Points	Baseline, %	Absolute Change (95% CI) Percentage Points	Baseline, %	Absolute Change (95% CI) Percentage Points
Age										
18–64 y	37.1	9.9 (5.2 to 14.6)	30.9	10.0 (0.8 to 19.2)	43.2	19.4 (8.7 to 30.1)	63.0	5.5 (0.8 to 10.2)	68.0	3.1 (–4.7 to 10.9)
65–75 y	58.5	9.6 (3.8 to 15.4)	41.3	13.1 (–0.2 to 26.4)	51.9	6.4 (–15.1 to 27.9)	63.7	7.3 (1.2 to 13.4)	62.2	–4.6 (–14.2 to 5.1)
Sex										
Men	39.6	14.0 (9.0 to 18.9)†	32.2	20.9 (9.8 to 31.9)†	45.8	10.4 (–1.8 to 22.5)	65.0	5.4 (–0.1 to 10.8)	71.5	–6.2 (–14.5 to 2.0)†
Women	47.3	5.9 (0.6 to 11.2)	35.8	3.1 (–7.2 to 13.4)	43.3	24.5 (10.3 to 38.7)	61.6	6.7 (1.5 to 11.8)	61.2	8.1 (–0.6 to 16.8)
Race or ethnicity										
Non-Hispanic white	48.2	7.7 (3.8 to 11.5)	36.0	10.8 (1.9 to 19.7)	44.5	12.9 (3.0 to 22.8)	61.7	6.9 (2.8 to 11.0)	67.9	2.4 (–5.5 to 10.4)
Other	35.3	13.5 (5.1 to 21.9)	29.5	12.1 (–1.7 to 26.0)	44.6	24.9 (6.1 to 43.7)	65.8	4.5 (–3.1 to 12.1)	63.4	–2.1 (–10.7 to 6.4)
Education										
<High school	46.8	23 (–4.9 to 9.5)†	23.6	23.1 (11.2 to 35.0)†	40.8	21.4 (6.3 to 36.4)	59.2	5.6 (–2.0 to 13.2)	61.4	2.1 (–8.5 to 12.6)

>High school	42.7	11.9 (7.3 to 16.4)	37.4	7.4 (−1.8 to 16.7)	45.9	15.9 (3.3 to 28.4)	64.4	6.2 (1.7 to 10.6)	69.3	0.2 (−7.4 to 7.9)
Insulin									
Yes	49.8	8.2 (1.3 to 15.1)	23.3	26.1 (15.5 to 36.7)†	44.1	18.6 (0.8 to 36.5)	74.9	6.5 (0.7 to 12.2)	61.2	−1.9 (−11.6 to 7.8)
No	40.7	10.4 (6.3 to 14.5)	38.7	4.8 (−4.9 to 14.5)	44.8	16.7 (5.8 to 27.6)	57.8	5.8 (1.1 to 10.6)	68.4	2.0 (−4.5 to 8.5)
Health Insurance									
Yes	45.6	10.2 (6.1 to 14.3)	31.3	14.5 (6.5 to 22.5)†	47.8	13.2 (3.9 to 22.5)	62.7	7.6 (3.6 to 11.5)	66.8	0.1 (−6.4 to 6.7)
No	29.1	7.2 (−5.1 to 19.4)	55.6	−14.7 (−38.7 to 9.3)	32.8	32.2 (7.7 to 56.6)	66.8	−4.5 (−18.3 to 9.3)	62.3	7.3 (−15.7 to 30.4)

*Predictive margins are calculated while controlled for confounders (age, sex race or ethnicity, education insulin use, and health insurance), LDL = low density lipoprotein.

†The percentage change difference in the 2 timeline-between comparison groups was scarifically significant.

‡LDL cholestrol was not examined by insulin use because insulin users in National Health and Nutrition Examination Survey, 1988–1994, were not asked to fast.

Source: Reprinted from Saaddine JB et al. (2006). Improvements in diabetes processes of care and intermediate outcomes: United States. *Annals of Internal Medicine* **144,** 465–74.

health plans (Trivedi et al. 2005, 2006), comparing each plan's absolute white-black disparity, adjusted for age and sex, with all other plans for each performance measure. From 1997 to 2002, racial disparities decreased for most measures, and blacks were within 2% of whites for eye examinations and for testing of glycemic and lipid control. Although there was a 7% difference between blacks and whites for LDL-C <130 mg/dL, the disparity had narrowed from 1997 by 6%, while the disparity for poor A1C levels increased from 4% to 7%. In a subsequent study more than 70% of the disparity was attributable to different outcomes for black and white individuals enrolled in the same health plan rather than selection of black enrollees into different health plans. Disparities between plans ranged from minimal to greater than 20%. The TRIAD (Translating Research into Action for Diabetes) study found few racial disparities among over 7456 patients in 10 geographically disparate health care plans that contracted with 68 provider groups (Brown et al. 2005). African Americans had lower rates (than whites) of A1C measurement (by 4.7%), lipid measurement (7%), and influenza vaccination (9.8%), but they had comparable or higher rates for nephropathy assessment, foot examination, dilated eye examinations, and aspirin advice or use. Latinos and Asians or Pacific Islanders had comparable or higher rates (versus whites) for all process measures. Lower socioeconomic position and education were associated with lower performance of dilated eye examinations. The absolute values of intermediate outcomes were higher in minorities. Mean A1C was higher among Latinos and Pacific Islanders (+0.3%) and African Americans (0.2%) than whites; LDL-C was higher (by 7 mg/dL) in African Americans than in whites. Inadequate blood pressure control (≥140/90 mm Hg) was more common in African Americans (55%) than whites (44.1%), while the rate for Latinos was 38.1%. In analyses to evaluate the intensity of medical management among subjects with suboptimal control of risk factors, such management was actually more aggressive for poorer, less educated, or minority patients. Within the Veterans Health Administration, a systematic review indicates differences in intermediate outcomes among different racial groups as well as between individuals with and without significant mental health conditions (Saha et al. 2008).

A body of literature also documents significant differences by sex, especially for management of cardiovascular risk factors on a population basis (Saaddine et al. 2006), in managed care (Bird et al. 2007; Chou et al. 2007), and in the Veterans Health Administration (Safford et al. 2003; Saha et al. 2008). Similar findings were reported within managed care settings within the TRIAD study (Ferrara et al. 2008; Saaddine et al. 2006).

The reasons for differences by race or sex in diabetes care remain unknown, but one possible causal factor of concern is discrimination. In a study by Trivedi and Ayanian of 54,968 participants in the 2001 California Health Interview Study, the authors found that 4.7% of the population (based on self-reports) had experienced discrimination in a health care setting during the previous 12 months (see Tables 18.7 and 18.8) (Trivedi and Ayanian 2006). Discrimination was more prevalent among most racial and ethnic minority groups, women, persons with Medicaid

TABLE 18.7 *Percentage of Individuals Reporting Use of Preventive Health Services by Race/Ethnicity, Gender, and Insurance Status before and after Adjusting for Perceived Discrimination*

	Preventive Health Service					
	Aspirin Use	Cholesterol Test	Foot Exam	HbA1C Test	Flu Shot	PSA Test
Race/ethnicity						
White (%)	39.5	79.7	70.3	89.6	69.8	50.1
African American (%)	33.0*	84.9*	79.9*	89.8	53.0*	45.8
OR† relative to whites	0.75	1.43	1.68	1.02	0.49	0.84
Adjusted OR†	0.76	1.46	1.74	1.03	0.50	0.85
Latino (%)	25.6*	72.6*	63.8*	76.4*	50.9*	29.5*
OR† relative to whites	0.53	0.68	0.74	0.38	0.45	0.42
Adjusted OR†	0.52	0.69	0.74	0.37	0.42	0.41
Asian (%)	29.5*	78.8	50.6*	85.2	71.2	28.9*
OR† relative to whites	0.64	0.95	0.43	0.67	1.08	0.41
Adjusted OR†	0.65	0.93	0.41	0.67	1.05	0.38
American Indian/Alaska Native (%)	30.2*	74.3	75.8	96.7*	64.9	33.4*
OR† relative to whites	0.66	0.73	1.32	3.35	0.80	0.50
Adjusted OR†	0.67	0.76	1.36	3.52	0.79	0.48
Gender						
Male (%)	39.4	78.5	70.5	88.2	68.7	N/A
Female (%)	31.7‡	79.4	64.9‡	83.3‡	66.5‡	N/A
OR† relative to males	0.71	1.06	0.77	0.67	0.91	N/A
Adjusted OR†	0.72	1.08	0.79	0.68	0.94	N/A
Insurance status						
Insured (%)	36.4	81.1	69.5	88.5	67.6	47.5

(continued)

TABLE 18.7   (*continued*)

	Preventive Health Service					
	Aspirin Use	Cholesterol Test	Foot Exam	HbA1C Test	Flu Shot	PSA Test
Uninsured (%)	26.3§	57.2§	50.3§	59.3§	38.8§	17.2§
OR† relative to insured	0.62	0.31	0.44	0.19	0.30	0.23
Adjusted OR†	0.64	0.32	0.44	0.19	0.31	0.23

*Different from whites ($P < .05$).
†OR indicates odds ratio. Adjusted OR indicated odds ratio after adjustment for perceived discrimination.
‡Different from males ($P < .05$).
§Different from insured ($P < .05$).
HbA1C, hemoglobin A1C; PSA, prostate specific antigen.

Source: Reprinted from: Trivedi AN, Ayanian JZ (2006). Perceived discrimination and use of preventive health services. *Journal of General Internal Medicine* **21**, 553–8.

TABLE 18.8   *Unadjusted and Adjusted Estimates of Preventive Health Services Use for Persons Reporting Discrimination Compared with those Reporting No Discrimination*

Preventive Health Service	Discrimination (%)	No Discrimination (%)	Adjusted Odds Ratio*	Adjusted P
Aspirin use	33.4	35.2	0.91 (0.76 to 1.10)	.32
Cholesterol testing	71.0	79.2	0.58 (0.48 to 0.71)	<.001
Foot exam	60.8	67.6	0.66 (0.45 to 0.96)	.03
Hemoglobin A1C testing	78.5	86.1	0.59 (0.39 to 0.89)	.01
Flu shot	61.6	67.3	0.73 (0.55 to 0.98)	.03
Prostate specific antigen testing	37.1	45.7	0.85 (0.61 to 1.17)	.32

Numbers of subjects for each service are weighted to reflect the adult population of California.
*Odds ratios adjusted for age, sex, race, income, education, number of doctor visits in the past year, self-reported health status, insurance status, marital status, citizenship status, English proficiency, rural vs. urban residence, comorbid medical conditions, and body mass index using propensity score methods.

Source: Reprinted from: Trivedi AN, Ayanian JZ (2006). Perceived discrimination and use of preventive health services. *Journal of General Internal Medicine* 21, 553–8.

or no insurance, persons of lower socioeconomic status, and those in fair or poor health. In unadjusted analyses persons who experienced discrimination were significantly less likely to receive A1C measurement and cholesterol testing, with absolute differences of 7.4% and 8.2%, respectively. After adjustment for demographic and clinical factors through the use of propensity scores, persons who experienced discrimination were significantly less likely to receive diabetic foot exams (odds ratio [OR] = 0.66, 95% confidence interval [CI] 0.45 to 0.96), A1C testing (OR 0.59, 95% CI 0.39 to 0.89), cholesterol testing (OR 0.58, 95% CI 0.48 to 0.71), and flu vaccination (OR 0.73, 95% CI 0.55 to 0.98). Uninsured adults had lower rates of all preventive health services than insured adults, but adjustment for perceived discrimination had minimal effect on the OR for these subgroups and services.

These and other studies suggest, then, that disparities can be minimized, but not eliminated, even within systems of care. Factors associated with disparities exist at the individual patient, provider, and systems levels; education and income remain factors in mediating disparities. TRIAD investigators recently reported that concerns about costs, low trust in one's physician, current smoking, and physical inactivity were independent predictors of poor control in that study, but they found that inclusion of these variables in a single model did not diminish associations of race/ethnicity or education with control of risk factors (Selby 2007). Most important, in a chronic disease like diabetes, patient preferences, health beliefs, and adherence and self-management behaviors play key roles.

Although disparities in long-term complications (such as lower-extremity amputations and end-stage renal disease) are well-known, understanding the causes for disparities and how to decrease and/or eliminate them remains less well understood. In part this is due to the general difficulty in collecting individual-level data over time with sufficient laboratory and self-reported variables to risk-adjust outcomes for key baseline covariates. Within the Kaiser Permanente system of health care, investigators found that hazard rates for amputation were not increased for African Americans versus whites, but African Americans had twice the risk borne by whites for end-stage renal disease defined by newly initiated treatments or deaths caused by renal failure (Karter et al. 2002b). One potential risk factor for unsatisfactory outcomes that has been poorly studied is mental health. In a large study of 114,890 veterans with diabetes who had completed a survey in 1999 using information from administrative and survey files, a 5% improvement in mental-health functioning correlated with a 5% lower rate of major amputations within the next year (Tseng et al. 2007b). The authors controlled for known risk factors involving the feet such as ulcers and vascular diseases as well as for demographics, body mass index (BMI), educational level, living arrangement, health insurance status, duration of diabetes, poor control of blood sugar, physical health functioning, health care utilization, and smoking.

In conclusion, while poverty and access to care remain important determinants of health care outcomes in diabetes, disparities by sex, race or ethnicity, and perhaps mental health persist even when socioeconomic factors and utilization of care are equalized. Therefore, some caution is necessary in making inferences that

outcomes necessarily represent differences in the "quality of care"
om a high-level perspective, it is clear that the quality of diabetes care
eet even minimal criteria for many Americans. Deficiencies in care have
despite numerous multidisciplinary efforts.

Public Health Preventive or Intervention Strategies

Challenges in Measuring Quality and Performance

The impact of measurement is contextual. For example, internal data can be used by physician groups, hospitals, and health care plans (Berwick et al. 2003) to prioritize and manage quality improvement efforts as well as for internal reimbursement. Public reporting of measures may affect the ratings of health care plans, and these plans can use these measures to market their services, while consumers can use them in making purchasing decisions. National report cards can best identify population-based needs (NCQA 2008). Consequently, as a general rule, those measures that will prioritize resources and will be used for pay for performance and/or public reporting (often referred to as accountability measures) require a greater strength of evidence that the intervention or treatment will have population benefit, that the measure has scientific soundness, and that the data are feasible to collect (NCQA 2008; U.S. Department of Health and Human Services 2007a). Specifically, measures must be able to distinguish that variations in adherence to a measure reflect differences between entities in the quality of care rather than in patient characteristics. This may require stratification of results and/or risk adjustment, but the process must be validated empirically. In contrast quality improvement measures may not be reliable enough to allow comparisons between providers and health plans, but they are sufficient to inform internal quality improvement within health care systems as well as assessment of public health (Berwick et al. 2003). We had previously noted that this was a major factor in the selection of accountability measures by DQIP (Fleming et al. 2001).

In this section we review the limitations of current quality measures, discuss challenges, and review recent research in the field, summarizing many of the themes and recommendations from a recent national conference on measurement of the quality of diabetes care sponsored by the Agency for Healthcare Research and Quality, the National Institutes of Health, and the Veterans Administration (Kerr 2006).

Limitations of Current Measure Sets

By definition, process measures (such as eye exams) are dichotomous (done or not done), but intermediate outcomes (A1C, blood pressure, and cholesterol) represent a continuous distribution. However, in the current "national measure sets," intermediate outcomes have been dichotomized as all-or-none threshold measures. Similarly, some measure sets include assessments of "good" and "poor control," such as A1C thresholds of <7% (good) or >9% (poor).

Dichotomous intermediate outcome measures, however, are not consistent with the clinical epidemiology of disease. For example the absolute risk reduction for A1C, blood pressure, and cholesterol is log linear, which means that the benefit— defined as fewer macrovascular and/or microvascular events—is proportional to the starting point (Baigent et al. 2005; DCCT Research Group 1993; Vijan and Hayward 2003). In addition benefit is continuous—a specific target goal does not need to be met to derive significant benefit; indeed, the marginal benefit may be minimal, close to the "goal." Furthermore, the balance of benefit and harms may differ for persons *not* included in clinical trials, who are often worse off than the study volunteers; for example, they may have specific or multiple physical and /or mental health conditions that would exclude them from the study or be unable to adhere to the study protocol for other reasons. Although easy to conceptualize, all-or-none intermediate measures for all persons have significant limitations in assessing population health and prioritizing quality improvement efforts (Hayward 2007; Kerr 2006; Pogach, Englegau, and Aron 2007a).

In addition for the purposes of comparisons, the IOM and the Agency for Healthcare Research and Quality have repeatedly indicated that a measure should either not be appreciably affected by any variables (covariates) outside of plan control or that any extraneous variables should be measured in order to calculate an adjusted result that corrects for the effects of covariates (Institute of Medicine 2001a, 2001b). However in the absence of validated methodologies for adjusting risk, a variety of recommendations have been made, such as using appropriate exclusionary criteria and stratifying target values (Pogach et al. 2007b).

Next-Generation Measures

The IOM recommends that initial measure sets for pay-for-performance include three cross-sectional dimensions of care—clinical (or technical) measures, patient-centered care, and (resource utilization) efficiency—but that they should move toward longitudinal and health-outcome measures as soon as that is feasible (Institute of Medicine 2006). A variety of efforts are already under way to develop a next generation of measures that will better reflect what is under the control of those being measured and will reward intensification of care and making progress towards a goal, rather than achieving an all-or-none or similar dichotomous measure.

Linked clinical action measures identify high-risk populations by the combination of a comorbid diagnosis and a poor intermediate outcome, and they evaluate processes of care involved with the initiation or intensification of pharmaceutical therapy (Kerr et al. 2003a). Credit is provided for either achieving the target goal or for providing appropriate medical management of patients for whom the goal is not achieved. As one example, among 1154 Veterans Administration patients with diabetes, 73% met a dichotomous LDL-C threshold of <130 mg/dL, while 87% met a linked action measure defined as LDL-C <130 mg/dL *or* an LDL-C ≥130 mg/dL on high-dose statin, *or* statin started or dose increased within 6 months of high LDL-C, *or* repeat LDL-C <130 mg/dL within 6 months of high LDL-C, *or* contraindications to a statin. This definition of a linked action measure illustrates the fact that in clinical practice many individuals are "not at goal" either because they cannot achieve goal given maximal treatment, have contraindications to intensifying treatment, or their physicians are using an appropriate incremental approach to intensifying treatment.

Clinical inertia, defined as the failure of providers to alter therapy in the face of clear indications for changes, has been demonstrated to affect control of risk factors (such as glycemic control, blood pressure, and cholesterol) (Phillips 2001; Rodondi et al. 2006). A recent study, however, found that in a managed health care plan, although 42% of patients not on insulin at baseline had A1C ≥8%, 58% had appropriate modifications to their therapy within 3 months, and 70% within 6 months.

A fundamental issue in the development of "tightly linked" clinical action measures is the definition of what constitutes appropriate action. The appropriate response may differ depending on how far control is from the goal, the intensity of current treatment, the presence of comorbid conditions, and patient preferences. For example, a 65-year-old patient with an A1C of 7.3% on maximum oral agents may choose not to take insulin. Similarly, if a patient is already on three or four antihypertensive medications but still has suboptimal blood pressure, one might consider that performance is adequate on the measure of clinical action (i.e., that no further intensification is necessary). Myalgias may impede intensification of statins. Failing to consider comorbid conditions, side effects, and low adherence to existing medications could lead to incorrect inferences regarding quality of care (Grant et al. 2007).

Barriers to the widespread implementation of linked measures include problems in collecting data because of the limited implementation in practice of electronic medical records, registries, and electronic prescribing, all of which make it difficult in practice to link claims data (for diagnoses), medications, and laboratory data. In addition it would be necessary to address other factors such as varying pharmaceutical benefits, medication adherence, and patients' involvement in self-management.

Measures Based on Individualized Targets and Progress to Goal

We have developed a conceptual model of the choice of an individual patient's target based on the six domains of quality outlined by the IOM (see Fig. 18.2). The model illustrates the complexity of the factors involved in the choice of something as seemingly simple as using shared decision making to negotiate an individualized target A1C. Pending the development of appropriate measures for these domains and their integration, a number of different approaches have been suggested. These include

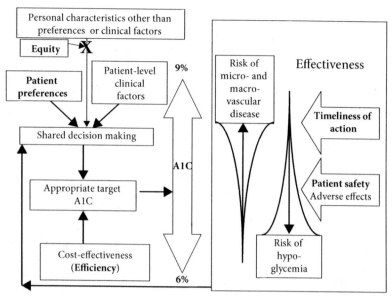

FIGURE 18.2. The choice of an appropriate target for hemoglobin a1c reflects shared decision making (patient centeredness) and cost-effectiveness (efficiency and effectiveness). Effectiveness (conceptualized as absolute risk reduction) involves timeliness of action and must also take into account the risk of adverse effects of treatment such as hypoglycemia (patient safety). Equity addresses patient-level factors related to race, ethnicity, and socioeconomic positioning. (From Aron and Pogach 2007.)

target stratification, use of exclusion criteria for particular measures, and continuous measures.

Based on systematic reviews of the evidence, multiple guidelines recommend stratification of A1C based on comorbidities, functional status, and life expectancy (Qaseem et al. 2007). One approach would be to use some assessment of functional status (Huang, Sachs, and Chin 2006), but such data are generally not available. Another, more feasible strategy would involve a single target but stratify by age and include exclusion criteria for individuals for whom the intervention is not appropriate (Pogach et al. 2007b). This approach was recently adopted by HEDIS (2008) for its proposed <7% good-control measure. However, the use of an all-or-none threshold measure approach does not address the issue raised earlier: for many patients who are reasonably close to an "optimal" target goal, intensification of medication is not undertaken because of personal choice, side effects of medications, or even costs.

To address the issue of making continuous progress toward a target goal, another recently proposed conceptual model is to address the population health benefit using continuous measurement of risk factors that is weighted by quality-adjusted life-years (QALYs) (Aron and Pogach 2007). A QALY is a year of life adjusted for its quality or its value, with a year in perfect health considered equal to 1.0 QALY. The value of a year in ill health would be discounted. For example, a year spent bedridden might have a value equal to 0.5 QALY. Because a QALY is a common denominator, several intermediate outcomes can be simultaneously compared for a single diabetic patient. For example, what would be the difference in absolute benefits (in terms of adding QALYs) of decreasing A1C, reducing LDL-C, or reducing blood pressure for an individual patient? Based on the results the clinician and patient can discuss what the best course of action would be. This approach recognizes that individual patients may have different preferences regarding the balance between short-term complications and long-term benefits of treatment of chronic diseases (Fleming et al. 1993).

This conceptual model has already been implemented in several ways in research studies. One approach is to use cumulative quality-adjusted life expectancy based on a summary measure of QALYs obtained from control of the three major intermediate outcomes: A1C, blood pressure, and LDL-C (Schmittdiel et al. 2007). This approach demonstrates that improving poor blood pressure is the dominant clinical strategy and that improvements in moderately controlled glycemia constitute the least effective strategy. This approach is supported by a recently reported study of post-interventional benefits in patients with type 2 diabetes after a 7.8-year multifactorial, intensive risk-reduction program with multiple drug combinations and behavior modification, with a follow-up of 13.3 years (Gaede, Lund-Andersen, and Parving 2008). The long-term effects of tight glycemic control (mean A1C achieved 7.7%) and therapy with aspirin, antihypertensive agents, and lipid-lowering drugs appeared to be additive. We may be on the cusp of new approaches for managing diabetes: a period of more intensive glucose control earlier in the disease when this is more obtainable, and more relaxed glycemic control values later in the course of the disease, coupled with maintenance of blood pressure and lipid management.

Another approach is to determine a "ceiling" (acceptable/not acceptable) and a "floor" (optimal goal) using two threshold values—for example, an A1C of 7% (floor) and 8% (ceiling), and assess improvement toward the goal (Pogach et al. 2007). This approach would be aligned toward quality improvement efforts in that it rewards intensive treatment of individuals markedly rather than marginally above target. The ceilings and floors could be established for different populations—for example, based on age, insulin use, or coexisting nephropathy. As is being done by HEDIS (2008) for A1C control, a measure of poor control (>9%) is still being kept to identify individuals who have the worst risk factor control. This approach has been applied to LDL-C and systolic blood pressure as well (Aron et al. 2006).

Disadvantages of QALY-weighted measures include the need to educate patients and providers about the concept and the necessity to emphasize the concept of progress toward risk reduction as opposed to meeting a target goal. There are also methodological issues that relate primarily to issues of the underlying foundation for QALYs in general and for using QALY weights for specific outcomes. Additional research is necessary to develop risk adjustment methods or to establish the proper denominator through use of exclusion criteria. Similarly, research is needed on methods of weighting measurement and predictive modeling (Engelgau 2005).

Patient Perspectives

Assessments of patient satisfaction with care are already widely used at the health plan level through the use of the CAHPS®-HP survey (Consumer Assessment of Health Plans Survey—health providers). However this survey does not capture important elements of how patients with chronic disease perceive the quality of the care they receive and particularly how they assess the support they get for improving self-management. Although the new CAHPS-CG (clinician group) survey focuses more on the physician–patient interaction, especially for patients with chronic illness, it still has only a few questions that relate directly to how well support for self-management is provided. Consequently, strong arguments have been made for the development of diabetes-specific, patient-centered measures (Glasgow, Peeples, and Skovlund 2008).

Nonetheless, substantial barriers to incorporating diabetes-specific, patient-centered measures exist, including the feasibility and cost of obtaining self-reported information from patients. There are methodological issues as well. Should the provision of diabetes education be a process measure, or should it be linked to outcomes—either intermediate outcomes such as A1C or so-called "patient-centered measures"—knowledge, behaviors, and satisfaction? For example, although diabetes education is a covered Medicare benefit, systematic reviews have demonstrated that diabetes education is often delivered in the context of other disease management tactics (i.e., education is bundled), and systematic reviews indicate that the benefit of educational interventions only modestly improves glycemic control and is proportional to the number of educational visits (Norris et al. 2001, 2002). The evidence for a widespread benefit of a widely recommended practice, self-monitoring of blood glucose in persons not on insulin, is minimal (Towfigh et al. 2008). Thus, measuring whether education or monitoring was provided or not would not necessarily improve outcomes, and it could increase costs without demonstrating benefit. Alternatively, one could assess patient knowledge. However, knowledge is affected by lower health literacy (Morris et al. 2006; Schillinger et al. 2002, 2006; Schillinger et al. 2002) and diabetes numeracy (Cavanaugh et al. 2008), both of which are correlated with lower socioeconomic status and may lead to less adherence to self-management and possibly worse glycemic outcomes. Thus, population health measures may need to account for or control for variation in socioeconomic status; alternatively, population health literacy could be an independent measure.

Both overall and provider-specific patient satisfaction have also been proposed as diabetes outcomes. However measurement of patient satisfaction is substantially affected by health status, and this effect is considerably greater for diabetes severity than for general physical functioning (Kerr et al. 2003b). Although participatory decision making is highly valued as a provider-level trait by patients and could improve satisfaction, its association with outcomes remains unclear (Epstein et al. 2004). In one study of patients with diabetes ratings of providers' effectiveness in communicating were more important than a participatory decision-making style in predicting diabetes self-management (Heisler et al. 2002). Further validation of instruments to measure these constructs is necessary if they are to be used for purposes of public reporting or payment.

■ Implications for Health Policy

In this chapter, we have argued that performance measurement should follow the recommendation of the IOM that "quality" is "the degree to which health services for individuals and populations increase the likelihood of desired health outcomes and are consistent with current professional knowledge." We have noted that although efficacy trials are sufficient for clinical guidelines and inform the development of accountability measures, technical considerations (bias, variability in practice, and definition of population at risk) must be considered in performance measurement systems. Although electronic health records may enable the next generation of diabetes measures to be linked to clinical actions, much work needs to be accomplished. In the interim policy makers need to consider benefits, harms, costs, and unintended behaviors for the relatively crude measures of process and intermediate outcomes in place today. Public health surveillance of adverse outcomes remains a critical function of federal and state agencies, but changes in rates may reflect the number and severity of illness in the denominator as well as outcomes in the numerator.

■ Areas of Uncertainty or Controversy

The evidence base for the control of risk factors in diabetes is rapidly changing. In the current year the ACCORD and ADVANCE studies and the Veterans Affairs Diabetes Trial have disproven the short-term benefit of tight glycemic control in terms of cardiovascular benefits for individuals with a longer duration of diabetes. Furthermore they have established serious hypoglycemia as a risk factor for cardiovascular mortality. On the other hand, long-term follow-up studies of intensive glucose control after recent-onset type 2 (Holman et al. 2008) and type 1 diabetes (Nathan et al. 2005) demonstrated extended and improved treatment benefits despite early post-trial loss of between-group glycemic differences. In a smaller study of type 2 diabetes post-interventional benefits were reported after a 7.8-year multifactorial, intensive risk-reduction program with multiple drug combinations and behavior modification, with a follow-up of 13.3 years. The long-term effects of tight glycemic control (mean A1C achieved 7.7%) and therapy with aspirin, antihypertensive agents, and lipid-lowering drugs appeared to be additive. A new paradigm to measuring quality of care for diabetes—one that can incorporate varying benefits of incremental improvement in multiple populations that differ by age, diabetes duration, and coexisting illness—will be necessary.

Economic Issues and Implications

Based on an American Diabetes Association analysis, the total estimated direct cost of diabetes in 2007 was $116 billion in excess medical expenditures. The largest components of medical expenditures were hospital inpatient care (50% of total cost), diabetes medication and supplies (12%), retail prescriptions to treat complications of diabetes (11%), and physician office visits (9%). People with diagnosed diabetes incurred average expenditures of $11,744 per year, of which $6,649 was attributed to diabetes. Decreasing these costs is therefore of societal importance.

However, the health care industry struggles with the sometimes conflicting imperatives to improve the delivery of "diabetes quality of care" while containing costs, that is, maximizing value, a subjective concept that can reasonably vary among different consumers. Indeed the IOM vaguely defines efficiency as "the highest possible quality given limited resources." Developers have not taken the cost-effectiveness of measures into account; nor have they considered their unintended consequences. For example there has been a marked increase in the costs of medication prescriptions for oral antiglycemic agents and insulin (Alexander et al. 2008). In another study, a cap on drug benefits was associated with lower drug consumption and unfavorable clinical outcomes, such as poorer adherence to drug therapy and poorer control of blood pressure, lipid levels, and glucose levels (Hsu et al. 2008). Therefore, developers of measures will need to increasingly consider costs to consumers and plans in the implementation of diabetes quality measures.

Developments over the Next 5 to 10 Years

In a recent editorial (Fisher 2006) it was noted that the IOM has emphasized "... that measures and rewards of performance should target multiple dimensions of care, initially including measures of technical quality, patient-centered care, and efficiency but moving toward longitudinal and health-outcome measures as soon as it is feasible. Because most Medicare beneficiaries receive care from multiple physicians in diverse institutional settings, the committee highlighted the need for measures and rewards that foster shared accountability and coordination of care." Efforts are under way by the National Quality Forum (2010) and Prometheus Payment, Inc. (2009), to develop "episodes of care" measures for diabetes.

It is clear that inferences regarding trends in outcomes—either intermediate risk factors or adverse events (such as amputations)—are limited by the use of cross-sectional population-level data in both public health and health care system settings. For example trending improvement in A1C using cross-sectional data overestimates improvement compared with using a fixed cohort. Conceptually this could be due to in-migration of patients with new onset—who would be easier to control; or out-migration of patients with higher A1C levels due to patient death or disenrollment due to dissatisfaction with care. The availability of multiple years of individual-level data minimizes attribution error, that is, differences in case mix attributed to difference in quality. This approach has been used to evaluate facility-level differences in A1C and health care outcomes such as amputation and dialysis (Karter et al. 2002a; Thompson et al. 2005). At this time, however, multiple methodological issues and the lack of availability of electronic health records still limit widespread adoption of longitudinal evaluations within health plans or for public health.

■ References

Action to Control Cardiovascular Risk in Diabetes Study Group (2008). Effects of intensive glucose lowering in type 2 diabetes. *New England Journal of Medicine* 358, 2545–59.

ACCORD Study Group (2010a). Effects of intensive blood-pressure control in type 2 diabetes mellitus. *New England Journal of Medicine* 362, 1575–85.

ACCORD Study Group (2010b). Effects of combination lipid therapy in type 2 diabetes mellitus. *New England Journal of Medicine* 362, 1563–74.

ADVANCE Collaborative Group (2008). Intensive blood glucose control and vascular outcomes in patients with type 2 diabetes. *New England Journal of Medicine* 358, 2560–72.

Ahmann AJ (2007). Guidelines and performance measures for diabetes. *American Journal of Managed Care* 13, S41–6

American Diabetes Association (2007). Economic costs of diabetes in the U.S. in 2007. *Diabetes Care* 31, 596–615.

American Medical Association. Participation tools: Medicare Physician Quality Reporting Initiative (PQRI). Available at http://www.ama-assn.org/ama/pub/category/17432.html. Accessed November 2, 2008.

Aron DC, Pogach LM (2007). One size does not fit all: a continuous measure for glycemic control in diabetes: the need for a new approach to assessing glycemic control. *The Joint Commission Journal on Quality and Patient Safety* 33, 636–43.

Aron DC, Pogach LM (2008). Using the Delphi method to inform performance measurement development: how should medical evidence be interpreted for policy decisions? *Quality & Safety in Health Care* 17, 315–7.

Aron DC, Rajan M, Pogach LM (2006). Summary measures of quality of diabetes care: comparison of continuous weighted performance measurement and dichotomous thresholds. *International Journal of Quality Healthcare* 19, 29–36.

Baigent C et al. (2005). Efficacy and safety of cholesterol-lowering treatment: prospective meta-analysis of data from 90,056 participants in 14 randomised trials of statins. *Lancet* 366, 1267–78.

Berwick D, James B, Coyne M (2003). Connections between quality measurement and improvement. *Medical Care* 41, I30–8.

Bird C et al. (2007). Does quality of care for cardiovascular disease and diabetes differ by gender for enrollers in managed care plans? *Women's Health Issues* 17, 131–8.

Brown A et al. (2004). Socioeconomic position and health among persons with diabetes mellitus: a conceptual framework and review of the literature. *Epidemiologic Reviews* 26, 63–77.

Brown A et al. (2005). Race, ethnicity, socioeconomic position, and quality of care for adults with diabetes enrolled in managed care: the Translating Research Into Action for Diabetes (TRIAD) study. *Diabetes Care* 28, 2864–70.

Cavanaugh K et al. (2008). Association of numeracy and diabetes control. *Annals of Internal Medicine* 148, 737–46.

Centers for Disease Control and Prevention (2007a). *Behavioral Risk Factor Surveillance System*. Atlanta: CDC.

Centers for Disease Control and Prevention (2007b). *National Health and Nutrition Survey*. Atlanta: CDC.

Chou A et al. (2007). Gender and racial disparities in the management of diabetes mellitus among medicare patients. *Women's Health Issues* 17, 150–61.

Davis T et al. (2001). Relationship between ethnicity and glycemic control, lipid profiles, and blood pressure during the first 9 years of type 2 diabetes: UK Prospective Diabetes Study (UKPDS 55). *Diabetes Care* 24, 1167–74.

Diabetes Control and Complications Trial (DCCT) Research Group (1993). The effects of intensive diabetes treatment on the development and progression of long-term complications in insulin-dependent diabetes mellitus. *New England Journal of Medicine* 329, 977–86.

Donabedian A (1966). Evaluating the quality of medical care. *Milbank Quarterly* 44, 166–206.

Donabedian A (1983). Quality, cost, and clinical decisions. *Annals of the American Academy of Political and Social Science* 468, 196–204.

Duckworth W (2008). VADT: Results. Presented at the American Diabetes Association Scientific Sessions, June 2008.

Engelgau MM (2005).Trying to predict the future for people with diabetes: a tough but important task. *Annals of Internal Medicine* 143, 251–64.

Epstein R, Alper B, Quill T (2004). Communicating evidence for participatory decision making. *JAMA* 291, 2359–66.

Ferrara A et al. (2008). Gender disparities in control and treatment of modifiable cardiovascular disease risk factors among patients with diabetes: translating research into action for diabetes (TRIAD). *Diabetes Care* 31, 69–74.

Fisher ES. (2006). Paying for performance—risks and recommendations. *New England Journal of Medicine* 355, 1845–7

Fleming B et al. (2001). The Diabetes Quality Improvement Project: moving science into health policy to gain an edge on the diabetes epidemic. *Diabetes Care* 24, 1815–20.

Fleming C et al. (1993). A decision analysis of alternative treatment strategies for clinically localized prostate cancer. Prostate Patient Outcomes Research Team. *JAMA* 269, 2650–8.

Gaede P, Lund-Andersen H, Parving H (2008). Effect of a multifactorial intervention on mortality in type 2 diabetes. *New England Journal of Medicine* 358, 580–91.

Geiss L et al. (2005). A national progress report on diabetes:success and challenges. *Diabetes Technology & Therapeutics* 7, 198–203.

Glasgow RE, Peeples M, Skovlund SE (2008). Where is the patient in diabetes performance measures? The case for including patient-centered and self-management measures. *Diabetes Care* 31, 1046–50.

Goldberg PA et al. (2006). "Glucometrics"—assessing the quality of inpatient glucose management. *Diabetes Technology & Therapeutics* 8, 560–9.

Grant RW et al. (2007). How doctors choose medications to treat type 2 diabetes: a national survey of specialists and academic generalists. *Diabetes Care* 30, 1448–53.

Harris MI (1996). Medical care for patients with diabetes. *Annals of Internal Medicine* 124, 117–22.

Harris MI (2002). Health care and health status and outcomes for patients with type 2 diabetes. *Diabetes Care* 23, 754–55.

Hays R et al. (1999). Psychometric properties of the CAHPS 1.0 survey measures. Consumer Assessment of Health Plans Study. *Medical Care* 37, MS22–31.

Hayward RA (2007). All-or-nothing treatment targets make bad performance measures. *American Journal of Managed Care* 13, 126–8.

Hayward RA et al. (2005). Reporting clinical trial results to inform providers, payers, and consumers. *Health Affairs* 24, 1571–81.

HEDIS®1 2009, Volume 2: Technical Update. Available at: http://www.ncqa.org/Portals/0/PolicyUpdates/HEDIS%20Technical%20Updates/2009_Vol2_Technical_Update.pdf. Accessed October 25, 2008.

Heisler M et al. (2002). The relative importance of physician communication, participatory decision making, and patient management. *Journal of General Internal Medicine* 17, 243–52.

Holman RR et al (2008). 10-year follow-up of intensive glucose control in type 2 diabetes. *New England Journal of Medicine* 359,1577–89.

Hsu J et al. (2006). Unintended consequences of caps on Medicare drug benefits. *New England Journal of Medicine* 354, 2349–59.

Huang ES, Sachs GA, Chin MH (2006). Implications of new geriatric diabetes care guidelines for the assessment of quality of care in older patients. *Medical Care* 44, 373–7.

Institute of Medicine (1990). *Medicare: A Strategy for Quality Assurance.* Washington, DC: National Academy Press.

Institute of Medicine (2001a). *Envisioning the National Healthcare Quality Report: Designing the National Healthcare Quality Report.* Washington, DC: National Academy Press.

Institute of Medicine (2001b). *Crossing the Quality Chasm: A New Health System for the 21st Century.* Washington, DC: National Academy Press.

Institute of Medicine (2002). *Unequal Treatment: Confronting Racial and Ethnic Disparities in Health Care.* Washington, DC: National Academy Press.

Institute of Medicine (2006). *Rewarding Provider Performance: Aligning Incentives in Medicare.* Washington, DC: National Academy Press.

Karter AJ et al. (2002). Ethnic disparities in diabetic complications in an insured population. *JAMA* 287, 2519–27.

Kerr EA et al. (2003a). Building a better quality measure: are some patients with 'poor quality' actually getting good care?. *Medical Care* 41, 1173–82.

Kerr EA et al. (2003b). The association between three different measures of health status and satisfaction among patients with diabetes. *Medical Care Research and Review* 60, 158–77.

Kerr EA et al. (2004). Diabetes care quality in the Veterans Affairs Health Care System and commercial managed care: the TRIAD study. *Annals of Internal Medicine* 141, 272–21.

Kerr EA, Agency for Research on Healthcare Quality, the National Institute for Diabetes and Digestive and Kidney Diseases, Veterans Administration Office of Quality and Performance (OQP) Conference (2006). *Assessing Quality of Care for Diabetes.* Ann Arbor, MI: Unpublished Report Submitted to AHRQ, NIDDK, and VA.

Kuo SL et al. (2005). Trends in care practices and outcomes among Medicare beneficiaries with diabetes. *American Journal of Preventive Medicine* 29, 396–403.

Landon BE et al. (2003). Physician clinical performance assessment: prospects and barriers. *JAMA* 290, 1183–9.

Landon B et al. (2007). Improving the management of chronic disease at community health centers. *New England Journal of Medicine* 356, 921–34.

Lohr KN, Eleazer K, Mauskopf K (1998). Health policy issues and applications for evidence-based medicine and clinical practice guidelines. *Health Policy* 46, 1–19.

Miller D, Pogach LM (2008). Utilizing longitudinal approaches to monitor quality and outcomes: Veterans Health Administration Diabetes Epidemiology Cohort. *Diabetes Science and Technology* 2, 24–32

Morris NS, MacLean CD, Littenberg B (2006). Literacy and health outcomes: a cross-sectional study in1002 adults with diabetes. *BMC Family Practice* 9, 7–49.

Mukhtar Q et al. (2006). Evaluating progress toward *Healthy People 2010* national diabetes objectives. *Preventing Chronic Disease* 3 (1), A11.

Nathan D et al. (2005) Intensive diabetes treatment and cardiovascular disease in patients with type 1 diabetes. *New England Journal of Medicine* 22, 2643–53.

National Committee for Quality Assurance (2007). *National Committee for Quality Assurance Report Cards,* Washington, DC: National Committee for Quality Assurance.

National Committee for Quality Assurance (2008) Desirable Attributes of HEDIS. Available at http://www.ncqa.org/tabid/415/Default.aspx. Accessed October 26, 2008.

National Committee for Quality Assurance (2009). *The State of Healthcare Quality 2007.* Washington, DC: National Committee for Quality Assurance.

National Committee for Quality Assurance. HEDIS 2009. Available at http://www.ncqa.org/tabid/784/Default.aspx. Accessed November 2, 2009.

National Quality Forum (2006). National Voluntary Consensus Standards for Adult Diabetes Care: 2005 Update. Available at http://www.qualityforum.org/publications/reports/diabetes_update.asp. Accessed November 2, 2008.

National Quality Forum (2010). Diabetes Measure Set: Value Based Episodes of Care. http://www.qualityforum.org/Projects/c-d/Diabetes_Measure_Set_Value-Based_ Episodes_of_Care/Comprehensive_Diabetes_Measure_Set__Value-Based_ Episodes_of_Care.aspx. Assessed May 3, 2010

Norris SL, Engelgau M, Narayan K (2001). Effectiveness of self-management training in type 2 diabetes: a systematic review of randomized controlled trials. *Diabetes Care* 24, 561–87.

Norris SL et al. (2002). Increasing diabetes self-management education in community settings. a systematic review. *American Journal of Preventive Medicine* 22, 39–66.

O'Connor P et al. (2005). Randomized trial of quality improvement intervention to improve diabetes care in primary care settings. *Diabetes Care* 28, 1890–7.

Oliver A (2007). The Veterans Health Administration: an American success story? *Milbank Quarterly* 85, 5–35.

Perlin JB, Pogach LM. (2006). Improving the outcomes of metabolic conditions: managing momentum to overcome clinical inertia. *Annals of Internal Medicine* 144, 525–7.

Phillips LS (2001). Clinical inertia. *Annals of Internal Medicine* 135, 825–34.

Pogach LM et al. (2004). Development of evidence-based guidelines for diabetes mellitus: the Veterans Health Administration-Department of Defense Guidelines Initiative. *Diabetes Care* 27, B82–9.

Pogach LM, Rajan M, Aron DM (2006). Aligning performance measurement with clinical epidemiology: comparison of weighted performance measurement and dichotomous thresholds for glycemic control in the Veterans Health Administration. *Diabetes Care* 29 (2), 241–6.

Pogach LM, Engelgau M, Aron D (2007). Measuring progress towards achieving A1c goals in diabetes care: pass/fail or partial credit. *JAMA* 297, 520–3.

Pogach LM et al. (2007). Should mitigating comorbidities be considered in assessing healthcare plan performance in achieving optimal glycemic control? *American Journal of Managed Care* 13, 133–40.

PROMETHEUS Payment® Inc. (2009). Available at http://www.prometheuspayment. org/playbook/chronic/diabetesECR.htm. Accessed May 3, 2010.

Qaseem A et al. (2007). Glycemic control and type 2 diabetes mellitus: the optimal hemoglobin A1c targets. A guidance statement from the American College of Physicians. *Annals of Internal Medicine* 147, 417–22.

Rodondi N et al. (2006). Therapy modifications in response to poorly controlled hypertension, dyslipidemia, and diabetes mellitus. *Annals of Internal Medicine* 144, 475–84.

Saaddine JB et al. (2002). A diabetes report card for the United States: quality of care in the 1990s. *Annals of Internal Medicine* 136, 565–74.

Saaddine JB et al. (2006). Improvements in diabetes processes of care and intermediate outcomes: United States. *Annals of Internal Medicine* 144, 465–74.

Safford M et al. (2003). Disparities in use of lipid–lowering medications among people with type 2 diabetes mellitus. *Archives of Internal Medicine* 163, 922–8.

Saha S et al. (2008). Racial and ethnic disparities in the VA Healthcare System. *Journal of General Internal Medicine* 23, 654–71.

Sanderson C, Dixon J. (2000). Conditions for which onset or hospital admission is potentially preventable by timely and effective ambulatory care. *Journal of Health Services Research & Policy* 5, 222–30.

Schillinger D et al. (2002). Association of health literacy with diabetes outcomes. *JAMA* 288, 475–82.

Schillinger D et al. (2006). Does literacy mediate the relationship between education and health outcomes? A study of a low-income population with diabetes. *Public Health Reports* 121, 245–54.

Schmittdiel J et al. (2007). Predicted quality-adjusted life years as a composite measure of the clinical value of diabetes risk factor control. *Medical Care* 45, 315–21.

Selby JV et al. (2007). Understanding the gap between good processes of diabetes care and poor intermediate outcomes: Translating Research into Action for Diabetes (TRIAD). *Medical Care* 45, 1144–53.

Sibthorpe B (2004). *A Proposed Conceptual Framework for Performance Assessment in Primary Health Care: a Tool for Policy and Practice.* Canberra: Australian Primary Health Care Research Institute.

Thompson W et al. (2005). Assessing quality of diabetes care by measuring longitudinal changes in hemoglobin A1c in the Veterans Health Administration. *Health Services Research* 40, 1818–35.

Towfigh A et al.(2008). Self-monitoring of blood glucose levels in patients with type 2 diabetes mellitus not taking insulin: a meta–analysis. *American Journal of Managed Care* 14, 468–75.

Trivedi AN, Ayanian JZ (2006). Perceived discrimination and use of preventive health services. *Journal of General Internal Medicine* 21, 553–8.

Trivedi AN et al. (2005). Trends in the quality of care and racial disparities in Medicare managed care. *New England Journal of Medicine* 353, 692–700.

Trivedi AN et al. (2006). Relationship between quality or care and racial disparities in Medicare health plans. *JAMA* 296, 1198–2004.

Tseng C et al. (2007a). Evaluation of regional variation in total, major, and minor amputation rates in a national health-care system. *International Journal for Quality in Health Care* 19, 368–76.

Tseng C et al. (2007b). The association between mental health functioning and nontraumatic lower extremity amputations in veterans with diabetes. *General Hospital Psychiatry* 29, 537–46.

UK Prospective Diabetes Study (UKPDS) Group (1998). Intensive blood-glucose control with sulphonylureas or insulin compared with conventional treatment and risk of complications in patients with type 2 diabetes (UKPDS 33). *Lancet* 352, 837–53.

U.S. Department of Health and Human Services (2000). *Healthy People 2010: With Understanding and Improving Health and Objectives for Improving Health.* 2nd ed. Washington, DC: U.S. Government Printing Office.

U.S. Department of Health and Human Services (2005). *National Healthcare Disparities Report.* Rockville, MD: Agency for Healthcare Research and Quality.

U.S. Department of Health and Human Services (2006). *Healthy People 2010: Midcourse Review.* Washington, DC: U.S. Government Printing Office.

U.S. Department of Health and Human Services (2007a). *AHRQ: Guide to Prevention Quality Indicators: Hospital Admission for Ambulatory Care Sensitive Conditions.* Version 3.1. Washington, DC: U.S. Government Printing Office.

U.S. Department .of Health and Human Services (2007b). *Ambulatory Care Quality Alliance Recommended Starter Set: Clinical Performance Measures for Ambulatory Care.* Washington, DC: U.S. Government Printing Office.

U.S. Department .of Health and Human Services (2007c). *National Health Care Quality Report.* Washington, DC: U.S. Government Printing Office.

U.S. Department of Health and Human Services. (2008a). Agency for Healthcare Research and Quality. Recommended Starter Set. The Ambulatory Care Quality Alliance. Clinical Performance Measures for Ambulatory Care. Available at: http://www.ahrq.gov/qual/aqastart.htm. Accessed November 2, 2008

U.S. Department of Health and Human Services (2008b). *Healthy People 2010: National Health Promotion and Disease Prevention Objectives.* Washington, DC: U.S. Government Printing Office.

U.S. Department of Health and Human Services (2008c). *Healthy People 2010: Midcourse Review.* Diabetes 5. Washington, DC: U.S. Government Printing Office. Available at *http://www.healthypeople.gov/data/midcourse/html/focusareas/ FA05Objectives.htm#5-10a.* Accessed October 25, 2008.

U.S. Department of Health and Human Services (2008d). *Healthy People 2010.* Available at http://www.healthypeople.gov/. Accessed October 25, 2008.

Van den Bergh G et al. (2001). Intensive insulin therapy in critically ill patients. *New England Journal of Medicine* 345, 1359–67.

Van den Bergh G et al. (2006). Intensive insulin therapy in the medical ICU. *New England Journal of Medicine* 354, 449–61.

Vijan S, Hayward RA. (2003). Treatment of hypertension in type 2 diabetes mellitus: blood pressure goals, choice of agents, and setting priorities in diabetes care. *Annals of Internal Medicine* 138, 593–602.

Wiener RS, Wiener DC, Larson RJ (2008). Benefits and risks of tight glucose control in critically ill adults: a meta-analysis. *JAMA* 300, 933–44.

Wilson C et al. (2005). Diabetes outcomes in the Indian health system during the era of the Special Diabetes Program for Indians and the Government Performance and Results Act. *American Journal of Public Health* 95, 1518–22.

19. Effectiveness of Interventions at the Health System, Provider, and Patient Levels to Improve the Quality of Diabetes Care

Catherine Kim, Hae Mi Choe, Yeong Kwok, and Jennifer Wyckoff

■ Main Public Health Messages

- Interventions can reduce hemoglobin A1C values on the order of 0.2 to 1.3 percentage points. Larger reductions in A1C are seen in patients with greater baseline values (≥9%).
- Interventions to improve diabetes care typically combine multiple features, but there is no consensus as to which features are most effective. Successful interventions usually involve multidisciplinary teams.
- A limitation of the existing literature on interventions is the focus on A1C rather than on other intermediate outcomes more closely related to cardiovascular events and mortality.
- Effective implementation of interventions may require resources that are beyond the scope of smaller organizations.
- Broader implementation of interventions may be challenging given the current fragmentation of the U.S. health care system and the unique requirements of local populations.

■ Introduction

The identification, treatment, and control of diabetes complications and the major risk factors for cardiovascular disease can reduce the morbidity and mortality associated with diabetes. As documented in the previous chapter, there is significant variation in the quality of diabetes care. Fortunately interventions to improve outcomes for persons with diabetes have increased in the past several years. A PubMed search of the terms "intervention" and "diabetes" and "quality" for the period of 1990–1995 yielded 35 studies; the same search conducted for 1995–2000 yielded 111 studies; and the same search for 2000–2007 yielded 518 studies. In an effort to consolidate this literature, multiple meta-analyses and systematic reviews have synthesized these reports.

In this chapter we review the results from different meta-analyses and reviews designed to address the effectiveness of different interventions. We organize these reviews by first describing interventions aimed at the health care system and health care providers, then interventions aimed at individuals, followed by features of these interventions associated with their success; finally, we look at implications for policy.

■ Interventions Aimed at the Health Care System and Providers

In this section we review interventions for health care systems and providers that are aimed at reducing hemoglobin A1C, followed by those aimed at process measures and intermediate outcomes. We then discuss issues of measuring effectiveness based on randomized trials as opposed to other study designs, and we review the health care organizational features associated with such interventions.

Reduction of Hemoglobin A1C

The vast majority of interventions for health care systems and providers have targeted A1C levels. We describe these interventions by using a meta-analysis that summarized these interventions. In 2006 Shojania and colleagues examined the impact of 11 types of strategies for quality improvement in adults with type 2 diabetes (Shojania et al. 2004, 2006); to be included in the meta-analysis, studies had to involve at least one component directed at changing providers or organizations. Box 19.1 describes these strategies in more detail. The definition of each strategy is broad, allowing for significant variation between studies. For example, quality improvement performed through "team changes" includes adding health care staff, use of multidisciplinary teams, and expanding the role of an existing health care provider.

Fifty-eight studies met the authors' inclusion criteria, which included type of design (randomized controlled trial [RCT]), quasiexperimental, and controlled before-after study) and report of A1C values pre- and postintervention. Interventions had a median duration of 13 months (interquartile range 6 to 18 months). Interventions involving *team changes* reduced A1C values by 0.33 percentage points more than interventions without such changes, and interventions involving *case management* reduced A1C by 0.22 percentage points more than

BOX 19.1 *Taxonomy Used to Classify Quality Improvement Strategies*

Audit and Feedback. Summary of clinical performance of health care delivered by an individual clinician or clinic over a specified period, which is then transmitted back to the clinician (e.g., the percentage of a clinician's patients who achieved a target glycosylated hemoglobin [HbA1C] level, or who have undergone a dilated-eye examination with a specified frequency).

Case Management. Any system for coordinating diagnosis, treatment, or ongoing patient management (e.g., arrangement for referrals, follow-up of test results) by a person or multidisciplinary team in collaboration with or supplementary to the primary care clinician.

Team Changes. Changes to the structure or organization of the primary health care team, defined as present if any of the following applied:

- Adding a team member or "shared care," e.g., routine visits with personnel other than the primary physician (including physician or nurse specialists in diabetic care, pharmacists, nutritionists, podiatrists).
- Use of multidisciplinary teams, i.e., active participation of professionals from more than one discipline (e.g., medicine, nursing, pharmacy, nutrition) in the primary, ongoing management of patients.
- Expansion or revision of professional roles (e.g., nurse or pharmacist plays more active role in patient monitoring or adjusting medication regimens).

Electronic Patient Registry. General electronic medical record system or electronic tracking system for patients with diabetes.

Clinician Education. Interventions designed to promote increased understanding of principles guiding clinical care or awareness of specific recommendations for a target condition or patient population. Subcategories of clinician education included conferences or workshops, distribution of educational materials, and educational outreach visits.

Clinician Reminders. Paper-based or electronic system intended to prompt a health professional to recall patient-specific information (e.g., most recent HbA1C value) or to perform a specific task (e.g., perform a foot examination). If accompanied by a recommendation, the strategy would be subclassified as decision support.

Facilitated Relay of Clinical Information to Clinicians. Clinical information collected from patients and transmitted to clinicians by means other than the existing medical record. Conventional means of correspondence between

(continued)

BOX 19.1 (*continued*)

clinicians were excluded. For example if the results of routine visits with a pharmacist were sent in a letter to the primary care physician, the use of routine visits with a pharmacist would count as a "team" change, but the intervention would not also be counted as "facilitated relay." If, however, the pharmacist issues structured diaries for patients to record self-monitored glucose values, which are then brought in person to office visits to review with the primary physician, then the intervention would count as "facilitated relay." Other examples include electronic or Web-based tools through which patients provide self-care data and which clinicians review, as well as point-of-care testing supplying clinicians with immediate HbA1C values.

Patient Education. Interventions designed to promote increased understanding of a target condition or to teach specific prevention or treatment strategies, or specific in-person patient education (e.g., individual or group sessions with diabetes nurse educator; distribution of printed or electronic educational materials). Interventions with patient education were included only if they also included at least one other strategy related to clinician or organizational change.

Promotion of Self-Management. Provision of equipment (e.g., home glucometers) or access to resources (e.g., system for electronically transmitting home glucose measurements and receiving insulin dose changes based on those data) to promote self-management. Interventions promoting patient self-management were included only if they also included at least one other strategy related to clinician or organizational change.

Patient Reminder Systems. Any effort (e.g., postcards or telephone calls) to remind patients about upcoming appointments or important aspects of self-care. Interventions with patient reminders were included only if they also included at least one other strategy related to clinician or organizational change.

Continuous Quality Improvement. Interventions explicitly identified as using the techniques of continuous quality improvement, total quality management, or plan-do-study-act, or any iterative process for assessing quality problems, developing solutions to those problems, testing their impacts, and then reassessing the need for further action.

Definitions of the 11 categories of quality improvement strategies were modified from the taxonomy used by the Cochrane Effective Practice and Organisation of Care (EPOC) group. The definition for "facilitated relay of clinical information" corresponds to the EPOC category "patient mediated interventions"; we chose a different name to avoid confusion with patient education, self-management, and patient reminders. A category for financial incentives was originally included, but no studies involving this strategy met our inclusion criteria.

(Reprinted with permission from Shojania and colleagues 2006.)

interventions that did not use case management. Such reductions constitute mild to moderate reductions in A1C. Case management interventions that empowered the nurse or pharmacist case manager to make medication changes were significantly more effective than those that did not (reduction of 0.96 percentage points, 95% confidence interval [CI] 0.52–1.41 percentage points) versus 0.41 percentage points (95% CI 0.20–0.62 percentage points). Similarly interventions involving multidisciplinary teams were more effective than team interventions without this feature. The largest reductions occurred among the patients with *poorest baseline control*, that is, patients with A1C levels greater than 9%.

Targeting Other Process Measures and Outcomes

Reductions in cardiovascular risk factors such as blood pressure and lipids are targeted less frequently than A1C. However, reductions in these risk factors are more effective in preventing cardiovascular mortality in patients with diabetes than are reductions in A1C (Vijan et al. 2003, 2004). In addition, diabetes interventions have been more successful at measuring process measures, for example, screening for risk factors or complications, and less successful at actually improving risk factor levels—specifically, intermediate outcomes such as blood pressure and lipid control. In the following section we describe interventions focusing on outcomes other than A1C reductions. First we describe the STENO-2 study, one of the few diabetes interventions to examine mortality as an outcome. Next we summarize the effectiveness of disease management for other macrovascular risk factors, such as blood pressure and lipids in persons with diabetes, by describing a meta-analysis by Knight and observational data from large managed-care studies and from initiatives at community health centers.

In an RCT of Dutch patients with type 2 diabetes and microalbuminuria, otherwise known as STENO-2 (named after the Steno Centre for Diabetes in Denmark), Gaede and colleagues found that an intervention also targeting macrovascular risk factors was feasible and could lead to reductions in cardiovascular mortality (Gaede et al. 2003). As with other programs for managing risk factors, the intervention included multiple features: a project team (doctor, nurse, dietician) who advanced behavioral and pharmacologic therapy in a stepwise manner and who worked separately from the patient's usual general practice physician, quarterly comprehensive individual consultations regarding risk factors, and counseling on diet and physical activity. All patients were eligible for courses on smoking cessation and the prescription of angiotensin-converting enzyme (ACE) inhibitors or angiotensin II-receptor antagonists irrespective of blood pressure level. The mean length of the intervention was longer than those of other similar interventions, lasting a mean of 7.8 years, with five patients needing to be treated for this length of time to prevent a single cardiovascular event, and with fewer than two patients needing to be treated for this length of time to reduce nephropathy, neuropathy, and retinopathy.

Accordingly, forward-thinking programs have attempted to incorporate other risk factors along with A1C reduction. In a 2005 meta-analysis of 24 studies by Knight and colleagues, disease management programs were associated with improvements in screening for retinopathy and foot lesions and A1C levels (for A1C, a decrease of 0.5 percentage points, 95% CI 0.3–0.6 percentage points). However, there were minimal improvements in control of blood pressure and lipids (Knight et al. 2005). Elements of these programs included systems- and provider-level components such as guidelines, protocols, care plans, and provider education. However, the authors comment on the relative lack of studies examining the non-glucose-related aspects of diabetes management, even though they included not only randomized trials but also nonrandomized studies with pre- and post-test comparisons and a control group.

Mangione and colleagues found that disease-management programs that included a greater number of quality improvement elements (such as physician reminders, performance feedback, and care management) were associated with better processes of care than programs that contained fewer elements (Mangione et al. 2006). In addition to measurement of A1C these process measures included measurement of lipid concentrations and proteinuria. As found in the meta-analysis by Knight, these interventions were not effective at actually improving lipid or blood pressure levels. Elsewhere, Fleming and colleagues noted that greater infrastructure (in the form of registries, automated reminders, academic detailing, and quality improvement work groups, etc.) was associated with better performance of diabetes-related Health Plan Employer Data Information Set (HEDIS) measures (Fleming et al. 2004). However, HEDIS measures are primarily targeted at measurement rather than control.

Similarly, examination of disease management initiatives based at community health centers improved process measures, but these initiatives did not improve intermediate outcomes such as A1C control or blood pressure (Landon et al. 2007).

Randomized Trial versus Other Study Designs

Nonrandomized trials reported greater improvements in physician behaviors than those observed in randomized trials, and nonrandomized studies reported significantly larger reductions in A1C levels as documented in the meta-analysis by Shojania and colleagues (Shojania et al. 2006). The more significant effects in nonrandomized studies suggest that more-motivated patients, physicians, and health systems engaged in interventions, and thus success from interventions in these studies reflects system-level biases in participation. Because these studies were not randomized, patients with greater baseline A1C may have enrolled in disease management programs, thus skewing any positive effects of the program. However, quality improvement interventions that use quasi-experimental designs generally apply to larger populations. In addition, randomized trials select a population that may represent a small percentage of those actually affected by diabetes and "cherry-pick" participants. Whatever the conclusion about which design is the more accurate representation of effectiveness, nonrandomized studies with null findings have a conservative bias. If intervention effects are not observed with nonrandomized designs, it is unlikely that effects will be observed with a randomized design. For example in the study reported by Landon and colleagues (Landon et al. 2007), which used a nonrandomized design, the lack of significant changes in intermediate outcome measures would likely persist with randomized assignment.

Organizational Features

The lesser influence of interventions on outcomes such as blood pressure and lipid levels has not slowed the growth of the disease management industry. The revenues of disease management companies reportedly increased from $85 million in 1997 to $600 million in 2002, and these numbers do not include the large number of disease management programs developed and operated internally by health plans (Casalino 2005). Such programs are generally aimed at patients, but, as noted in the meta-analyses, they combine elements of health system and provider-directed change.

The adoption of key features of disease management has been slower at the provider-group level, reflecting the smaller organizations and perhaps more limited resources. In 2003 Casalino and colleagues surveyed 1104 provider groups about their use of disease registries, case management, physician feedback, clinical practice guidelines, and self-management skills and found that most groups employed at least one of these features and that informational technology and the presence of financial incentives at the provider group level were associated with adoption (Casalino et al. 2003). Therefore, health care organizational systems with greater infrastructure and financial resources may be more conducive to diffusion of disease management (Kim et al. 2004).

■ Strategies for Individual Patients

Diabetes interventions targeting the patient, as opposed to health care systems or providers, fall into several categories: education in self-management, self-monitoring of blood glucose, adherence to antidiabetic medications, and psychological interventions. In the following section we summarize interventions aimed at the individual by using available meta-analyses and systematic reviews organized by category. As with interventions including one component of provider or organizational change, the majority of interventions for individual patients also address reductions in A1C levels and, less commonly, other intermediate outcome measures, with the greatest improvement in outcomes observed in participants with the greatest margin for improvement. Reviews disagree about key features of the interventions, with several supporting specific modalities (such as group vs. individual learning or face-to-face vs. distance learning) and others refuting these features, and so these areas are covered in further detail in the following section.

Education in Self-Management

Interventions focusing on diabetes self-care skills, or self-management, are the most common type of intervention targeting individuals. We discuss the effectiveness of these interventions through review of four meta-analyses. These reviews demonstrate that interventions aimed at improving self-management can lead to reductions in A1C, but no single intervention type is superior, and the types of interventions range widely.

A 2002 review by Norris and colleagues included 31 RCTs of education in diabetes self-management (Norris et al. 2002). Studies involving pre- and postcomparisons or nonrandom assignment were excluded. The authors noted that self-management improved A1C levels by 0.76 percentage points (95% CI 0.34–1.18) more than in the control group, but effects tended to wane slightly over time. Interventions included didactic and participatory sessions, group support along with individual activities, collaborative education by health workers or patients, use of flash cards, dietician visits, weight management, telephone calls, computerized assessments, home visits, and demonstrations of recommended meals. No specific feature of intervention was more associated with greater improvements in A1C than any of the other features. Of note, study participants had poor glycemic control at baseline, with A1C levels averaging 9%.

Warsi and colleagues published a similar meta-analysis in 2004, which examined 16 studies in the same time frame as the review conducted by Norris and colleagues (Warsi et al. 2004). Warsi and associates also included nonrandomized studies if a concurrent control group was evaluated. They observed moderate effects, with reductions in A1C on the level of 0.45 percentage points (95% CI 0.17–0.74 percentage points). Specific features such as program duration, number of sessions, and conceptual model were not associated with significant reductions. Of note, this review also included programs geared at hypertensive patients and patients affected by arthritis, and so the power to detect associations with these features was high.

In a 2004 meta-analysis of 28 studies of diabetes patient education, using similar search terms as those employed by Norris and colleagues, Ellis and co-workers focused on several different qualitative aspects, including face-to-face delivery of the intervention, the use of cognitive reframing as a teaching method, and the inclusion of exercise, all of which were associated with greater impact and were associated with 44% of the variance in control (Ellis et al. 2004). The criteria required that all of the studies be RCTs, thus excluding pre- and post-test comparisons as well as quasi-randomized studies. Of note, group versus individual setting; having a dietician as the provider; intensity of intervention, including duration and number of educational contacts; provision of team support; and content, that is, adherence to medications versus self-monitoring of blood glucose, exercise, and psychosocial aspects, did not have independent effects. Whatever the subtype of intervention, the authors concluded that diabetes education resulted in reductions in A1C of approximately 0.32 percentage points (95% CI 0.069–0.571 percentage points) more than those seen in control groups.

In another meta-analysis from 2005 Chodosh and colleagues also attempted to identify the elements of the programs most responsible for the benefits obtained (Chodosh et al. 2005). In their meta-analysis, which included 26 RCTs involving diabetes as well as 14 RCTs on hypertension and 13 on osteoarthritis, they examined the effects of tailoring and of a group setting, feedback, a psychological emphasis, and medical care, that is, delivery of the intervention directly by their medical providers. In these studies, feedback was defined as some form of individual review of the participant's progress with the provider of the intervention, as distinct from interventions where no such review exists (this type of feedback to the patient is distinct from feedback to the provider on her/his performance). The presence of "tailoring" describes interventions modified to patients' specific needs and/or circumstances. The degree of tailoring could range from design of race- or gender-specific materials to review of individual progress and adjustment of goals on a continuous basis. Along with reduction in A1C, the authors examined interventions whose endpoint was weight loss.

In this study, diabetes self-management interventions had no significant effect on weight reduction, while significant reductions were seen in fasting blood glucose (–17 mg/dL) and in A1C (–0.81 percentage points). Within the diabetes studies, the use of feedback to the individual patient affected diabetes outcomes. However, none of the components mentioned above were effective across the other disease conditions examined, most notably hypertension. Further examination of highly successful studies did not reveal any common elements. The authors found evidence of publication bias and concluded that this may have led to the "positive" identification of key elements in previous studies, and they concluded that a priori identification of the necessary components of a chronic disease management program would not be evidence based. Intervention effects were most powerful for diseases responsive to medication, and the authors speculated that increased adherence to medication could be responsible for much of the change.

Two meta-analyses appearing in 2003 examined self-care interventions (educational or behavioral) in the subset of patients with type 2 diabetes and a further subset of older minority adults with type 2 disease (Gary et al. 2003). The studies were all RCTs. The authors found modest declines in A1C (0.43 percentage points, 95% CI 0.08–0.96 percentage points) resulting from behavioral interventions as well as improved adherence to medication and from self-monitoring of blood glucose, although again one particular type of intervention was not necessarily more effective than others. Changes in weight were not significant, and there was a lack of association between duration of the interventions and effectiveness.

Sarkisian and colleagues examined 12 self-care interventions for older adults who were members of ethnic minorities (Sarkisian et al. 2003); the interventions were most successful in patients with poor glycemic control and where they included tailoring by culture or age, group-delivery modalities, and adult family members. Although a single pooled point estimate could not be calculated because of the study's heterogeneity, the improvements in A1C were modest across studies. This review included RCTs but also nonrandomized studies, and the authors note that this may have led to an overstating of the effects. Participants with high baseline A1C (>11%) had the most dramatic reductions.

Adherence to Antidiabetic or Antihypoglycemia Medications

Although the majority of interventions have focused on education, some have been directed elsewhere, including adherence to medication. Unfortunately, interventions aiming to improve such adherence specifically have shown inconsistent and small effects. We review these studies through the discussion of a 2005 meta-analysis (Vermeire et al. 2005).

Vermeire and colleagues reviewed 21 studies assessing interventions aimed at improving adherence to recommendations on medication, as opposed to recommendations on exercise or diet (Vermeire et al. 2005). A broad range of studies were eligible, including RCTs but also controlled trials, pre- and postinterventions, and prospective cohort studies that assessed changes in adherence. Interventions were generally aimed at improvements in A1C and included nurse interventions, home aides (mailed reminders or ancillary staff visits), diabetes education programs, pharmacist-led interventions, and manipulations for dosing and frequency. Although declines in A1C existed, and improvement was noted in the expected process measures, the effects were generally small and could not be attributed to the intervention. Two of the obstacles the authors encountered were the missing definitions of adherence and the absence of an actual measurement of adherence, which was sometimes not specified. The authors concluded that focusing solely on adherence to medication might not be adequate to improve outcomes.

Self-Monitoring of Blood Glucose

Efforts to encourage self-monitoring of blood glucose among individuals not using insulin have had underwhelming results, and here we review two meta-analyses on this topic.

Self-monitoring is standard among patients already dependent on insulin, and to study this practice in a randomized fashion would be difficult if not ethically impossible. In 2005 Welschen and colleagues found that six randomized trials evaluating the effect of self-monitoring of blood glucose led to reductions in A1C (Welschen et al. 2005a, 2005b). Because the studies were heterogeneous, it was not possible to pool the data to obtain a single estimate, but the two largest studies suggested an effect, although these studies had some methodological limitations. Overall, the quality of the evidence was poor to moderate, and an accompanying note to the Cochrane review (Welschen et al. 2005b) disagreed with the conclusion that self-monitoring improved A1C results. Although Welschen and colleagues eventually concluded that self-monitoring might be helpful, it was only marginally so, and the studies lacked data on other outcomes that might be affected, including quality of life and satisfaction. Of note, in a clinical setting, self-monitoring of blood glucose is generally not applied to nonusers of insulin unless they use the data to alter their behavior.

Physiological Interventions

Because of the high prevalence of depression among patients with diabetes, reportedly three times as common in people with diabetes as in healthy controls for an estimated prevalence of about 15% (Gavard et al. 1993), researchers have attempted to improve glycemic control through effective psychological therapy (counseling, cognitive behavior therapy, or psychodynamic therapy). We review interventions with this focus by discussing two meta-analyses on this topic (Ismail et al. 2004; Winkley et al. 2006).

Ismail and colleagues examined 25 RCTs testing such interventions in persons with type 2 diabetes (Ismail et al. 2004). The pooled mean difference in A1C was 0.76 percentage points (95% CI 0.18–1.34 percentage points) and was accompanied by lower levels of psychological distress. Other outcomes, such as weight control, were not affected. No specific type of therapy was more effective than another, although the patient populations were difficult to compare. Although greater effects were expected in patients with greater psychological distress, such changes were not seen.

In 2006, the same research group examined the effects of such interventions among persons with type 1 diabetes and found slightly different results (Winkley et al. 2006). Interventions were more successful in children and adolescents, with reductions seen in A1C levels and in distress, but the interventions did not have similar effects in adults. Although the researchers did not comment on the possible reasons for differences from their previous meta-analysis of patients with type 2 diabetes, they noted that the therapy focused primarily on cognitive behavior therapy. Only one study focused on patients with existing psychological problems rather than those meeting criteria by a particular scale, meaning that patients could have symptoms even if by strict definition they did not qualify as having a psychological disorder.

■ Key Features of the Interventions

Group-Based versus Individual Learning

Interventions delivered in a group rather than an individual setting offer several theoretical advantages. Participants may be able to offer each other social support and reinforce the messages delivered in the group by the interventionist, and such delivery might also be more cost-effective. On the other hand individual interventions might be more tailored to the individual participant and more effectively address that person's unique barriers. In the meta-analyses by Norris et al. (2002), Chodosh et al. (2005), and Gary et al. (2003), group support was not associated with additional improvements in A1C. Wens and colleagues noted in a 2007 meta-analysis that the studies comparing group-based learning to individual learning that were included in the 2001 Cochrane meta-analysis were too limited by their designs to draw any strong conclusions (Wens et al. 2008).

In contrast a 2005 meta-analysis of RCTs and controlled clinical trials by Deakin and colleagues found that among persons with diabetes, group-based education programs reduced A1C by 1.4 percentage points (95% CI 0.8–1.9 percentage points) at 4–6 months and by 1.0 percentage points (95% CI 0.3–3 percentage points) at 2 years, lowered fasting glucose levels, reduced body weight by 1.6 kg, improved diabetes knowledge, lowered systolic blood pressure by 5 mm Hg (95% CI 1–10 mm Hg), and reduced the need for diabetes medication (Deakin et al. 2005). The primary difference between this meta-analysis and the other reviews was that Deakin's analysis purported to examine the effects of group support versus individual counseling, whereas other reviews of a group versus individual patients were post hoc comparisons. Therefore in the comparisons of Chodosh and colleagues (in their meta-analysis examining diabetes along with hypertension and osteoarthritis), group effects could have been confounded by the other intervention elements, such as tailoring, as well as by unnamed confounders. The difference is revealing, as it shows that an intervention delivered to a group may be more effective in the absence of other interventions but perhaps less powerful in settings where multiple quality improvement attempts are already occurring. An alternate explanation is that the inclusion of controlled trials in addition to randomized trials in the analyses by Deakin and colleagues and Sarkisian and associates exaggerated the effects of group education.

Face-to-Face versus Distance Learning

Interventions delivered at a distance, such as by telephone, offer several advantages. First they could reduce barriers of transportation that might prohibit effective participation in face-to-face models. Second they may be more receptive to participants' concerns about time and scheduling. Third they might be more cost-effective than face-to-face models. On the other hand face-to-face methods might more powerfully reinforce the intervention's messages by leveraging the greater interventionist-participant contact. In the meta-analyses by Warsi et al. (2004) and Ellis et al. (2004), face-to-face delivery was more effective than other types of learning. In a more recent meta-analysis Wens and colleagues (Wens et al. 2008) noted that design issues limited the strength of this conclusion. Distance-learning methods may be more effective, however, for participants who are selected for reduced access to care. Shea and colleagues (Shea et al. 2006) found that telemedicine significantly reduced not only A1C levels but also systolic and diastolic blood pressures and low-density lipoprotein cholesterol levels even among groups that already had moderate glycemic control; participants were those living in federally designated medically underserved areas of New York State.

Newer distance learning such as Web-based technologies might offer the advantages of distance learning but with greater flexibility than telephone-based management. For example McMahon and colleagues (McMahon et al. 2005) tested a Web-based intervention that offered education, explicit instructions on care management, uploading of current glucose logs, allowing for review by a care manager, and internal messaging that allowed communication with the care manager. Reductions in A1C were 1.9 percentage points versus 1.4 percentage points in usual care, a significant difference, and hypertensive participants also experienced significantly greater reductions in blood pressure and increases in high-density lipoprotein cholesterol than usual care groups. Elsewhere, Verhoeven and colleagues conducted a meta-analysis that specifically examined teleconsultation or videoconferencing interventions aimed at improving diabetes care (Verhoeven et al. 2007). Although they did not find that teleconferencing led to improvements in A1C, videoconferencing was associated with significant improvements in A1C ranging from 0.3 to 1.3 percentage points, although the studies were too heterogeneous to be combined into a single estimate.

Intensity of Intervention

A greater amount of contact between the interventionist and the participant would be expected to produce greater intervention effects, and, in fact, Norris and colleagues found that more intensive contact was associated with better outcomes (a decrease of 1 percentage point in A1C per 24 hours of contact) (Norris et al. 2002). In contrast Warsi and colleagues (Warsi et al. 2004), Ellis and associates (Ellis et al. 2004), and Ismail and co-workers (Ismail et al. 2004) did not find that program duration or number of sessions was associated with better outcomes. Ellis et al. speculate that this lack of effect, particularly for intensity of the intervention, may have been due to lack of variation in the "dose" of the interventions, and there may have been an inadequate number of studies to capture this effect.

In the United States most insurers pay for approximately 10 hours of diabetes education. Therefore, most interventions that involve patient-education components incorporate at least this amount of education. In addition 40% of the control groups in the review by Ismail (Ismail et al. 2004) had some level of interventions involving diabetes education that led to a statistically significant reduction in A1C (from pre- to postintervention) among these groups. For the psychological distress interventions that Ismail and colleagues investigated, the association between the duration and number of sessions with the outcomes was low, perhaps due to the short duration of follow-up or the higher rates of dropout associated with longer therapies.

Number of Strategies Employed

The majority of studies employed several strategies to improve their outcome, regardless of the outcome chosen or the level of the intervention. Indeed, in a Cochrane review published in 2001, Renders and colleagues documented multifaceted interventions in all of the studies (Renders et al. 2001). Strategies were not used in isolation, and interactions may have existed between strategies. In the meta-analysis by Shojania and colleagues (Shojania et al. 2006), a greater number of strategies per study was not associated with greater reductions in A1C. This may reflect the fact that the interventions were already complex rather than that multifaceted interventions were less successful than simpler interventions.

■ Implications for Health Policy and Areas of Uncertainty

The burgeoning need to address deficits in the quality of care combined with the fragmented nature of the U.S. health care delivery system makes implementation of uniform policy guidelines difficult. Drivers for change include the rising prevalence of diabetes and the failure of the existing health system to prevent and treat the complications of diabetes. The federal government has engaged in this debate by funding an examination of disease management programs; these programs are directed at the patient and operate independently of existing health care delivery systems.

In 2005, the Centers for Medicare & Medicaid Services (CMS) began a disease management initiative that involved the funding of large RCTs to examine regional programs to improve care for chronically ill beneficiaries in traditional Medicare fee-for-service. If the programs are successful in improving quality and reducing costs in these trials, CMS may expand them nationally if the magnitude of effects equals or exceeds those discussed earlier in this chapter, and contracting with private disease management companies and pressure to fund their services with public resources will increase. If the effects are more limited, alternate solutions need to be explored. The lack of uniformly effective approaches for other risk factors such as lipid control and hypertension suggests that current programs, or at least reports of these programs, may not adequately focus on these alternate outcomes. Although these programs could potentially be improved with minimal effort, the current literature does not suggest that the desired reductions in morbidity and mortality would occur.

The typical duration of diabetes quality-of-care interventions, changes over time in the effectiveness of these interventions, and the difficulties of maintaining such programs are generally not reported in the literature. Several features, particularly disease registries and other electronic-system reminders, require considerable financial resources for implementation but much less effort to maintain. Other features, such as ongoing case management, usually require at least the salary for staff to maintain such programs. Such ongoing costs may dictate that the nature of disease management programs changes over time. Difficulties with ongoing patient participation, rather than sustainability of the program itself, are usually the focus of reports. Not surprisingly, formal evaluations of cost-effectiveness and the features associated with cost-effectiveness are lacking.

The federal CMS has also prepared to implement legislation for pay-for-performance, but the exact nature of such programs and their cost-effectiveness remain unspecified. These programs attempt to harness pecuniary concerns to motivation for quality improvement, and they may affect more than 80% of persons enrolled in managed care (Rosenthal et al. 2006). Such initiatives have been in part based on conceptual models and work from the 1980s suggesting that fee-for-service schemes are associated with more frequent ordering of tests and reflect principal-agent economic theory (Epstein et al. 1986), which holds that the presence of incentives for a behavior will lead to greater performance of the behavior.

Such straightforward associations between payment scheme and outcomes have not been consistently documented, however. Fee-for-service reimbursement, or reimbursement by service with no incorporation of a particular set of quality measures, seems to be associated with *poorer* or *equivocal* measurement of quality measures when comparisons are made with salaried reimbursement (Ettner et al. 2006; Keating et al. 2004; Kim et al. 2007). The lack of association between the reimbursement for a procedure and the performance of the procedure reflects the presence of mitigating factors on incentives, particularly capitation, rewards for satisfaction, culture, and clinical indications. In a review conducted in 2003, Rosenthal and Frank examined the success of quality payment schemes in health care as well as other areas such as school performance (Rosenthal and Frank 2006). The results were notable for having minimal impact beyond better documentation.

More recent reports of pay-for-performance programs suggest that modest effects may exist, with incentives tied to general quality improvement initiatives and usually linked to diabetes process rather than outcome measures (Levin-Scherz, DeVita, and Timbie 2006; Mehrotra et al. 2007; Young et al. 2007). As noted earlier, addressing process measures only may not necessarily result in improved control of risk factors, but measurement of these risk factors is generally more responsive to such initiatives. A review by Rosenthal and Dudley suggests that the key features that will need to be considered are the target of the incentive (the physician versus the provider group), the amount, which measures should be targeted and what the target should be, and how risk stratification should occur (Rosenthal and Dudley 2007). As with disease management and other approaches for quality improvement, solutions may need to be tailored for the specific health care setting and the unique mix of patients and providers in that setting.

■ **References**

Casalino L (2005). Disease management and the organization of physician practice. *JAMA* **293**, 485–8.

Casalino L et al. (2003). External incentives, informational technology, and organized processes to improve health care quality for patients with chronic diseases. *JAMA* **289**, 434–41.

Chodosh J et al. (2005). Meta-analysis: chronic disease self-management programs for older adults. *Annals of Internal Medicine* **143**, 427–38.

Deakin T et al. (2005). Group based training for self-management strategies in people with type 2 diabetes mellitus. *Cochrane Database of Systematic Reviews* **2**, CD003417.

Ellis S et al. (2004). Diabetes patient education: a meta-analysis and meta-regression. *Patient Education and Counseling* **52**, 97–105.

Epstein AM, Begg CB, McNeil BJ (1986). The use of ambulatory testing in prepaid and fee-for-service group practices. Relation to perceived profitability. *New England Journal of Medicine* **314**, 1089–94.

Ettner S et al. (2006). Are physician reimbursement strategies associated with processes of care and patient satisfaction for patients with diabetes in managed care? *Health Services Research* **41**, 1221–41.

Fleming B et al. (2004). The relationship between organizational systems and clinical quality in diabetes care. *American Journal of Managed Care* **10**, 934–44.

Gaede P et al. (2003). Multifactorial intervention and cardiovascular disease in patients with type 2 diabetes. *New England Journal of Medicine* **348**, 383–93.

Gary T et al. (2003). Meta-analysis of randomized educational and behavioral interventions in type 2 diabetes. *Diabetes Educator* **29**, 488–501.

Gavard J, Lustman P, Clouse R. (1993). Prevalence of depression in adults with diabetes. An epidemiological evaluation. *Diabetes Care* **16**, 1167–78.

Ismail K, Winkley K, Rabe-Hesketh S (2004). Systematic review and meta-analysis of randomised controlled trials of psychological interventions to improve glycaemic control in patients with type 2 diabetes. *Lancet* **363**, 1589–97.

Keating N et al. (2004). The influence of physicians' practice management strategies and financial arrangements on quality of care among patients with diabetes. *Medical Care* **42**, 829–39.

Kim C et al. (2004). Managed care organization and the quality of diabetes care. *Diabetes Care* **27**, 1529–34.

Kim C et al. (2007). Physician compensation from salary and quality of diabetes care. *Journal of General Internal Medicine* **22**, 448–52.

Knight K et al. (2005). A systematic review of diabetes disease management programs. *American Journal of Managed Care* **11**, 242–50.

Landon B et al. (2007). Improving the management of chronic disease at community health centers. *New England Journal of Medicine* **356**, 921–34.

Levin-Scherz J, DeVita N, Timbie J (2006). Impact of pay-for-performance contracts and network registry on diabetes and asthma HEDIS measures in an integrated delivery network. *Medical Care Research and Review* **63**, 14S–28S.

Lindenauer P et al. (2007). Public reporting and pay for performance in hospital quality improvement. *New England Journal of Medicine* **356**, 486–96.

Mangione C et al. (2006). The association between quality of care and the intensity of diabetes disease management programs. *Annals of Internal Medicine* **145**, 107–16.

McMahon G et al. (2005). Web-based care management in patients with poorly controlled diabetes. *Diabetes Care* **28**, 1624–9.

Mehrotra A et al. (2007). The response of physician groups to P4P incentives. *American Journal of Managed Care* **13**, 249–55.

Norris SL et al. (2002). Self-management education for adults with type 2 diabetes. *Diabetes Care* **25**, 1159–71.

Rosenthal MB, Dudley RA (2007). Pay-for-performance: will the latest payment trend improve care? *JAMA* **297**, 740–4.

Rosenthal MB, Frank RG (2006). What is the empirical basis for paying for quality in health care? *Medical Care Research Review* **63**, 135–57.

Rosenthal MB et al. (2006). Pay for performance in commercial HMOs. *New England Journal of Medicine* **355**, 1895–902.

Sarkisian CA et al. (2003). A systematic review of diabetes self-care interventions for older, African-American, or Latino adults. *Diabetes Educator* **29**, 467–9.

Shea S et al. (2006). A randomized trial comparing telemedicine case management with usual care in older, ethnically diverse, medically underserved patients with diabetes mellitus. *Journal of the American Medical Informatics Association* **13**, 40–51.

Shojania K et al., eds. (2004). *Closing the quality gap: a critical analysis of quality improvement strategies*. In Volume 1—*Series Overview and Methodology*. Rockville, MD: Agency for HealthCare Research and Quality. AHRQ Publication No. 04-0051-1.

Shojania K et al. (2006). Effects of quality improvement strategies for type 2 diabetes on glycemic control: a meta-regression analysis. *JAMA* **296**, 427–40.

Verhoeven F et al. (2007). The contribution of teleconsultation and videoconferencing to diabetes care: a systematic literature review. *Journal of Medical Internet Research* **9**, e37.

Vermeire E et al. (2005). Interventions for improving adherence to treatment recommendations in people with type 2 diabetes mellitus. *Cochrane Database of Systematic Reviews* **2**, CD003638.

Vijan S, Hayward RA (2003). Treatment of hypertension in type 2 diabetes mellitus: blood pressure goals, choice of agents, and setting priorities in diabetes care. *Annals of Internal Medicine* **138**, 593–602.

Vijan S, Hayward RA (2004). Pharmacologic lipid-lowering therapy in type 2 diabetes mellitus: *Annals of Internal Medicine* **140**, 650–8.

Warsi A et al. (2004). Self-management education programs in chronic disease. *Archives of Internal Medicine* **164**, 1641–9.

Welschen LM et al. (2005a). Self-monitoring of blood glucose in patients with type 2 diabetes who are not using insulin: a systematic review. *Diabetes Care* **28**, 1510–7.

Welschen LM et al. (2005b). Self-monitoring of blood glucose in patients with type 2 diabetes mellitus who are not using insulin. *Cochrane Database of Systematic Reviews* **2**, CD005060.

Wens J et al. (2008). Educational interventions aiming at improving adherence to treatment recommendations in type 2 diabetes: a sub-analysis of a systematic review of randomised controlled trials. *Diabetes Research and Clinical Practice* **79**, 377–88.

Winkley K et al. (2006). Psychological interventions to improve glycaemic control in patients with type 1 diabetes: systematic review and meta-analysis of randomised controlled trials. *British Medical Journal* **333**, 65.

Young G et al. (2007). Effects of paying physicians based on their relative performance for quality. *Journal of General Internal Medicine* **22**, 872–6.

20. Economic Costs of Diabetes and the Cost-Effectiveness of Interventions to Prevent and Control This Disease

Ping Zhang and Rui Li

■ Main Public Health Messages

- Diabetes imposes a large economic burden on the national health care system and affects not only national economies but also individuals and their families.
- The estimated direct medical cost of diabetes worldwide in 2007 was as much as US$421.7 billion.
- The economic burden of diabetes will continue to increase in the near future. Globally, the estimated annual direct medical cost for this disease could reach US$558.6 billion by 2025.
- Worldwide, the indirect cost of diabetes, as measured by lost productivity, is also large.
- Diabetes substantially reduces quality of life for those who have this disorder.
- With limited health care resources, policy makers at the national and local levels need to prioritize intervention programs in diabetes.
- Cost-effectiveness analysis can assist in the setting of priorities for programs in diabetes.
- The cost-effectiveness of interventions to prevent or control diabetes varies greatly.
- Those interventions that strong evidence indicates are either cost saving, very cost-effective, or cost-effective should be adopted.
- More research is needed to evaluate those interventions for which the current evidence on cost-effectiveness is weak.

■ Introduction

In addition to exerting a negative impact on health, diabetes imposes a large economic burden on the national health care system. Correspondingly, it stresses national economies as well as individuals and their families. Even so, many interventions are available for reducing the burden of this disease that can be adopted in either clinical or public health settings. In this chapter we first briefly describe the economic burden of diabetes, and then we focus on the prioritization of different interventions based on the framework of cost-effectiveness analysis (CEA). We conclude with a summary and some implications for policy.

■ Economic Burden of Diabetes

The economic burden of diabetes can be measured in terms of direct medical, indirect, and intangible costs. Direct medical costs include resources used to treat the disease. Indirect costs include lost productivity caused by morbidity, disability, or premature mortality. Intangible costs refer to the reduced quality of life for people with diabetes that is brought about by stress, pain, and anxiety.

Direct Medical Costs

For 2007, the 1-year direct medical cost of diabetes worldwide for persons aged 20 to 79 years was estimated to be US$232 billion but may have been as high as US$421.7 billion. Measured in international dollars (ID), which correct for differences in purchase power across countries, the estimated costs in 2007 were between 286.1 billion and 518.9 billion. These costs will no doubt rise substantially in years to come, with published estimates for the year 2025 of US$302.5 to US$558.6 billion and $381.1 to $701.2 billion (ID) (International Diabetes Federation 2006). Most of these estimated direct medical costs will be in developed countries, with the United States alone accounting for more than half. Overall, direct health care costs of diabetes range from 2.5% to 15% of annual health care budgets, depending on the local prevalence of diabetes and the sophistication of the treatment available (International Diabetes Federation 2006).

On a per capita basis, a person with diabetes incurs medical costs that are two to five times as high as those of a person without diabetes (International Diabetes Federation 1999). Globally the International Diabetes Federation predicted that in 2007 the average expenditure per person was US$505 or $725 (2007 ID) (International Diabetes Federation 2006). Not unexpectedly, expenditures varied substantially across geographical regions and countries. By region, a person with diabetes in Africa spent the least (US$71 or $180 [ID]), whereas a European person spent the most (US$1228 or $1561 [ID]). By country per capita yearly medical expenditure ranged from a low of $25 (ID) in Somalia to a high of more than $6000 (ID) in the United States.

Not surprisingly the direct medical costs of managing the complications of diabetes exceed those for managing diabetes itself. For example, of the estimated US$116 billion in total direct medical costs for diabetes in the United States in 2007, $27 billion was for directly treating the disease, $58 billion was for treating diabetes-related chronic complications, and $39 billion was for excess costs for general medical care among people with diabetes (American Diabetes Association 2008). In China the cost of managing diabetes complications is four times as much as that for managing diabetes by itself (Tang et al. 2003). In that country, hospital costs account for a majority of the total direct medical costs. In the United States hospitalizations attributable to diabetes cost $58 billion in 2007, or 50% of the total direct medical expenditure for diabetes in that year (American Diabetes Association 2008). In Latin America and the Caribbean 53% of the total direct medical costs in 2000 were for drugs and hospitalization (Barcelo et al. 2003).

In many countries a significant proportion of the direct medical costs for diabetes is paid by the patient or her/his family. Indeed, in some countries, a sizable portion of the family's entire income may be spent for diabetes care. In India, for example, families at the middle- and low-income levels spent 15% and 25%, respectively, of their family income on diabetes care if the family had an adult with type 1 diabetes (Shobhana et al. 2002).

Indirect and Intangible Costs

For the world as a whole (or by region) there is no information on the indirect costs of diabetes, but estimates from individual countries indicate that such costs are quite large. For example in the United States in 2007 the estimated indirect cost was US$58 billion, or about one-third of the total economic cost of diabetes in this country (American Diabetes Association 2008). In developing countries the indirect cost is as least as much as or even higher than direct medical costs and will continue to increase in the next three decades, as the largest predicted rise in the number of people with diabetes in those countries will be in the economically productive age groups of 20–40 years and 45–64 years (King, Aubert, and Herman 1998).

Diabetes lowers a person's quality of life by compromising physical, psychological, and social functioning (Polonsky 2000). The demands of self-care can be burdensome, frustrating, and overwhelming, and adjustment to the disease is often accompanied by negative emotional responses, including anger, guilt, frustration, denial, and loneliness. The impact of long-term complications such as heart disease, stroke, and kidney failure can be severe, leading to major changes in a patient's ability to function in daily life. The ongoing threat of complications can be worrisome and depressing, and social relationships may be severely affected. Using a value of 1 to reflect full health and 0 to stand for death, a study of a national representative sample of 38,678 persons in the United States showed that the 2778 persons with diabetes had a mean value of 0.75, and without considering its related complications, diabetes alone would lower the quality of life by 0.04 on the scale described (Sullivan and Ghushchyan 2006). Using a financial standard to measure the impact of diabetes on a person's quality of life is, not surprisingly, quite difficult.

■ Cost-Effectiveness of Interventions for Prevention and Control of Diabetes

With limited health care resources and an increased availability of public health and clinical interventions, health policy makers at the national and local levels increasingly seek guidance on how to prioritize intervention programs. Each intervention has its own costs, health benefits, and risks. CEA is one of the tools that can help decision makers sort through alternatives and decide which ones should be chosen from the point of view of economic efficiency. CEA is designed to determine which means of attaining particular health goals are the most efficient; choosing those health programs or interventions that have the least cost for a given outcome would lead to a more efficient use of health care resources. Those resources that are saved through more cost-effective approaches can be devoted to expanding existing programs or to developing other important health and social endeavors.

Applying Cost-Effectiveness Analysis to Decisions on Resource Allocation

CEA is an analytic tool in which the costs and effects of a program and at least one alternative are calculated and presented in a ratio of incremental cost to incremental effect (Gold et al. 1996). The cost-effectiveness ratio (CER), the typical expression of the results of CEA, is calculated as the difference in cost between two interventions divided by the difference in health benefit obtained (Drummond et al. 2005). For example in assessing the cost-effectiveness of an intensive lifestyle intervention for preventing type 2 diabetes among high-risk individuals by using a standard lifestyle intervention as the basis of comparison, the CER can be estimated as:

$$\frac{C_I - C_s}{B_I - B_s}$$

where C_I = net cost of the intensive lifestyle intervention, C_S = net cost of the standard lifestyle intervention, B_I = net health benefit of the intensive lifestyle intervention, and B_S = net health benefit of the standard lifestyle intervention. The net cost associated with an intervention is the difference between costs and savings associated with the intervention. For example the net cost of the intensive lifestyle intervention equals the cost of the intervention program plus any induced costs such as additional expenses to purchase healthier food minus the medical costs saved from treating a smaller number of patients with diabetes. The net health benefit of an intervention is the sum of health gained or lost because of the intervention. In this example the net benefits (also called effectiveness) of the intensive lifestyle intervention are the gain in health as a result of better quality of life from losing body weight and the cases of diabetes prevented minus any health loss associated with adverse events such as injury from the intensive exercise program.

The costs of an intervention are always measured with a monetary term, whereas health effects are measured in either natural units of health, such as a case of diabetes prevented, a year of life saved, or a quality-adjusted life year (QALY) gained. When QALY is used as the effectiveness measure, the CEA is given another name, cost-utility analysis (CUA). A QALY is a year of life adjusted for impairments in health-related quality of life, and thus it represents a year lived with full health. In contrast to CEA, which uses natural units of health to measure the effect of interventions, CUA can facilitate a comparison of broader intervention categories such as those used for preventing or treating different health conditions, because the effects of different interventions are all measured in QALY. When the effectiveness of intervention is measured in a natural health unit, the comparison of different interventions is necessarily restricted to those that produce that same natural unit.

CEA can assist with decisions on public health policy or clinical practice by showing the relative efficiency of different intervention options. In a simple case of two alternative comparisons, program A versus program B, there are four possible scenarios: (1) A is more effective but costs more than B; (2) A is less effective and costs more than B; (3) A is less effective and costs less than B; and (4) A is more effective and costs less than B. The choices of B under scenario (2) and A under scenario (4) are clear and straightforward. The choices under the other two scenarios are less clear, however. There, a threshold CER is required for determining whether A or B should be adopted. If the CER for A, compared with B, is below the threshold, A should be adopted, and vice versa.

Selecting such a cost-effectiveness threshold, however, is both difficult and controversial. In fact the choice of this threshold depends on many factors, such as who is making the decision, what the purpose of the analysis is, how the decision maker values health, money, and risk, and what the available resources are (Owens 1998).

Although the CEA can provide very valuable information for making a sound decision, it is not and should not substitute for a complete decision-making process. Indeed, in determining whether to offer a specific intervention, economic efficiency is only one of many factors to consider. In truth, there may be good reasons to offer an inefficient intervention, and there may be good reasons not to offer an efficient intervention. These reasons include concerns about fairness and justice that are not fully captured in the sum of QALYs or in the ways that the costs are valued, the existence of benefits and costs that are outside the realm of health factors, and the feasibility of implementation (Gold et al. 1996).

Cost-Effectiveness of Interventions to Prevent or Control Diabetes

Methods for Compiling the Evidence

We compiled the current evidence on the cost-effectiveness of interventions used for the prevention and control of type 1 or type 2 diabetes by conducting a systematic review. We included all published studies in English during the period of January1985 to December 2005 and followed the steps recommended by the Cochrane Collaboration (Alderson et al. 2004) in conducting our review. After selecting the studies and extracting information from them, we adjusted the CERs, expressing them in the same year and same currency. We then divided the studies by type of intervention and study population (U.S. and non-U.S.) and classified the cost-effectiveness of each intervention on the basis of its CER. Finally, we ranked the interventions based on the strength of the evidence and the level of cost-effectiveness.

We took several steps to select the studies and extract relevant information. First we searched seven bibliographic electronic databases (MEDLINE, EMBASE, CINAHL, PsychInfo, Soc Abs, Web of Science, and Cochrane Library) by using key words to indicate diabetes (26 words), costs (4 words), effectiveness (4 words), and CEA (3 words) and then obtained the abstracts of the relevant articles. Second two reviewers applied the criteria for inclusion and exclusion to independently determine the eligibility of each article by reading its abstract first, then the full article. When there was disagreement about inclusion, consensus was achieved through discussion or with the help of a third reviewer. Finally, information from each selected article was extracted using a standard form. The form included the study type, intervention evaluated and its comparators, population to which it was applied, perspective, analytical time horizon, methods for deriving the results, health risk, benefits and costs of the intervention and its comparators, discounting rates used, CERs, sensitivity analyses, and conclusion reached. The reference lists of all included articles were screened for additional citations. The journal *Diabetes Care* was manually searched, as it was expected to be highly relevant.

We included in our review only those studies that were rated as being either "good" or "excellent" in quality. We used a 13-item quality assessment tool from the *British Medical Journal* author's guide for economic studies (Drummond 1996) to rate the quality of each study. This tool considers four items—categories of costs, sources of the cost data, categories of benefits, and sources of benefit-specific data—as the necessary components for any CEA. Studies that missed any of the four items were considered as being "low quality" and excluded. Ratings for the other nine items on the tool were based on a "yes" or "no" answer for the following questions (i.e., whether certain things were done): the analytical horizon was reported, the study perspective was reported, the model was clearly described, currency and year of costs were reported, the cost was discounted, the benefits were discounted, the CERs were reported, and the sensitivity analyses were performed. The study received one point for each "yes" answer and zero for each "no." The quality of a study was rated as "fair" if the total score was 1–3, "good" for 4–6, and "excellent" for 7–9.

We reported the CERs in 2005 ID instead of U.S. dollars because the former are more comparable across countries. To do so, first, we inflated the costs in all CERs to reflect 2005 currency by using the consumer price index (CPI) of the country in which the CER was originally reported. For the U.S. studies we inflated the cost of the CER by using the medical care component of the CPI (Bureau of Labor Statistics 2008). Then we converted the cost of the CER into ID using each country's 2005 purchase power parity rate (International Monetary Fund 2004). If a study did not report the year of currency for the CER, we assumed that the currency year was 1 year prior to the publication date. In addition we used the CER value that was associated with the health care system perspective and for which both the cost and benefits of the intervention were discounted. If the CER was reported in other perspectives or undiscounted in the main analysis, we searched for this information from the sensitivity analyses.

We grouped interventions into several categories: diabetes prevention, screening for undiagnosed type 2 diabetes, managing the glucose level of patients with diabetes, managing the risk factors for diabetes complications, screening for and treating diabetes-related complications, and multicomponent interventions. Within each category we grouped interventions together if the content of the intervention and the population to which it was applied were similar. When there was more than one study that evaluated exactly the same intervention for the same population, we reported the range of CERs. Because the cost-effectiveness of an intervention could depend on the health care delivery and payment system, we reported the study results by two regions: United States and other regions (included mainly Australia, Canada, and Western Europe). There were no cost-effectiveness studies from developing countries at the time of this review.

We ranked interventions by their cost-effectiveness and the strength of the evidence to derive the cost-effectiveness. Following Laupacis and colleagues (Laupacis et al. 1992) and other literature (Klonoff and Schwartz 2000), we classified cost-effectiveness into five levels based on their CERs: cost saving, very cost-effective, cost-effective, marginally cost-effective, and not cost-effective. The CERs per QALY or life year gained were negative if the intervention was cost saving, less than $25,000 if very cost-effective, greater than or equal to $25,000 but less than $50,000 if cost-effective, greater than or equal to $50,000 but less than $100,000 if marginally cost-effective, and more than $100,000 if not cost-effective.

The strength of the evidence for assessing cost-effectiveness was either strong or weak. We considered evidence to be strong if it met either of two multipart criteria: Criterion 1: The cost-effectiveness of the intervention was evaluated by at least two studies *and* these studies were rated as "good" or "excellent" *and* the short-term effectiveness of the interventions has been demonstrated by good-quality randomized clinical trials *and* the long-term health and economic consequences of the intervention were derived from a validated diabetes disease simulation model *and* the studies produced similar CERs; Criterion 2: Only one study evaluated the cost-effectiveness of the intervention *and* that study was rated as "excellent" in quality *and* the clinical effectiveness of the intervention had been shown by large, multicenter, randomized clinical trials such as Diabetes Prevention Program, Study to Prevent NIDDM (STOP-NIDDM Trial), the Diabetes Control and Complications

Trial (DCCT), the United Kingdom Prospective Diabetes Study (UKPDS), and the Scandinavian Simvastatin Survival Study (4S). We considered evidence for a cost-effectiveness assessment to be weak if only one study evaluated the cost-effectiveness of the intervention *and/or* the estimate of an intervention's effectiveness was based on epidemiologic data or data from trials that were small or not randomized, was simulated by diabetes disease models only, or was assessed by studies rated as "fair" in quality. All studies that aimed at evaluating public policy and screening recommendations for diabetes and its complications were included in the "weak" evidence category.

Combining the five levels of cost-effectiveness with two levels of strength of evidence yielded 10 categories into which an intervention could fall. We labeled those interventions with strong evidence by adding the word "clearly" and those interventions with weak evidence by adding the word "possibly" before each level of cost-effectiveness.

Cost-Effectiveness of the Interventions

Table 20.1 summarizes the results of the studies in the United States. In all there were 21 studies that had evaluated 30 different interventions. The intervention populations included persons at high risk for type 2 diabetes, persons with undiagnosed type 2 diabetes, or persons with diagnosed type 1 or type 2 diabetes. The analytical time frame ranged from a 3-year within-trial analysis to lifetime simulation modeling. The CERs varied from cost saving to more than $100,000 per QALY. All but one of the studies were rated as of excellent quality.

Using a lifestyle intervention to prevent type 2 diabetes among people with impaired glucose tolerance (IGT), one study showed that within the 3 years of the Diabetes Prevention Program, the intervention cost $19,000 per additional case of diabetes prevented. Per QALY gained the cost was $30,000 if the intervention was implemented at the individual level; for delivery in a group setting the cost was $6000 per additional case of diabetes prevented or $11,000 per additional QALY gained (The Diabetes Prevention Program Research Group 2003). The two other studies (Eddy, Schlessinger, and Kahn 2005; Palmer et al. 2004c) showed that, over a long period of time, the same intervention cost a range of $1400 to $78,000 per additional QALY gained if it was delivered at individual levels and was cost saving or cost less than $15,000 per additional QALY gained when delivered in a group setting. Using metformin to prevent diabetes in the same population, within the 3 years of the Diabetes Prevention Program the intervention cost $39,000 with a brand-name drug and only $14,000 using a generic drug for an additional case of diabetes prevented within the 3-year clinical trial period. Over a lifetime, metformin cost about $39,000 to $44,000 with the brand-name drug and just $2000 with the generic drug per an additional QALY gained.

The cost-effectiveness of screening for undiagnosed type 2 diabetes was evaluated by two studies (CDC Diabetes Cost-Effectiveness Study Group 1998;

TABLE 20.1 *Cost-Effectiveness from the Health Care System Perspective of Interventions for the Prevention and Control of Diabetes, 2005 International Dollars, the United States*

Author and Year of Study	Intervention	Comparison Intervention	Study Population	Analytical Time Frame	Cost-Effectiveness Ratio ($/QALY)*	Quality of the Study	Comments
Preventing type 2 diabetes							
Diabetes Prevention Program (DPP) Study Group, 2004	Lifestyle modification	Standard care	Adults with impaired glucose tolerance	3 years	$19,000/diabetes case avoided	Excellent	Within-trial analysis. Did not include long-term benefits and costs.
	Individual				$6000/ diabetes case avoided		
	Group	Standard care					
	Metformin						
	Brand name				$39,000/diabetes case avoided		
	Generic				$14,000/diabetes case avoided		
Herman et al. 2005; Eddy et al. 2005	Lifestyle modification	Standard care or no intervention	Adults with impaired glucose tolerance	Lifetime or 30 years	$1400–$78,000	Excellent, excellent	Used a disease progression model; included the long-term health benefits and costs.
	Individual						
	Group				Cost saving: –$15,000		
	Metformin	Standard care or no intervention					
	Brand name				$39,000–$44,000		
	Generic				$2000		

(continued)

TABLE 20.1 *(continued)*

Screening for undiagnosed type 2 diabetes

Author and Year of Study	Intervention	Comparison Intervention	Study Population	Analytical Time Frame	Cost-Effectiveness Ratio ($/QALY)*	Quality of the Study	Comments
CDC 1998	One-time opportunistic screening for all	No screening	Adults	Lifetime	Overall, $82,800. Ranged from $20,000 to over $200,000, depending on age	Excellent	CDC study considered only microvascular complications.
Hoerger et al. 2004	One-time opportunistic screening for all	No screening	Adults	Lifetime	$48,000–$126,000 depending on age	Excellent	Hoerger et al. considered both microvascular and macrovascular complications.
	One-time opportunistic screening, persons with hypertension	No screening			$31,000–$87,000 depending on age		
	One-time opportunistic screening for all	Screening for persons with hypertension			$144,000–$467,000 depending on age		

Managing glucose level

DCCT 1996	Intensive glucose control	Standard care	Adults with type 1 diabetes	Lifetime	$44,000	Excellent	Used a disease progression model based on data from the DCCT
Eastman et al. 1997; CDC 2002	Intensive glucose control: sulfonylurea or insulin	Standard care	Adults with newly diagnosed type 2 diabetes	Lifetime	$48,000–$57,000 depending on studies	Excellent	Used disease progression model with data mainly from US DCCT or UKPDS.
Eddy et al. 2005	Lifestyle modification + medication for standard care	Medication for standard care	Adults with onset of type 2 DM	30 years	$30,000	Excellent	Used a disease progression model to model the continued DPP lifestyle invention after persons with IGT get DM.

Managing risk factors for diabetes-related complication

Herman et al. 1999	Simvastatin for cholesterol control	Placebo	Adults with type 2 diabetes with dyslipidemia with CVD	5 years	Cost saving	Excellent	Within-trial analysis of the Scandinavian Simvastatin Survival Study (4S)

(continued)

TABLE 20.1 *(continued)*

Author and Year of Study	Intervention	Comparison Intervention	Study Population	Analytical Time Frame	Cost-Effectiveness Ratio ($/QALY)*	Quality of the Study	Comments
Grover 2001	Simvastatin for cholesterol control	Placebo	Adults with type 2 diabetes with dyslipidemia, no CHD	Lifetime	Men: $7000–$19,000/LYG; Women: $18,000–$32,000/ LYG	Good	Used cardiovascular disease life expectancy model
CDC 2002	Pravastatin for intensive cholesterol control:	Standard care	Adults with type 2 diabetes with dyslipidemia	Lifetime	$72,000	Excellent	Used disease progression model with data mainly from US DCCT or UKPDS
Elliot 2000; CDC 2002	Tight hypertension control with goal of less than 130/85 mm Hg	Standard care	Type 2 diabetes adults with hypertension	Lifetime	Cost saving	Excellent, excellent	Used a disease progression model with data from literature
Earnshaw 2002	Smoking cessation	Standard care	Adults with newly diagnosed type 2 diabetes	Lifetime	$14,000	Excellent	Used type 2 disease progression model with data mainly from UKPDS

Study	Intervention	Comparator	Population	Time horizon	Cost	Quality	Comments
Martzel et al. 2003	Orlistat + one oral antidiabetes agent + weight management using ADA guideline	One oral antidiabetes agent + weight management using ADA guideline	Overweight and obese adults with type 2 diabetes	11 years	$10,000/diabetes complication-free year	Excellent	Used a simple type 2 disease progression model with data mainly from UKPDS

Screening for and early treatment of diabetes-related complications

Study	Intervention	Comparator	Population	Time horizon	Cost	Quality	Comments
Javitt et al. 1994	Screening for and early treatment of retinopathy at different intervals: 2, 3, or 4 years plus 6-, 12-, 18-month follow-up checkup if having advanced retinopathy	No screening	Adults with type 2 diabetes	Lifetime	Cost saving	Excellent	Used a diabetes disease progression model. Federal budgetary perspective
Vijan et al. 2000	Screening for diabetes retinopathy every 5, 3, 2, 1 year	No screening	Adults with type 2 diabetes with different A1C level	Lifetime	20,000–37,000	Excellent	Used a type 2 diabetes disease progression model. More cost-effective with a higher A1C level
	Screening annually	Screening every 2 years			$108,000		
	Every 2 years	Screening every 3 years			$50,000		
	Every 3 years	Screening every 5 years			$30,000		

(*continued*)

TABLE 20.1 (*continued*)

Author and Year of Study	Intervention	Comparison Intervention	Study Population	Analytical Time Frame	Cost-Effectiveness Ratio ($/QALY)*	Quality of the Study	Comments
Dong et al. 2004	Screening for and treating microalbuminuria with ACE inhibitor	Standard care	Adults with type 1 diabetes	Lifetime	$35,000	Excellent	Used a type 1 diabetes disease progression model. More cost-effective with a higher A1C level
Golan et al. 1999	Treating all with ACE inhibitor	Screening for and treating proteinuria	Adults aged 50 years and older with type 2 diabetes	Lifetime	Cost saving	Excellent	Used type 2 disease progression model.
	Screening and treating microalbuminuria with ACE inhibitor	Screening for and treating proteinuria			Cost saving		More cost-effective with younger age groups.
	Treating all with ACE inhibitor	Screening for and treating microalbuminuria with ACE inhibitor			$10,000		

Study	Intervention	Comparator	Population	Time horizon	Cost	Quality	Comments
Palmer et al. 2004	Irbesartan starting at the state of microalbuminuria	Standard care	Adults with type 2 diabetes	25 years	Cost saving	Excellent	Used type 2 disease progression model. Did not include the cost of detection of microalbuminuria and overt nephropathy.
	Irbesartan starting at the state of overt nephropathy	Standard care			Cost saving		
	Irbesartan starting at the state of microalbuminuria	Irbesartan starting at the state of overt nephropathy			Cost saving		
Treating diabetes complications							
Rosen et al. 2005	Medicare coverage for ACE inhibitors	Medicare coverage for ACE inhibitors in 2006	Persons with diabetes in the Medicare program	Lifetime	Cost saving	Excellent	Medicare perspective.
Shama et al. 2001	Immediate vitrectomy for treating hemorrhage secondary to diabetic retinopathy	Delayed vitrectomy	Diabetes patients with diabetic retinopathy	Lifetime	$2000	Excellent	

(continued)

TABLE 20.1 *(continued)*

Author and Year of Study	Intervention	Comparison Intervention	Study Population	Analytical Time Frame	Cost-Effectiveness Ratio ($/QALY)*	Quality of the Study	Comments
Douzdjia et al. 1998	Dialysis	No treatment	Type 1 diabetes patient with end-stage renal disease	5 years	$438,000	Excellent	Simple decision model.
	Transplant of kidney from a cadaver	No treatment			$216,000		
	Transplant of kidney from a living donor	No treatment			$171,000		
	Simultaneous transplant of pancreas and kidney	No treatment			$141,000		
	Transplant of kidney from living donor	Dialysis; transplant of kidney from a cadaver; dialysis			Cost saving		
	Simultaneous pancreas-kidney transplant	(Kidney transplant from cadaver)			Cost saving		
	Simultaneous pancreas-kidney transplant	Kidney transplant from a living donor			30,000		

*Cost-effectiveness ratio is in international dollars per QALY, or otherwise as indicated.

ACE, angiotensin-converting enzyme; ADA, American Diabetes Association; CHD, coronary heart disease; CVD, cardiovascular disease; DCCT, Diabetes Control and Complications Trial; DM, diabetes mellitus; DPP, Diabetes Prevention Program; IGT, impaired glucose tolerance; LYG, life year gained; QALY, quality-adjusted life years; UKPDS, United Kingdom Prospective Diabetes Study.

Hoerger et al. 2004). Compared with no screening, opportunistic screening among all U.S. adults cost $20,000 to over $200,000 per additional QALY gained, depending on age group and study. If the screening targeted those with hypertension, the intervention would cost $31,000 to $87,000 per additional QALY gained. In a comparison with the targeted screening, opportunistic screening cost $144,000 to $467,000 per additional QALY gained.

In a comparison with standard care, intensive insulin therapy among type 1 diabetes patients was estimated to cost $44,000 per additional QALY gained (DCCT Research Group 1996). Intensive glycemic control in conjunction with sulfonylurea or insulin treatment among type 2 patients was estimated to cost between $48,000 and $57,000 per QALY among those newly diagnosed with diabetes (Eastman 1998). Intensive lifestyle intervention cost $30,000 per QALY (versus standard care) among those with newly developed diabetes (Eddy, Schlessinger, and Kahn 2005).

In three studies in which intensive control of cholesterol was evaluated (CDC Diabetes Cost-effectiveness Group 2002; Grover et al. 2001; Herman et al. 1999), the CERs varied from negative (cost saving) to $72,000 per additional life year gained, depending on the drug therapies and the study population. Intensive control of blood pressure using angiotensin-converting enzyme (ACE) inhibitors was cost saving based on results from two well-conducted studies (CDC Diabetes Cost-effectiveness Group 2002; Elliott, Weir, and Black 2000). One study estimated that a smoking cessation program among persons with diabetes cost $14,000 per additional QALY gained (Earnshaw et al. 2002). Orlistat therapy cost about $10,000 per additional year gained of no diabetes complications, compared with placebo, among overweight or obese type 2 diabetes patients (Lamotte et al. 2002; Maetzel et al. 2003).

Two studies (Javitt et al. 1994; Vijan, Hofer, and Hayward 2000) estimated the value of screening and early treatment for diabetic retinopathy at different screening intervals among persons with type 2 diabetes. Screening for retinopathy was found to be cost saving or to cost from 20,000 to 37,000 per QALY gained compared with no screening. The CERs fell as the screening interval increased. Screening for retinopathy at a frequency of every 2 years cost $50,000 per QALY gained compared with a 3-year screening interval. Annual screening for diabetic retinopathy cost more than $100,000 per additional QALY gained compared with screening every 2 years. Screening for and treating microalbuminura with ACE inhibitors compared with standard care among type 1 diabetes patients cost $35,000 per additional QALY gained (Dong et al. 2004). In another study for persons with newly diagnosed type 2 diabetes, screening for and treating microalbuminuria with either ACE inhibitors or irbesartan was cost saving compared with screening for and treating proteinuria with the same drug treatment (Golan, Birkmeyer, and Welch 1999; Palmer et al. 2004a). Treating every patient with newly diagnosed type 2 diabetes using ACE inhibitors cost $10,000 per additional QALY gained compared with screening for microalbuminuria and treating with ACE inhibitors those who tested positive (Golan, Birkmeyer, and Welch 1999). Medicare coverage for ACE inhibitors for diabetes patients was cost saving compared with having patients pay for the medications out of their own pockets (Rosen et al. 2005).

Two studies evaluated the cost-effectiveness of treating the complications of diabetes (Sharma et al. 2001). Immediate vitrectomy for treating eye hemorrhage among persons with diabetic retinopathy cost $2000 per additional QALY gained compared with victrectomy when symptoms appeared (Sharma et al. 2001). All treatments, including dialysis and kidney transplant among persons with end-stage renal disease, cost more than $100,000 per additional QALY gained (Douzdjian, Ferrara, and Silvestri 1998). However, kidney transplant from a living donor was cost saving compared with dialysis or a kidney transplant from a cadaver. Simultaneous pancreas-kidney transplant cost $30,000 per additional QALY gained compared with kidney transplant alone from a living donor (Douzdjian, Ferrara, and Silvestri 1998).

Table 20.2 summarizes the results of studies in developed countries outside the United States; in all, 32 studies assessed 38 discrete interventions in 17 different countries. Most of the studies were in western European countries, with the United Kingdom having the highest number. The intervention population included people at risk for type 2 diabetes and people with diagnosed type 1 or type 2 diabetes but not people with undiagnosed diabetes. Compared with the United States, a high number of studies evaluated the cost-effectiveness of pharmacological therapies. Two studies also assessed the cost-effectiveness of multicomponent interventions. Similar to the studies for the United States, the analytical horizon varied from a within-trial analysis to modeling of disease progression over the patient's lifetime. The CERs ranged from cost saving to costing more than $100,000 per additional QALY gained.

Three studies (Caro et al. 2004; Palmer et al. 2004c; Segal, Dalton, and Richardson 1998) showed that individual-based intensive lifestyle intervention among people with IGT was either cost saving or cost less than $8000 per additional life year gained, depending on the country, in a comparison with standard care (brief counseling). Group-based lifestyle intervention was more cost-effective than individual-based intervention. Metformin for preventing diabetes among people with IGT was cost saving in Canada, Australia, France, Germany, and Switzerland and cost $7000 per additional life year gained in the United Kingdom (Caro et al. 2004; Palmer et al. 2004c). Using acarbose to prevent diabetes among persons with IGT was cost saving in Canada (Caro et al. 2004), but it cost $1000 per additional case of diabetes prevented in Sweden (Quilici et al. 2005). However the same intervention would be cost saving in that country if it were applied to people with both IGT and cardiovascular disease (Quilici et al. 2005).

In nine studies (Almbrand et al. 2000; Clarke et al. 2001, 2005; Coyle, Palmer, and Tam 2002; Gray et al. 2000; Neeser et al. 2004; Palmer et al. 2004b; Scuffham and Carr 2003; Wake et al. 2000) that evaluated the cost-effectiveness of glucose management, the CERs ranged from cost saving to $54,000 per additional life year gained, depending on the specific therapy, comparison group, and country setting. For type 1

TABLE 20.2 *Cost-Effectiveness of Interventions for the Prevention and Control of Diabetes, Health Care System Perspective, in Selected Developed Countries,* in 2005 International Dollars*

Authors, Year of Study, and Country	Interventions	Comparison Intervention	Study Populations	Analytical Time Frame	Cost-Effectiveness Ratios ($/QALY)†	Quality of the Study	Comments
Preventing type 2 diabetes							
Segal et al. 1998, Australia	Lifestyle modification for seriously obese persons with IGT	Standard care	Adults with IGT or overweight or seriously obese adults or with CVD risk factor	25 years	Cost saving	Good	Used a simulation model with data from published literature.
	Group course for lifestyle modification for overweight men	Standard care			Cost saving		
	Media campaign plus community support	No campaign			Cost saving		
	Surgery for BMI ≥40 (kg/m²) with IGT	Standard care			$3000/LYG		
	Physician advice for BMI ≥27 with CVD risk factor	Standard care			$1000/LYG		
Caro et al. 2004, Canada	Individual lifestyle modification	Standard care	Adults with IGT	10 years	$1000/LYG	Excellent	Used a disease progression model with data from the DPP and UKPDS; included the long-term health benefits and costs.
	Metformin	Standard care			Cost saving		
	Acarbose	Standard care			Cost saving		
	Individual lifestyle modification	Metformin			$7000/LYG		
	Individual lifestyle modification	Acarbose			$8000/LYG		
	Acarbose	Metformin			$2000/LYG		

(continued)

TABLE 20.2 *(continued)*

Authors, Year of Study, and Country	Interventions	Comparison Intervention	Study Populations	Analytical Time Frame	Cost-Effectiveness Ratios ($/QALY)[†]	Quality of the Study	Comments
Palmer et al. 2004, Australia and European counties	Individual lifestyle modification	Standard care	Adults with IGT	Lifetime		Excellent	Used a disease progression model with data from the DPP and UKPDS; included the long-term health benefits and costs.
	Australia				Cost saving		
	France				Cost saving		
	Germany				Cost saving		
	Switzerland				Cost saving		
	United Kingdom				$8000/LYG		
	Metformin	Standard care					
	Australia				Cost saving		
	France				Cost saving		
	Germany				Cost saving		
	Switzerland				Cost saving		
	United Kingdom				$7000/LYG		
Quilici et al. 2005, Sweden	Acarbose, persons with high-risk diabetes	Standard care	Adults at high risk for type 2 diabetes and cardiovascular disease	3.3 years	$1000/diabetes case avoided	Excellent	Within-trial analysis.
	Acarbose, persons with high-risk diabetes and cardiovascular diseases	Standard care			Cost saving		

Managing glucose level

Scuffham et al. 2003, United Kingdom	Insulin pump	Insulin needle injection	Type 1 diabetes	8 years	$20,000	Excellent	Used a disease progression model with data from literature.
Palmer et al. 2004, United Kingdom	Insulin detemir-based basal-bolus	Protamine hagedorn human insulin-based Basal-bolus	Type 1 diabetes	Lifetime	$52,000	Excellent	Used a disease progression model with data from literature.
Gray et al. 2000, United Kingdom	Intensive glucose control (sulfonylurea or insulin) in the trial setting Intensive glucose control (sulfonylurea or insulin) in a routine clinic setting	Standard care (primarily diet)	Adults with type 2 diabetes	10 years	Cost saving $2000/ diabetes complication free year	Excellent	Within-trial analysis of UKPDS.
Almbrand et al. 2000, Sweden	Intensive insulin treatment	Standard care	Diabetes patients (either type 1 or type 2) with myocardial infarction	5 years	$9000	Excellent	Within-trial analysis of the Diabetes Mellitus Insulin Glucose Infusion in Acute Myocardial Infarction trial.

(continued)

TABLE 20.2 (*continued*)

Authors, Year of Study, and Country	Interventions	Comparison Intervention	Study Populations	Analytical Time Frame	Cost-Effectiveness Ratios ($/QALY)[†]	Quality of the Study	Comments
Wake et al. 2000, Japan	Multiple insulin injections for intensive glucose control	Conventional insulin injection	Adults with type 2 diabetes	10 years	Cost saving	Excellent	Within-trial analysis of the Kumamoto study.
Clark et al. 2001, United Kingdom	Metformin for intensive glucose control	Standard care (primarily diet)	Overweight adults with newly diagnosed type 2 diabetes	11 years	Cost saving	Excellent	Within-trial analysis of UKPDS.
Clark et al. 2005, United Kingdom	Intensive glucose control (sulfonylurea or insulin)	Standard care (primarily diet)	Adults with newly diagnosed type 2 diabetes	Lifetime	$10,000	Excellent	Used a disease progression model with data from UKPDS; included the long-term health benefits and costs.
	Intensive glucose control (metformin)		Metformin for the overweight subgroup		Cost saving		
Neeser et al. 2004, Gemany	Pioglitazone + metformin	Sulfonylurea + metformin	Overweight adults with onset of type 2 DM	Lifetime	$54,000/LYG	Excellent	Used a disease progression model with data from UKPDS and other clinical trials; included the long-term health benefits and costs.
	Pioglitazone + metformin	Acarbose + metformin			$15,000/LYG		
	Pioglitazone + sulfonylurea	Sulfonylurea + metformin			$24,000/LYG		
	Pioglitazone + sulfonylurea	Acarbose + metformin			$11,000/LYG		

Study	Intervention	Comparison	Population	Time horizon	Cost-effectiveness	Quality	Comments
Coyle et al. 2005, Canada	Pioglitazone, Pioglitazone, Pioglitazone	Glibencalmide, Metformin, Diet + exercise	Adults with onset of type 2 DM	Lifetime	$36,000/LYG, $45,000/LYG, $23,000/LYG	Excellent	Used a disease progression model with data mainly from UKPDS; included the long-term health benefits and costs.

Managing risk factors for diabetes-related complications

Study	Intervention	Comparison	Population	Time horizon	Cost-effectiveness	Quality	Comments
UKPDS 1998, United Kingdom	Tight hypertension control with β blocker or ACE inhibitor; Trial setting; Routine clinic setting	Standard care	Adults with newly diagnosed type 2 diabetes with hypertension	8 years [not sure]	Cost saving; $2000/diabetes complication-free year	Excellent	Within-trial analysis of UKPDS.
Gray et al. 2001, United Kingdom	Tight hypertension control using β blocker (atenolol)	Tight hypertension control using ACE inhibitor (captopril)	Adults with type 2 diabetes with hypertension	8 years	Cost saving	Excellent	Within-trial analysis of UKPDS. The two drugs were same in effectiveness but different in costs.
Clark et al. 2005, United Kingdom	Tight hypertension control using β blocker or ACE inhibitor	Standard care	Adults with newly diagnosed type 2 diabetes with hypertension	Lifetime	$1000	Excellent	Used a disease progression model with data from UKPDS; included the long-term health benefits and costs.
Mason et al. 2005, United Kingdom	Specialist nurse–led clinics for lipid or blood pressure control	Standard care	Adults with newly diagnosed type 2 diabetes with hypertension or hyperlipidemia	Lifetime	$12,000 for hypertension control; $60,000 for lipid control	Excellent	Used a disease progression model with data from UKPDS, heart protection study.

(continued)

TABLE 20.2 (*continued*)

Authors, Year of Study, and Country	Interventions	Comparison Intervention	Study Populations	Analytical Time Frame	Cost-Effectiveness Ratios ($/QALY)†	Quality of the Study	Comments
Jonsson et al. 1999, European countries	Simvastatin for intensive cholesterol control: Sweden Denmark Norway Finland United Kingdom Germany France Italy Portugal Belgium Spain	Standard care	Adults with diabetes and myocardial infarction and/or angina	5.4 years	$3000/LYG $<1000/LYG Cost saving $5000/LYG $4000/LYG $2000/LYG Cost saving $2000/LYG $3000/LYG Cost saving $2000/LYG	Good	Used data from Scandinavian Simvastatin Survival Study. Costs were estimated as the net of the increase in drug and outpatient visits and savings from a lower hospitalization rate.
Grover et al. 2001, Canada, European countries	Simvastatin for intensive cholesterol control: Canada France Germany Italy United Kingdom	Standard care	Adults with diabetes without myocardial infarction and/or angina	Lifetime	Men: $2000-$13,000/LYG; Women: $3000-$24,000/LYG, depending on age and country	Good	Used a cardiovascular disease life expectancy model.

Feher et al. 2003, United Kingdom	Fenofibrate for intensive cholesterol control	Pravastatin	Adults with type 2 diabetes	5	$4000/LYG	Excellent	Used a disease simulation model with data from published clinical trials.
Lamotte et al. 2002, Belgium	Adding orlistat to the standard treatment for persons with Hyperlipidemia Hypertension Hyperlipidemia and hypertension Neither hyperlipidemia nor hypertension	Standard treatment with metformin as implemented in the UKPDS	Overweight and obese adults with no pre-existing diabetes complication	10	$10,000/LYG $10,000/LYG $5000/LYG $26,000/LYG	Excellent	Used a disease simulation model with data from published clinical trials.

Screening for and early treatment of diabetes-related complication

Borch-Johnsen et al. 1993, Germany	Annual screening for and treating of microalbuminuria with anti-hypertension medication	No treatment until development of macroproteinuria	Adults with type 1 diabetes	Lifetime	Cost saving	Good	Diabetes disease progression simulation model.
Kiberd et al. 1995, Canada	Screening for and treating microalbuminuria with ACE inhibitor	Screening for hypertension and macroproteinuria	Adults with type 1 diabetes	Lifetime	$55,000	Good	Diabetes disease progression simulation model.

(continued)

TABLE 20.2 *(continued)*

Authors, Year of Study, and Country	Interventions	Comparison Intervention	Study Populations	Analytical Time Frame	Cost-Effectiveness Ratios ($/QALY)[†]	Quality of the Study	Comments
Tennval et al. 2001, Sweden	Optimal foot ulcer prevention, including annual foot exams, appropriate footwear, appropriate treatment for non-ulcerative pathology, and patient education for persons at three levels of neuropathy	Standard care	Adults with type 2 diabetes and neuropathy risk: high risk = previous foot ulcer or amputation; moderate risk = CVD and/or foot deformity; low risk = no specific risk factors.	Lifetime	Cost saving for high risk; Cost saving: $6000 for moderate risk; >$100,000 for low risk.	Excellent	Used a disease simulation model with data from published clinical trials.
Ortegan et al. 2004, The Netherlands	Optimal foot care (OFC), including professional foot care, education, regular inspections, identifying high-risk patients, and treating ulcerative lesions.	Standard care	Newly diagnosed type 2 diabetes	Lifetime	$16,000 for OFC	Excellent	Assuming that the intervention reduced foot lesions by 90%.
	Multidisciplinary treatment of established foot ulcers plus intensive glycemic control (IGC).				$41,000 for IGC		
	OFC + IGC				$10,000 for OFC + IGC		

Treating diabetes complications

Study	Intervention	Comparator	Population	Time horizon	Result	Quality	Model
Clark et al. 2002, Canada	Publicly funding ACE inhibitors	No-payment strategy	Type 1 diabetes patients with microproteinuria	21 years	Cost saving	Excellent	Decision-tree analysis.
Scouchet et al. 2003, France; Szucs et al. 2004, Switzerland	Losartan therapy	Placebo	Type 2 diabetes patients with nephropathy	4 years	Cost saving	Excellent	Decision-tree analysis.
Palmer et al. 2003 Belgium and France; Palmer et al. 2004, UK	Irbesatan therapy	Amlodipine Placebo	Type 2 diabetes with hypertension and nephropathy	10 years	Cost saving	Excellent	Diabetes disease progression model.

Multidimensional diabetes management

Study	Intervention	Comparator	Population	Time horizon	Result	Quality	Model
Palmer et al. 2000, Switzerland	C (conventional insulin therapy) +EYE C+ACE C+EYE+ACE Where: EYE = annual screening for treating retinopathy; ACE = annual screening for and treating microalbuminuria	C	Type 1 diabetes patients	Lifetime	Cost saving Cost saving Cost saving	Excellent	Diabetes disease progression model.

(continued)

TABLE 20.2 *(continued)*

Authors, Year of Study, and Country	Interventions	Comparison Intervention	Study Populations	Analytical Time Frame	Cost-Effectiveness Ratios ($/QALY)[†]	Quality of the Study	Comments
Gozzoli et al. 2001, Switzerland	EP	Standard treatment with 50% of patients on insulin, 10% on oral antidiabetic agents, and 5% on diet, regular blood and urine glucose self-monitoring.	Type 2 diabetes patients	Lifetime	$7000/LYG	Excellent	Diabetes disease progression model.
	EP+NS				Cost saving		
	EP+NS+RS				Cost saving		
	Where: EP = educational program, NS = nephropathy screening, RS = retinopathy screening						

[*]Countries included were Australia, Belgium, Canada, Denmark, Finland, France, Germany, Italy, Japan, The Netherlands, Norway, Spain, Sweden, Switzerland, and United Kingdom, and the selection was based on study availability.

[†]Cost-effectiveness ratio is in international dollars per QALY, or otherwise as indicated.

ACE, angiotensin-converting enzyme; BMI, body mass index; CVD, cardiovascular disease; DM, diabetes mellitus; DPP, Diabetes Prevention Program; IGT, impaired glucose tolerance; LYG, life years gained; QALY, quality-adjusted life years; UKPDS, United Kingdom Prospective Diabetes Study.

patients, use of an insulin pump cost $20,000 per additional QALY compared with needle injections (Scuffham and Carr 2003). Insulin detemir-based basal-bolus therapy cost $52,000 per additional QALY compared with protimine-hagedorn-human-based basal-bolus therapy (Palmer et al. 2004b). For type 2 patients intensive glycemic control using insulin, sulfonylureas, or metformin to reduce A1C (glycosylated hemoglobin) levels to less than 7% was estimated to cost less than $10,000 per additional life year gained or QALY among people with newly diagnosed diabetes in the United Kingdom (Almbrand et al. 2000; Clarke et al. 2001, 2005; Gray et al. 2000; Wake et al. 2000). But using metformin for intensive glucose control among those with newly diagnosed diabetes who were also overweight would be cost saving (Clarke et al. 2001; Gray et al. 2000). In Germany use of pioglitazone as a first-line antidiabetic drug cost less than $55,000 per additional life year gained in a comparison with glyburide, metformin, or diet and exercise (Neeser et al. 2004), and in Canada, using pioglitazone as a second-line antidiabetic drug cost less than $45,000 per additional life year gained in a comparison with metformin or acarbose (Coyle, Palmer, and Tam 2002).

In three studies that examined intensive control of blood pressure using either ß blockers or an ACE inhibitor, the drugs were cost saving or cost less than $1000 per life year gained in the United Kingdom, depending on the intervention setting and comparators, among people with diabetes and hypertension (Clarke et al. 2005; Gray et al. 2001; UK Prospective Diabetes Study Group 1998). A nurse-led intervention to control blood pressure cost $12,000 per additional QALY gained in a comparison with standard care (Mason et al. 2005). In all western European countries among diabetes patients using drugs, intensive control of cholesterol cost less than $24,000 per additional life year gained for both primary and secondary prevention of cardiovascular disease (Feher, Langley-Hawthorne, and Byrne 2003; Grover et al. 2001; Jonsson, Cook, and Pedersen 1999). Independent of the country cholesterol control was more cost-effective among men than among women (Grover et al. 2001). A nurse-led lipid control program cost $60,000 per additional QALY gained in a comparison with standard care (Mason et al. 2005). In Belgium orlistat among overweight or obese type 2 diabetes patients cost less than $26,000 per additional life year gained in a comparison with metformin (Lamotte et al. 2002).

In Germany screening for microalbuminuria and treating with ACE inhibitors those who tested positive was estimated to be cost saving among type 1 patients in a comparison with no screening and no treatment until the patient developed macroproteinuria (Borch-Johnsen et al. 1993). In Canada this same intervention would cost $55,000 per additional QALY in a comparison with screening for and treating proteinuria (Borch-Johnsen et al. 1993; Kiberd and Jindal 1995). Elsewhere optimal prevention of foot ulcers based on the recommended guideline was estimated to be cost saving among diabetes patients at high risk of such ulcers and, relative to standard care, cost $6000 among those at moderate risk but more than $100,000 per additional QALY among those at low risk (Tennvall and Apelqvist 2001). In another study, optimal foot care alone or optimal foot care plus intensive glucose control cost less than $16,000 per additional QALY in a comparison with standard care (Ortegon, Redekop, and Niessen 2004).

Using losartan and irbesartan to prevent diabetic nephropathy in patients with type 2 diabetes was estimated to be cost saving compared with either placebo or amlodipine therapy in Switzerland, France, Belgium, and the United Kingdom (Palmer et al. 2003; Souchet et al. 2003). Public insurance payment for ACE inhibitors for diabetes patients was cost saving compared with having patients pay for the medications out of their own pockets in Canada (Clark et al. 2000). In Switzerland multicomponent interventions, a combination of patient and physician educational programs, various forms of blood glucose management, and interventions to lower the risk of diabetes-related complications such as cardiovascular diseases, eye diseases, and renal disease through early diagnosis and appropriate treatments could be either cost saving or cost less than $10,000 per additional life year gained for persons with type 1 or type 2 diabetes (Gozzoli et al. 2001; Palmer et al. 2000).

Ranking the Cost-Effectiveness of the Interventions

Table 20.3 summarizes the interventions by their level of cost-effectiveness, strength of evidence, and study region. In the United States two interventions were clearly cost saving, two were clearly very cost-effective, four were clearly cost-effective, two were clearly marginally cost-effective, and no intervention was clearly not cost-effective. In addition, eight interventions were possibly cost saving, five were possibly very cost-effective, five were possibly cost-effective, two were possibly marginally cost-effective, and one was possibly not cost-effective. Without considering the strength of evidence, of the 30 interventions being evaluated, 83% were either cost saving, very cost-effective, or cost-effective; 13% were marginally cost-effective; and only 3% were not cost-effective. In developed countries outside the United States seven interventions were clearly cost saving and six were clearly very cost-effective. No intervention was classified as being clearly cost-effective, clearly marginally cost-effective, or clearly not cost-effective. Seven interventions were possibly cost saving, 12 were possibly very cost-effective, 3 were possibly cost-effective, 3 were possibly marginally cost-effective, and 1 was possibly not cost-effective. Combining all interventions without considering the strength of evidence, of the 38 interventions being evaluated, 92% were cost saving, very cost-effective, or cost-effective, and 8% were marginally cost-effective or not cost-effective.

■ Summary and Implications for Policy

The economic burdens imposed by diabetes are large, and this disorder substantially reduces the quality of life of those who have it. Fortunately, many interventions are available that can be used to reduce the burden of diabetes, but their cost-effectiveness varies greatly.

TABLE 20.3 Ranking the Interventions for the Prevention and Control of Diabetes Based on their Cost-Effectiveness Ratios: United States and Other Developed Countries, 1985–2005

Cost-Effectiveness	Interventions in United States	Interventions in Other Developed Countries
Clearly cost saving	• ACE inhibitors or beta-blocker treatment for intensive hypertension control among type 2 diabetes patients. • Simvastatin for preventing CVD among type 2 diabetes patients with dyslipidemia with history of CHD, compared with placebo.	• Metformin for preventing type 2 diabetes among persons with IGT except in United Kingdom. • Acarbose for preventing diabetes and CVD among persons with IGT and CVD risk factors. • Metformin for intensive glucose control among persons with type 2 diabetes and overweight. • Multiple insulin injections for intensive glucose control compared with single insulin injection among patients with type 2 diabetes. • ACE inhibitors or β-blocker treatment for intensive hypertension control among persons with newly diagnosed type 2 diabetes. • Intensive hypertension control using atenolol compared with captopril among persons with type 2 diabetes and hypertension. • Losartan and irbesartan for slowing progression of nephropathy compared with placebo among persons with type 2 diabetes and nephropathy.
Clearly very cost-effective: less than $25,000 per additional QALY or LYG.	• Generic metformin for preventing type 2 diabetes among persons with IGT. • Intensive group-based lifestyle intervention for preventing type 2 diabetes among persons with IGT.	• Metformin for preventing type 2 diabetes among persons with IGT in United Kingdom. • Acarbose for preventing diabetes among persons with IGT. • Intensive group-based lifestyle intervention for preventing type 2 diabetes among person with IGT. • Intensive individually based lifestyle intervention for preventing type 2 diabetes among persons with IGT. • Intensive glycemic control using insulin, sulfonylureas, or metformin targeting an A1C level of less than 7% among type 2 diabetes patients. • Simvastatin treatment for preventing CVD among type 2 diabetes patients with dyslipidemia and history of CHD.

(continued)

TABLE 20.3 (*continued*)

Cost-Effectiveness	Interventions in United States	Interventions in Other Developed Countries
Clearly cost-effective: $25,000 to $50,000 per additional QALY or LYG.	• Brand-name metformin for preventing type 2 diabetes among persons with IGT. • Intensive individually based lifestyle intervention for preventing type 2 diabetes among persons with IGT. • Intensive insulin therapy among type 1 diabetes patients. • ACE inhibitor treatment for all newly diagnosed type 1 diabetes compared with screening for and treating microalbuminuria.	
Clearly marginally cost-effective: $50,000 to $100,000 per additional QALY or LYG.	• Intensive glycemic control using sulfonylurea or insulin for type 2 diabetes patients. • Pravastatin for intensive cholesterol control for type 2 diabetes patients.	
Clearly not cost-effective: more than $100,000 per additional QALY or LYG.	• No interventions in this category.	
Possibly cost saving	• Screening for and treating microalbuminuria with ACE inhibitors or irbesartan for type 2 diabetes compared with screening for and treating proteinuria • Treat all people with ACE inhibitor compared with screening for and treating proteinuria among those aged 50 years or more with type 2 diabetes • Government paying for ACE inhibitors for all Medicare beneficiaries with diabetes • Irbesartan starting at the state of microalbuminuria compared with routine care • Irbesartan starting at the state of overt nephropathy compared with routine care • Irbesartan starting at the state of microalbuminuria compared with irbesartan starting at the state of overt nephropathy	• Media campaign plus community support for weight loss. • Intensive glycemic control among type 1 diabetes patients. • Optimal foot care for persons with previous foot ulcer or amputation. • Canadian provincial government paying for ACE inhibitors for persons with type 1 diabetes and overt nephropathy. • Screening for and treating microalbuminuria with anti-hypertension medications compared with no treatment until patients develop macroproteinuria for type 2 diabetes patients. • Conventional insulin therapy, plus screening for and treating retinopathy, and screening for and treating microalbuminuria compared with conventional insulin therapy alone for type 1 diabetes patients. • Educational program, plus screening for and treating retinopathy, and screening for and treating microalbuminuria compared with standard antidiabetic care for type 2 diabetes patients.

Possibly very cost-effective: less than $25,000 per additional QALY or LYG

- Kidney-alone transplants from a living donor compared with dialysis or transplant from a cadaver for persons with type 1 diabetes at the stage of ESRD

- Orlistat for losing weight for obese type 2 diabetes patients
- Simvastatin for preventing CVD among type 2 diabetes patients with dyslipidemia but without CHD history compared with placebo
- Smoking cessation among type 2 diabetes
- Treat all people with ACE inhibitor compared with screening for and treating microalbuminura among those aged 50 years or more with type 2 diabetes
- Early vitrectomy for treating various eye hemorrhages compared with late vitrectomy

- Surgery for BMI ≥ 40 (kg/m^2) with IGT.
- Physician advice for BMI ≥ 27 with CVD risk factor.
- Pioglitazone as a first-line antidiabetic drug compared with diet and exercise among overweight persons with type 2 diabetes.
- Insulin pump compared with using insulin needle among persons with type 1 diabetes.
- Intensive hypertension control for persons with type 2 diabetes in specialist nurse-led clinics.
- Adding orlistat for losing weight compared with metformin treatment alone among overweight or obese type 2 diabetes patients.
- Simvastatin for preventing CVD among type 2 diabetes patients with dyslipidemia but without CHD history.
- Fenofibrate for cholesterol control compared with pravastatin for primary prevention of CVD among type 2 diabetes patients.
- Intensive insulin therapy, plus screening for and treating retinopathy, and screening for and treating microalbuminuria compared with conventional insulin therapy alone for type 1 diabetes.
- Optimal foot care for preventing foot ulcers among persons with neuropathy and peripheral vascular disease or deformity.
- Guideline-based optimal foot care among persons with newly diagnosed type 2 diabetes.
- Good wound care plus standard antidiabetic care for treating foot ulcers comparing with standard care alone.

(continued)

TABLE 20.3 *(continued)*

Cost-Effectiveness	Interventions in United States	Interventions in Other Developed Countries
Possibly cost-effective: $25,000 to $50,000 per additional QALY or LYG	• Lifestyle modification compared with standard care among persons with onset of type 2 diabetes • Eye screening every 1,3,5 years and treating retinopathy for type 2 diabetes patients compared with no screening • Annual eye screening and treating retinopathy for type 2 diabetes patients with poor glycemic control or in younger age group, or with insulin-treated diabetes compared with screening every other year. • Cholesterol control using pravastatin for primary preventing CVD • Simultaneous pancreas-kidney transplants from a living donor compared with kidney transplant alone for persons with ESRD	• Pioglitazone as a first-line antidiabetic drug compared with glyburide and metformin among overweight persons with type 2 diabetes. • Insulin detemir compared with protamin hagedorn human insulin among type 1 patients. • Screening for and treating microalbuminuria with ACE inhibitors for type 1 diabetes patients compared with treatment with ACE inhibitors in patients with hypertension, macroproteinuria, or both.
Possibly marginally cost-effective: $50,000 to $100,000 per additional QALY or LYG	• Opportunistic screening for undiagnosed type 2 diabetes among all adults • Target screening for undiagnosed type 2 diabetes among persons with hypertension	• Pioglitazone as a first-line antidiabetic drug compared with sulfonylurea among overweight persons with type 2 diabetes. • Intensive lipid control for persons with type 2 diabetes and hypercholesterolemia by specialist nurse-led clinics.
Possibly not cost-effective: more than $100,000 per additional QALY or LYG	• Universal screening for undiagnosed type 2 diabetes compared with targeting screening	• Optimal foot care for preventing foot ulcer among persons with no neuropathy and peripheral vascular disease or foot ulcer or amputation.

*ACE, angiotensin-converting enzyme; BMI, body mass index; CHD, coronary heart disease; CVD, cardiovascular disease; ESRD, end-stage renal disease; IGT, impaired glucose tolerance; LYG, life years gained; QALY, quality-adjusted life years.

Interventions backed by strong evidence that they are either cost saving, very cost-effective, or cost-effective represent a good use of health care resources and should be adopted. For both the United States and the other developed regions, these interventions include (1) intensive lifestyle interventions (either individual or group based) and metformin (either brand name or generic) treatment for preventing type 2 diabetes among high-risk individuals; (2) ACE inhibitors and beta-blockers for intensive control of hypertension among type 2 diabetes patients; and (3) simvastatin for preventing cardiovascular disease among type 2 patients with dyslipidemia and a history of coronary heart disease. Additional region-specific interventions that should be adopted in the United States include (1) intensive glucose control among type 1 patients, and (2) treatment with ACE inhibitors for all newly diagnosed type 1 patients.

In the other developed regions outside the United States, the desirable interventions were (1) acarbose for preventing diabetes among persons with IGT (with and without additional risk factors for cardiovascular disease), (2) multiple insulin injections for intensive glucose control among type 2 users of insulin, (3) losartan and irbesartan for slowing the progression of nephropathy among persons with type 2 diabetes and nephropathy, and (4) intensive glycemic control (target A1C of 7% or less) using insulin, sulfonylureas, or metformin among type 2 patients.

Interventions with strong evidence to support the conclusion that they are marginally cost-effective represent a relatively less efficient use of health care resources and should be adopted with great caution. In the United States, such interventions include intensive glycemic control targeting an A1C of 7% for type 2 patients and pravastatin therapy for intensive control of cholesterol, also for type 2 patients. In the other developed regions no interventions were found to be marginally cost-effective. Interventions with strong evidence to support the conclusion that they are not cost-effective do not represent a good use of health care resources and should not be adopted.

Regarding the many interventions where the evidence was weak and the finding was that they were possibly cost-effective, as well as the small number with weak evidence that were found to be either possibly marginally cost-effective or possibly not cost-effective, clearly, more research is needed. Future research should focus on those interventions that are currently ranked as being possibly cost saving, possibly very cost-effective, or possibly not cost-effective. The first two categories would represent a very good use of health care resources and would be given the highest priority if current results were confirmed. In contrast the last category represents inefficient use of health care resources, and those interventions should not be adopted if the results are confirmed.

In addition, more studies are needed to estimate the cost-effectiveness of the multi-component interventions, of changes in health policy, and of translation of research on how to implement interventions in a real-world public health or clinical setting. Many patients would be likely to receive multicomponent diabetes treatment simultaneously rather than through a single intervention. These multicomponent interventions could include intensive glycemic control, intensive control of hypertension, treatment with ACE inhibitors for diabetic nephropathy, screening for diabetic retinopathy, and more. Translational interventions at the population level, particularly policy changes, are very important tools to improve the health of the population with diabetes in a particular country or region. Without further evidence, the CEA is limited in its ability to say whether interventions in this category should be adopted. Policy and clinical decisions on adopting these interventions should take into consideration, in addition to cost-effectiveness, such factors as expert opinion, health benefits beyond the diabetes-related outcomes, the ease with which the intervention could be adopted, the availability of other alternatives, and other social objectives.

Several potential limitations of the analysis should be considered before we may draw any conclusions from this chapter. First, the costs of interventions may have changed since the studies were performed. For example brand-name drugs used in older studies may have been replaced by lower-cost generic versions or newer and more effective brand-name drugs. Second, many of the studies are based on disease progression models and are thus dependent on the assumptions of the model employed. Third, the CER of an intervention depends on the specific comparison group used, and thus it is important to look at what comparison group was used to derive the CER of interest. For example, intensive glycemic control to an A1C $\leq 7.0\%$ is cost-effective relative to a baseline control value of $\geq 9.0\%$, but it may not be cost-effective relative to a baseline of $\geq 7.5\%$. Finally, some publication bias may exist for the interventions included in our review. In brief, some interventions that do not end up being cost-effective may not get published.

Caution should be taken when applying the results from our review to public health and clinical decisions. First both our current ranking of the interventions and the summaries of the studies' conclusions were based on evidence that is currently available to us. These rankings and conclusions may change as new evidence becomes available in the future. Second the cost-effectiveness studies included in our review were quite heterogeneous, which made the process of synthesizing the results a very difficult task. Although we have made numerous efforts to "standardize" the results across studies, some of the difference in CERs could be a result of intrinsic heterogeneity across studies. Heterogeneity could have many sources, including the different assumptions used cross the studies, the data sources and structure of the disease simulation model used, specific benefits and costs included for a given intervention, the analytical horizon, and so on. Finally, CEA as a tool for public policy and clinical decisions has limitations in its own right, including (1) having only a limited ability to describe the distribution of the benefits and costs of an intervention, (2) having no information on society's or individuals' willingness to pay for such an intervention or on the social and legal aspects of the intervention, and (3) the failure to consider the ethical issues. All these aspects are important for determining whether a cost-effective intervention can be successfully implemented in the real-world setting.

■ References

Alderson P et al. (2004). *Cochrane Reviewers' Handbook 4.2.2* [updated March 2004]. Oxford: The Cochrane Collaboration.

Almbrand B et al. (2000). Cost-effectiveness of intense insulin treatment after acute myocardial infarction in patients with diabetes mellitus; results from the DIGAMI study.[see comment]. *European Heart Journal* **21**(9), 733–9.

American Diabetes Association (2008). Standards of Medical Care in Diabetes-2008. *Diabetes Care* **31**, S12–54.

Barcelo A et al. (2003). The cost of diabetes in Latin America and the Caribbean. *Bulletin of the World Health Organization* **81**, 19–27.

Borch-Johnsen K et al. (1993). Is screening and intervention for microalbuminuria worthwhile in patients with insulin dependent diabetes? *British Medical Journal* **306**, 1722–5.

Bureau of Labor Statistics (2008). Consumer Price Index for All Urban Consumers (CPI-U): U.S. City Average, by Medical Care. Washington, DC: Bureau of Labor Statistics.

Caro JJ et al. (2004). Economic evaluation of therapeutic interventions to prevent Type 2 diabetes in Canada. *Diabetic Medicine* **21**, 1229–36.

CDC Diabetes Cost-Effectiveness Group (2002). Cost-effectiveness of intensive glycemic control, intensified hypertension control, and serum cholesterol level reduction for type 2 diabetes. *JAMA* **287**, 2542–51.

CDC Diabetes Cost-Effectiveness Study Group (1998). The cost-effectiveness of screening for type 2 diabetes. *JAMA* **280**, 1757–63.

Clark WF et al. (2000). To pay or not to pay? A decision and cost-utility analysis of angiotensin-converting-enzyme inhibitor therapy for diabetic nephropathy. *Canadian Medical Association Journal* **162** (2), 195–8.

Clarke P et al. (2001). Cost-effectiveness analysis of intensive blood-glucose control with metformin in overweight patients with type II diabetes (UKPDS No. 51). *Diabetologia* **44**, 298–304.

Clarke PM et al. (2005). Cost-utility analyses of intensive blood glucose and tight blood pressure control in type 2 diabetes (UKPDS 72). *Diabetologia* **48**, 868–77.

Coyle D, Palmer AJ, Tam R (2002). Economic evaluation of pioglitazone hydrochloride in the management of type 2 diabetes mellitus in Canada. *Pharmacoeconomics* **20**, 31–42.

DCCT Research Group (1996). Lifetime benefits and costs of intensive therapy as practiced in the diabetes control and complications trial. *JAMA* **276**, 1409–15.

Diabetes Prevention Program Research Group (2003). Within-trial cost-effectiveness of lifestyle intervention or metformin for the primary prevention of type 2 diabetes. *Diabetes Care* **26**, 2518–23.

Dong FB et al. (2004). Cost effectiveness of ACE inhibitor treatment for patients with type 1 diabetes mellitus. *Pharmacoeconomics* **22**, 1015–27.

Douzdjian V, Ferrara D, Silvestri G (1998). Treatment strategies for insulin-dependent diabetics with ESRD: a cost-effectiveness decision analysis model. *American Journal of Kidney Diseases* **31**, 794–802.

Drummond MF (1996). Guidelines for Authors and Peer Reviewers of Economic Submissions to the *BMJ*. *British Medical Journal* **313**, 275–83.

Drummond MF et al. (2005). *Methods for the Economic Evaluation of Health Care Programmes*. New York: Oxford University Press.

Earnshaw SR et al. (2002). Optimal allocation of resources across four interventions for type 2 diabetes. *Medical Decision Making* **22**, S80–91.

Eastman RC (1998). Cost-effectiveness of treatment of type 2 diabetes. *Diabetes Care* **21**, 464–5.

Eddy DM, Schlessinger L, Kahn R (2005). Clinical outcomes and cost-effectiveness of strategies for managing people at high risk for diabetes. *Annals of Internal Medicine* **143**, 251–64.

Elliott WJ, Weir DR, Black HR (2000). Cost-effectiveness of the lower treatment goal (of JNC VI) for diabetic hypertensive patients. Joint National Committee on Prevention, Detection, Evaluation, and Treatment of High Blood Pressure. *Archives of Internal Medicine* **160**, 1277–83.

Feher MD, Langley-Hawthorne CE, Byrne CD (2003). Cost-outcome benefits of fibrate therapy in type 2 diabetes. *British Journal of Diabetes & Vascular Disease* **3**, 124–30.

Golan L, Birkmeyer JD, Welch HG (1999). The cost-effectiveness of treating all patients with type 2 diabetes with angiotensin-converting enzyme inhibitors. *Annals of Internal Medicine* **131**, 660–7.

Gold MR et al. (1996). *Cost-Effectiveness in Health and Medicine*. New York: Oxford University Press.

Gozzoli V et al. (2001). Economic and clinical impact of alternative disease management strategies for secondary prevention in type 2 diabetes in the Swiss setting. *Swiss Medical Weekly* **131**, 303–10.

Gray A et al. (2000). Cost effectiveness of an intensive blood glucose control policy in patients with type 2 diabetes: economic analysis alongside randomised controlled trial (UKPDS 41). United Kingdom Prospective Diabetes Study Group. *British Medical Journal* **320**, 1373–8.

Gray A et al. (2001). An economic evaluation of atenolol vs. captopril in patients with type 2 diabetes (UKPDS 54). *Diabetic Medicine* **18**, 438–44.

Grover SA et al. (2001). How cost-effective is the treatment of dyslipidemia in patients with diabetes but without cardiovascular disease? *Diabetes Care* **21**, 45–50.

Hoerger TJ et al. (2004). Screening for type 2 diabetes mellitus: a cost-effectiveness analysis. *Annals of Internal Medicine* **140**, 689–99.

International Diabetes Federation (1999). *Diabetes Health Economics: Facts, Figures, and Forecasts*. Brussels, Belgium IDF.

International Diabetes Federation (2006). *Diabetes Atlas*. Brussels, Belgium: IDF.

International Monetary Fund (2004). *World Economic Outlook Database*. New York: IMF.

Javitt JC et al. (1994). Preventive eye care in people with diabetes is cost-saving to the federal government. Implications for health-care reform. *Diabetes Care* **17**, 909–17.

Jonsson B, Cook JR, Pedersen TR (1999). The cost-effectiveness of lipid lowering in patients with diabetes: results from the 4S trial. *Diabetologia* **42**, 1293–301.

Kiberd BA, Jindal KK (1995). Screening to prevent renal failure in insulin dependent diabetic patients: an economic evaluation. *British Medical Journal* **311**, 1595–9.

King H, Aubert RE, Herman WH (1998). Global burden of diabetes, 1995–2025: prevalence, numerical estimates, and projections. *Diabetes Care* **21**, 1414–31.

Klonoff DC, Schwartz DM (2000). An economic analysis of interventions for diabetes. *Diabetes Care* **23**(3), 390–404.

Lamotte M et al. (2002). A health economic model to assess the long-term effects and cost-effectiveness of orlistat in obese type 2 diabetic patients. *Diabetes Care* **25**, 303–8.

Laupacis A et al. (1992). How attractive does a new technology have to be to warrant adoption and utilization? Tentative guidelines for using clinical and economic evaluations. *Canadian Medical Association Journal* **146**, 473–81.

Maetzel A et al. (2003). Economic evaluation of orlistat in overweight and obese patients with type 2 diabetes mellitus. *Pharmacoeconomics* **21**, 501–12.

Mason JM et al. (2005). Specialist nurse-led clinics to improve control of hypertension and hyperlipidemia in diabetes: economic analysis of the SPLINT trial. *Diabetes Care* **28**, 40–6.

Neeser K et al. (2004). Cost effectiveness of combination therapy with pioglitazone for type 2 diabetes mellitus from a German statutory healthcare perspective. *Pharmacoeconomics* **22**, 321–41.

Ortegon MM, Redekop WK, Niessen LW (2004). Cost-effectiveness of prevention and treatment of the diabetic foot: a Markov analysis. *Diabetes Care* **27**, 901–7.

Owens DK (1998). Interpretation of cost-effectiveness Analyses. *Journal of General Internal Medicine* **13**, 716–7.

Palmer AJ et al. (2000). The cost-effectiveness of different management strategies for type I diabetes: a Swiss perspective. *Diabetologia* **43**, 13–26.

Palmer AJ et al. (2003). An economic evaluation of irbesartan in the treatment of patients with type 2 diabetes, hypertension and nephropathy: Cost-effectiveness of Irbesartan in Diabetic Nephropathy Trial (IDNT) in the Belgian and French settings. *Nephrology Dialysis Transplantation* **18**, 2059–66.

Palmer AJ et al. (2004a). Cost-effectiveness of early irbesartan treatment versus control (standard antihypertensive medications excluding ACE inhibitors, other angiotensin-2 receptor antagonists, and dihydropyridine calcium channel blockers) or late irbesartan treatment in patients with type 2 diabetes, hypertension, and renal disease. *Diabetes Care* **27**, 1897–903.

Palmer AJ et al. (2004b). Cost-effectiveness of detemir-based basal/bolus therapy versus NPH-based basal/bolus therapy for type 1 diabetes in a UK setting: an economic analysis based on meta-analysis results of four clinical trials. *Current Medical Research and Opinion* **20**, 1729–46.

Palmer AJ et al. (2004c). Intensive lifestyle changes or metformin in patients with impaired glucose tolerance: modeling the long-term health economic implications of the diabetes prevention program in Australia, France, Germany, Switzerland, and the United Kingdom. *Clinical Therapeutics* **26**, 304–21.

Polonsky WH (2000). Understanding and assessing diabetes-specific quality of life. *Diabetes Spectrum* **13**, 29.

Quilici S et al. (2005). Cost-effectiveness of acarbose for the management of impaired glucose tolerance in Sweden. *International Journal of Clinical Practice* **59**, 1143–52.

Rosen AB et al. (2005). Cost-effectiveness of full medicare coverage of angiotensin-converting enzyme inhibitors for beneficiaries with diabetes. *Annals of Internal Medicine* **143**, 89–99.

Scuffham P, Carr L (2003). The cost-effectiveness of continuous subcutaneous insulin infusion compared with multiple daily injections for the management of diabetes. *Diabetic Medicine* 586–93.

Segal L, Dalton AC, Richardson J (1998). Cost-effectiveness of the primary prevention of non-insulin dependent diabetes mellitus. *Health Promotion International* **13**, 197–209.

Sharma S et al. (2001). The cost-effectiveness of early vitrectomy for the treatment of vitreous hemorrhage in diabetic retinopathy. *Current Opinions in Ophthalmology* **12**, 230–4.

Shobhana R et al. (2002). Costs incurred by families having type 1 diabetes in a developing country—a study from Southern India. *Diabetes Research and Clinical Practice* **55**, 45–8.

Souchet T et al. (2003). An economic evaluation of Losartan therapy in type 2 diabetic patients with nephropathy: an analysis of the RENAAL study adapted to France. *Diabetes & Metabolism* **29**, 29–35.

Sullivan PW, Ghushchyan V (2006). Preference-based EQ-5D index scores for chronic conditions in the United States. *Medical Decision Making* **4**, 410–20.

Tang L et al. (2003). Assessing the impact of complications on the costs of type 2 diabetes in urban China. *Chinese Journal of Diabetes* **11**, 238–41.

Tennvall GR, Apelqvist J (2001). Prevention of diabetes-related foot ulcers and amputations: a cost-utility analysis based on Markov model simulations. *Diabetologia* **44**, 2077–87.

UK Prospective Diabetes Study Group (1998). Cost effectiveness analysis of improved blood pressure control in hypertensive patients with type 2 diabetes: UKPDS 40. *British Medical Journal* **317**, 720–6.

Vijan S, Hofer TP, Hayward RA (2000). Cost-utility analysis of screening intervals for diabetic retinopathy in patients with type 2 diabetes mellitus. *JAMA* **283**, 889–96.

Wake N et al. (2000). Cost-effectiveness of intensive insulin therapy for type 2 diabetes: a 10-year follow-up of the Kumamoto study. *Diabetes Research & Clinical Practice* **48**, 201–10.

21. Adult Diabetes and Quality of Life, Psychosocial Issues, and Sexual Health

Roger T. Anderson, Manjiri D. Pawaskar, Fabian Camacho,
and Rajesh Balkrishnan

■ Main Public Health Messages

- Diabetes is a leading cause of morbidity and mortality in the United States.
- Diabetes has a significant impact not only on physical health but also on the psychological and social well-being of men and women.
- The high risk of functional impairment and depression associated with diabetes can reduce average levels of quality of life.
- The prevention and control of diabetes need to include enhancing and supporting personal well-being and productivity.
- The rising epidemic of diabetes in adults of all ages will significantly decrease the health-related quality of life of those affected.
- The effectiveness and benefit of public health programs in diabetes control can be evaluated in terms of gains in health-related quality of life and the productivity of groups or populations.

■ Introduction

Diabetes mellitus is the seventh-leading cause of mortality in the United States and in 2005 afflicted approximately 20.8 million Americans, or 7% of the overall population in that year (Heron 2007). The toll from diabetes poses an immense economic burden on the health care system, with a recent estimate of $174 billion for a single year, made up of $116 billion in direct medical costs and $58 billion in reduced productivity (American Diabetes Association 2007). Although these societal or public health costs of diabetes are well noted, such estimates cannot completely describe the total costs associated with the diabetes epidemic. This is because diabetes significantly impairs health-related quality of life (HRQL) among those with this condition. Diabetes may be thought of as a "complex chronic disease," which is defined as a disease involving multiple morbidities and including physical and mental health conditions with ongoing self-management behaviors and needs for social support (Sevick et al. 2007). Epidemiologic studies show that a large proportion of individuals with either type of diabetes (type 1 or type 2) are at risk of suffering significant decrements in dimensions of HRQL, including symptom distress such as excessive thirst, frequent urination, fatigue, and neuropathies (Testa and Simonson 1998); functional limitations; restrictions in normal activities; work limitations; poor general health; depression; anxiety; and social withdrawal that are directly or indirectly caused by diabetes (Aubert et al. 1995; Egede 2004; Geiss et al. 1995; Rubin and Peyrot 1999; Songer 1995). In addition, the daily burden of self-managing diabetes with lifestyle and medical therapies may significantly reduce HRQL (Anderson et al. 2004, 2009).

In summary, a focus on diabetes and HRQL in public health is essential to: (1) develop, or propose, models for health care systems that may effectively support diabetes "survivorship" issues; (2) provide a focus on preventing avoidable negative health outcomes with diabetes, both by controlling disease progression and by supporting patient needs at all points along the continuum of care; and (3) more appropriately weigh the true cost of diabetes and its treatment options to patients and to society, and in doing so identify effective preventive and therapeutic regimens that produce the largest momentum toward improved well-being.

■ Background/Historical Perspective

Health-Related Quality of Life and Diabetes: General View

The term "quality of life" has gained considerable importance in research on medical care and outcomes over the last two decades (Patrick 1990; Shumaker, Anderson, and Czajkowski 1990; Ware, Kosinski, and Keller 1996). HRQL is generally defined as "those attributes valued by patients, including their resultant comfort or sense of wellbeing; the extent to which they are able to maintain reasonable physical, emotional, and intellectual function; and the degree to which they retain their ability to participate in valued activities within the family, in the work place, and in the community" (Shumaker et al. 1990). This is a conceptual extension of the World Health Organization's (World Health Organization 1952) definition of "health" as comprising physical, emotional, and social well-being. HRQL is thus an individual's perception about his or her potential to live a subjectively fulfilling life. Accordingly, the generic effects of disease and its management on an individual's HRQL include the following dimensions:

- *Physical functioning* is the ability to conduct a variety of activities ranging from self-care to more challenging and vigorous activities that require mobility, strength, or endurance that individuals perform in their daily lives for autonomy. Diabetes can exert profound limitations with impact ranging from ambulation to fine motor skills from its potential for symptoms such as fatigue and complications leading to large- and small-vessel disease. *Functional limitations* are at the level of the whole person, such as restrictions in basic physical and mental actions, such as ambulation, reaching, stooping, and climbing stairs (Verbrugge and Jette 1994). Other limitations are in the performance of social roles and organized tasks within a sociocultural context such as work, household management, personal care, hobbies, active recreation, or leisure (Nagi 1976). Thus, a range of physical well-being may be indexed by the ability to walk, rise, or bend; engage in purposeful activities such as self-care, generally classified as basic "activities of daily living" (ADL), such as self-care and ambulation; "instrumental activities of daily living" (IADL), such as cooking, performing light and moderate household activities, managing money, and functioning in the community; and advanced activities of daily living (AADL), such as more strenuous tasks. At the level of behavior, physical impairment may translate to disability by disrupting social roles, or individual self-care and autonomy. To appropriately weigh the impact of diabetes on physical health, a broad-spectrum measure is needed to allow the clinical researcher to assess the range of physical behaviors and roles an individual routinely performs with little or no difficulty and how long or intensely an individual experiences a specified reduction in physical health within a period of time or demand. A challenge in assessing perceived physical health is how to handle individual adaptation, or physical compensation, to overcome deficits in physical functioning (Stewart and Painter 1997; Stewart et al. 1989).

- *Psychological well-being* refers to the individual's emotional health and is another major dimension of general health that can be affected greatly by chronic conditions like diabetes. Negative affective states such as general distress or "demoralization" (Frank 1974) can be assessed as depressive affect, the subject's general sense of fatigue (Berwick et al. 1991; Ware et al. 2000), or outlook on life such as feeling hopeful or discouraged or experiencing health worry. Similarly, it is important to consider positive aspects of emotional functioning such as joy, vigor, and hopefulness for the future (Bradburn 1969; Kercher 1992; Zautra 1995) that may result from the successful management of diabetes.

- *Social functioning* refers to a person's ability to sustain interactions with family, friends, and the community. A key aspect of social functioning is the person's self-appraised performance in her or his social roles and valued activities; satisfaction with one's social life is also important. An illness and its treatment may be perceived as having less negative impact on HRQL if the person is able to maintain valued social role functions such as caring for children or grandchildren, engaging in social activities with friends, or remaining active in the community. Other effects from diabetes as a complex chronic disease that may limit social functioning include anxiety or reluctance to use insulin in public settings (Nafes et al. 2006; Cefalu et al. 2008) or potential weight gain, limitations in time or schedule from difficult self-management regimens, or physical discomfort or disability. These problems may lead to a diminished sense of well-being or a feeling that life is not meaningful, setting in motion further decline from being more sedentary (Eaton et al. 1996; Rubin and Peyrot 1999; Anderson et al. 2001). Social functioning may also be sensitive to early perceptions of physical and emotional disturbances from disease. Kou et al. (2004) found in a study of elderly community-dwelling diabetes patients enrolled in the Medicare Managed Care program with no ADL disability at baseline that loss in social functioning on the Medical Outcomes Study Short Form-36 (SF-36) measure was an early indicator of subsequent disability over a 2-year period.

- *Perceived health* is different from clinical assessments because it is an overall appraisal by the individual using her or his own reference point. Because HRQL is subjective, the perception of health is usually a stronger predictor of HRQL than are objective measures and provides valuable information on patient risk beyond that determined from clinical risk factors alone (Curtis et al. 1997; Hayes et al. 2008). Although clinical measures are useful to describe disease activity, they do not capture the patient's experience with diabetes, such as depression or frustration with self-care and disease management.

Health-Related Quality of Life: An Expanded View

Although there is broad agreement on the core HRQL dimensions, which comprise physical, psychological, and social functioning, other dimensions of HRQL may be important to consider with a disease such as diabetes that can have far-reaching effects on patient functioning. This more comprehensive evaluation of HRQL allows the clinical researcher to more precisely weigh the burden of diabetes on the lives of patients, as it is empirically experienced, to target therapeutic strategies and to monitor outcomes.

Personal productivity extends the focus of the effects of disease or illness on functioning to include paid and unpaid activities. Measures can include the amount of paid employment for a given period (for instance, number of days with full pay or hours worked per week), productivity in performing household tasks, and the extent of volunteer or community activities. In younger populations, the focus may shift to school attendance and performance in school activities.

Intimacy and sexual functioning refer to one's ability to form and maintain close personal relationships and aspects of sexual relationships. Although not included in many generic measures of HRQL, sexual functioning and satisfaction are core humanistic qualities affected by disease and illness, including diabetes. Measures of sexual functioning may include items regarding a person's emotional and physical ability to perform and/or participate in sexual activities, the types of sexual activities in which a person engages, the frequency with which such activities occur, and people's satisfaction with their sexual functioning or level of activity.

Sleep disturbance may be generated from depression and anxiety, which are often a consequence of chronic diseases like diabetes, as well as from bodily discomfort such as pain, respiratory symptoms, and frequent urination. Survey items assessing sleep habits may examine factors such as sleep patterns (e.g., ability to fall asleep at night, number of times awakened during the night, waking up too early in the morning or difficulty in waking up in the morning, and number of hours slept during a typical night) and sleep quality.

Pain is another commonly assessed dimension of HRQL. Apart from a global assessment of pain, measures may include the degree of pain related to specific physical activities, such as bending, reaching, or walking upstairs, as well as the type of pain, such as throbbing, shooting, or aching.

■ Diabetes and Health-Related Quality of Life

Within the general framework of HRQL above, the impact of diabetes and its treatment upon individual functioning and well-being may be characterized as effects on basic physical, psychological, and social dimensions of health and more extensive effects on personal productivity, sexual functioning, and overall life satisfaction. Diabetes may have *direct effects* on HRQL both from the disease process itself that causes impairment and from having to live with diabetes as a chronic illness and thus a source of psychosocial strain or distress. Also to be considered are effects associated with *diabetes treatment*, which may be either adverse or beneficial. Diabetes type, duration, and disease severity and treatment can all be conceptualized as important mediators or moderators of the impact diabetes may have on HRQL. Finally it is important to distinguish diabetes effects on HRQL from factors that are not part of the disease itself, such as older age, lower education, and lower income, all of which are associated with worse HRQL (Keinänen-Kiukaanniemi et al. 1996).

General Effects of Diabetes

Because of the large variability in severity of diabetes symptoms and rates of complications, persons with diabetes can have an overall HRQL that is notably lower than persons with no chronic illness but more similar to persons with other chronic illnesses (Alonso et al. 2004; Rubin and Peyrot 1999; Sprangers et al. 2000). In a population study Stewart and colleagues (1989) found that the quality-of-life summary ratings for diabetes were lower than those for a control sample with no chronic conditions but were higher than those of patients with conditions such as congestive heart failure, myocardial infarction, arthritis, chronic lung problems, gastrointestinal disorder, back problems, or angina. Brown and colleagues (2004) found in a study of adults aged 50 years or older that persons with diabetes reported nearly twice as many unhealthy days (physical or mental) as those without diabetes. Similarly older adults with diabetes were significantly more likely to report 14 or more unhealthy days (physical or mental). These findings are supported by Egede (2004), who analyzed findings from the National Health Interview Survey and found that approximately 58% of adults with diabetes had one or more functional deficits or physical disabilities (based on self-report), versus only 24% of adults without diabetes. Finally, a longer duration of diabetes was associated with lower energy and mobility, decreased physical functioning, and worse sexual functioning in a community sample of patients (Camacho et al. 2002; Glasgow et al. 1997; Klein, Klein, and Moss 1998).

A consistent association of diabetes and psychiatric disorders is found in the literature, but its nature is uncertain (Anderson et al. 2001). Persons with diabetes have been shown to have twice the risk for having a diagnosis of depression as those without diabetes (Eaton et al. 1996) and are more likely to have deficits in cognitive function (Wandell, Brorsson, and Aberg 1998; Wandell 1999). A meta-analysis of 39 diabetes studies estimated that diabetes doubles the odds of depression (Anderson et al. 2001). Gavard and colleagues (1993) found that major depression was present in 14.7% of diabetic patients and elevated symptoms of depression in 26%. There is also evidence from population studies that depression and reduced physical functioning are mutually synergistic, such that either one can intensify the effects of the other (Camacho et al. 1991; Harris, Cronkite, and Moos 2006). The role of glycemic control in association with depression and psychosocial status is subject to debate. Depression might contribute to poorer glycemic control through direct biological effects such as those mediated through humoral or neurophysiologic mechanisms (de Groot et al. 2001; Geringer et al. 1988). However, few studies have explored the possibility that diabetes-related emotional distress may be recursive and play a significant role in glycemic control (Jacobson et al. 1994; Weinger and Jacobson 2001). Regardless of causal direction, depression is an important "fellow traveler" of diabetes that worsens the impact of diabetes on HRQL and raises challenges regarding its treatment.

Effects of Glycemia and Complications

The relation between metabolic control and HRQL in diabetes is not well understood and is inconsistent. Studies have found that better glycemic control favors a better quality of life by relieving the negative symptoms of hyperglycemia (Rubin and Peyrot 1999; Testa and Simonson 1998; Van der Does et al. 1996; Weinberger et al. 1994). Similarly in the UKPDS (United Kingdom Prospective Diabetes Study Group) study dimensions of HRQL such as tension and total mood disturbance were associated with number of hypoglycemic episodes (UKPDS Group 1999). Evidence for glycemic effects on HRQL seems to be stronger when diabetes-specific HRQL indices are used, although null findings from general measures have also been reported (Ahroni et al. 1994; Anderson et al. 1997; UKPDS Group 1999). Two of the largest and most noted diabetes trials, the Diabetes Control and Complications Trial (DCCT) and the UKPDS, did not show appreciable gains in HRQL through improved glycemic control from intensive treatment of type 1 (DCCT 1996, 2000) and type 2 diabetes (UKPDS 1999). However in each of these two trials, a potential for benefit from improved glycemia may have been countered or even cancelled by side effects of medications, or demands and complexity of the regimen, factors that were not measured. However some investigators have found only a poor association with metabolic control due to hypoglycemia, experienced as fatigue and lethargy (Peyrot and Rubin 1997; Wikblad, Leksell, and Wibel 1996). It is likely that exposures such as duration, number of events, and intensity affect the strength of associations of glycemia and metabolic control on physical or mental well-being.

Diabetic complications have a well-documented effect on HRQL. Complications such as limb discomfort, impaired vision, physical function, fatigue, and complaints associated with microvascular disease for both type 1 and type 2 diabetes have been shown to be associated with significant HRQL impairment (de Groot et al. 1999; UKPDS Group 1999). Camacho and colleagues (2002) reported that HRQL was significantly associated with complaints relating to symptoms of the legs and feet and with impaired vision (Camacho et al. 2002; Gulliford and Mahabir 1999). Wandell and colleagues (1998) and Glasgow et al. (1997) found that the number of comorbid conditions and diabetes-related complications were the strongest predictors of diminished physical and role functioning. Microvascular conditions such ,as microalbuminuria that are often asymptomatic have not been shown to have a substantial impact on HRQL (Glasgow et al. 1997). Studies by Anderson and colleagues (1997) and Jacobson, de Groot, and Samson (1994) have reported a significant decrease in all SF-36 scale scores, representing domains of physical, social, and emotional well-being, as the number of complications increases. Specific concerns such as the frequency and severity of diabetic symptoms, complications and comorbid conditions, and health worries are significant associated with HRQL in diabetes (Luscombe 2000; Polonsky 2002). The strength and consistency of the results in this literature strongly support the conclusion that symptom distress in diabetes is a primary factor in determining the quality of life in diabetes (Testa and Simonson 1998).

Diabetes and Sexual Health/Function

Sexual dysfunction is a highly prevalent complication of diabetes ranging in male patients from 10% to 52% and among women patients from 25% to 63% (Grover 2006; Heiman 2002; Jackson 2004; Penson and Wessells 2004). Persons with diabetes are at increased risk for both organogenic and psychogenic sexual dysfunction (Thomas and LoPiccolo 1994) and significantly reduced HRQL, especially in emotional domains such as those in the SF-36 (Litwin, Nied, and Dhanani 1998) and other generic health measures. For example, in a large study of diabetes clinics, De Berardis and colleagues (2002) reported a dramatic increase in the prevalence of severe depressive symptoms, lower scores in the mental components of the SF-36 associated with sexual dysfunction, and a less satisfactory sexual life. Interestingly, a majority of the patients surveyed reported that their sexual problems had not been investigated or discussed by their physicians, making this deficit perhaps one of the most hidden HRQL consequences of diabetes.

Men with diabetes are three times as likely to develop erectile dysfunction (ED) as men without diabetes (Heiman 2002), including sexual dysfunction, disorders of libido, and ejaculatory problems, and ED can significantly reduce quality of life (De Berardis et al. 2002; Enzlin et al. 2003; Penson et al. 2003). According to the National Ambulatory Medical Care Survey (NAMCS), in 1999 approximately 22 of every 1000 men in the United States sought medical attention for ED (Skaer et al. 2001). Not surprisingly, the incidence of ED increases with age. Chronic ED affects about 5% of men in their 40s and 15%–25% of men by the age of 65. Transient ED and inadequate erection affect as many as 50% of men between the ages of 40 and 70 years (Johannes et al. 2000). Penson and co-workers (Penson et al. 2003) found that men with diabetes reported significantly worse ED and satisfaction with intercourse than those without diabetes. Rance and colleagues also looked at the impact of ED on HRQL; these authors found that men with diabetes reported that ED had a significant impact on their lives and stated that it needed to be treated as similar to other complications associated with diabetes (Rance et al. 2003). The authors also conducted a survey to determine the relative importance of treating ED versus other complications of diabetes. Men with ED recorded this problem as the third most important complication of diabetes. In addition, men with diabetes with or without ED reported that they were willing to pay more to avoid ED than other complications of diabetes except kidney disease and blindness.

ED has been associated with longer duration of diabetes, poor metabolic control, and the presence and number of diabetic complications (Fedele et al. 2000). Not surprisingly, ED may have a deleterious impact on marital relationships, self-esteem, and quality of life. ED was associated with higher levels of diabetes-specific health distress and worse psychological adaptation to diabetes, both of which were also related to worse metabolic control. Erectile problems were also associated with a dramatic increase in the prevalence of severe depressive symptoms, lower scores in the mental components of the SF-36, and a less satisfactory sexual life in a longitudinal study of type 2 diabetes (De Berardis et al. 2002; Enzlin et al. 2003) and has been associated with age, body mass index (BMI), duration of diabetes, and diabetic complications in men (Enzlin et al. 2003). Despite a significant negative effect on their quality of life, some men may be reluctant to mention the problem to their physicians, and physicians may feel reluctant to ask their patients about sexual dysfunction.

The extent of sexual dysfunction in women with diabetes has been a controversial subject for over 30 years (Schreiner-Engel et al. 1987). Some studies have reported that diabetes is associated with sexual dysfunction in women (Enzlin et al. 1998; Laumann, Paik, and Rosen 1999), whereas others have not. In one study the incidence of sexual dysfunction was 18% in women with type 1 diabetes and 42% in women with type 2 disease (Enzlin et al. 1998). Some women with diabetes have less interest in sex because they are depressed, tired due to high blood glucose levels, or have vaginal dryness that causes intercourse to be painful. Women with diabetes have double the risk of disturbed lubrication, dyspareunia, and decreased sexual desire than seen in the general population (LeMone 1996; Rosen et al. 1993).

The most common sexual dysfunction in women with diabetes has been decreased sexual arousal with slow and/or inadequate lubrication (Enzlin 2002). An earlier study also noted that women with diabetes may experience decreased sexual desire and more pain with intercourse, but problems with orgasm are not more frequent (Enzlin et al. 1998). Diabetes further deteriorates women's sexual expression, self-esteem, and sexual satisfaction and hampers marital relationships (LeMone 1996). Women with diabetes may also experience recurring cystitis or vaginal yeast infections.

In women, depression and the quality of the partner relationship was a significant predictor of sexual dysfunction (Enzlin et al. 2003). Newman and Bertelson (1986) found women with diabetes to be more likely to be depressed and less satisfied with their sexual relationships than those without diabetes. Their study also noted a complete absence of orgasm in 35% of women with diabetes, whereas only 6% of nondiabetic women had a similar complaint. A qualitative study evaluated the impact of diabetes on sexual intimacy in women; the study noted that women experienced guilt, shame, and embarrassment associated with the disease, which affected sexual functioning (Sarkadi and Rosenqvist 2003). Patients with diabetes are generally reluctant to discuss their sexual problems with health care professionals, and thus it is essential to provide professional attention for any sexual disturbances experienced by these patients.

Diabetes as a Chronic Stressor

Diabetes may be considered a major life-altering event that leads to significant psychological distress (Dalewitz, Khan, and Hershey 2000; Rubin and Peyrot 1992). The basis for this hypothesis comes from psychological stress theory (Bradburn 1969; Dohrenwend et al. 1980; Frank 1974; Lazarus 1977; Lazarus and Folkman 1984; Pearlin and Schooler, 1978), which indicates that feelings of constant challenges and feeling overwhelmed psychologically may produce generalized distress and demoralization. Long-term management of diabetes can require continuous use of medication, with an increased emphasis on self-care and self-management. Patients with diabetes commonly face issues related to the burden of self-management on their lifestyle, and they often are unable to complete diabetes self-care tasks (Rubin, Peyrot, and Siminerio 2006). Patients with diabetes requiring more intensive or complex management become emotionally distressed or overwhelmed due to complex disease management and the load of daily self-care demands (Polonsky et al. 2002; Keers et al. 2004). A study of lower-income patients with diabetes from over 15 communities found that as many as one-fifth reported significant hassles with self-care, such as having to avoid certain foods, having to schedule the demands of their daily lives around medications, and having symptoms interfere with their everyday activities (Anderson et al. 2003). More directed self-care behaviors such as checking blood glucose and taking medications as prescribed were difficult for approximately one-third to one-half of respondents (39% to 46%).

A link between coping and perceived difficulties with the impact of diabetes on HRQL has been made in several studies. In a study of adolescents with type 1 diabetes, Grey and colleagues (Grey et al. 1998) found that subjects who reported more worry about diabetes were more depressed, had lower self-efficacy toward managing their diabetes, and found coping with diabetes both harder and more upsetting. The combination of depression and challenges coping with the diabetes accounted for 48% of the variance in the impact of diabetes on quality of life. Coelho and colleagues (2003) examined the relationship between coping with diabetes and HRQL in a study of 123 patients with non-insulin-dependent diabetes; they found, overall, that avoidance styles of coping were related to worse quality of life than were active or confrontative coping styles. Similarly, Watkins and colleagues (2000) reported that diabetes-specific health behaviors were related to an increased sense of burden that was negatively associated with quality of life in a study of 296 adults aged 20–90 years with type 1 or 2 diabetes. However, there is also evidence that stress reduction leads to improved self-management and successful glycemic control (Surwit et al. 2002).

In summary, diabetes may present a continued source of life stress, leading to lower HRQL through psychological distress that may compound more direct effects of diabetes on HRQL such as limited role function. Much of the variability in stress appears to be associated with coping styles, patient support, and treatment complexity. These issues, although important as potential mediators or moderators in conceptual models of HRQL, also suggest opportunities for patient care and support in health care systems. It should be noted that for some patients diabetes is a lifelong disorder, begun in childhood. Thus, one may also need to consider the impact of diabetes and its treatment on the HRQL of children as they develop (McCarthy et al. 2002), but this discussion goes beyond the effects that are the focus of this chapter.

Effects of Medical Treatment on Health-Related Quality of Life

Models of HRQL with diabetes are not complete without consideration of treatment effects. This is because much of the use of HRQL information is aimed at understanding the benefit to the patient or to society of lifelong treatment. Although preventing diabetes complications is itself an important goal, the overall benefit of treatment must be determined from long-term studies that include assessments of patient well-being. There are several medication- or therapy-related factors that affect HRQL in patients, including complexity of the regimen, hypoglycemic events, inconvenience of administration, social stigma, and having a troublesome dosing schedule (Hunt, Valenzuela, and Pugh 1997; Korytkowski 2002; Peyrot et al. 2003). Additionally, some treatment regimens or diabetes medication classes have been associated with notable side effects such as weight gain (Lawson et al. 1999; Stratton et al. 2000), peripheral edema, gastrointestinal disturbances, and, more recently, cardiovascular complications (Nissen and Wolski 2007). Jacobson and colleagues (1994), using the diabetes quality of life (DQOL) instrument, reported decreased

HRQL for patients with type 2 diabetes as the complexity of the treatment regimen increased.

Some studies have found that insulin therapy was associated with an increase in psychological disturbances and stress (Hanninen et al. 1998), but other studies have suggested no deleterious effect of treatment intensification with insulin in type 2 patients. A conceptual difficulty in clarifying the effects of the treatment agent or regimen on HRQL is potential confounding by disease severity. Patients who are being treated with insulin or other agents have likely failed previous therapies or may have suffered progression of their disease. In addition, studies have not routinely collected all of the medication side-effect data needed to relate to HRQL outcomes.

The UKPDS conducted two randomized controlled trials to investigate the influence of therapies for metabolic control on HRQL and concluded that quality of life for type 2 patients does not appear to be affected by intensive policies to improve blood pressure or glucose control (UKPDS 1999). Similar results have been obtained by others (Gilden et al. 1990; Parkerson et al. 1993). Whether intensified treatments cancelled out benefits from better symptom control is uncertain in these studies. Other investigators have shown that intensive insulin management can be cost-effective and associated with an improvement in health outcomes and quality of life (Ristic and Bates 2003). Another large study, the ACCORD trial, was able to determine the relative HRQL benefits of intensive glycemic control relative to treatment burden, although there was no evidence of diminished treatment satisfaction related to treatment burden (Personal Communication from unpublished data, R. Anderson July 2010). To date, there are insufficient data on the unique effects of medical treatment on HRQL in the context of glycemic control—whether beneficial or adverse. If, on balance, the burdens of intensive management of glycemia are wholly compensated by benefits to HRQL from optimal glycemic control, one might ask how long this equilibrium might last. And can more effective treatment approaches be developed that may result in a net gain to HRQL over the longer course?

Adherence to Pharmacotherapy

Research on the correlation of satisfaction with diabetes treatment suggests that patients may form preferences for diabetes regimens based on degree of complexity, convenience, ability to integrate the regimen in daily life, efficacy in controlling blood glucose levels (Bradley and Speight 2002; Lewis et al. 1998; Peyrot and Rubin 2005; Witthaus, Stewart, and Bradley 2001), and manner or method of delivery (Anderson et al. 2004; Sampson et al. 2007). Thus the manner of treatment, the patient or "operator" needed to successfully adhere, and the potential for side effects could have a direct effect upon HRQL in study populations of diabetes patients and an indirect effect through suboptimal self-management of diabetes. Poor adherence to medications in patients with diabetes has been associated with the development of complications, disease progression, hospitalizations, depression, and premature disability and mortality. Despite these known consequences, adherence rates to oral antidiabetic medications in the United States were found to be significantly low, ranging from 36% to 93%, as they were for insulin therapy, varying from 62% to 64% (Cramer 2004; Pladevall et al. 2004). There is ample evidence that depression reduces adherence to pharmacologic treatment of diabetes and by this mechanism contributes to poorer glycemic control (Ciechanowski, Katon, and Russo 2000; de Groot et al. 1999; Lustman et al. 2003). However, depression may also make diabetes patients less likely to seek medical care, which may in turn make them less likely to engage in appropriate self-care.

■ Psychosocial Interventions and Health-Related Quality of Life

The high risk for functional impairment, depression, and overall lower HRQL with diabetes challenges conventional public health models of diabetes prevention and control and leads us to reframe diabetes care as a system of supportive care management at multiple levels within the community (Wagner et al. 2005). Increased levels of family support, cohesion, and organization have been shown to improve adherence and result in better glycemic control, whereas family conflict and dysfunction is a predictor of difficulties with adherence (Glasgow et al. 1997). Nontraditional approaches to patient education and support may be beneficial. For instance, Ellis and colleagues (2004) demonstrated that interventions such as goal setting, cognitive reframing, and problem solving were more effective than didactic education in producing and maintaining changes in behavior. A recent meta-analysis of six randomized trials in diabetes tentatively concluded that social support interventions positively affect patient self-care and outcomes (Van Dam et al. 2005). In a synthesis of the literature, Marks and colleagues (2005) showed that incremental goal setting, self-monitoring and self-appraisal, problem solving, and modeling were effective in improving behavioral and clinical outcomes in a variety of patient populations. Similarly, a benefit of guided educational interventions on HRQL was found in a meta-analysis of five randomized studies in diabetes patients (Zhang et al. 2007).

Other nontraditional interventions shown to be effective with diabetes in the literature include psychosocial support and reinforcement (Jones et al. 2003; Piette, Weinberger, and McPhee 2000; Steed et al. 2005), training in coping skills (Grey et al. 1998), cognitive behavior therapy (Fosbury et al. 1997), family behavior therapy (Anderson et al. 1999; Wysocki et al. 2000), and psychological counseling for patients with self-management difficulties, which can successfully improve HRQL (Glasgow, Fisher, and Anderson 1999; Snoek and Skinner 2002). Collaborative goal setting has been found to be effective in interventions to enhance diabetes self-management (Fisher et al. 2005) and reduce health risks (Alexy 1985; Puczynski et al. 2005). Taken together, the evidence on behavioral strategies for patient support suggests that conventional medical interventions aimed at achieving optimal A1C outcomes can be promoted with more intensive cognitive and behavioral interventions. Unfortunately the relative clinical value of assessing patient barriers to self-management and HRQL deficits and including behavioral strategies in the context of intensive therapy (e.g., targeting A1C levels below 7%) on HRQL, glycemic control, and adverse events has been underused as an intervention and approach to diabetes management.

■ Conclusion

In summary, diabetes can affect an individual's HRQL from pathways involving impairment and disease progression, having a lifelong illness that requires lifestyle restrictions, and from being on medical therapies that impose side effects and possible treatment burdens. These pathways were discussed as being relevant to a complex chronic disease model. In this light the treatment of diabetes demands special attention to optimize long-term management and HRQL outcomes. Needed are the development and testing of interventions with a multidisciplinary approach that involves health care professionals, including physicians, nurse educators, pharmacists, behavioralists, and dietitians, as well as the patients themselves.

■ References

Ahroni JH et al. (1994). The health and functional status of veterans with diabetes. *Diabetes Care* **17**, 318–21.

Alexy B (1985). Goal setting and health risk reduction. *Nursing Research* **34**, 283–8.

Alonso J et al. (2004). IQOLA Project Group: Health-related quality of life associated with chronic conditions in eight countries: results from the International Quality of Life Assessment (IQOLA) Project. *Quality of Life Research* **13**, 283–98.

American Diabetes Association (2007). Standards of medical care in diabetes—2007. *Diabetes Care* **30**, s4–41.

Anderson BJ et al. (1999). An office-based intervention to maintain parent-adolescent teamwork in diabetes management: impact on parent involvement, family conflict, and subsequent glycemic control. *Diabetes Care* **22**, 713–21.

Anderson RJ et al. (2001). The prevalence of comorbid depression in adults with diabetes: a meta-analysis. *Diabetes Care* **24**, 1069–78.

Anderson RM et al. (1997). A comparison of global versus disease-specific quality-of-life measures in patients with NIDDM. *Diabetes Care* **20**, 299–305.

Anderson RT et al. (2003). Patient-centered outcomes of diabetes self-care. Associations with satisfaction and general health in a community clinic setting. *North Carolina Medical Journal* **64**, 58–65.

Anderson RT et al. (2004). Development and validation of the insulin treatment satisfaction questionnaire. *Clinical Therapeutics* **26**, 565–78.

Anderson RT et al. (2009). Diabetes Medication Satisfaction Tool: a focus on treatment regimens. *Diabetes Care* **32**(1), 51–3.

Aubert RE et al. (1995). Diabetes-related hospitalization and hospital utilization. In: Harris MI et al., eds. *Diabetes in America*, 2nd ed., pp 553–70. Washington, DC: U.S. Government Printing Office. National Institutes of Health Publication No. 95–1468.

Berwick DM et al. (1991). Performance of a five-item mental health screening test. *Medical Care* **29**, 169–76.

Bittner B (2008). Intensive Glucose-Lowering Arm of Diabetes Study Halted Early: Increased Death Rate Sparks Concern. Available at http://www.aafp.org/online/en/home/publications/news/news-now/clinical-care-research/20080225accordstudy.html. Accessed April 15, 2008.

Bradburn NM (1969). *The Structure of Psychological Wellbeing*. Chicago: Aldine.

Bradley C, Speight J (2002). Patient perceptions of diabetes and diabetes therapy: assessing quality of life. *Diabetes/Metabolism Research and Reviews* **18**, S64–9.

Brown DW et al. (2004). Diabetes mellitus and health-related quality of life among older adults. Findings from the behavioral risk factor surveillance system (BRFSS) *Diabetes Research and Clinical Practice* **65**, 105–15.

Camacho FT et al. (2002). Investigating correlates of health related quality of life in a low-income sample of diabetics. *Quality of Life Research* **11**, 783–96.

Camacho T et al. (1991). Physical activity and depression: evidence from the Alameda County Study. *American Journal of Epidemiology* **134**, 220–31.

Cefalu WT et al. (2008). Patients' perceptions of subcutaneous insulin in the OPTIMIZE study: A multicenter follow-up study *Diabetes Technology & Therapeutics* **10**(1), 25–38.

Ciechanowski PS, Katon WJ, Russo JE (2000). Depression and diabetes: impact of depressive symptoms on adherence, function, and costs. *Archives of Internal Medicine* **160**, 3278–85.

Coelho R, Amorim I, Prata J (2003). Coping styles and quality of life in patients with non-insulin-dependent diabetes mellitus. *Psychosomatics* **44**, 312–8.

Cramer JA (2004). A systematic review of adherence with medications for diabetes. *Diabetes Care* **27**, 1218–24.

Curtis JR, Martin DP, Martin TR (1997). Patient-assessed health outcomes in chronic lung disease. *American Journal of Respiratory and Critical Care Medicine* **156**, 1032–9.

Dalewitz J, Khan N, Hershey CO (2000). Barriers to control of blood glucose in diabetes mellitus. *American Journal of Medical Quality* **15**, 16–25.

De Berardis G et al. (2002). Erectile dysfunction and quality of life in type 2 diabetic patients: a serious problem too often overlooked. *Diabetes Care* **25**, 284–91.

de Groot M et al. (1999). Glycemic control and major depression in patients with type 1 and type 2 diabetes mellitus. *Journal of Psychosomatic Research* **46**, 425–35.

de Groot M et al. (2001). Association of depression and diabetes complications: a meta-analysis. *Psychosomatic Medicine* **63**, 619–30.

Diabetes Control and Complications Trial/Epidemiology of Diabetes interventions and Complications Research Group (2000). Retinopathy and nephropathy in patients with type 1 diabetes four years after a trial of intensive therapy. *New England Journal of Medicine* **342**, 381–9.

Dohrenwend BP et al. (1980). Nonspecific psychological distress and other dimensions of psychopathology. Measures for use in the general population. *Archives of General Psychiatry* **37**, 1229.

Eaton WE et al. (1996). Depression and risk of onset of type II diabetes: a prospective population-based study. *Diabetes Care* **20**,1097–102.

Egede LE (2004). Diabetes, major depression and functional disability among U.S. adults. *Diabetes Care* **27**, 421–8.

Ellis SE et al. (2004). Diabetes patient education: a meta-analysis and meta-regression. *Patient Education and Counseling* **52**, 97–105.

Enzlin P et al. (1998). Diabetes mellitus and female sexuality: a review of 25 years' research. *Diabetic Medicine* **15**, 809–15.

Enzlin P at al. (2002). Sexual dysfunction in women with type 1 diabetes: a controlled study. *Diabetes Care* **25**, 672–7.

Enzlin P et al. (2003). Prevalence and predictors of sexual dysfunction in patients with type 1 diabetes. *Diabetes Care* **26**, 409–14.

Fedele D et al. (2000). Erectile dysfunction in type 1 and type 2 diabetics in Italy. *International Journal of Epidemiology* **29**, 524–31.

Fisher EB et al. (2005). Ecological approaches to self-management: the case of diabetes. *American Journal of Public Health* **95**, 1523–35.

Fosbury JA et al. (1997). A trial of cognitive analytic therapy in poorly controlled type I patients. *Diabetes Care* **20**, 959–64.

Frank JD (1974). Psychotherapy: the restoration of morale. *American Journal of Psychiatry* **131**, 3.

Gavard JA, Lustman PJ, Clouse RE (1993). Prevalence of depression in adults with diabetes: an epidemiological evaluation. *Diabetes Care* **16**, 1167–78.

Geiss S et al. (1995). Mortality in non-insulin-dependent diabetes. In: Harris M et al., eds. *Diabetes in America*, 2nd ed., pp 133–55. Washington, DC: U.S. Government Printing Office, National Institutes of Health Publication No. 95–1468.

Geringer ES et al. (1988). Depression and diabetic neuropathy: a complex relationship. *Journal of Geriatric Psychiatry and Neurology* **1**, 11–5.

Gilden JL et al. (1990). Effects of self-monitoring of blood glucose on quality of life in elderly diabetic patients. *Journal of the American Geriatric Society* **38**, 511–5.

Glasgow RE et al. (1997). Quality of life and associated characteristics in a large national sample of adults with diabetes. *Diabetes Care* **20**, 562–7.

Glasgow RE, Fisher EB, Anderson BJ (1999). Behavioral science in diabetes. Contributions and opportunities. *Diabetes Care* **22**, 832–43.

Grey M et al. (1998). Short-term effects of coping skills training as adjunct to intensive therapy in adolescents. *Diabetes Care* **21**, 902–8.

Grover SA et al. (2006). The prevalence of erectile dysfunction in the primary care setting: importance of risk factors for diabetes and vascular disease. *Archives of Internal Medicine* **166**, 213–9.

Gulliford MC, Mahabir D (1999). Relationship of health-related quality of life to symptom severity in diabetes mellitus: a study in Trinidad and Tobago. *Journal of Clinical Epidemiology* **52**, 773–80.

Hanninen J, Takala J, Keinänen-Kiukaanniemi S. 1998. Quality of life in NIDDM patients assessed with the SF-20 questionnaire. *Diabetes Research and Clinical Practice* **42**, 17–27.

Harris A, Cronkite R, Moos R (2006). Physical activity, exercise coping, and depression in a 10-year cohort study of depressed patients. *Journal of Affective Disorders* **93**, 79–85.

Hayes AJ et al. (2008) Can self-rated health scores be used for risk prediction in patients with type 2 diabetes? Diabetes Care **31**, 795–7.

Heiman JR (2002). Sexual dysfunction: overview of prevalence, etiological factors, and treatments. *Journal of Sex Research* **39**, 73–8.

Heron MP (2007). *Deaths: Leading Causes for 2004.* National vital statistics reports, vol. 56. Hyattsville, MD: National Center for Health Statistics.

Hunt LM, Valenzuela MA, Pugh JA (1997). NIDDM patients' fears and hopes about insulin therapy. The basis of patient reluctance. *Diabetes Care* **20**, 292–8.

Jackson G (2004). Sexual dysfunction and diabetes. *International Journal of Clinical Practice* **58**, 358–62.

Jacobson AM et al. (1994). Psychosocial aspects of diabetes. In: Kahn Cr, Weir G, eds. *Joslin's Diabetes Mellitus,* 13th ed., pp 431–50. Philadelphia: Lea & Febiger.

Jacobson MJ, de Groot M, Samson JA (1994). The evaluation of two measures of quality of life in patients with type 1 and type 2 diabetes. *Diabetes Care* **17**, 267–74.

Johannes CB et al. (2000). Incidence of erectile dysfunction in men 40 to 69 years old: longitudinal results from the Massachusetts Male Ageing Study. *Journal of Urology* **163**, 460–3.

Jones H et al. (2003). Changes in diabetes selfcare behaviors make a difference in glycemic control: the Diabetes Stages of Change (DiSC) study. *Diabetes Care* **26**, 732–7.

Keers JC et al. (2004). Do diabetologists recognise self-management problems in their patients? *Diabetes Research in Clinical Practice* **66**, 157–61.

Keinänen-Kiukaanniemi S et al. (1996). Health related quality of life in diabetic patients measured by the Nottingham Health profile. *Diabetic Medicine* **13**, 382–8.

Kercher K (1992). Assessing subjective wellbeing in the old-old. *Research on Aging* **2**, 131–68.

Klein BE, Klein R, Moss SE (1998). Self-rated health and diabetes of long duration. The Wisconsin Epidemiologic Study of Diabetic Retinopathy. *Diabetes Care* **21**, 236–40.

Korytkowski M (2002). When oral agents fail: practical barriers to starting insulin. *International Journal of Obesity and Related Metabolic Disorders* **26** (Suppl. 3), S18–24.

Kovacs M et al. (1990). Psychological functioning of children with insulin-dependent diabetes mellitus: a longitudinal study. *Journal of Pediatric Psychology* **15**, 619–32.

Laumann EO, Paik A, Rosen RC (1999). Sexual dysfunction in the United States: prevalence and predictors. *Journal of the American Medical Association* **281**, 537–44.

Lawson ML et al. (1999). Effect of intensive therapy on early macrovascular disease in young individuals with type 1 diabetes: a systematic review and meta-analysis. *Diabetes Care* **22**, B35–9.

Lazarus RS, Folkman S (1984). Coping and adaptation. In: Gentry WD, ed. *The Handbook of Behavioral Medicine,* pp 282–325. New York: Guilford.

Lazarus RS (1977). Psychological stress and coping in adaptation and illness. In: Lipowski NZ, Lipsi DR, Whybrow PC, eds. *Psychosomatic medicine: current trends.* New York: Oxford University Press.

LeMone P (1996). The physical effects of diabetes on sexuality in women. *Diabetes Educator* **22**, 361–6.

Lewis KS et al. (1988). A measure of treatment satisfaction designed specifically for people with insulin-dependent diabetes. *Diabetic Medicine* **5**, 235–42.

Litwin MS, Nied RJ, Dhanani N (1998). Health-related quality of life in men with erectile dysfunction. *Journal of General Internal Medicine* **13**, 159–66.

Luscombe FA (2000). Health-related quality of life measurement in type 2 diabetes. *Value Health* **3**, 15–28.

Lustman PJ et al. (1997). The course of major depression in diabetics. *General Hospital Psychiatry* **19**, 138–43.

Lustman PJ et al. (2003). Depression and poor glycemic control: a meta-analytic review of the literature. *Diabetes Care* **23**, 934–42.

Marks R, Allegrante JP, Lorig K (2005). A review and synthesis of research evidence for self-efficacy-enhancing interventions for reducing chronic disability: implications for health education practice (Part II). *Health Promotion Practice* **6**, 148–56.

McCarthy AM et al. (2002). Effects of diabetes on learning in children. *Pediatrics* **109**, E9.

Nafees B et al. (2006). How diabetes and insulin therapy affects the lives of people with type 1 diabetes. *European Diabetes Nursing* **3**(2), 292–7.

Nagi SZ (1976). Epidemiology of disability among adults in the United States. *Milbank Memorial Fund Quarterly* **54**, 439–66.

Newman AS, Bertelson AD (1986). Sexual dysfunction in diabetic women. *Journal of Behavioral Medicine* **9**, 261–70.

Nissen SE, Wolski K (2007). Effect of rosiglitazone on the risk of myocardial infarction and death from cardiovascular causes. *New England Journal of Medicine* **356**, 2457–71.

Norris SL, Engelgau MM, Narayan KMV (2002). Effectiveness of self management training in type 2 diabetes: a systematic review of randomized controlled trials. *Diabetes Care* **24**, 561–87.

Norris SL et al. (2002). Self-management education for adults with type 2 diabetes: a meta-analysis of the effect on glycemic control. *Diabetes Care* **27**, 1159–71.

Parkerson GR et al. (1993). Disease-specific versus generic measurement of health-related quality of life in insulin dependent diabetic patients. *Medical Care* **31**, 629–39.

Patrick DL (1990). Measurement of health status in the 1990s. *Annual Review of Public Health* **2**, 165–83.

Pearlin LI, Schooler C (1978). The structure of coping. *Journal of Health and Social Behavior* **19**, 2–21.

Penson D, Wessells H (2004). Erectile dysfunction in diabetic patients. *Diabetes Spectrum* **17**, 225–30.

Penson DF et al. (2003). Do impotent men with diabetes have more severe erectile dysfunction and worse quality of life than the general population of impotent patients? Results from the Exploratory Comprehensive Evaluation of Erectile Dysfunction (ExCEED) database. *Diabetes Care* **26**, 1093–9.

Peyrot M et al. (2003). An international study of psychological resistance to insulin use among persons with diabetes. *Diabetologia* **46**(2), A89.

Peyrot M, Rubin RR (1997). Levels and risks of depression and anxiety symptomatology among diabetic adults. *Diabetes Care* **20**, 585–90.

Peyrot M, Rubin RR (2005). Validity and reliability of an instrument for assessing health-related quality of life and treatment preferences: the Insulin Delivery System Rating Questionnaire. *Diabetes Care* **28**, 53–8.

Piette JD, Weinberger M, McPhee SJ (2000). The effect of automated calls with telephone nurse follow-up on patient-centered outcomes of diabetes care: a randomized, controlled trial. *Medical Care* **38**, 218–30.

Pladevall M et al. (2004). Clinical outcomes and adherence to medications measured by claims data in patients with diabetes. *Diabetes Care* **27**, 2800–5.

Polonsky WH (2002). Emotional and quality-of-life aspects of diabetes management. *Current Diabetes Reports* **2**, 153-9.

Puczynski S et al. (2005). Collaborative goal setting to improve lifestyle behaviors: lessons learned from NOPCRN. *Annals of Family Medicine* **3** (Suppl. 2), S60–2.

Radloff LS (1977). The CES-D Scale: a self-report depression scale for research in the general population. *Applied Psychological Measures* **1**, 385–401.

Rance J et al. (2003). How much of a priority is treating erectile dysfunction? A study of patients' perceptions. *Diabetic Medicine* **20**, 205–9.

Ristic S, Bates PC (2003). Effects of rapid-acting insulin analogs on overall glycemic control in type 1 and type 2 diabetes mellitus. *Diabetes Technology & Therapeutics* **5**, 57–66.

Rosen RC et al. (1993). Prevalence of sexual dysfunction in women: results of a survey study of 329 women in an outpatient gynecological clinic. *Journal of Sex and Marital Therapy* **19**, 171–88.

Rubin RR, Peyrot M (1992). Psychosocial problems and interventions in diabetes. A review of the literature. *Diabetes Care* **15**, 1640–57.

Rubin RR, Peyrot M (1999). Quality of life and diabetes. *Diabetes/Metabolism Research and Reviews* **15**, 205–18.

Rubin RR, Peyrot M, Siminerio LM (2006). Health care and patient-reported outcomes: results of the cross-national Diabetes Attitudes, Wishes and Needs (DAWN) study. *Diabetes Care* **29**, 1249–55.

Sampson MJ et al. (2007). A national survey of in-patient diabetes services in the United Kingdom. *Diabetic Medicine* **24**, 643–9.

Sarkadi A, Rosenqvist U (2003). Intimacy and women with type 2 diabetes: an exploratory study using focus group interviews. *Diabetes Educator* **29**, 641–52.

Schreiner-Engel P et al. (1987). The differential impact of diabetes type on female sexuality. *Journal of Psychosomatic Research* **31**, 23–33.

Sevick MA et al. (2007). Patients with complex chronic diseases: perspectives on supporting self-management. *Journal of General Internal Medicine* **22** (Suppl. 3), 438–44.

Shumaker SA, Anderson R, Czajkowski SM (1990). Psychological tests and scales. In: Spilker G, ed. *Quality of Life Assessments in Clinical Trials*, pp 95–113. New York: Raven Press.

Skaer T et al. (2001). Trends in the rate of self-report and diagnosis of erectile dysfunction in the United States 1990–1998: was the introduction of sildenafil an influencing factor? *Disease Management & Health Outcomes* **9**, 33–41.

Snoek FJ, Skinner TC (2002). Psychological counseling in problematic diabetes: does it help? *Diabetic Medicine* **19**, 265–73.

Songer T (1995). Disability in diabetes. In: Harris MI et al., eds. *Diabetes in America*, 2nd ed., pp 259–82. Washington, DC: U.S. Government Printing Office. National Institutes of Health Publication No. 95–1468.

Sprangers MA et al. (2000). Which chronic conditions are associated with better or poorer quality of life? *Journal of Clinical Epidemiology* **53**, 895–907.

Steed L et al. (2005). Evaluation of the UCL diabetes self-management programme (UCL-DSMP): a randomized controlled trial. *Journal of Health Psychology* **10**, 261–76.

Stewart AL et al. (1989). Functional status and well-being of patients with chronic conditions. Results from the Medical Outcomes Study. *JAMA* **262**, 907–13.

Stewart AL, Painter PL (1997). Issues in measuring physical functioning and disability in arthritis patients. *Arthritis Care and Research* **10**, 395–405.

Stratton IM et al. (2000). Association of glycaemia with macrovascular and microvascular complications of type 2 diabetes (UKPDS 35): prospective observational study. *British Medical Journal* **321**, 405–12.

Surwit RS et al. (2002). Stress management improves long-term glycemic control in type 2 diabetes. *Diabetes Care* **25**, 30–4.

Testa MA, Simonson DC (1998). Health economic benefits and quality of life during improved glycemic control in patients with type 2 diabetes mellitus: a randomized, controlled, double-blind trial. *Journal of the American Medical Association* **280**, 1490–6.

Thomas A, LoPiccolo J (1994). Sexual functioning in persons with diabetes: issues in research, treatment and education. *Clinical Psychology Review* **14**, 1–86.

UK Prospective Diabetes Study Group (1999). Quality of life in type 2 diabetic patients is affected by complications but not by intensive policies to improve blood glucose or blood pressure control (UKPDS 37). *Diabetes Care* **22**, 1125–36.

Van Dam HA et al. (2005). Social support in diabetes: a systematic review of controlled intervention studies. *Patient Education and Counseling* **59**, 1–12.

Van der Does FE et al. (1996). Symptoms and wellbeing in relation to glycemic control in type 2 diabetes. *Diabetes Care* **19**, 204–10.

Verbrugge LM, Jette AM (1994). The disablement process. *Social Science & Medicine* **38**, 1–14.

Wagner EH et al. (2005). Finding common ground: patient-centeredness and evidence-based chronic illness care. *Journal of Alternative and Complementary Medicine* **11** (Supp. 1), S7–15.

Wandell PE (1999). The health-related quality of life in diabetic patients with psychiatric disorders. *Practical Diabetes International* **16**, 174–8.

Wandell PE, Brorsson B, .Aberg H (1998). Quality of life among diabetic patients in Swedish primary health care and in the general population: Comparison between 1992 and 1995. *Quality of Life Research* **7**, 751–60.

Ware J, Kosinksi M, Gandek B (2000). *SF-36® Health Survey: Manual & Interpretation Guide*. Lincoln, RI: Quality Metric Incorporated.

Watkins KW et al. (2000). Effect of adults' self-regulation of diabetes on quality-of-life outcomes. *Diabetes Care* **23**, 1511–5.

Weinberger M et al. (1994). The relationship between glycemic control and health-related quality of life in patients with non-insulin-dependent diabetes mellitus. *Medical Care* **32**, 1173–81.

Weinger K, Jacobson AM (2001). Psychosocial and quality of life correlates of glycemic control during intensive treatment of type 1 diabetes. *Patient Education and Counseling* **42**, 123–31.

Wikblad K, Leksell J, Wibel L (1996). Health-related quality of life in relation to metabolic control and late complication in patients with insulin dependent diabetes mellitus. *Quality of Life Research* **5**, 123–30.

Witthaus E, Stewart J, Bradley C (2001). Treatment satisfaction and psychological wellbeing with insulin glargine compared with NPH in patients with Type 1 diabetes. *Diabetic Medicine* **18**, 619–25.

World Health Organization (1952). *Constitution of the World Health Organization*. In: *Handbook of Basic Documents*, 5th ed., pp 3–20. Geneva: WHO.

Wysocki T et al. (2000). Randomized, controlled trial of behavior therapy for families of adolescents with insulin-dependent diabetes mellitus. *Journal of Pediatric Psychology* **25**, 23–33.

Zautra AJ (1995). Arthritis and perceptions of quality of life: an examination of positive and negative effect in rheumatoid arthritis patients, *Health Psychology* **5**, 399–408.

Zhang X et al. (2007). The effects of interventions on health-related quality of life among persons with diabetes: a systematic review. *Medical Care* **45**, 820–34.

SECTION 4

DIABETES CONTROL
PROGRAMS AND POLICIES

22. The Diabetes Prevention and Control Programs in the United States and Public Health Law and Policy

Patricia Thompson-Reid and Kristina L. Ernst

■ Key Public Health Messages

- Evidence-based public health practice is essential for reducing the social and economic burden of diabetes, and it is integral to the translation of science into practical applications at the community level.
- Policy initiatives that provide resources to support development, and integration at all levels of operation, are important elements for program growth. These factors, coupled with a competent workforce possessing the skills to provide leadership, technical assistance, and information to all partners, are essential for success.
- It is not sufficient to translate clinical research into policy and practice; there should also be efforts to optimize public health practice through research at the community level or at the level where services are delivered.
- Strategic partners play an integral role in the successful implementation of programs at the national, state, and local level.
- Increasing access to care and the delivery of interventions to vulnerable populations are major challenges in public health.
- Guidelines, evaluation, and training must be adapted and implemented to support the successful expansion of program activities.
- Primary, secondary, and tertiary prevention are important components of reducing the burden of diabetes in disparate populations, but in the long term, primary prevention may have the most significant impact in lowering medical, psychosocial, and economic costs.

■ Introduction

The Diabetes Prevention and Control Program, which is funded by the Centers for Disease Control and Prevention (CDC), operates through 59 state and territorial health departments. The program's development has been influenced greatly by diabetes advocates, health care professionals, people with diabetes, professional organizations such as the American Diabetes Association (ADA) and the American Association of Diabetes Educators (AADE), visionary leaders at the CDC, and policy makers. Early on, there was particular concern about the health and education of persons with diabetes; more recently, advocates and policy makers have focused concern on the health and wellness of all Americans with chronic diseases (National Institutes of Health 2005).

■ Background/Historical Perspective

In 1974 the U.S. Congress passed Public Law 93-354, the National Diabetes Mellitus Research and Education Act. This act paved the way for the development of chronic disease prevention and control programs and, more specifically, established a National Commission on Diabetes with a mandate to increase the visibility and funding for diabetes-related activities through development of a long-range plan that would organize national resources to accomplish this goal. The commission made the following recommendations as part of its long-range plan:

1. Federal leadership and resources were needed to facilitate the evaluation and dissemination of research on the epidemiology, etiology, and prevention and control of diabetes.
2. The CDC should undertake a community education, health care, and disease control program.
3. A National Diabetes Advisory Board (NDAB) should be established to oversee and track implementation of the recommendations of the Commission.
4. Diabetes Research and Training Centers should be established.

Over the 15 years of its existence the NDAB advised Congress, the National Institutes of Health (NIH), CDC, and all other federal agencies involved in diabetes-related activities (Genuth 1994; The National Diabetes Advisory Board 1988). Most relevant was the recommendation to establish state diabetes control programs under the primary responsibility of the CDC, programs that would involve community education, health care, and disease control. Other important actions were the establishment of the Model Diabetes Program for the Indian Health Service, the Diabetes Data Group, the Diabetes Research and Training Centers, and the implementation of the Diabetes Control and Complications Trial to answer questions about hyperglycemia and its relationship to the development of diabetes complications. In 1987 the NDAB recommended the "establishment of a Diabetes Translation Center at the CDC, to plan, conduct, and coordinate national efforts to transfer diabetes research more rapidly into patient care" (Ring 1988). This recommendation was carried out with congressional support, and it had a major impact on the development and implementation of what were then named the State Diabetes Control Programs.

The Changing Paradigm at the CDC

In 1970 the Public Health Service changed the name of CDC's predecessor, the Communicable Disease Center, to the Center for Disease Control to reflect the agency's vision of expanding its focus from communicable diseases to include the prevention and control of chronic diseases and related risk factors (Ethridge 1992). There was also growing concern about the increasing burden of diseases related to "lifestyle" (Foege 1981). In the First National Health and Nutrition Examination Survey (NHANES I), conducted between 1971 and 1974, the prevalence of diabetes in the United States was found to be 3.2%. Data from NHANES I and NHANES II showed that the highest prevalence of diabetes was among persons with the lowest incomes (Kanjilal et al. 2006) and that persons with diabetes had a higher risk of death, lower survival, and lower life expectancy than persons without diabetes (Gu et al. 1998). In 1976 NHANES II showed that only about half of people with diabetes knew that they had the disease.

Earlier, results from the National Health Interview Survey in 1974 revealed that persons with diabetes were more frequent users of the medical care system, both ambulatory care and in-hospital services, than persons without diabetes. The majority of patients with diabetes visited the physician's office, but approximately 30% of those aged 20 years or older had used the emergency room or outpatient clinic as a source of care during the last 12 months, compared with approximately 19% of the general population without diabetes who had used those service sites (Harris 1985). Differences in these behaviors between the populations examined were even more alarming when analyzed by race and income (Drury 1981).

In addition, only about 4% of all visits made by persons with diabetes to a physician's office involved physicians whose specialty was diabetes or endocrinology. For diabetes patients aged 45 and older, the proportion of visits to cardiovascular specialists was identical to that for patients without diabetes in the general population. The proportion visiting an ophthalmologist was lower for persons with diabetes than for persons without diabetes (Harris 1985). The 1977 National Ambulatory Medical Care Survey found that in visits where diabetes was the primary diagnosis, drugs were prescribed for 62% of patients, diet modification for 37%, and blood pressure checks for 67%, but in only 3% of visits did patients have their eyes checked. Persons with diabetes had fewer visits to the dentist than did persons without diabetes. Gum disease, a complication of diabetes, is less likely to occur if one makes recommended visits to the dentist.

In brief, such data demonstrated that many persons with diabetes were not receiving adequate preventive care. Even with the use of available treatment options, however, health care providers and individuals with diabetes would also need appropriate policies to support a health care delivery system that would provide access to information and treatment for all persons with diabetes. These options would require the assurance of a workforce to deliver health promotion, patient care, and in-service training for health professionals in order to motivate behavioral changes in both providers and patients for achieving positive health outcomes.

In the 1970s the CDC underwent an extensive strategic planning process in which it solicited recommendations for what it should do to improve the health of the nation. The result was a prioritization of programs and activities; diabetes was listed as a preventable "*Health Problem of Noteworthy Significance*" under the subheading of *Unnecessary Morbidity and Mortality* (Foege 1981).

■ The Diabetes Control Demonstration Projects

State Partners and the CDC Diabetes Control Program

In keeping with the recommendations of the NDAB, the groundwork was initiated for the establishment of a CDC Diabetes Control Program in state health departments, the traditional and strategic partners of the CDC. These entities carried out their mandate for health promotion and health protection through the three core functions of public health: assessment, assurance, and policy development. At that time there was little documentation about effective interventions for diabetes control at the community level. In 1977 the Diabetes Control Activity, initially housed in the Bureau of Epidemiology at the CDC, provided one million dollars to fund 10 community pilot projects through competitive grants to the states to reduce diabetes morbidity and mortality. In addition to providing services focused on secondary and tertiary prevention, these cost-reimbursement contracts provided resources for building infrastructure, or administrative capability, at the state level to enable the State Diabetes Control Programs to carry out activities to improve access to affordable, high-quality diabetes care and services to high-risk populations (Drury et al. 1981; Genuth 1994; Ring 1988).

Grantees were charged to "use basic epidemiologic principles and methods to identify and implement appropriate interventions to reduce diabetes-related morbidity and mortality" (Murphy et al. 2004). The states funded were South Carolina, Colorado, Georgia, Illinois, Maine, Nebraska, New York, Rhode Island, Michigan, and Mississippi (Centers for Disease Control 1980; Ring 1988). The original contracts outlined broad goals for disease outcomes and provided the CDC with the experience and opportunity that eventually led to what is now called the cooperative agreement (Public Law 95-224) (Pomeroy et al. 1986). This legal instrument outlined the relationship between the federal government, CDC, and the state or other local entities, and allowed substantial involvement of the CDC through-out the implementation of these projects. The activities of the pilot projects were divided into phases (Centers for Disease Control 1980; Ring 1988). Phase 1, or the first year of the program, was devoted to assessment and planning, while Phase 2 (year 2) became the implementation or intervention phase. Most Diabetes Control Programs focused their activities in three categories: professional education, patient education, and health care delivery. They also worked to maintain and improve their epidemiology and surveillance capacity developed in Phase 1.

The Diabetes Advisory Boards

The Diabetes Control Programs also established Diabetes Advisory Boards, or com-mittees made up of representatives from professional and voluntary organizations, academic institutions, hospitals, and medical centers, experts in diabetes, primary care providers, and local leaders. Membership in the advisory boards committees in the initial 10 states, plus Ohio and Washington, added in 1979 ranged from 9 to 45 persons. ADA affiliates were represented in all states' advisory bodies, and the Juvenile Diabetes Foundation was represented in most states. Local and county health departments and Diabetes Research and Training Centers (supported by the National Institute of Diabetes and Digestive and Kidney Diseases) were also repre-sented on the board in some states. Information sharing and providing guidance to the Diabetes Control Programs were the primary roles of the advisory committees in Phase 1 of the pilots. These committees were also a link between the program and the communities served. The advisory boards reviewed the findings from Phase 1 and proposed specific interventions and programmatic guidance for Phase 2. Advisory committees provided opportunities for partnerships, diabetes advocacy, and addi-tional manpower to carry out Diabetes Control Program activities (CDC 1983).

Because of the strategies and focus of the State Diabetes Control Program and its partnerships at the state level, it was separated from the other chronic disease programs housed in the Center for Environment Health at CDC, and it moved to the Center for Prevention Services, where it eventually became a separate division (Ring 1988; Center for Disease Control 1978, 1980). Simultaneously, the Center for Health Promotion and Health Education at the CDC brought together all the personal health and lifestyle programs. This Center, renamed in 1988 the National Center for Chronic Disease Prevention and Health Promotion, is where CDC's Division of Diabetes Translation currently resides.

■ A New Way of Working with CDC Partners:
   The Cooperative Agreement

In 1980 the CDC became the Centers for Disease Control that included six Centers (Foege 1981). The 1979 Surgeon Generals Report on Health Promotion and disease

Prevention was released, and it signaled a trend at the CDC toward focus on health promotion, disease prevention, and "lifestyle related diseases" (The Surgeon General's Report on Health Promotion and Disease Prevention, 1979). The State Diabetes program grew to 20 states as eight additional states were funded with cooperative agreements for a 5-year project period. These new states, California, Kentucky, Louisiana, Minnesota, Missouri, New Jersey, Pennsylvania, and Utah, were funded through an approach that fostered collaboration or an "assistance transaction," now referred to as the cooperative agreement. As of 1980 all 20 Diabetes Control Programs were funded through this cooperative mechanism (Center for Disease Control 1980; Pomeroy et al. 1986). Public Health Advisors were assigned by the CDC to these states, and they operated with substantial involvement in assisting the state programs to plan and implement diabetes control activities. Essential to this new style of working with state partners was the requirement for accountability from both the CDC and its partners and the expectation that the CDC continue to be good stewards of public funds while collaborating continuously with the states in the implementation of the program. This platform provided the flexibility for incorporating strategically, the developing science of diabetes into program activities. It was co-learning environment that gave the CDC an opportunity to provide leadership in the development and implementation of public health strategies for reducing the burden of a chronic disease at several levels of public health practice. Diabetes was the first chronic disease program to use the cooperative agreement, and this funding mechanism and technical assistance approach became the model for chronic disease and other CDC programs that continue to this day.

In fiscal year 1981, supplemental funds were awarded to 8 of the 20 state projects to carry out short-term projects aimed at increasing knowledge about diabetes care and practice at the community level, appropriate evaluation methodologies, epidemiologic investigations, and strategies for translation and dissemination of diabetes knowledge and science (Berlin et al. 1986). In 1983, the NDAB released the National Standards for Diabetes Patient Education, developed in collaboration with the CDC, the AADE, the Diabetes Research and Training Centers, the International Diabetes Center, the Juvenile Diabetes Foundation, and the National Diabetes Information Clearinghouse. In promoting these standards, the NDAB noted the barriers to the widespread availability of preventive approaches to self-care, lack of patient and provider knowledge about diabetes, inadequate reimbursement policies, and lack of coordination among key components of the health care system. Evaluation of the pilot for this program also found that the recognition program could have a positive impact in fostering third-party reimbursement for ambulatory diabetes education programs (Centers for Disease Control 1981). In addition, the NDAB, NIH, and the CDC collaborated to develop and publish *The Prevention and Treatment of Five Complications of Diabetes: A Guide for Primary Care Practitioners,* which provided standards of care and gave support to the activities implemented by the State Diabetes Control Programs (Genuth 1994). During this period, interventions were designed to reduce diabetes-related complications through assurance of services or the improved availability of quality diabetes care and diabetes education services. These interventions were based on the provision of direct services with a focus on secondary and tertiary prevention, but this approach had a limited impact. The premise that education alone would lead to behavior change was unsubstantiated, and there were not enough resources to serve all of the population in need. The CDC program and many state projects were also involved in activities seeking third-party reimbursement in support of educational efforts. Their efforts were focused on reimbursement for diabetes education and were directed toward the three main third-party payers: Medicare, Medicaid, and Blue Cross and Blue Shield (Centers for Disease Control 1981). Insurance coverage for persons with diabetes eventually became an urgent issue.

The next several phases of the program were influenced by new science and technology (see Appendix 22.1), and by efforts to translate the best available knowledge into effective clinical and public health practice at the community level (Pomeroy et al. 1986; Center for Disease Control 1980; Narayan et al. 2000). The discovery of photocoagulation therapy in 1981, for example, underscored the need for early detection of eye disease and other complications of diabetes in order to prevent progression to more serious outcomes. The findings of the Early Treatment of Diabetic Retinopathy Study Research Group were published in 1991; this landmark study demonstrated the importance of regular dilated eye exams and of early detection and treatment of diabetic retinopathy. The State Diabetes Control Programs, for their part, began to communicate the benefits of annual eye exams to people with diabetes and to health care professionals (Javitt and Aiello 1996).

Building on partnerships at the state and local levels, efforts were made to reach underserved and uninsured populations and to track screened persons to ensure that they received recommended treatment (Murphy et al. 2004). For example the Harris County Hospital District in Houston, Texas, an intervention site of the state's Diabetes Control Program (Baker 1993), developed an interdisciplinary intervention for reducing the complications of diabetes and preventing premature mortality. This project was supported by a patient and professional education component and served a large, low-income, high-risk population in nine community health centers. The program established partnerships with the Baylor College of Medicine in Houston for the development of protocols for eye disease, while it worked with the Ben Taub Orthopedic Foot Clinic in developing protocols focused on lower-extremity complications.

Activities were also implemented for the development of protocols targeting the early detection, diagnosis, treatment, and management of hypertension and dyslipidemia and the detection, treatment, and control of type 1 and type 2 diabetes. A culturally sensitive curriculum for patients and self-study kits for providers were among the educational tools produced. In addition incentives were given to nurses who became diabetes educators. An evaluation showed positive results in screening, detection, and treatment of diabetes-related visual impairments, hypertension, and patient knowledge.

The Houston example was typical of most State Diabetes Control Program interventions during this period. The majority of implementation activities focused on five areas identified as contributing to excessive diabetes morbidity and mortality: inadequate patient education and self-care; inadequate knowledge and proficiency among health care providers; lack of third-party reimbursement for diabetes education in the ambulatory setting; inadequate planning, coordination, and evaluation of health services and resources for persons with diabetes; and lack of adequate data on morbidity and mortality. A Diabetes Program Handbook was developed by the CDC and distributed to program managers in 1983; it was a useful reference for organizing and operating a Diabetes Control Program based on the experience of the state programs to address the areas above (Pomeroy et al. 1986).

In 1982, in keeping with the recommendations of the NADB, the multicenter Diabetes Control and Complications Trial was initiated (The National Diabetes Advisory Board 1988). The purpose of this study was to compare the effects of conventional treatment and tight glycemic control on vascular complications in persons with type 1 diabetes. Also started during the latter part of this period was Project DIRECT, a community diabetes demonstration project in an African American population that was funded primarily by the CDC (www.cdc.gov/dm/projects). DIRECT stands for "Diabetes Intervention Reaching and Educating Communities Together." Designed to develop, implement, and evaluate strategies that could be incorporated into state-based diabetes prevention and control programs nationwide, DIRECT has developed and sustained partnerships with the community of Southeast Raleigh, North Carolina; the Division of Public Health in the North Carolina Department of Health and Human Services; Wake County (North Carolina) Human Services; and the CDC.

In 1988, the Translation Advisory Committee for the Diabetes Prevention and Control Programs (TAC) was established; the TAC met twice a year and advised the Director of the Division of Diabetes Translation on policies and strategies related to the achievement of program goals (CDC 2000). Based on the recommendations of the 1987 National Long Range Plan to Combat Diabetes, the CDC Diabetes Translation Center developed "Diabetes Today" (The National Diabetes Advisory Board 1988; CDC DM Projects 2008), a two-tiered training program for health professionals on how to plan and implement community-based programs for persons with diabetes. This 5-day training program began with health professionals who after completing the training would prepare and deliver a 2-day training course with community leaders for planning diabetes related activities at the community level. The basic tenets were empowerment, applied epidemiology, community organization and development, self-evaluation, and intervention development. The course was evaluated through case studies focused on the "Diabetes Today" interventions in five pilot states; "Diabetes Today" was found to be successful in organizing community members and increasing the awareness of community members about diabetes and its complications. This framework was used in developing interventions that ranged from community walking clubs to interventions involving managed care and work sites.

By the early 1990s there were 29 states and one territory with Diabetes Control Programs (Ring 1988). The pilots became programs with a growing emphasis on comprehensive, evidence-based public health approaches targeting specific complications of diabetes instead of the provision of direct service. Diabetes was firmly established as a serious public health problem (Vinicor 1994), and there was ongoing discussion about health reform and managed care. Health departments were moving away from direct services and more toward the three core functions of public health: assessment, assurance, and policy development (The Institute of Medicine 1988).

In summary, this phase of the national diabetes program was influenced by the growing concern for the burden of the disease in the population, the development of an adequate surveillance system for diabetes, policy initiatives, and the development of science and technology. The resources for implementing strategies at the community level were limited; even so, Diabetes Control Programs collaborated with state and national agencies to develop numerous consensus guidelines for preventing and treating the complications of diabetes, for patient education, and for reimbursement initiatives (Ring 1988). They were also able to establish local partnerships that laid the groundwork for building an infrastructure at the state level for diabetes control activities (Murphy 2004). Collectively, the Diabetes Control Programs were part of an information-gathering system to support program development for diabetes control and a model for the translation of science into public health practice and for chronic disease in general. In addition, they were developing a template for providing public health services to populations in need, through efforts to convene and work with disparate partners in the health delivery system; it was a good beginning.

■ The Emerging Science of Diabetes and Development of New Partnerships

In 1993 the NIH released the results of the Diabetes Control and Complications Trial (DCCT); the study found that good glycemic control reduced diabetic eye disease by 76%, kidney disease by 50%, and nerve damage by 60% (The Diabetes Control and Complications Trial Research Group 1993). In response to the study's findings, the national diabetes program moved from a complication-specific approach to a more integrated and coordinated systems-based approach to diabetes care. In addition, the program model became more oriented to community-level, systems-based interventions and less focused on direct clinical services. The results of the United Kingdom Prospective Diabetes Study (UKPDS) (UKPDS Group 1998) confirmed for type 2 diabetes many of the findings of the DCCT (for insulin-dependent diabetes) and that lowering blood pressure was as important as lowering glucose levels.

Economic Issues

The Lewin-VHI study, released in 1994, found that the total cost of health care in the United States for people with diabetes exceeded $105.2 billion in 1992. Costs per person with diabetes were estimated to be more than four times as great as for persons without diabetes. This study included the full range of costs, including hyperglycemia and comorbidities (Rubin et al. 1992). Dissemination of this information led to increased awareness among policy makers of the social and economic costs associated with diabetes and its complications.

As of July 1995 there were 40 state programs funded to continue work on developing infrastructure, expertise, and leadership at the state level, and two states, Michigan and Minnesota, were given additional funds to demonstrate a statewide model for Diabetes Control Programs. The overall program model focused on defining the burden, developing new approaches, implementing effective programs, and coordinating efforts with the health system. New approaches were expressed in giving information to the community, technical assistance, social action, and health systems approaches, including policy-based initiatives and legislative advocacy (Anderson et al. 1995).

The HMO Group

In 1996 the CDC (in collaboration with the HMO Group) held a meeting in Atlanta, Georgia, to bring together HMOs, CDC, and Diabetes Control Programs to discuss opportunities for collaboration at the local level. The keynote address was presented by the Speaker of the U.S. House of Representatives, Newt Gingrich of Georgia, who became a diabetes champion. This was a testimony to the work of the Diabetes Control Programs and diabetes advocates in raising the level of awareness about the social and economic burden of diabetes. Attendees included representatives from the states' Diabetes Control Programs, quality improvement organizations, health care professionals, and other health care providers with a specialty or an interest in diabetes education and care management. The components of change and specific collaborative opportunities in the areas of data systems, disease/case management, and outreach were identified and discussed. Here began the discussion around a new focus for public health practice for chronic diseases—from care delivery to the strategic influence of partners and stakeholders in the planning and delivery of services. The challenge to the national Diabetes Control Program was to develop a strategy to influence federal, state, and local partners to support efforts in control and prevention. During this meeting the Minnesota Diabetes Control Program presented Project IDEAL (Improving Diabetes Care through Empowerment, Active Collaboration, and Leadership), a population-based intervention and a model of collaboration between the Diabetes Control Program and managed care. It developed and implemented processes that facilitated improvements in diabetes care by identifying the need for changes within primary care clinics and then created a plan to make these changes happen. During the pilot stage of IDEAL, the frequency of eye exams, foot exams, and microalbumin testing increased substantially, and these results were replicated in the intervention phase. Within 2 years average hemoglobin A1C values for participants decreased from 9.2% to 7.7%. Four states formed a collaborative to work with HMOs in New England; the group's purpose was the collective sharing of information and strategies for marketing diabetes messages, promoting provider relations, and developing measures for defining success in the region.

The Latino Diabetes Initiative for Action

In 1995 the CDC convened the National Hispanic/Latino Expert Consultant Group to make recommendations on approaches to impact the burden of diabetes in Hispanic/Latino populations. This led to the creation of the National Hispanic/Latino Diabetes Initiative for Action (NH/LDIA). This Initiative outlined a framework of interdisciplinary, culturally relevant approaches to control diabetes and its complications in the U.S. Latino/Hispanic populations.

These recommendations led to the development of several ongoing projects and policies such as the U.S.–Mexico Border Project, the Community Health Worker Position Statement, and the publication of guidelines and culturally relevant and linguistically appropriate health promotion materials for Hispanic/Latino populations.

■ The Development of National Program Objectives

With additional funding in 1997, the program developed into the National Diabetes Program. In 1999 the program adopted a set of national program objectives, which supported those of *Healthy People 2010* (National Center for Health Statistics 1998):

- By 2004, demonstrate success in achieving an increase in persons with diabetes who receive foot exams, eye exams, vaccination, and A1C testing.
- By 2004, demonstrate progress in establishing linkages for the promotion of wellness, including physical activity for persons with diabetes.
- By 2004, demonstrate progress in reducing health disparities for high-risk populations with respect to diabetes prevention and control.

With more awareness of the economic cost of caring for persons with diabetes, coupled with the compelling science for preventing diabetes, the national program began a new focus on preventive care services. Substantial and compelling evidence indicated that the complications and disability associated with diabetes could be prevented or delayed in both type 1 and type 2 disease (The Diabetes Control and Complications Trial Research Group 1993; The UK Prospective Diabetes Study

[UKPDS] Group 1998). Thus the National Diabetes Program began to design, implement, and evaluate multidimensional and multidisciplinary approaches to population-based prevention and control.

■ The Model of Influence

The Model of Influence (Fig. 22.1) is a systems-based change model in which the Diabetes Control Programs engaged in activities to convene and collaborate with strategic partners in the state in order to reduce the medical and psychological, social, and economic burden of diabetes. Coordination and activation of the larger diabetes community, including advocating for policy and environmental changes, began to emerge.

The Model of Influence is operationalized through several capacity-building activities: (1) community interventions such as community mobilization training; (2) health communications (such as an influenza campaign); and (3) health systems change such as the implementation of the Chronic Care Model and the development and promulgation of statewide guidelines. Because some state programs do not have sufficient resources to implement all three efforts simultaneously, growth levels in these three areas were gradual. Resource limitations have necessitated the expansion of partnerships at the federal and national and local level, with the aim

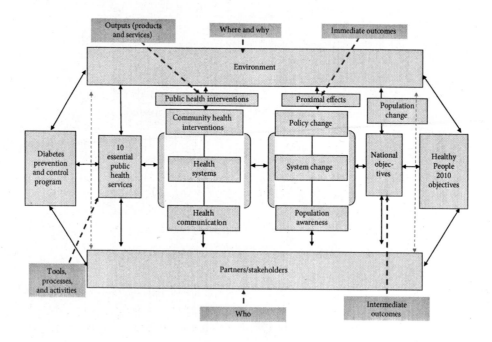

FIGURE 22.1. The Model of Influence. Division of Diabetes Translation

of achieving synergy across organizations and agencies in order to affect change in communities and health systems (Murphy et al. 2004).

Examples of the Model of Influence

Health Systems

The Washington State Diabete Control Program. In Washington State the Diabetes Control Program worked with various strategic partners to implement case management efforts focused on "redesigning" primary care to meet the needs of those with chronic diseases like diabetes. Efforts included: (1) establishment of a diabetes registry; (2) development of a diabetes Outcome Measurement Task Force and support for collaborative self-management via chronic care clinics; (3) conferences and lifestyle programs; and (4) statewide dissemination of evidence-based guidelines and protocols for optimum delivery of diabetes care.

Diabetes Management: Making the Business Case. In 1997 Washington Business Group on Health (WBGH) and the CDC joined forces to initiate a dialogue on diabetes management between the business community and public health. After a survey of the membership of 165 large private and public employers and with the help of a team of experts, WBGH and the CDC convened "Diabetes Management: Making the Business Case" (WBGH 1999). The result was that collaborations with local employers were implemented in State Diabetes Control Programs as part of their health systems approaches for reducing the burden of diabetes. Elsewhere the California Diabetes Control Program worked in partnership with the Pacific Business Group on Health to promote the establishment statewide guidelines, and the Michigan Program worked with General Motors to promote diabetes wellness programs.

The Diabetes Collaborative. During 1998 the Division of Diabetes Translation entered into a partnership with the Health Resources and Service Administration (HRSA) on the Diabetes Health Disparities Collaborative. This interagency, public-private partnership between the National Diabetes Control Program and HRSA's Bureau of Primary Health Care and the Institute for Health Care Improvement used proven quality improvement and care practices to improve the health care and health status of people with diabetes who use community health centers. The state Diabetes Control Programs provided technical assistance in performance measurement, professional education, and minigrants to support data entry and diabetes education support services.

An example of a health system change resulting from quality improvements is illustrated in the June 2007 issue of *Health Services Research*. A university-based team led by Elbert S. Huang reported on a relatively inexpensive effort to improve the process of care at 17 Midwestern Federally Qualified Health Centers that participated in the Diabetes Health Disparities Collaborative. Improved processes of care included regular testing for hemoglobin A1C, assessment of blood lipid levels, eye exams, and blood pressure checks with appropriate follow-up. Also included were preventive treatments such as using angiotensin-converting enzyme (ACE) inhibitors and aspirin. These improvements added very little expense. The program cost about $700 per patient the first year, $600 the second year, $500 the third, and leveled off at $378 annually beginning in year four. The clinics also implemented the Chronic Care Model, using a multidisciplinary team and employing electronic registries to track clinical outcomes with quarterly reporting to primary providers. Because of this frequent electronic reporting, health care providers became more focused on making adjustments in therapy, which led to improvements in A1C, lipids, and blood pressure within a relatively short time. Education in self-management and goal setting by individual patients was incorporated into each visit, and frequent "Plan, Do, Study, Act" cycles resulted in sustained improvements in care practices.

As a result of these initiatives the average 1-year reduction in A1C values for patients enrolled in the electronic registries was from >8% to 7.5%. At less than $500 per patient each year, this modest quality improvement effort can potentially reduce the incidence of major complications such as end-stage kidney disease, which can cost $44,000 per patient each year (Huang et al. 2007).

Community Interventions

"The Healthy Hair Starts with a Healthy Body". The "Healthy Hair Starts with a Healthy Body" is a salon-based campaign developed in Michigan to educate African American men and women about their diabetes and risk of kidney disease and to motivate preventive behaviors is another example of the community intervention component of the Model of Influence. The centerpiece of this salon intervention is the "health chat" offered by stylists. This motivational appeal highlights disease risk factors faced by African Americans and asks clients to take one or more steps: improve diet, increase exercise, stop smoking, or take medication and seek follow-up for their disease from a health care provider (Madigan, Smith-Wheelock, and Krein 2007).

The Appalachian Diabetes Today Project. Using the CDC *"Diabetes Today"* program as the planning translation model, the Appalachian Diabetes Prevention project works to enhance local leadership, develop policies, and create partnerships at the community level to address the burden of diabetes. This includes activities to assure collection of local data for the development of community-based efforts for reducing the burden of diabetes in the Appalachian region. Activities such as training and data collection are coordinated in the region, which follows the spine of the Appalachian Mountains and spans the 13 states; all of West Virginia and parts of Alabama, Georgia, Kentucky, Maryland, Mississippi, New York, North

Carolina, Ohio, Pennsylvania, South Carolina, Tennessee, and Virginia are currently involved with this project. The program collaborates with the Appalachian Regional Commission and the Center for Rural Health at Marshall University, West Virginia.

Health Communications

The Flu Campaign. The Division of Diabetes implemented a Flu Campaign in 1998 in collaboration with the National Immunization Program. This is an example of the Model of the Influence at work engaging public and private partners in an effort to improve vaccination rates among people with diabetes. Through a social marketing approach, this public service campaign encouraged people with diabetes to get influenza and pneumococcal vaccinations, and it promoted awareness that people with diabetes are at greater risk of dying from the flu or pneumonia. Over the past 10 years vaccination rates for people with diabetes have risen significantly. Since 1999 increasing the rates of influenza and pneumococcal vaccinations has remained a major focus of the State Diabetes Control Programs. Many programs now routinely achieve consensus among a variety of stakeholders to improve vaccination rates and to track improvements.

Other Examples: The CDC Native Diabetes Wellness Program

The Native Diabetes Wellness Program (Wellness Program) was established by CDC's Division of Diabetes Translation in 2004, replacing the National Diabetes Prevention Center. The Balanced Budget Act of 1997 Special Diabetes Program for the Indians Grant Program has provided one-third of the budget for the Wellness Program; the rest is provided by the Division of Diabetes Translation. The mission of this program is to work with a growing circle of partners to address the health inequities so starkly revealed by diabetes in Indian Country. With social justice and respect for Native and Western science as grounding principles, the Wellness Program strives to support community efforts to promote health and prevent type 2 diabetes.

The objectives are to: (1) support sustainable, evaluable ecological approaches to promote the use of traditional foods in American Indian and Alaska Native communities; (2) share messages through stories and art about survival and traditional ways of health that are remembered, retold, and talked about in homes, schools, and communities; (3) share and evaluate Native and Western science-based programs, including community outreach, talking circles, community-based interventions, and diabetes education in schools; and (4) support meaningful tribal consultation at state and federal levels. Tribal leaders guided the program to view traditional culture as a source of health, with a focus on youth. Accomplishments include developing and disseminating the award-winning "Eagle Books" series, and establishing cooperative agreements with tribes and tribal organizations for promoting environmental interventions to promote health and prevent diabetes. The Eagle Books are a series of four stories about wise animal characters who engage Rain That Dances, Simon, Little Hummingbird, and Thunder Cloud in the joy of physical activity, eating healthy foods, and learning from their elders about health and diabetes prevention.

In 2005 the Wellness Program awarded 3-year grants to eight tribes or tribal organizations. Interventions included policy changes that affected community members across multiple generations, including school-menu and vending-machine options, community-wide health promotion messages, and the extension of walking trails. A 5-year cooperative agreement (2009–2013) focusing on traditional foods and sustainable ecological approaches was awarded to 11 tribes or tribal organizations in 2008, and an additional six in 2009. The purpose of the program is to: (1) support community use of traditional foods and sustainable ecological approaches for diabetes prevention and health promotion in American Indian and Alaska Native communities; and (2) engage communities in identifying and sharing the stories of healthy traditional ways of eating, being active, and communicating health information and support for diabetes prevention and wellness (Wilson and Satterfield 2007).

The Essential Public Health Services

The identification and assessment of existing data on the incidence, prevalence, and complications of diabetes and on available health care resources were the first steps in developing a system-wide plan to coordinate and activate the larger diabetes community to increase access to care in all of the project states. This was achieved by first conducting an assessment of the Essential Public Health Services (EPHS) between 2004 and 2006 (Nelson et al. 2002). See Figure 22.2. This assessment sought to: (1) document the magnitude of diabetes problems in the state in order to set policy and priorities; (2) identify geographic areas and populations at risk of morbidity and mortality from complications of diabetes; (3) develop baseline data for further evaluation of program activities; (4) identify the need for epidemiologic or special studies to further define diabetes problems or provide information about appropriate strategies for interventions; (5) assess the availability and accessibility of resources needed to address identified problems; and (6) link this information with available health care resources to identify where program activities might be targeted.

Based on input from the states' advisory boards and analyses of the EPHS assessments, each state identified needs and problems related to access to care and the delivery of diabetes care and education. These local problems were rated according to their importance and amenability to intervention, and each state then developed implementation activities based on its particular identified need, resources, advisory board interests, and staff expertise and experience.

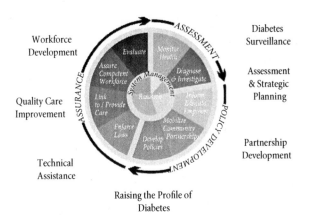

FIGURE 22.2. The ten essentials of public health. The National Public Health Performance Standard Program, 1994.

■ Diabetes Prevention and the Current Structure of the Diabetes Prevention and Control Programs

In 2002 the Diabetes Prevention Program (DPP) Study found that among persons with prediabetes, lifestyle changes, such as improvements in diet and engaging in daily physical activity, can prevent or delay the onset of type 2 diabetes. Participants who engaged in such lifestyle changes reduced their risk of developing diabetes by 58% (Bowman et al. 2003). The State Diabetes Control Programs were renamed the Diabetes Prevention and Control Programs (DPCP) to better reflect the dual-pronged approach of prevention and care. With this name change, primary prevention was added to the existing secondary and tertiary prevention efforts of the National Diabetes Program.

In 1997 in accordance with the Balanced Budget Act of 1997, Medicare benefits were expanded to include diabetes education effective February 2001 (http://aops-mas-iis.od.cdc.gov/Policy/Doc/policy475.htm). This significant change responded to the collaborative efforts of the members of national diabetes organizations, including the AADE and ADA, and their advocates. The DPCPs also played a major role in the education of policy makers that eventually resulted in the passing of state reimbursement for diabetes supplies and services, which was important in improving access and care for persons with diabetes. As part of a Medicare and Medicaid benefits improvement act, Congress added a medical nutrition therapy benefit for diabetes and renal disease effective January 2002. In 2007, 46 states and the District of Columbia had third-party reimbursement for diabetes education services and supplies.

In 2004 the National Diabetes Program had 59 State Diabetes Prevention and Control Programs; these programs have a solid presence in all 50 states, the District of Columbia, and eight U.S. jurisdictions. The DPCPs were organized as follows: 32 capacity-building programs that provide basic programmatic and surveillance functions with small-scale projects that are implemented in specific areas of the state, and 27 basic-implementation DPCPs with more elaborate infrastructure and staffing. Basic implementation programs have enhanced capacity in program surveillance, epidemiology, and evaluation.

Systems Dynamics Modeling

A major focus of the DPCPs is the development of strategic partners for achieving program goals. The progression from healthy to at-risk status, to disease, and ultimately death is not always understood or agreed on from a population perspective, and thus program planners for national efforts like the National Diabetes Prevention and Control Program need decision support tools to help them not only advise but also explain their preferred set of interventions to constituent groups, or potential partners. The systems modeling approach, a computer-based model of outcomes from various program interventions, improves our (and our partners') understanding of the "futures" that are likely to be generated by examining the impact of a range of alternative assumptions and interventions on the system. "System dynamics modeling shows why interventions to protect against chronic diseases have only gradual effects on prevalence. Simulation modeling enables planners and policy makers to explore for themselves the plausible short- and long-term consequences of historic trends and to compare the effects of alternative interventions before committing limited resources" (Milstein et al. 2007).

As emerging science revealed the cost-effectiveness of preventing diabetes, the National Diabetes Program embarked on new population-focused interventions. In 2004, CDC's Division of Diabetes Translation began exploring the issues associated with implementing diabetes prevention in the public health system. These issues include identifying methods for determining the prevalence of prediabetes among the general population, raising awareness among health care providers and high-risk populations about the risk factors associated with prediabetes, and determining which partnerships need to be formed to implement effective interventions.

The Diabetes Prevention Initiative

In 2005 the Diabetes Primary Prevention Initiative (DPPI) was established as a CDC-funded project; DPPI involves five state DPCPs, CDC staff, and contractors collaborating in three areas: interventions, surveillance, and systems modeling. The DPPI states (California, Massachusetts, Michigan, Minnesota, and Washington) (Ernst 2008) were charged with creating an action plan for federal, state, and local public health to significantly impact the incidence of type 2 diabetes via primary prevention. Approaches included exploration of data sources to identify people with prediabetes and an effort to engage them in preventive strategies in community settings. Surveillance activities included testing the sensitivity and specificity of several new Behavioral Risk Factor Surveillance Survey and HealthStyles questions to assess the awareness and estimated prevalence of prediabetes among U.S. adults. Interventions were focused on engaging at-risk populations in lifestyle behaviors aimed at reducing modifiable risk factors for type 2 diabetes.

Since the onset of the DPPI, five stakeholder groups representing health care systems, community organizations, businesses and employers, county and state policy makers, consumers, and special populations have become partners in the interventions. The five state DPCPs funded to work on the DPPI had existing relationships and previous experience working with these stakeholder groups for the promotion of clinical practice guidelines, work-site wellness, and policy development.

Since the implementation of the DPPI, the DPCPs have been successful in building capacity to address prediabetes within health systems or organizations and establishing new or strengthened partnerships among key stakeholders in the prevention of type 2 diabetes. The states involved in the DPPI were able to recruit and retain a range of partners, including other health department programs, hospitals, employers, health plans, and policy makers. Health systems interventions were implemented with a focus on awareness of prediabetes , screening activities, lifestyle interventions, and health policies related to prediabetes. Nonclinical interventions included the development of statewide screening and treatment guidelines and institutionalizing screening for prediabetes in detection, treatment, or other health promotion initiatives. The DPCPs were successful in increasing prediabetes detection and treatment awareness among health care providers, individuals at risk, and employers. In addition, peer support attained during group delivery of lifestyle education was found to have the potential for individual sustainment of behavior change related to healthy eating and daily physical activity.

In January 2006, the *New York Times* ran a series of articles on diabetes (Ubina 2006) describing the possible complications, lack of access to care, and how lifestyle-based interventions to control diabetes can result in positive outcomes.

Today, two-thirds of the state DPCPs collaborate with employers to improve the health of employees and to potentially reduce employees' health care costs by shifting the emphasis of benefits from acute care to prevention. By translating scientific evidence and providing guidance to employers, benefit language and policies were developed to implement a comprehensive preventive services program within the employers' medical plans. Employers now recognize that individuals who are in low-risk categories and who practice preventive behaviors have few medical claims in all categories and have less absenteeism (Campbell et al. 2006). Some wellness programs have also added incentives such as time off for physical activity, as well as provision for healthy-living classes at work. Insurance companies have responded to this trend. In the spring of 2007 WellPoint Inc., a large health insurer, began intensive promotion of preventive practices such as immunizations and diabetes-management tools to its insured members nationwide.

Between the mid-1990s and the present, the quality of diabetes care has improved substantially. Nationally gains have been identified in control of cholesterol and in regular exams of the eyes, feet, and teeth in persons with diabetes. Improvements have also been noted in the use of aspirin, influenza and pneumococcal vaccines, and in regular exams of the eyes, feet, and teeth in persons with diabetes. In addition, the number of people with diabetes who monitor their blood glucose has increased (Saaddine et al. 2006). The Diabetes Control Programs have contributed greatly to national improvements in the delivery and use of preventive care practices. All 59 programs strongly emphasize and influence improvements in the quality of diabetes care within their state health care system This includes the promotion of the use of evidenced-based standards of care and the Chronic Care Model for the delivery of care. Raising awareness among populations with or at risk for diabetes through the use of evidenced based materials from the National Diabetes Education Program has also complemented the efforts of the DPCPs in this area of concern.

The activities of CDC will continue to depend on the experiences, expertise, and commitment of state and territorial health departments. In 1977 widely disparate views existed among health professionals concerning standards of patient care and education, criteria for diagnosis, and optimal treatment and case management. This situation and the lack of an integrated provider system contributed to the problems of inadequate patient education and provider knowledge. A major accomplishment of the State DPCPs in the ensuing years has been the development of a network of public and private organizations concerned with the problems of diabetes. Many groups that previously worked in isolation, or who were once adversaries, have now formed a broad-based coalition mobilized toward the common goal—the reduction of the medical, social, and economic effects of diabetes. In their role as conveners of various diabetes-related partners and collaborators in the larger health delivery system, the state-based DPCPs have helped to bring about the implementation of a coordinated disease management approach to diabetes using the Chronic Care Model. This has proved to be effective in improving glycemic control and the delivery of preventive screenings for microvascular and macrovascular disease. Patient outcomes have been further improved by promoting education on self-management. In addition, the DPCPs have had great success in engaging and mobilizing communities to take action around diabetes. This action includes support for the building of community infrastructure for the sustainment of behavior change in the areas of physical activity, access to care, and education and self-efficacy. Collaboration with the nonfederal task force charged with developing the *Community Guide to Preventive Services* led to recommendations and supportive evidence for disease management in health care systems, self-management in the home for children with type 1 diabetes, and self-management education in community gathering places for adults with diabetes (Task Force on Community Preventive Services 2001). In 2006 several states surpassed the Healthy People objective for self-monitoring of glucose levels (Pan et al. 2007). Researchers found that the percentage of adults with diabetes who checked their blood glucose levels at least once a day increased by over 22% between 1997 and 2006.

Today, state DPCPs engage in the surveillance of clinical indicators of diabetes and the evaluation of interventions to improve the delivery of diabetes care within the state with a focus on facilitating the adoption of the six components of the Chronic Care Model by health systems: (1) effective self-management where patients have an active role in determining their care; (2) treatment decisions based on explicit, proven evidence-based guidelines; (3) an efficient care delivery system that incorporates standardized procedures and includes up-to-date patient information; (4) a clinical information system or registry that can track individual patient as well as populations of patients; (5) creation of environments in health care systems where quality improvement efforts flourish; and (6) developing alliances and partnerships with state community agencies, faith organizations, clubs, and businesses (Wagner 1998).

■ The Future

When the DPCPs were conceived, many felt that these programs would eventually become self-sustaining. However, because of the rapid growth in the risk factors for the development of this disease in the U.S. population and the emerging science for prevention of diabetes, there is now even greater need for continuing to support the CDC's efforts in directing this national program. There is widespread recognition that the interventions to correct root causes associated with increases in the prevalence of the disease lie outside of the clinical setting; therefore, the program will consider the social determinants of health and factors associated with them, in efforts to implement a program for the primary prevention of diabetes, as well as ongoing efforts for controlling the complications of the disease for persons with diabetes.

A clear vision, strong leadership, and strategic partners at the national and local levels have been instrumental in the growth and development of the program. This was driven and supported by a solid surveillance system, the science of diabetes, health system and policy interventions, and the collaboration of partners in the public, nonprofit, and private sectors.

As we move forward and incorporate primary prevention of diabetes into the CDC program model, there will be a need for resources to support translational research that identifies effective practices for delivering health services, for promoting healthy life style choices, and for evaluating our efforts in this area.

The integration of activities with other chronic disease programs that is now being executed will facilitate the sharing of experiences and tools, the implementation of multidisciplinary research, and the collaboration with nontraditional partners. This will help us to answer some of the hard questions about public health practice at the community level. There will be a need for more relevant training to assure a competent public health workforce armed with the knowledge and leadership skills to identify, develop, and maintain strategic partners for achieving program goals and to advocate for the development of policies that are more upstream and far-reaching in their ability to enhance healthy behaviors in populations of people.

Another major challenge for achieving success in reducing the burden of this disease is the implementation of culturally appropriate messages, interventions, and the assurance of access to effective services to vulnerable and underserved populations at risk for diabetes, or who already have the disease. Until we can achieve this, we will not reduce disparities, no matter how well designed our programs are or how capable we are of delivering quality clinical services. The lack of policies and systems that facilitate access and follow-up at all three levels of prevention, for all segments of the population, is a major challenge to public health for reducing disparities and the social and economic burden of this disease.

The Division of Diabetes completed a strategic planning process in 2008 and identified four aspirational, goals for the National Diabetes Program: (1) prevent diabetes; (2) prevent complications, disabilities, and burden associated with diabetes; (3) eliminate health disparities; and (4) maximize organizational capacity to achieve the National Diabetes Program goals. These goals and the 10 Essential Services of Public Health are the basis for the framework that will guide the national program, and the activities of the DPCPs over the next 5 years and beyond (see Fig. 22.3).

Finally, the DPCPs and the CDC cannot do this alone. Ongoing coordination and integration activities involving other federal agencies, and the public, private, and nongovernmental organizations at the national, state, and community levels are needed. Successful collaboration such as this would enable us to leverage scarce resources across a variety of sectors and to advocate for policies that support and facilitate the implementation of crosscutting activities with other programs that have similar goals—programs such as physical activity, nutrition, smoking and health, cardiovascular disease, arthritis, oral health, and others to reduce the burden of diabetes, its related comorbidities, and to improve the health and quality of life of the general public as well as people with and at risk for diabetes.

National Diabetes Program Framework

Essential Public Health Services (How)	Goals			
	1. Prevent diabetes.	2. Prevent complications, disabilities, and burden associated with diabetes.	3. Eliminate diabetes related health disparities.	4. Maximize organizational capability to achieve the NDP goals
1. Monitor health status				
2. Diagnose and investigate health problems				
3. Inform, educate and empower people				
4. Mobilize community partnerships and action				
5. Develop policies and plans				
6. Enforce laws and regulations				
7. Link people to needed personal health services				
8. Assure competent workforce.				
9. Evaluate effectiveness, accessibility, and quality				
10. Research for new insights and innovative solutions				

FIGURE 22.3. The National Diabetes Program framework

APPENDIX 22.1 *Response of the National Diabetes Prevention and Control Programs to Scientific Findings*

Phase	Scientific Finding	Context for Translation	Response	Intended Effects	Results
1	Education on diabetes management can lead to sustained changes in behavior.	No public health infrastructure for prevention of chronic disease.	Funds to build state program infrastructure; guidelines for educational interventions.	At local level, develop and maintain resources to implement effective diabetes control strategies in patient and professional education.	Development of 5 state programs and early partnerships for education.
2	Diabetic Retinopathy Study: Photocoagulation treatment can prevent blindness, and regular screening examination can identify persons in need of treatment.	Symptom-less disease; large disparities in access to insurance and care among high-risk groups.	Screening, referral, and follow-up services targeted to vulnerable uninsured persons.	Reduce morbidity and mortality by direct delivery of services to vulnerable uninsured persons.	Development of partnerships for service delivery with health professionals and community-based organizations.
3	Diabetes Control and Complications Trial: control of blood glucose can reduce eye, kidney, and foot disease.	National health care reform, changing role of public health from care delivery to influence.	Population-based intervention; system change through models of influence; national objectives for key preventive services.	Increase access to care by providing diabetes care in mainstream health care systems; reduce morbidity and mortality by changing environment, policy, and systems.	Establishment of 59 grant programs and of national objectives; identification of 3 methods of influence; development of partnerships for system, policy, and environmental change.

(continued)

APPENDIX 22.1 (*continued*)

Phase	Scientific Finding	Context for Translation	Response	Intended Effects	Results
4	Diabetes Prevention Program: Primary prevention works.	Reduced resources; varied levels of access to health care; racial and ethnic disparities in health care; Expansion of strategic partnerships.	Awareness messages and tools; pilot projects; system links to support lifestyle change.	Increase awareness; identify barriers and opportunities for translation at the community level.	Change of program name; development of public health model for primary prevention and translation of DPP to public health practice; pilots in 5 States.

Source: Adapted from Murphy D, et al. (2004). *Annals of Internal Medicine* **140**, 978–84.

■ References

Anderson L, Bruner LA, Satterfield D (1995). Diabetes control programs: new directions. *Diabetes Educator* **21**, 432–8

Baker SB et al. (1993). A diabetes control program in a public health care setting. *Public Health Reports* **108**, 596–604.

Berlin N et al. (1986). National standards for diabetes patient education programs: pilot study results and implementation plan: a report by the National Standards Steering Committee of the National Diabetes Advisory Board. *Diabetes Educator* **12**, 292–6.

Bowman BA et al. (2003).Translating the science of primary, secondary, and tertiary prevention to inform the public health response to diabetes. *Journal of Public Health Management and Practice* November (Suppl.), S8–14.

Campbell KP et al., eds. (2006). *A Purchaser's Guide to Clinical Preventive Services: Moving Science into Coverage.* Washington, DC: National Business Group on Health.

Centers for Disease Control (1978). *The Diabetes Control Demonstration Projects 1978: Assessment Summary Phase 1,* issued 1979. Atlanta, GA: Department of Health, Education, and Welfare.

Centers for Disease Control (1980). *The Diabetes Control Program: UPDATE 1980.***1**(1), 1–8. Atlanta, GA: U.S. Department of Health and Human Services.

Centers for Disease Control (1981). *The Diabetes Control Program: UPDATE December 1981.* **2**(3), 1–8. Atlanta, GA: U.S. Department of Health and Human Services.

Centers for Disease Control (1982). *The Diabetes Control Program: UPDATE 1982.* **3**(3–4), 1–12. Atlanta, GA: U.S. Department of Health and Human Services.

Centers for Disease Control and Prevention (1997a). Diabetes management: making the business case. Report of a consultation with Business and Health Leaders.

Centers for Disease Control and Prevention (1997b). Evaluation of "Diabetes Today" Course Effectiveness, Task 16, Westat Inc. Unpublished Report.

Diabetes Control and Complications Trial Research Group (1993). The effect of intensive treatment of diabetes on the development and progression of long-term complications in insulin-dependent diabetes mellitus. *New England Journal of Medicine* **329**, 777–86.

Division of Diabetes Translation, Centers for Disease Control and Prevention (2007). Historical review: CDC's Diabetes Program 1977–2007, DDT internal document. Atlanta, GA: U.S. Department of Health and Human Services, Centers for Disease Control and Prevention.

Drury TF, Harris MI, Lipsett LF (1981). Prevalence and management of diabetes. In: *Health US 1981,* pp 25–32. Hyattsville, MD: National Institutes of Health. DHHS Publication No. (PHS) 82-1232.

Ethridge EW (1992). *Sentinel for Health. A History of the Centers for Disease Control Program.* Berkeley: University of California.

Foege WH (1981). Centers for Disease Control. *Journal of Public Health Policy* **2**, 8–18.

Genuth SM (1994). The role of the National Diabetes Advisory Board in diabetes management. *Diabetes Care* **17**, 28–31.

Gu K, Cowie CC, Harris MI (1998). Mortality in adults with and without diabetes in a national cohort of the U.S. population, 1971–1993. *Diabetes Care* **21**, 1138–45.

Harris MI (1985). Ambulatory medical care for diabetes. In: National Diabetes Data Group, eds. *Diabetes in America*, 1st ed., chapter XXV, pp 1–13. Bethesda, MD: National Institutes of Health. NIH Publication No. 85–1468.

Healthy People—The Surgeon General's Report on Health Promotion and Disease Prevention (1979). Available at: http://profiles.nlm.nih.gov/NN/B/B/G/K/segments.html. Accessed October 30, 2008.

http://aops-mas-iis.od.cdc.gov/Policy/Doc/policy475.htm. Accessed May 10, 2007.

http://diabetes.niddk.nih.gov/dm/pubs/preventionprogram/index.htm.

Huang ES et al. (2007). The cost-effectiveness of improving diabetes care in U.S. federally qualified community health centers. *Health Services Research* **42**, 2174–93.

Institute of Medicine, Committee for the Study of the Future of Public Health, Division of Health Care Services (1988). *The Future of Public Health*. Washington, DC: National Academy Press.

Javitt JC, Aiello LP (1996). Cost-effectiveness of detecting and treating diabetic retinopathy. *Annals of Internal Medicine* **124**, 164–9.

Kanjilal S et al. (2006). Socioeconomic status and trends in disparities in 4 major risk factors for cardiovascular disease among US adults, 1971–2002. *Archives of Internal Medicine* **166**, 2348–55.

Kovar G, Harris MI, Hadden WC (1987). The scope of diabetes in the United States. *American Journal of Public Health* **77**, 1549–50.

Madigan ME, Smith-Wheelock L, Krein SL (2007). Healthy hair starts with a healthy body: hair stylists as lay health advisors to prevent chronic kidney disease. *Preventing Chronic Disease* **4** (3), A64.

Milstein B et al. (2007). Charting plausible futures for diabetes prevalence in the United States: a role for system dynamics simulation modeling. *Preventing Chronic Disease* **4** (3), A52. Available at http://www.cdc.gov/pcd/issues/2007/jul/07. Accessed December 30, 2008.

Murphy D, Chapel T, Clark C (2004). Moving diabetes care from science to practice: the evolution of the National Diabetes Prevention and Control Program. *Annals of Internal Medicine* **140**, 978–84.

Narayan KM et al. (2000).Translation research for chronic disease: the case of diabetes. *Diabetes Care* **23**, 1794–8.

National Center for Health Statistics (2010). Healthy people 2010 . Available at: www.cdc.gov/nchs/hphome. Accessed February 19, 2008.

National Diabetes Advisory Board (1988). *The National Long Range Plan to Combat Diabetes 1987*. Bethesda, MD: U.S. Department of Health and Human Services, NIH Publication No. 88-1587.

National Institutes of Health (2005). *Report of the National Institutes of Diabetes and Digestive and Kidney Diseases, Diabetes Centers 2005 Directors Meeting*. Bethesda, MD: National Institutes of Health.

Nelson JC et al. (2002). *The Public Health Competency Handbook: Optimizing Individual and Organizational Performance for Public Health.* Atlanta, GA: Center for Public Health Practice of the Rollins School of Public Health.

Pan L, Mukhtar Q, Geiss LS (2007). Self monitoring of blood glucose among adults with diabetes United States, 1997–2006. *MMWR Morbidity and Mortality Weekly Report* **56**, 1133–7.

Pomeroy S et al. (1986). Centers for Disease Control State—Based Diabetes Control Programs, pp 584–90. In: Davidson JK, ed. *Clinical Diabetes Mellitus: A Problem Centered Approach.* New York: Thieme, Inc.

Ring A (1988). Bridging the gap between research and practice: the CDC Translation Center. *Diabetes Spectrum* **1**, 147–52.

Rubin RJ, Alman WM, Mendelson DN (1992). 1994 Health care expenditures for people with diabetes mellitus. *Journal of Clinical Endocrinology and Metabolism* **78**, 809A–F.

Saaddine JB et al. (2006). Improvements in diabetes processes of care and intermediate outcomes: United States, 1988–2002. *Annals of Internal Medicine* **144**, 465–74.

Solber LI et al. (1997). Using continuous quality improvement to improve diabetes care in populations: the IDEAL model. Improving care for Diabetics through Empowerment Active collaboration and Leadership. *Joint Commission Journal on Quality Improvement* **23**, 581–92.

State Success Stories. Available at: www.chronicdisease.org. Accessed June 20, 2007.

Task Force on Community Preventive Services (2001). Strategies for reducing morbidity and mortality from diabetes through health-care system interventions and diabetes self-management in community settings. *MMWR Recommendations and Reports* **50** (RR16), 1–15.

Ubina I (2006). Rising Diabetes Threat Meets a Falling Budget and Cost and Effect (2006). *New York Times* May 2006.

UK Prospective Diabetes Study (UKPDS) Group (1998). Intensive good-glucose control with sulphonylureas or insulin compared with conventional treatment and risk of complications inpatients with type 2 diabetes (UKPDS33). *Lancet* **352**, 837–51.

U.S. Public Health Service. Office of the Surgeon General, DHEW(PHS) (1979). Publication No. 79-55071 Washington, DC: U.S. Public Health Service.

Vinicor F (1994). Is diabetes a public health disorder? *Diabetes Care* **17** (S1), 22–7.

Wagner EH et al. (2001). Improving chronic illness care translation; evidence into action. *Health Affairs* **20** (6), 64–78.

Wilson KM, Satterfield DW (2007). Where are we to be in these times? The place of chronic disease prevention in community health promotion. *Preventing Chronic Disease* **4** (3), A74. Available at: http://www.cdc.gov/pcd/issues/2007/jul/07. Accessed February 13, 2008.

www.cdc.gov/dm/projects. Accessed February 13, 2008.

23. NATIONAL DIABETES EDUCATION PROGRAM AND THE ROLE OF PARTNERSHIP IN THE PREVENTION AND MANAGEMENT OF DIABETES

Jane Kelly, Joanne M. Gallivan, and Charles M. Clark Jr.

■ Main Public Health Messages

- The National Diabetes Education Program (NDEP) translates research findings of major public health impact into practice by increasing awareness of diabetes and related research findings.
- NDEP involves public and private partners in improving treatment and outcomes for people with diabetes, promoting early diagnosis, and preventing or delaying the onset of diabetes.
- Since the inception of the NDEP in 1997, the program has grown in its partnerships, diversity of educational materials, support for community interventions, and outreach to populations suffering from disparities in health.
- NDEP has created three major outreach efforts, entitled "Control Your Diabetes. For Life," "Be Smart About Your Heart. Control the ABCs of Diabetes: A1C, Blood Pressure and Cholesterol," and "Small Steps. Big Rewards. Prevent Type 2 Diabetes." The first two campaigns were subsequently combined to emphasize the importance of comprehensive control of cardiovascular risk factors coupled with attention to blood pressure and lipids as well as glycemic control.
- Its partnership network has been essential to NDEP's success. These partners provide direction; identify gaps, challenges, and opportunities; participate in the development of appropriate health education materials; and provide trusted venues for outreach.
- Process measures indicate the broad reach of NDEP's media campaigns, and pilot testing confirms the accurate delivery of its health communications messages.

■ Introduction

Purpose

The National Diabetes Education Program (NDEP) was initiated in 1997; it was given the mission of translating the science of diabetes control and prevention into messages that would improve awareness of the disease and increase the potential to prevent both its complications and the disease itself. NDEP's overall purpose is to mobilize a critical mass of public and private sector organizations at the national, state, and community levels to improve treatment and outcomes for people with diabetes, promote early diagnosis, and prevent the onset of diabetes.

■ Background/Historical Perspective

NDEP was initially formed to translate the findings of the Diabetes Control and Complications Trial Research Group (DCCT 1993) into a health communications initiative; this landmark trial, sponsored by the National Institutes of Health (NIH), demonstrated that improved glycemic control reduces diabetes complications. Since that time, however, the program has become more comprehensive.

Sponsors

The Division of Diabetes Translation (DDT) of the Centers for Disease Control and Prevention (CDC) and the National Institute of Diabetes and Digestive and Kidney Diseases (NIDDK) of the NIH, part of USDHHS, jointly sponsor the NDEP with the participation of over 200 private and public partner organizations. This CDC/NIH partnership differs from other educational programs (e.g., blood pressure, cholesterol, asthma, eye) that are led solely by CDC or NIH. The NDEP joint initiative reflects each agency's unique contribution—NIH as a supporter of the basic research underlying campaigns and CDC's translational research with support for the dissemination of infrastructure through state programs and cooperative agreements with national minority organizations.

NDEP is the leading federal public education program in the promotion of diabetes prevention and control. NDEP began in 1997 with one message, that diabetes is serious, common, costly, but controllable. Similarly, NDEP began with one product—a video that introduced NDEP to potential partners. Over the decade since 1997 NDEP has developed more than 100 materials and tools, four Web sites, and one newsletter. Ten years after its inception, NDEP has built a Coordinating Committee of over 35 public and private partner organizations to advise it on its work and collaborate in strategic planning. NDEP is predicated on the concept of building an effective partnership network and implements its strategic plan through the activities of 10 Work Groups. The public and private organizations that comprise NDEP's 10 Work Groups include associations of health profession-als, health-related organizations, state Diabetes Prevention and Control Programs, and community-based consumer groups with trusted outreach to special popula-tions with diabetes. NDEP offers an opportunity for these diverse organizations to work together on health communications, wide dissemination of collaboratively developed NDEP messages, and continued partnership growth. The program's sponsorship by two major federal health organizations provides a firm basis of credibility, commitment, and resources as well as links to state and local public health agencies nationwide.

Need

Current scientific evidence demonstrates that much of the morbidity and mortality of diabetes can be prevented or delayed by comprehensive treatment with diet, exer-cise, and new pharmacological treatments directed toward normalization of blood glucose levels, blood pressure, and lipids. Further, research now shows that type 2 diabetes can be prevented or delayed in people with prediabetes through modest weight loss and regular physical activity. In 2007, according to the CDC National Diabetes Fact Sheet: 2007, an estimated 57 million Americans had prediabetes and thus were at high risk for the disease.

Unfortunately, a wide gap still exists between current and desired diabetes care (Saaddine 2002), even though the disease is one of the leading causes of death and disability in the United States—affecting an estimated 23.6 million Americans in 2007, including almost 6 million who had not been diagnosed (CDC 2008).

Goals and Objectives

The goal of the NDEP is to reduce the illness and death associated with diabetes and its complications through five principal objectives:

1. To increase awareness of the seriousness of diabetes, its risk factors, and strategies for preventing diabetes and its complications among high-risk groups.
2. To improve understanding about diabetes and its control and to promote better self-management behaviors among people with diabetes.
3. To improve health care providers' understanding of diabetes and its control and to promote an integrated approach to care.
4. To promote health care policies that improve the quality of diabetes care and access to such care.
5. To reduce disparities in health in racial and ethnic populations disproportionately affected by diabetes.

The program's goals and objectives support a major federal government public health initiative, *Healthy People 2010*, which has established health objectives for reducing the burden of diabetes in the first decade of the 21st century.

Organizational Structure

NDEP's organizational structure consists of a Coordinating Committee composed of approximately 35 representatives of mostly nongovernmental organizations that determines overall program direction, an Operations Committee composed of the chairs and vice chairs of all NDEP work groups, an Executive Committee (composed of CDC and NIH leadership plus three nonfederal representatives), and multiple special-populations work groups (see Fig. 23.1). The NDEP Executive Committee Chair is appointed by NIH and CDC and is selected for leadership ability, in-depth understanding of diabetes science, commitment to the participatory collaborative process, and broad appreciation of the issues in diabetes control and prevention at multiple levels. The NDEP Operations Committee Chair is selected

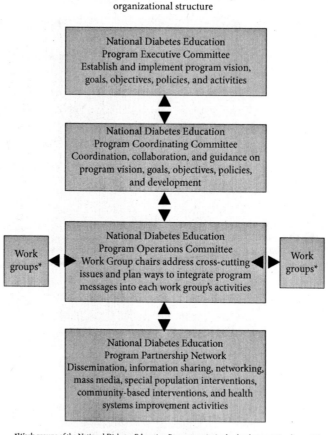

*Work groups of the National Diabetes Education Program assist in the development, implementation, and/or evaluation of specific program components.

FIGURE 23.1. NDEP organizational structure

from among existing work group chairs and vice chairs to represent them as a group at the Executive Committee.

The Coordinating Committee provides coordination, collaboration, and guidance on the program's vision, goals, objectives, policies, and overall product development. In addition, Coordinating Committee members promote the NDEP and share information about NDEP materials, messages, and activities with their own organizations' staffs and memberships.

The Executive Committee oversees the development of the NDEP strategic plan. CDC and NIH are the federal agencies on this committee and have fiduciary responsibility for all NDEP appointments and expenditures. The final responsibility for fund allocation remains with these federal agencies. Financial and staff resources from each agency are used to determine program activities.

The goals of the Operations Committee are to address cross-cutting issues related to NDEP activities and to implement the NDEP strategic plan.

NDEP Work Groups

Individual NDEP work groups have been developed to address the needs of special populations, to help NDEP understand how to reach health professional and business audiences, and to help translate diabetes messages for specific consumer and health professional entitles. Some NDEP work groups were brought together for a specific task (e.g., to create the *Team Care* document) and then dissolved; others are ongoing. At this writing (2009) there are 10 NDEP work groups:

- African American/African Ancestry
- American Indian/Alaska Native
- Asian American/Pacific Islander
- Business Health Strategy
- Children and Adolescents
- Evaluation
- Health Care Professionals
- Hispanic/Latino
- Older Adults
- Pharmacy, Podiatry, Optometry, and Dental (PPOD) Professionals.

NDEP conducts extensive formative research in planning a campaign and tailoring materials. By examining what has worked in other health communications programs and through discussion of the results of NDEP's focus groups with work group member organizations, NDEP tailors campaigns and messages to develop targeted educational materials. All NDEP materials are pretested to ensure the messages are appropriate and that qualitative data from focus groups inform the development of new tools for community interventions.

Epidemiology and Clinical Trials

NDEP is grounded in science developed through clinical trials and epidemiologic research. These findings are presented elsewhere in this volume.

■ Public Health Preventive Intervention Strategies

Program Strategies

Five strategies guide the NDEP's information and education activities:

1. Develop and implement ongoing diabetes awareness and education activities.
2. Identify, develop, and disseminate educational tools and resources for people with diabetes and those at risk, including materials that address the needs of special populations.
3. Disseminate guiding principles that promote quality diabetes care.
4. Promote policies and activities to improve the quality of diabetes care and access to such care.
5. Create program partnerships with other organizations concerned about diabetes and the health status of their constituents.

NDEP's Main Campaigns and Key Messages

NDEP's main campaigns are based on the broad dissemination to its target audiences of major scientific findings in diabetes and their implications. The *Control Your Diabetes. For Life* campaign, NDEP's first campaign, focused on communicating the message of the importance of glycemic control. As new science demonstrated the key role of blood pressure and lipid control, and in recognition that heart disease accounts for two-thirds of diabetes deaths, a new NDEP campaign (*Be Smart About Your Heart, Control the ABCs of Diabetes: A1C, Blood Pressure and Cholesterol*) was developed with a focus on cardiovascular disease (CVD). The original *Control* and *Be Smart* campaigns have since been merged into one comprehensive approach (see Fig. 23.2). NDEP now has two major campaigns:

- *Control Your Diabetes. For Life.* The campaign focuses on educating people with diabetes about the importance of controlling their diabetes to avoid or delay its serious complications, including heart disease, stroke, blindness, nerve damage, kidney disease, and lower-limb amputations.
- *Small Steps, Big Rewards. Prevent Type 2 Diabetes.* The key message for the *Small Steps* campaign is based on the findings of the Diabetes Prevention Program (Knowler et al. 2002): People at high risk for diabetes can prevent or delay onset of the disease by losing 5%–7% of their body weight through

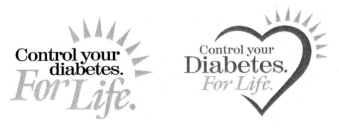

FIGURE 23.2. Original and revised NDEP control logo messages

modest lifestyle changes such as making lower-fat/-calorie food choices and engaging in 30 minutes of moderate-intensity physical activity at least 5 days a week. The campaign is targeted at delaying or preventing the onset of type 2 diabetes in adults at increased risk.

Both campaigns have components that integrate NDEP's five major objectives with outreach using the program strategies described above, some involving cross-collaboration among work groups. Direct-to-consumer diabetes control materials are consistently among the most frequently requested NDEP materials, along with a few select primary prevention materials for those at risk. These materials were developed and undergo continuous revision through the coordination of review feedback from the diverse organizations represented in NDEP work groups to incorporate advances in thinking within medical and behavioral science, ensure cultural appropriateness where pertinent, and improve readability by using clear language.

By involving partners from the earliest stages of campaign and educational product development, all five strategies are employed to reach NDEP goals. The participatory process enhances partnership. Broad expertise is harnessed through the NDEP Partnership Network to develop general and targeted diabetes awareness tools and activities. Dissemination and implementation opportunities are maximized through outreach by these partner organizations, which are trusted sources for NDEP target audiences (community members, health care professionals, employers, and policy makers). NDEP provides a forum to foster consensus for guiding principles in diabetes care among the major health care professional and diabetes organizations in the United States. Policy in changing health care systems, access to health care, and the provision by health plans of diabetes supplies and services are influenced by NDEP's Web sites www.BetterDiabetesCare.nih.gov and www.DiabetesAtWork.org. Other examples of integration by NDEP of the major objectives using these strategies include:

- NDEP booklet *4 Steps to Control Your Diabetes. For Life*—A popular general educational product for people with diabetes, *4 Steps* was developed and is continually revised with input from the NDEP Health Care Professional and PPOD work groups and reviewed by other work groups for tailoring its messages. The Hispanic/Latino and Asian American/Pacific Islander work groups have developed translations into Spanish and 15 Asian or Pacific

Islander languages. The Children and Adolescents Work Group developed a series of tip sheets for children and later for teens in English and Spanish, presenting much of the information from *4 Steps* in a format more appealing to youth. The principles from *4 Steps* were also brought into the *Power to Control Diabetes Is in Your Hands* materials created by the Older Adults Work Group to focus on diabetes control and Medicare benefits.

- Some very innovative approaches have evolved through NDEP's commitment to a participatory process with community-based organizations. NDEP Hispanic/Latino Work Group member organization National Latina Health Network uses *teatros*, an improvisational community theater approach, to communicate NDEP messages to various audiences. The NDEP African American/African Ancestry Work Group uses the NDEP music CD/DVD *Step By Step* (*New Beginning*) in its faith-based outreach working with parish nurses, and it works with NDEP partners (e.g., National Coalition of Pastors' Spouses and National Urban League) to encourage physical activity in people with diabetes and those at risk.

- Partners enhance NDEP's reach in the use of local media and by incorporating NDEP into existing initiatives. The American Indian/Alaska Native Work Group developed billboards based on the NDEP *Small Steps, Big Rewards. Prevent Type 2 Diabetes* campaign for use in rural areas with a large proportion of Native Americans. Black Women's Health Imperative adapted NDEP's *Power to Prevent: A Family Lifestyle Approach to Diabetes Prevention* for use in its all-women health promotion program. The Department of Health for the Country of Mexico, a member of the NDEP Hispanic/Latino work group, uses NDEP product *Movimiento Por Su Vida* in training *promotores de salud* (community health workers) and in collaboration with the U.S./Mexico Border Project in diabetes interventions.

- In June 2008, the PPOD Professionals Work Group released a series of podcasts (accessible at www.cdc.gov/podcasts) that address guiding principles of team care, raise awareness of the seriousness of diabetes and the action steps needed for preventing complications, and promote better self-management by addressing the diabetes ABCs (A1C, blood pressure, and cholesterol) to both health care professionals and people with diabetes. Two of these podcasts (*Preventing Vision Loss* and *Living with Vision Loss and Diabetes*) represent further partnership collaborative efforts via recorded interviews with the National Federation of the Blind.

Target Audiences

NDEP's target audiences are the following groups:

- People with diabetes and their families, with special attention to Hispanics/Latinos, African Americans, Asian Americans, Pacific Islanders, American Indians, Alaska Natives, children with diabetes, and older adults.

- People at increased risk for type 2 diabetes, especially those with prediabetes, ethnic populations at high risk, older adults, and women who have experienced gestational diabetes.
- Health care professionals, with an emphasis on outreach to all members of the health care team.
- Health care payers, purchasers, and policy makers.

NDEP's Key Components

NDEP's comprehensive approach is built on five key components:

- Awareness campaign—NDEP's major health communications campaigns seek to raise awareness and rely on other components to provide support for the action steps promoted.
- Special populations—NDEP seeks to address the needs of special populations such as racial and ethnic minorities and those with special concerns (e.g., children with diabetes).
- Community interventions—NDEP develops tools for use in community interventions and supports partner organizations in implementing programs in diabetes prevention and control.
- Health systems—A major focus of the NDEP Health Care Professional Work Group is health systems change, and tools for implementing change are provided through the NDEP-sponsored Web site www.betterdiabetescare. nih.gov.
- Partnership network—Considered the keystone for NDEP's effectiveness, the partnership network consists not only of the organizations collaborating with NDEP on work groups but also of all the organizations and volunteers who use NDEP materials in programs and individual efforts in diabetes prevention and control.

Figure 23.3 illustrates the NDEP logic model depicting these goals, objectives, audiences, campaigns, strategies, and key components.

Results/Accomplishments

NDEP's broad reach can be seen in the process measures described below.

Web Site Communications

The reach of NDEP's public education campaigns has been extensive, resulting in news stories that have reached more than 1 billion readers and more than 3.1 million publications distributed via the National Diabetes Information Clearinghouse. Limited numbers of all NDEP materials are free, may be ordered or downloaded from the NDEP Web site, and may be reproduced or reprinted at no cost, furthering

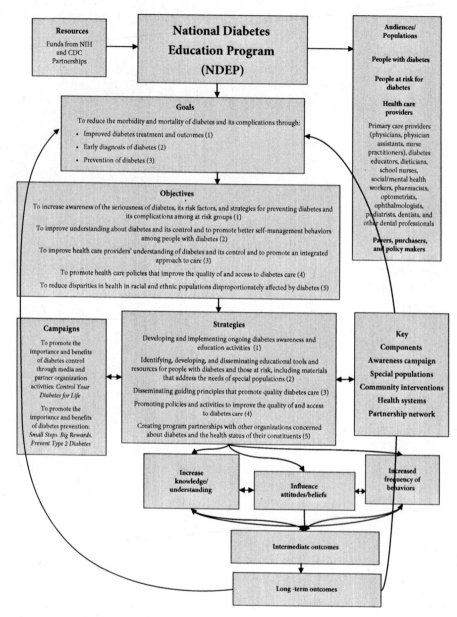

FIGURE 23.3. NDEP logic model

the effective distribution of the educational products and health promotion materials to NDEP audiences.

In 2007 the total number of visits to www.ndep.nih.gov increased by 14%, a total of more than 2.7 million visits. In 2007 the total number of visits to the *BetterDiabetesCare.nih.gov* Web site increased by 11%, from over 126,000 to over 140,000. The total number of visits to the *Diabetesatwork.org* Web site was over 23,000 in 2007. NDEP continues to work on developing marketing strategies to promote the availability of these resources to employers, health care professionals, and health care systems managers.

Media Communications

NDEP considers media—newspapers, magazines, television, radio, and the Internet—critical to awareness efforts. Articles in mainstream publications such as *Parade* magazine and *Fitness*, as well as journals for health care professionals, feature NDEP as a key educational resource. NDEP-sponsored radio media tours (RMT) in 2007 that addressed specific listener audiences are estimated to have reached more than 10 million listeners through national airings on Black Radio Network, CNN Radio Noticias, Metro Source, Metro Source Español, Radio Lazer, SRN News, and USA Radio Network. In May 2007 NDEP conducted a "Diabetes Education in Older Adults" RMT that reached an estimated 13 million listeners. National airings included Metro Source and American Urban Radio Network. Airings also included the Missouri statewide network, the number one news-talk station in San Francisco–Oakland–San Jose, California, and the number one news station in the Washington, DC, area.

NDEP has developed television and radio public service announcements (PSAs) for several different audiences (including older adults and ethnic minorities that are disproportionately affected by diabetes) as well as live-read radio PSA scripts that are available for downloading on the NDEP Web site. NDEP partner organizations further NDEP's reach by using these PSAs as is or by tailoring them using local public figures as voices.

Overall, NDEP media outreach process measures (see Fig. 23.4) estimate:

- News stories reaching more than 1 billion readers.
- Television and radio PSAs valued at more than $30 million.
- Print PSAs reaching more than 53 million readers.

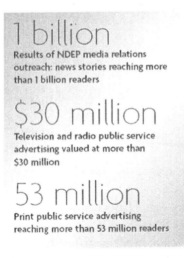

FIGURE 23.4. NDEP media outreach

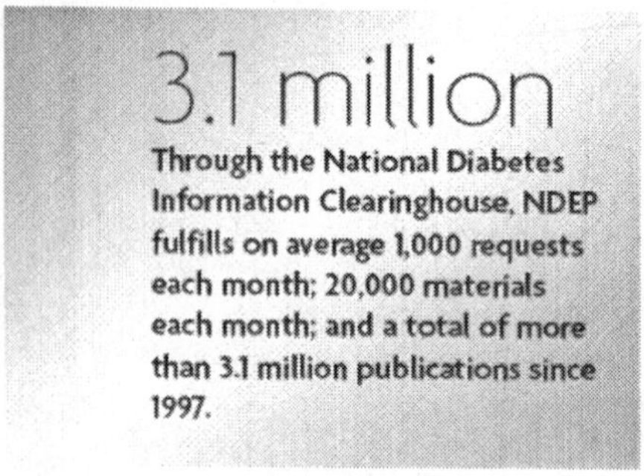

3.1 million

Through the National Diabetes Information Clearinghouse, NDEP fulfills on average 1,000 requests each month; 20,000 materials each month; and a total of more than 3.1 million publications since 1997.

FIGURE 23.5. NDEP dissemination of educational materials

NDEP Publications

The NDEP develops publications for a broad array of audiences, including people with diabetes and their family members, health care professionals, people at risk for diabetes, school personnel, parents of children with diabetes, community organizations and leaders, business leaders, and policy makers in the health care system. More than 3.1 million publications have been distributed (see Fig. 23.5). Partner organizations reprint NDEP products; all are copyright-free and may be reproduced without permission.

Outreach to Diverse Populations

NDEP special population work groups collaborate with NDEP to tailor messages and develop culturally and linguistically appropriate patient education materials for high-risk populations. NDEP conducts formative research to identify knowledge, attitudes, and self-reported behaviors as well as perception of diabetes risk and self-efficacy. All NDEP materials are pretested with target audiences. NDEP has adapted materials for all campaigns for a wide diversity of audiences. For example, the NDEP work groups adapted the primary prevention message to appeal to specific high-risk audiences, resulting in a general audience campaign (*Get Real*) as well as tailored educational materials:

1. *More Than 50 Ways to Prevent Diabetes* (African American).
2. *We Have the Power to Prevent Diabetes* (American Indian/Alaska Native).
3. *Two Reasons to Prevent Diabetes: My Future and Theirs* (Asian/Pacific Islander).
4. *It's Not Too Late to Prevent Diabetes. Take Your First Step Today* (Older Adults).
5. *Prevengamos La Diabetes Tipo 2 Paso a Paso* (Let's Prevent Type 2 Diabetes Step by Step) (Hispanic/Latino).
6. *It's Never Too Early to Prevent Diabetes* (women who have had gestational diabetes mellitus).

Health Disparities

NDEP supports reduction of health disparities among diverse populations by funding six to eight national organizations through cooperative agreements in 3- to 5-year cycles to provide outreach to high-risk, ethnically diverse populations using NDEP materials and community interventions. In the most recent funding cycle (2005–2010) over 60 applications were examined in an objective panel review, with eight organizations eventually selected. NDEP provides a total of $3 million per year in funding support for this 5-year project period through cooperative agreements with the following eight national organizations:

- Association of American Indian Physicians
- Black Women's Health Imperative
- Khmer Health Advocates
- Latina Health Network
- National Alliance for Hispanic Health
- National Association of School Nurses
- National Medical Association
- Papa Ola Lokahi (serving Native Hawaiian and Pacific Islanders)

Activities of the Black Women's Health Imperative and National Latina Health Network using NDEP materials were mentioned earlier in this chapter. Examples of activities involving two other organizations in the list above, Association of American Indian Physicians (AAIP) and Papa Ola Lokahi, are as follows:

- The AAIP supported implementation of a kit called *Move It! And Reduce Your Risk of Diabetes*, which is designed for creating physical activity programs in school settings. By offering *Move It* minigrants to schools with a high proportion of American Indians/Alaska Natives, AAIP supported the development of programs that have been sustained beyond the initial funding.
- During outreach activities in Hawaii and the Pacific Island territories, Papa Ola Lokahi conducted focus groups, adapted NDEP materials, and offered technical assistance to diabetes prevention and control programs as well as community groups on use of the materials in health communications and community interventions. The Pacific Diabetes Education Program is a trusted source of adapted and translated NDEP materials for Native Hawaiians and Pacific Islanders.

A description of each of these organizations' collaborative plans with NDEP can be found at www.cdc.gov/diabetes/ndep.

Data and Trends on Impact/Evaluation

NDEP's evaluation efforts are guided by the CDC's Framework for Program Evaluation in Health. NDEP's overall logic model (see Fig. 23.3) guides steps and outcomes measures, and several NDEP work groups have developed individual logic models to focus their work. For reasons of time and resource constraints, NDEP uses independent national and regional surveys such as NHANES (National Health and Nutrition Examination Survey), BRFSS (Behavioral Risk Factor Surveillance System), Roper, and others to guide the program on the state of the nation's knowledge, attitudes, and behaviors. The American surveys provide the core data. NDEP partners, including the American Diabetes Association, American Academy of Nurse Practitioners, and American Association of Diabetes Educators, have shared results of public, health care professional, and member surveys. Federal agencies, including the Veterans Administration, and the TRIAD (Translating Research into Action for Diabetes) program track health data and have shared results through published data.

It is difficult to measure the impact of NDEP's campaign messages and materials that is independent of the effect of other educational efforts delivered to the public or to patients through their health care providers. NDEP tracks process measures to identify the reach of public service advertising, media relations, and the number of materials downloaded or ordered. NDEP carefully pretests materials to assess their potential effectiveness and works closely with partners to monitor the impact of materials when they are put to use. This section highlights some findings from these national and regional datasets and will then move to a discussion of NDEP-specific surveys.

Federal and Partner-Conducted Surveys

Various national surveys give conflicting results on the fraction of the population that is aware of hemoglobin A1C. Certainly any changes in awareness cannot be attributed solely to NDEP, but it is useful to understand the baseline awareness in recent years. The first NDEP campaign, *Control Your Diabetes. For Life,* launched in 1998, focused on the importance of glycemic control and knowing one's A1C value. According to the BRFSS, a random-digit telephone survey, the percentage of people with diabetes who had heard of the A1C test was 26% in 1997, 28% in 1998, and 30% in 1999 (BRFSS 1997, 1998, 1999). According to the ADA-sponsored Roper Global Diabetes Program, U.S. Diabetes Patient Market Survey, the proportion of people with diabetes who had heard of the hemoglobin A1C test or HbA1C (now referred to as A1C) increased from 31% in 1998 to 50% in 2000 and 60% in 2004, providing evidence for a possible impact of the *Control Your Diabetes* campaign in increasing awareness of the A1C test (see Fig. 23.6) (ADA Roper ASW Survey 2007).

The NDEP *Be Smart about Your Heart: Know the ABCs of Diabetes* emphasizes the importance of knowing one's A1C number as well as the importance of blood pressure and cholesterol control. According to the Roper Global Diabetes Program, U.S. Diabetes Patient Market Survey, the proportion of people with diabetes who have had an A1C test within the past 12 months has increased, but not dramatically

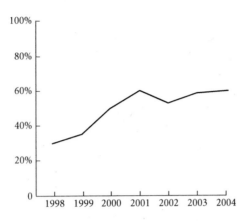

FIGURE 23.6. Knowledge of A1C testing among people with diabetes (answered "yes" to question "Prior to today, have you ever heard of Hemoglobin A1C or HbA1C test?")

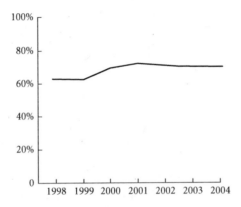

FIGURE 23.7. Percentage of people with diabetes who have had an A1C test in the past year, 1998–2004 (answered "yes" to the question "In the past 12 months, have you had an HbA1C test?")

(see Fig. 23.7) (Roper Global Diabetes Program, U.S. Diabetes Patient Market Survey 2007).

Among health care professionals there has also been an increasing awareness of the importance of comprehensive care of diabetes. This includes an increase in awareness of the "ABCs" message (see Fig. 23.8) (ADA Physician Study 2002, 2005; American Association of Nurse Practitioners Survey 2005).

NDEP-Conducted Surveys

NDEP collects feedback during pilot testing and evaluates the impact of specific NDEP products through a variety of means such as Web-based continuing education programs and partner-supported community interventions using NDEP products. NDEP also conducts a biannual Partner Survey to gather information from

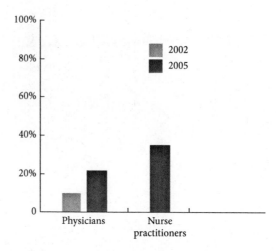

FIGURE 23.8. Percentage of health care professionals who have heard of the "ABCs of Diabetes," 2002 and 2005 (answered "yes" to the question "Are you familiar with the 'ABCs of Diabetes'?")

partners on their activities using NDEP materials and campaigns, including any evaluation data obtained.

In March 2006 NDEP conducted its first "Survey of Public Attitudes, Knowledge and Practices Related to Diabetes" (NDEP 2007), whose purpose was to provide insight into areas of motivation for target audiences as well as the public's perception of risk, knowledge, attitudes, and practices related to NDEP's goals and objectives. Although awareness of the seriousness of diabetes has increased, only modest changes in health outcomes have occurred. The results of the first NDEP survey served as a baseline to assess change in knowledge, attitudes, and behaviors. The NDEP survey, repeated in 2008, confirmed the findings from the 2006 survey. Most notably, having a family history of diabetes continues to be the most identifiable risk factor for developing type 2 diabetes in all populations and NDEP has revised its prevention materials to emphasize this risk factor.

A national random-digit telephone survey of people over 45, the NDEP survey included a total of 1763 people, including:

- People with diabetes (374)
- People with prediabetes (181)
- People at high risk for diabetes (730)
- Others (478)

The survey over-sampled African Americans (397) and Hispanics (498). Data were collected by computer-assisted telephone interviews lasting 15 minutes that were conducted in English or Spanish. Participants reflected the larger population—16% had diabetes, and more than 50% had been told that they had prediabetes or were at high risk of developing diabetes based principally on their weight and age (Box 23.1).

> **BOX 23.1   *Terms Used to Express Diabetes Risk***
>
> - A *person with diabetes* is defined as one who answers "Yes" to the following question: "[Other than during pregnancy,] has a doctor or other health professional ever told you that you have diabetes or sugar diabetes?"
> - A *person with prediabetes* is defined as one who answers "Yes" to one or more of the following: "Have you ever been told by a doctor or other health professional that you have: Prediabetes? Impaired fasting glucose? Impaired glucose tolerance? Borderline diabetes? Or high blood sugar?"
> - A *person at high risk for diabetes* is defined as one who, by self-reported height and weight, has a body mass index (BMI) of 25 or greater and/or has been told by a doctor or other health professional that he or she is at high risk for diabetes and/or has ever been told by a health care provider that she had gestational diabetes or high blood sugar during pregnancy.

General public awareness of the seriousness of diabetes rose from just 8% in 1998 (as reported by the Roper Starch Survey performed for the ADA) to 89% in 2006 according to the NDEP survey. In 2006 45% of the population had heard of the term "prediabetes," including 41% of men and 48% of women. African Americans (31%) and Hispanics (31%) were less likely than whites to have heard of prediabetes (50%).

The 2006 NDEP survey also examined perception of risk relative to the prevention of diabetes and revealed multiple gaps in knowledge. Reasons given for feeling at risk for diabetes included having a family history of diabetes (60%), being overweight (22%), and having poor dietary habits (13%). Fewer than 5% of participants gave their age as a reason for feeling at risk, and fewer than 1% gave their race or ethnic background as a reason. Although the low rates of perceived risk for many established risk factors are troubling, the strong link in the public mind between risk for diabetes and family history represents an opportunity for health communication. Of people identified in the survey as at high risk for diabetes, 54% of those with a family history of diabetes (defined as mother, father, brother, or sister having the disease) reported feeling at risk for diabetes, compared with 16% of those with no family history. As part of an ongoing process, NDEP is reviewing its many primary prevention materials for possible revisions in view of these findings about perceived risk. Repeating this survey, and completing it with qualitative research to help understand its messages and outreach strategies, is a key priority for NDEP's evaluation. NDEP uses survey information such as this to tailor efforts in health communications directed to health care professionals and the development of tools to facilitate health care professionals' communications with patients.

Partnership Building

NDEP partner organizations collaborate to develop educational materials that are culturally and linguistically appropriate but also to create consensus around critical issues. For example the NDEP Children and Adolescents with Diabetes Work Group brought together key stakeholders in developing the NDEP product *Helping the Student with Diabetes Succeed at School: A Guide for School Personnel* (also known as the NDEP *School Guide*). This document helps to promote safety and equal educational opportunities for students with diabetes. By providing recommendations regarding a team approach that involves school personnel, health care professionals, the child, and his or her family, the NDEP *School Guide* seeks to eliminate discrimination in the school on the basis of diabetes. The opportunity for collaboration via the NDEP work group was critical for bringing together diverse partner organizations to endorse the NDEP *School Guide*, such as the American Academy of Pediatrics, AADE, ADA, American Medical Association, Juvenile Diabetes Research Foundation International, National Association of Elementary School Principals, National Association of Secondary School Principals, National Association of School Nurses, and U.S. Department of Education.

Partnership is at the center of NDEP's success. Partnership between NDEP and the ADA fostered collaboration and a synergistic approach to simultaneous promotion of the NDEP *Be Smart About Your Heart* campaign, which targeted consumers, and the ADA *Make The Link* campaign targeting health care professionals, which concerned diabetes and CVD. As described above, NDEP partners share the results of surveys and evaluations, often seeking NDEP's input on data-collection questions of interest. State-Based Diabetes Prevention and Control Programs evaluate NDEP materials as part of programmatic assessments at state and regional levels. NDEP partners offer trusted access to at-risk populations and pilot-test NDEP materials to ensure that their products resonate with target audiences.

NDEP's partnerships have provided new venues and innovative outreach using NDEP products. For example, the Pan American Health Association now features on its Web site a low-impact aerobics video using the music from *Movimiento Por Su Vida*, an NDEP product promoting physical activity. *Movimiento* has been used in training promotores (community health workers) at the U.S.–Mexico border, in work-site interventions to promote employee wellness, and in community health events such as *Dia de la Mujer Latina* (where salsa dancers demonstrated culturally appropriate ways to have fun with physical activity). In addition it is being reproduced by other partners such as the ADA, State-Based Diabetes Prevention & Control Programs, and the Ministry of Health of the country of Mexico. State- and U.S. Territory-Based Diabetes Prevention and Control Programs have tailored and adapted NDEP materials to promote NDEP's campaign messages in movie theaters, billboards, and mass transit ads; to use in health systems interventions in the Bureau of Primary Health Care Health Disparities Collaborative; and to be part of community interventions in collaboration with programs such as REACH (Racial and Ethnic Approaches to Community Health).

For a complete list, including membership in the individual work groups, see the NDEP Progress Report posted at *http://www.ndep.nih.gov/diabetes/pubs/NDEP_ ProgressRpt07.pdf.*

Many more examples of partnership in action are provided on www.ndep.nih. gov and www.cdc.gov/diabetes/ndep.

Implications for Health Policy

NDEP does not set policy, but it does have materials that inform policy makers. Examples include:

- The NDEP publication *Silent Trauma* discusses the importance of CLAS (Culturally and Linguistically Appropriate Standards) in providing appropriate interpreter services.
- *NDEP Guiding Principles for Diabetes Care: For Health Care Professionals* provides an overview of the key elements of early and intensive clinical diabetes care and prevention. They form the basis of NDEP's public and professional awareness programs and are based on the best level of evidence available.
- The NDEP Web site www.diabetesatwork.org describes workplace policies that promote diabetes control and prevention and promotes inclusion of health plan benefits for diabetes supplies.
- The NDEP's BetterDiabetescare.nih.gov Web site is focused on how to improve the way health care professionals deliver diabetes care and on how the health care delivery system can be designed to innovate and improve care, rather than the clinical care itself. NDEP believes that systems change is essential to provide the type of evidence-based, patient-centered care needed to effectively manage diabetes and prevent the serious complications associated with the disease. The Web site's content is based on current, peer-reviewed literature and evidence-based practice recommendations.
- *Helping the Student with Diabetes Succeed: a Guide for School Personnel* informs policy makers of antidiscrimination laws in the school setting and provides tools to support implementation of policy change.

Economic Issues and Implications

In the NDEP Strategic Plan, the Coordinating Committee has prioritized understanding and communicating the cost-effectiveness of diabetes prevention and control. The NDEP Health Care Professional and Business Health Strategy work groups are collaborating to review the findings of cost-effectiveness studies for translation to NDEP target audiences. NDEP promotes interventions that are evidence based and cost-effective, such as the lifestyle intervention of the Diabetes Prevention Program, and has developed tools to translate these interventions to multiple settings and for different populations.

NDEP has not performed a cost-effectiveness evaluation of its materials that are used in interventions, but it relies on several principles. According to the Oxford Health Alliance 2006 publication *Chronic Disease: An Economic Perspective*, "The results of society-level interventions [in chronic disease control and prevention] have been mixed, with the greatest success attributable to programmes with long-term, multi-sectoral, collaborative approaches that engage different parts of society—especially the public and private sectors together—and reinforce key messages through multiple outlets" (p. 44).

NDEP's partnership approach reflects these concepts. Future directions for NDEP include greater emphasis on "making the economics case" by identification of cost-effective clinical and public health interventions in diabetes control and prevention. A few tools are currently available to raise awareness of the cost-effectiveness of diabetes control and prevention in various venues. For example one of the NDEP products, a Web site for business and managed care leaders (www.diabetesatwork.org), includes an interactive assessment tool for employers to compare the predicted economic burden of poorly controlled diabetes. By entering the demographics of the workforce, the tool calculates the likely economics burden of diabetes by using current prevalence data with average health care costs. The site then provides suggestions for selecting appropriate health plan benefits, materials and recommendations for work-site wellness interventions, and information on the impact of chronic disease (including comorbid conditions such as depression) on worker productivity and absenteeism.

■ Areas of Uncertainty or Controversy

Usefulness of Diabetes Education in Preventing and Managing the Disease

The NDEP was established to disseminate information regarding diabetes control and translate scientific knowledge into terms understandable by the general public. At present, however, information is limited on the impact of knowledge in changing behavior relative to preventing and controlling diabetes. NDEP employs the concepts inherent in the Health Belief Model (that perceived severity, susceptibility, benefits, and barriers affect action) and Social Cognitive Theory (awareness, benefits, and self-efficacy in the adoption of health behaviors) in creating educational materials (Hampson 2001; NCI 2008; Warsi 2004).

According to the Oxford Health Alliance *Chronic Disease: An Economic Perspective* (Suhrcke 2006), there is some evidence to support mass media campaigns and education in diabetes prevention. The authors of a World Bank study in the Pacific Islands conclude that mass media education is cost-effective compared to secondary prevention of obesity if the intervention reaches a large-enough population and if the prevalence of obesity and other targeted diseases is high (World Bank 2000).

There is evidence to suggest that "self-management diabetes education" is cost-effective for prevention of diabetes. Some research also points to diet and physical activity (lifestyle) changes as very cost-effective for prevention of diabetes. In a cost-effectiveness analysis of lifestyle modification in the DPP, diet and exercise counseling cost about $8800 per quality-adjusted life-year saved compared with no prevention, with a favorable cost-effectiveness profile at any adult age studied.

Using these principles, NDEP has developed tailored media campaign materials as well self-management "how-to" tools for promoting a healthy diet and increasing physical activity.

- NDEP materials have clear action steps. Examples of such materials include:
  - *4 Steps to Control Your Diabetes. For Life* brochures.
  - *Small Steps, Big Rewards. Prevent Type 2 Diabetes* multicultural primary prevention tip sheets.
- NDEP products strive for self-management support, for example,
  - *Tips on Helping the Person With Diabetes.*
  - *New Beginnings: A Guide to Living Well With Diabetes.*
- NDEP tools for health care professionals reflect the health communications literature, which indicates that "I recommend … " statements are more effective than third-person statements (e.g., "ADA recommends … "):
  - *GAME PLAN* tool kit.
  - Patient education poster developed by the PPOD Work Group.
- Recent NDEP products have had more emphasis on self-management support for diabetes control and prevention.
  - The *GAME PLAN* tool kit for people at risk for type 2 diabetes provides behavior change tools based on the experience of the Diabetes Prevention Program study.
  - *Power To Prevent: A Family Lifestyle Approach to Diabetes Prevention* uses the NDEP *GAME PLAN* tool kit materials in a support-group-like setting to help people set goals, monitor food and physical activity, and report accountability to a peer group with a lay facilitator.
  - *Road to Health/El Camino Hacia La Buena Salud* tool kit supports community health workers in outreach using motivational interviewing techniques to provide self-management support for diabetes prevention.
  - *New Beginnings: Living Well with Diabetes* discussion guide builds from a motivational film produced by an independent filmmaker to guide people in dealing with the emotional barriers to behavioral change for diabetes control.

A major barrier to effective care is a health care system that is poorly designed to care for chronic disease. The Institute of Medicine's (IOM's) *Crossing the Quality Chasm: A New Health System for the 21st Century* (Institute of Medicine 2001) reports and identifies major gaps in the quality of today's health care organizations. The IOM report asserts that achieving improvement will require redesign of these health care organizations (microsystems) and suggests three comprehensive redesign principles: that care should be (1) knowledge based, (2) patient centered, and (3) systems minded. In consideration of these recommendations and others the NDEP Health Care Professional Work Group developed a health systems change Web site, www.betterdiabetescare.nih.gov. This Web site was developed to help health care providers and organizations change the way they deliver care so that they could improve diabetes outcomes by assessing the need for change, developing strategies, implementing innovative tools, and evaluating changes in systems of care. The Web site also provides tools for health care professionals for supporting patient self-management. Some examples of the Web-based materials are the following:

- Information on the effectiveness of patient education that focuses on skills in troubleshooting, self-management, goal setting, and disease management.
- Video clips of interactions between diabetes educators and patients demonstrating support for self-management and motivational interviewing skills.
- Templates and tools used in various systems of care to track and monitor diabetes control and behavior change.

Effective models of diabetes care have implemented one or more of the proposed interventions: system changes, patient education, and physician education. NDEP strives to support all three.

■ Success and Limitations

Partnership

The keystone in NDEP's success is its partnership network. Organizational partners help to identify gaps, recommend needed formative research, contribute to development of creative products, support pilot testing, contribute to revision, and ultimately act as trusted dissemination points to audiences that NDEP wants to reach. NDEP's partnership network provides a venue for organizations that might not otherwise meet with each other to collaborate. Ultimately the NDEP structure that creates evidence-based materials developed by the participatory process with its partners increases NDEP's reach as partners reproduce materials, implement NDEP-based programs, adapt products to local needs, and perform evaluation. Maintaining partnerships is, however, resource intensive.

Consensus

The NDEP participatory approach uses a consensus process among its diverse members to develop core program messages. Consensus adds value in that the target audiences receive consistent messages on diabetes prevention and control from all NDEP partners. Developing materials via a consensus process takes additional time, however, which some partners find discouraging.

Increased Awareness

Recognition of diabetes as a serious disease has greatly increased since NDEP's inception. *Small Steps, Big Rewards. Prevent Type 2 Diabetes* is the first national campaign to promote awareness of diabetes prevention. The broad adoption and adaptation of NDEP messages by national, state, and local organizations attests to NDEP's success in providing tools and messages for increased awareness.

Outreach to Special Populations

NDEP partner organizations represent trusted access to reach special populations that may have historical mistrust of the government. Some NDEP materials were revised by partner organizations to be more culturally appropriate. Examples include:

- Translation and adaptation by the Ethiopian Community Development Council of NDEP materials into Amharic, Somali, Arabic, and French for African immigrants.
- Revision of NDEP *Small Steps, Big Rewards* brochure and the *4 Steps* booklet by Papa Ola Lokahi for Native Hawaiians to include more tailored images, activities, and motivational concepts.
- National Coalition of Pastors' Spouses and Black Women's Health Imperative have both adapted NDEP materials developed for African Americans to complement their intervention programs.

Limitations of Materials Accessible Only on the Internet

NDEP strives to provide the general public with free printed hard copies of all materials, but resource limitations have led to some products being offered only online. The hardest-to-reach audiences may not have access to these materials unless partner organizations download and print the materials. To reach these audiences the NDEP disseminates and promotes its materials and products to local community organizations and agencies that provide services to hard-to-reach audiences. Although more homes have personal computers today than ever before, many people, especially in lower-income groups or older adults with limited interest in learning computer skills, are unable or unwilling to use the Internet to access NDEP educational products or information. Many homes and public libraries provide Internet access by slower dial-up only, which makes downloading large or graphically complex materials impracticable. Although NDEP provides HTML versions for many products that are more easily downloaded by dial-up Internet access, graphics designed to appeal to specific target audiences are necessarily lost in downloading HTML. Internet access in some U.S. Pacific Island territories requires an international phone call, limiting the usefulness of online availability to this population.

Continued Challenge of Developing Innovative, Motivational Research

NDEP is aware that raising awareness and increasing knowledge is not enough to change behavior. Accordingly, it plans to incorporate new information on how to effectively facilitate self-care and behavior change in people at risk for and with diabetes and assist health care professionals in working effectively with patients to make these lifestyle changes.

Need for more Effective Marketing to the Business and Managed Care Audience

NDEP's Web site www.diabetesatwork.org continues to have a relatively low number of visitors (48,638 in 2005). NDEP collaborated with the Washington Business Group on Health (now known as the National Business Group on Health) to place www.diabetesatwork.org on that group's server in the hope that the target audience would be more likely to visit the site on that server. There were some challenges in this approach, however. As NDEP had no direct control over posting to the Web site, there were delays in making changes to the site and repairing broken links. Although these challenges have been resolved, the number of visitors is still low. In 2008, www.diabetesatwork.org had 19,982 visits and 66,869 pageviews. The NDEP Business Health Strategy Work Group is developing additional content to attract business and managed care, such as case studies of return on investment and the economics required to "make the business case" of diabetes prevention and control.

Infrastructure Challenges and Opportunities

As NDEP grew, so did the need for increased communication across work groups for improved collaboration. This led to the development of the Operations Committee and to several successful cross-collaborative projects among work groups (e.g., between PPOD and the Hispanic/Latino Work Group in the development of the Spanish PPOD poster). NDEP is still exploring varied approaches to the composition of its work groups. For example, since 2005 the Hispanic/Latino Work Group has involved the Diabetes Prevention and Control Programs from the states with the 10 highest Hispanic/Latino populations as *ad hoc* members. Other work groups have been considering different approaches to involving the Diabetes Prevention and Control Programs. Providing flexibility for composition of the work groups within a framework has been accomplished through the development of individual work group models, approved by both the individual work group and the NDEP Executive Committee, to guide decisions on recruiting new members.

Role of Volunteers

Members of NDEP's work groups are volunteers who receive travel support to attend in-person meetings but not honoraria or other compensation for their work with NDEP. Some of the challenges NDEP has experienced in working with a large volunteer base include the need to clarify roles of volunteers versus paid NDEP staff, the difficulties in engaging volunteers, maintaining energy and commitment, and differing views on the level of organizational infrastructure needed (e.g., levels of approval for decisions). Regardless, NDEP has shown great success in maintaining continued participation by key organizational partners despite staff turnover.

■ Lessons Learned

Partnership Is Key

- From its inception, NDEP identified the need for consensus to avoid duplicative, competing messages that can confuse the public.
- NDEP's Partnership Network is predicated on the concept that its partners have a special understanding of the needs, knowledge, attitudes, and perceptions of the constituency they serve that can contribute to the development of effective messages and interventions.
- Partners advise NDEP of the need for adapting messages:
  - Both the Asian American/Pacific Islander (AAPI) and American Indian/Alaska Native (AI/AN) work groups indicated that the "Control" message may not resonate as such with the AAPI and AI/AN audiences. In the AAPI case, it was better to translate "Control the ABCs" to "Take Care of Your Heart." For AI/AN, the word "Control" was changed to "Manage."
  - The Hispanic/Latino Work Group expressed concern about a cultural attitude of fatalism that would limit the effectiveness of the "Control" message. In focus groups, diabetes control was perceived by some as challenging "God's will." The NDEP adapted the *Control Your Diabetes. For Life* message in the "*Thunder and Lightning*" campaign in which a lightning bolt provides a dramatic backdrop to the statement "There are some things in life you cannot control. Luckily, diabetes is not one of them."
  - The cultural competency of the weight-loss message was called into question among some ethnic populations who view a larger body habitus as more attractive or powerful. Research has shown (Liburd 1999) that African American women shown silhouettes of female figures consistently choose larger figures as more attractive. Among Pacific Islanders,

large body size has been traditionally revered as a mark of power. Both the African American/African Ancestry and AAPI work groups expressed concern that a simple message of "lose weight if you are overweight" would be ineffective in these populations, which do not necessarily perceive themselves as overweight at the BMI risk standard. The issue is compounded by the fact that the BMI standard for increased risk varies with racial/ethnic group. At-risk BMI for non-Asian Americans is ≥25, for Asian Americans, it is ≥23, and for Pacific Islanders, it is ≥26.

- NDEP has used this information to focus on achieving a "healthy weight," indicating the BMI cutoffs for increased risk of type 2 diabetes and CVD rather than using terms such as "overweight" and "obese," which can be viewed as cultural constructs. In addition, the at-risk charts for diabetes in the *GAME PLAN* tool kit and AAPI prevention tip sheet have different cutoff points for Asian American and Pacific Islander populations.

- The NDEP Partner Survey tool provides feedback for program improvement. NDEP conducts its biannual Partner Survey to gather information on the activities of its work group members and feedback on NDEP products, campaigns, and activities. It has provided feedback for program improvement from its closest organizational partners and contributes to the development of NDEP's strategic planning. New tools, revisions to materials, and new approaches to dissemination and promotion have evolved from the responses to the Partner Survey. Individualized progress reports of the work groups, which summarize the responses of the work groups' members to the Partner Survey as well as data on the number of work group-specific products ordered or downloaded from NDEP, help the work groups assess their achievement of strategic goals, plan strategies and goals for the future, and track overall progress for the program.

- There is a need for community intervention tools as well as awareness campaigns. NDEP Partner Surveys have repeatedly asked for tools that could be used in community interventions, support groups, diabetes prevention or education classes, and with a variety of community-based partners. Partners have also asked NDEP for "how-to" kits using NDEP materials to help patients learn to manage their diabetes and make lifestyle changes.

- Since its inception, NDEP has created media campaign tools for partners, but in recent years several work groups have developed multiple component kits or modular curricula for clinical and community interventions. Some of these kits are:
  - *GAME PLAN* tool kit for health care providers and patients.
  - *The Power to Control Diabetes Is in Your Hands* kit on Medicare benefits for older adults with diabetes.
  - *Power to Prevent: A Family Lifestyle Approach to Diabetes Prevention*—A 12-module curriculum that uses other NDEP materials to help people develop healthy behavioral skills in the areas of food, physical activity, and diabetes self-management.

■ Developments over the Next 5 to 10 Years

From the beginning NDEP has implemented a strategic planning process that incorporates obtaining input and guidance from the program's Coordinating Committee and work group members on future directions and priority activities. In 2008 NDEP has adopted a new Strategic Plan, which calls for increased use, reach, and evaluation of existing NDEP messages, materials, and products; increased partnership outreach and promotional activities to reach target audiences; and increased cross-collaboration among work groups.

NDEP is interested in going beyond awareness to support partners in program implementation with the creation of "how-to" kits using NDEP materials, such as the *Power to Prevent* curriculum, which uses multiple other NDEP tools in a primary prevention behavioral change approach, and the development of train-the-trainer materials to augment effectiveness of new NDEP products such as the *Road to Health* tool kit.

NDEP materials undergo continuous review and revision. A cross-cutting group from several work groups is currently planning review of NDEP materials for opportunities to include more information on the impact of depression and other psychosocial conditions on diabetes outcomes. NDEP has also been exploring the topic of facilitating behavior change to improve care for people at risk for and with diabetes. The NDEP has recently produced the "Support for Behavior Change Resource," an online searchable database of research articles, tools, and programs that address the "how to" of psychosocial issues, lifestyle, and behavior change that can help individuals or groups cope with diabetes and make and sustain behavior change.

At this time, NDEP continues to commit resources to primary prevention as well as to diabetes control.

■ Applicability to International Settings

NDEP materials are available in English, Spanish, and 15 Asian or Pacific Islander languages. NDEP partners have taken steps to translate NDEP materials into additional languages and adapt them to other cultural audiences. NDEP has received feedback about NDEP materials being used in Africa, Asia, Australia, Europe, South America, and the Pacific Islands as well as by our North American neighbors.

In addition to the activities of the Hispanic/Latino Work Group (which includes partnership with the Pan American Health Organization as a work group member organization), the NDEP has developed several successful unfunded collaborative efforts with the International Diabetes Federation, specifically with the South and Central American (IDF-SACA) Region to identify opportunities to facilitate scientific exchange between diabetes associations in that region and to identify, discuss, and act on diabetes issues affecting Latin America. Technical assistance has been provided by NDEP staff members to the International Diabetes Foundation to increase capacity building and training in areas such as diabetes awareness, media training, and the use of NDEP campaigns and materials. In return, NDEP has received insightful information about the needs of the Latino population in the areas of diabetes educational materials, products, and campaigns.

■ Summary

In its single decade of existence the NDEP has become the focal point for those looking for scientifically valid information about diabetes and its treatment, as reflected by the steady increases in numbers of visitors to NDEP Web sites. NDEP has also become a unique forum for those nongovernmental organizations with constituencies that have diabetes or are at risk for having the disease. The emergence of diabetes as a recognized public health problem and the increase in those who believe it to be serious can be viewed as a measure of the success in realizing NDEP's major objective in this area. Other NDEP goals, such as reducing disparities, still have a long way to go. Although NDEP plans to continue work on increasing public awareness, its biggest challenges for the next decade will be to examine and enhance the ability of the health care system to efficiently and effectively deal with people with diabetes and to enhance the self-care abilities of people with diabetes, especially those who are disadvantaged people. NDEP believes that the participatory model using a wide variety of partners and a wide spectrum of approaches is effective, but it recognizes that its work has just begun.

■ References

ADA Physician Study (2002, 2005) and American Association of Nurse Practitioners Survey (2005). Reported in the National Diabetes Education Program Progress Report 1997–2007. Available at http://www.ndep.nih.gov/diabetes/pubs/NDEP_ProgressRpt07.pdf. Accessed June 29, 2008.

ADA Roper ASW Survey (2002, 2003, 2004). Reported in the National Diabetes Education Program Progress Report 1997–2007. Available at http://www.ndep.nih.gov/diabetes/pubs/NDEP_ProgressRpt07.pdf. Accessed June 29, 2008.

ADA-sponsored patient survey (1998–2004). Reported in the National Diabetes Education Program Progress Report 1997–2007. Available at http://www.ndep.nih.gov/diabetes/pubs/NDEP_ProgressRpt07.pdf. Accessed June 29, 2008.

Behavioral Risk Factor Surveillance System (1997, 1998, 1999, 2003). Available at http://www.cdc.gov/brfss/technical_infodata/surveydata.htm. Accessed September 28, 2007.

Centers for Disease Control and Prevention (2008). National diabetes fact sheet: general information and national estimates on diabetes in the United States, 2007.

Atlanta, GA: U.S. Department of Health and Human Services, Centers for Disease Control and Prevention. Available at http://www.cdc.gov/diabetes/pubs/pdf/ ndfs_2007.pdf. Accessed June 29, 2008.

Committee on Quality of Health Care in America, Institute of Medicine (2001). *Crossing the Quality Chasm: A New Health System for the 21st Century.* Washington, DC: National Academies Press.

Diabetes Control and Complications Trial Research Group (1993). The effect of intensive treatment of diabetes on the development and progression of long-term complications in insulin-dependent diabetes mellitus. *New England Journal of Medicine* **329**, 977–86.

Hampson S et al. (2001). Effects of educational and psychosocial interventions for adolescents with diabetes mellitus: a systematic review. *Health Technology Assessment* **5** (10), 1–79.

Healthy People 2010 (2005). Available at http://www.healthypeople.gov/Publications/. April 15, 2010.

Herman WH et al. (2005). The cost-effectiveness of lifestyle modification or metformin in preventing type 2 diabetes in adults with impaired glucose tolerance. *Annals of Internal Medicine* **142**, 323–32.

Knowler WC et al. (2002). Reduction in the incidence of type 2 diabetes with lifestyle intervention or metformin. *New England Journal of Medicine* **346**, 393–403.

Making Health Communications Work, National Cancer Institute (2008). Available at http://www.cancer.gov/pinkbook. Accessed June 29, 2008.

NDEP (2007). Survey of public attitudes, knowledge, and practices related to diabetes. *NDEP Newsletter* **9** (1). Available at http://www.ndep.nih.gov. Accessed January 30, 2009

Saadine JB et al. (2002). A diabetes report card for the United States: quality of care in the 1990s. *Annals of Internal Medicine* **136**, 565–74.

Suhrcke M et al. (2006). *Chronic Disease: An Economic Perspective.* London: Oxford Health Alliance. Also available at www.oxha.org. Accessed January 30, 2009.

Warsi A et al. (2004). Self-management education programs in chronic disease: a systematic review and methodological critique of the literature. *Archives of Internal Medicine* **164**, 1641–9.

SECTION 5

DIABETES IN DEVELOPING COUNTRIES

24. Prevalence/Incidence, Risk Factors, and Future Burden of Type 1, Type 2, and Gestational Diabetes in Developing Countries

Chittaranjan S. Yajnik, Terrence Forrester, Kaushik Ramaiya,
Nikhil Tandon, Shailaja Kale, and Marshall Tulloch-Reid

■ Main Public Health Messages

- Developing countries have a disproportionately high burden of diabetes, and it is rapidly increasing. In 2025 two of three diabetes patients worldwide will be from developing countries, and one in three will be from India or China.
- The public health agenda for developing countries includes the unenviable double burden of grappling with nutritional deficiency and infectious diseases while also tackling the rapidly increasing noncommunicable diseases. Rapid socioeconomic transition and unequal distribution of benefits contribute to the double burden.
- In developing countries, diabetes manifests at a younger age and lower body mass index and progresses faster than in Europeans. These characteristics may be related to intrauterine nutritional experiences that compromise growth and promote adiposity.
- Rapid childhood growth is an additional risk factor for type 2 diabetes, suggesting a biphasic nutritional etiology.
- Treatment of diabetes and its complications places a huge burden on the economy of the developing countries that may impair their growth and development.
- Control of the epidemic will involve joint action by individuals, families, societies, and nations. Societal and political actions may be crucial.
- Novel approaches to prevention must take account of the "life-course" evolution of diabetes risk. Urgent research is required in this field.

Special thanks to Smita R Kulkarni, Gaurvika Nayyar, and Parag Yajnik for their help in writing the manuscript.

553

■ Introduction

Diabetes is fast becoming the leading cause of morbidity and mortality worldwide. Traditionally considered a disease of affluence, it is now occurring at an alarming rate in poor, developing countries, where more than 80% of the world population lives. Today the prevalence of diabetes in many developing countries is higher than that reported in developed countries. In addition, many of these developing countries are facing the double burden of a high prevalence of infectious diseases and undernutrition at the same time that the noncommunicable diseases are emerging. Health systems of the developing world are ill equipped to deal with this complex scenario, and the combined effect of diabetes, cardiovascular disease, malaria, tuberculosis, and HIV could have a catastrophic effect on the health and economy of many developing nations, negating some of the accumulated gains of development.

The rise in prevalence of diabetes in the last few decades has been so rapid, the number of individuals affected so large, and the morbidity and fatal consequences so severe, that this epidemic threatens to be the largest the world has ever faced. The current strategies of treatment and prevention may prove inadequate, and the cost of implementing them could overwhelm the existing public health systems in most countries. In addition to effective translation of the current knowledge we need to test new ideas in treatment and prevention. The expanding epidemic is not explained by Mendelian genetic factors, which have remained stable in the recent evolutionary past, but instead presumably by rapid environmental changes, which influence the expression of the susceptibility genes (epigenetics). Comparative studies of such mechanisms in the high- and low-incidence populations are likely to provide important information on the prevention of type 2 diabetes.

We will discuss some of the issues related to the three most common types of diabetes (type 1, type 2, and gestational diabetes [GDM]) that are particularly relevant to the developing countries. Our main focus will be on type 2 diabetes, which constitutes over 90% of all diabetes worldwide.

We have labeled North America and Western Europe as the developed world and countries in Asia, Africa, Latin America, and the Caribbean as the developing world. In this chapter we present published data from these developing countries but particularly from India and Asia because of the lead author's experience.

■ Background/Historical Perspective

Burden of Diabetes and Related Disorders

The growing problem of diabetes and related disorders in developing countries has only recently been appreciated because of a paucity of standardized data over time. Many of these studies have not been nationally representative and may involve survey data from communities or regions within a country. They predominantly involve adults and do not always distinguish type 1 from type 2 diabetes. They are also difficult to identify through the usual Internet search engines, particularly those published in Spanish or Portuguese (Royle, Bain, and Waugh 2005). In addition changes in diagnostic criteria often make it difficult to make direct comparisons between studies done over long time intervals. However, despite their limitations, these studies have provided valuable insight into the changing epidemiology of the disease in the developing world.

The epidemic of diabetes in the developing countries was heralded by studies in migrants from their countries to the developed countries. Thus, the Southall Survey in London raised the alarm when it showed that the age-adjusted prevalence for migrant Asians was 3.8 times as high as in Europeans (Mather and Keen 1985). Serial prevalence studies in South India have documented a rise in the prevalence of diabetes from approximately 2% in the 1970s to approximately 18% in 2007 (Ramachandran A 2005; Mohan et al. 2006; Ramachandran A et al. 2008). The National Urban Diabetes Survey in 2001 showed an average prevalence of about 12% in adults in six metropolitan cities (Ramachandran A et al. 2001). In the Caribbean cross-sectional surveys of adult Trinidadians and Jamaicans found a prevalence of diabetes in the 1960s of <2% in persons of African descent (Poon-King 1968; Tulloch 1961). However 30 years later the estimated prevalence of diabetes in adults ranged from 9% to 18% (Hennis et al. 2002; Ragoobirsingh, Lewis-Fuller, and Morrison 1995; Wilks et al. 1999). In Africa, diabetes was considered a rare disease up until the mid-1980s in most regions of the continent with the exception of South Africa. The five countries in sub-Saharan Africa with a significantly higher prevalence of diabetes have considerable variation economically: Nigeria, South Africa, Democratic Republic of Congo, Ethiopia, and Tanzania (Mbanya, Kengne, and Assah 2006). Racial differences in disease prevalence have been noted in all of these populations, with persons of Southeast Asian origin having a higher prevalence of the disease than those of African origin (Sobngwi et al. 2001).

Based on available data from population-based surveys that used World Health Organization (WHO) criteria for diagnosis of diabetes and mortality projections from developed countries, WHO (Wild et al. 2004) and the International Diabetes Federation (IDF) (International Diabetes Federation 2006) have reported on the estimated burden of diabetes across the world and projected it for the next three decades. Table 24.1 lists the 10 countries with the largest number of diabetic patients in 2007 and the number projected for 2025. In 2007 there were an estimated 246 million diabetic patients worldwide, with 165 million of them living in the developing world. Globally the number of patients with diabetes is projected to increase to 380 million by 2025. Because the prevalence of diabetes increases with age, the greatest increase in prevalence is expected in the regions that will have the biggest gain in life expectancy. A 50% increase in the current prevalence of diabetes has been projected, with 276 million in the developing world, including 70 million in India and 59 million in China. Thus, two in three patients will be from a developing country, and one in three will be either Indian or Chinese.

TABLE 24.1 *Top 10 Countries: Number of People with Diabetes (20–79 Years) and Impaired Glucose Tolerance 2007 and 2025*

	Number of People with Diabetes				Number of People with IGT			
	Country (2007)	Persons (Millions)	Country (2025)	Persons (Millions)	Country (2007)	Persons (Millions)	Country (2025)	Persons (Millions)
1	India	40.9	India	69.9	China	64.3	China	79.1
2	China	39.8	China	59.3	India	35.9	India	56.2
3	USA	19.2	USA	25.4	Russian Federation	17.8	Indonesia	20.6
4	Russian Federation	9.6	Brazil	17.6	Indonesia	14.1	Russian Federation	17.8
5	Germany	7.4	Pakistan	11.5	Japan	12.9	United States of America	16.5
6	Japan	7.0	Mexico	10.8	United States of America	12.4	Japan	12.7
7	Pakistan	6.9	Russian Federation	10.3	Brazil	8.4	Brazil	11.5
8	Brazil	6.9	Germany	8.1	Bangladesh	6.8	Pakistan	11.0
9	Mexico	6.1	Egypt	7.6	Pakistan	6.4	Bangladesh	10.6
10	Egypt	4.4	Bangladesh	7.4	Ukraine	6.0	Mexico	7.7

In developing countries, diabetes occurs at a younger age, with the majority of people with diabetes being 45–64 years old, unlike the distribution in developed countries, where most people with diabetes are aged 65 or over. In addition the prevalence of impaired glucose tolerance (IGT) in some of these regions such as Africa and Southeast Asia is often two to three times the prevalence of diabetes—a large pool from which additional cases can develop. Although worldwide there does not appear to be a difference by gender in the prevalence of diabetes, surveys in the Caribbean and Latin America have demonstrated a higher prevalence of diabetes in women, who tend to be more obese (Martorell et al. 1998).

Data on GDM is relatively sparse and heterogeneous because of different methods and approaches used for diagnosis. In the relatively low-risk, rural Chinese provinces the rate is approximately 2%, whereas in relatively affluent Hong Kong it is 14% (Ko et al. 2002). The rates in urban India have increased from <2% to approximately 16% in the last decade (Seshiah et al. 2004, 2007), while they doubled in China and South Africa over the same period. In Mexico the rates were already in double figures in the last decade.

Diabetes affects all systems of the body and leads to chronic and debilitating complications that reduce life expectancy by many years. In low- and middle-income countries chronic noncommunicable diseases (including diabetes) accounted for 50% of the disease burden in 2005 (Reddy et al. 2005). In India diabetes and cardiovascular disease are estimated to have contributed 31% of 10.3 million deaths and 12% of 291 million disability-adjusted life years (DALYs) lost in 2005 (Abegunde et al. 2007). The impact of diabetes on these two measures is expected to rise rapidly in India. Although effective treatment is available for many diabetic complications (laser for retinopathy, dialysis for kidney failure, angioplasty and bypass surgery for heart disease), it is very expensive and beyond the reach of many patients. The estimated direct cost for treating diabetes and its complications is more than the current total health budget in many developing countries, and where these costs are borne by the government, they can constitute a substantial portion of that country's gross domestic product (GDP). For example, in an economic analysis of the cost of diabetes in four Caribbean islands (Jamaica, the Bahamas, Barbados, and Trinidad and Tobago), the cost (direct plus indirect) of diabetes if adequately treated ranged from 0.5% of GDP in the Bahamas to 5.21% of GDP in Trinidad and Tobago (Abdulkadri, Cunningham-Myrie, and Forrester 2009). Difficulty obtaining data on age- and gender-specific diabetes prevalence and mortality, the costs associated with diabetes treatment, as well as indirect costs resulting from complications and premature mortality often make calculating the economic burden of diabetes in developing countries difficult (Cunningham-Myrie et al. 2008). Estimates from the few studies available in developing countries suggest that unmitigated morbidity and premature mortality due to diabetes will jeopardize the economic development of many of these nations.

The demonstration in clinical trials that the onset of diabetes may be postponed by intensive lifestyle management focused on modifying diet and physical activity is welcome news (Gillies et al. 2007), as are reports that intensive control of glycemia, blood pressure, and lipid levels reduces the rate of vascular complications and mortality in diabetic patients (Gaede et al. 2003, 2008). However, despite the burden that diabetes will have on the developing world and the potential benefits of prevention programs using changes in lifestyle, only two published randomized trials of nutritional primary prevention have been conducted in developing countries, one in China (Pan et al. 1997) and the other in India (Ramachandran A et al. 2006). In addition the health systems of the developing world, still struggling to cope with infection and malnutrition, are unable to translate this evidence effectively, thus contributing another barrier to the control of the diabetes epidemic.

■ Transition (the Price of Progress)

In the 1970s, Omran proposed the concept of the "epidemiological transition" to describe the changing profile of disease during economic development (Omran 1971), a concept that has been more recently elaborated by others (Popkin 2004; Yusuf et al. 2001a, 2001b). Economic development has been universal, but a rapid rate of economic growth is associated with adverse health effects. Europe underwent the transition at a slower pace, which perhaps allowed the population to adapt adequately. However many developing countries, especially in Asia, have undergone very rapid economic development, which appears to have been associated with some adverse health consequences. Seven of the 10 fastest-growing economies of the world are Asian, and together they contributed 42% of the increase in world GDP during the period 1975–1992. India has emerged as the fastest-growing creator of wealth in the world but has seen a quintupling of its diabetes prevalence over the past 30 years.

One effect of economic development is a reduction in early-life mortality and an increase in life expectancy. In India in the last three decades, infant mortality has fallen from 120 to below 60 per 1000 live births, mortality under age 5 years has been reduced from over 200 to 70 per 1000 live births, and life expectancy has risen from 50 to 64 years (UNDP India 1998). In 1970, 49% of Indians were older than 18 years, and in 2005 this number had increased to 57% (see Fig. 24.1). Nutritional-deficiency disorders (for example, kwashiorkor-marasmus, vitamin A deficiency blindness) and infectious diseases (smallpox, diphtheria, polio myelitis) are gradually being replaced by lifestyle-related and degenerative diseases (obesity, diabetes, cardiovascular disease, osteoporosis, cancer, dementias) (Gopalan 1997). However, the two coexist, resulting in a double burden of disease. This is prominently seen in India, China, Southeast Asia, South America, and the more developed countries of Africa (such as South Africa, Nigeria, and Tanzania). Intriguingly, the double burden may be seen in the same family (undernourished child and obese parents, as described in slums in Brazil) (Sawaya et al. 1995) and in the same individual

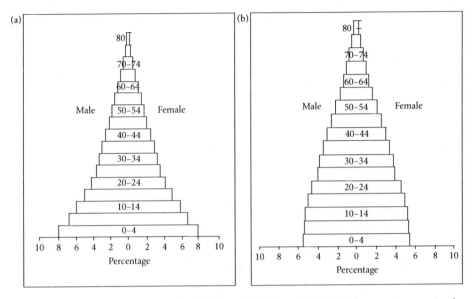

FIGURE 24.1. Population pyramids of India in (a) 1970 and (b) 2005 show an increase in the population belonging to middle and older age, thus increasing the population at risk for type 2 diabetes

during her/his lifetime: undernutrition in early life but overnutrition and obesity later (Yajnik 2004a).

Within a specific country the educated and the affluent benefit more from economic development, but they also suffer more from obesity and diabetes than do the poor. This is exemplified by reported rural-urban differences (obesity and diabetes are more prevalent in the urban setting, nutritional deficiency and infectious diseases more common in rural areas) (Ramachandran A. et al. 2008; Yajnik et al. 2008a). With advancing development, the earlier beneficiaries (affluent) start showing a delay in the age of degenerative diseases (cardiovascular disease in the United States and Europe) (Yusuf et al. 2001a, 2001b). In the foreseeable future however, the predictions for type 2 diabetes and cardiovascular disease in the developing countries are for relentless progression.

One of the contributors to the emergence of the chronic disease epidemic is dietary change. In South Korea, between the 1960s and the 1990s the proportion of plant food in the diet decreased from 97% to 79%, intake of carbohydrate energy decreased from 81% to 64%, while energy from fat increased from 6% to 19% (Kim, Moon, and Popkin 2000). A recent analysis of national consumer expenditure surveys in India over the last five decades has shown a progressive reduction in household expenditures on food in all income groups because of the low cost of cereals, which are the staple food for the population (Ramachandran P 2008). Despite a decline in expenditure there is a small increase in cereal intake, especially in low-income groups. Conversely, there is a decrease in the consumption of pulses (edible seeds from various crops such as peas or lentils) because of a prohibitive increase in their cost. The consumption of fats and oils has increased, especially in urban areas, although they contribute less than 15% of total energy.

In the last decade there has been a small decrease in total energy consumption, although there is a progressive increase in obesity. Although data on this question are scarce and inconclusive, first principles lead us to hypothesize that these changes in dietary intake are accompanied by changes in patterns of physical activity. The presumption is that there is a decrease in physical activity due to mechanization, at home, at work, and during leisure time. This presumption, in turn, rests on the widespread appearance of labor-saving devices in domestic, office, and agricultural environments, resulting in a reduction in energy expenditure through physical activity. Mechanized transport has no doubt had a major impact on activity as well (7.8 million motorbikes and scooters sold in India last year, and the cheapest four-wheeler yet, Nano, is waiting to enter the market). These changes might have led to a cumulative positive energy balance, increasing obesity and type 2 diabetes. Increased energy expenditure on physical activity in the sub-Saharan populations (except South Africa) is associated cross-sectionally with lower levels of overweight and obesity. Leanness and increased fitness from increased energy expenditure through physical activity may contribute to the lower prevalence of glucose intolerance in these populations.

Urbanization

A major indicator of transition is the rate of urbanization. At the time of India's independence (1947), 14% of the population lived in cities. This increased to 30% by the year 2000 and is expected to reach 42% by 2021 (Registrar General and Census Commissioner 2006). Less than 5% of rural but up to a third of urban Indian adults are overweight (BMI > 25, as calculated by weight in kilograms divided by height in meters squared) (Yajnik 2004b). Diabetes is four times as common in urban Indians as in their rural counterparts, and rates are even higher in those who have migrated to the West. The recent wave of rapid urbanization in India is partly fueled by increased job availability, for example by outsourcing of jobs from developed countries (globalization). The young employees in the call centers earn a substantial salary, spend long, stressful hours in their sedentary occupations, eat fast food, and display a pattern of increased consumption. Rapid growth in cities has led to haphazard construction, which discourages physical activity and relaxation. Such a lifestyle would predispose to weight gain, obesity, and diabetes, including GDM. Additionally concerns about safety and traffic make exercise difficult. The National Urban Diabetes Survey 2001 reported diabetes in 2.4% and IGT in 11.5% of those aged 20–29 years (Ramachandran A et al. 2001), and 15% of urban pregnant women were found to have GDM in a recent survey (Seshiah et al. 2007); the rates are considerably lower in the agricultural rural population.

Urban–rural differences are also reported in Africa (Sobngwi et al. 2001) and in Latin America (Aschner 2002), with higher rates of obesity and diabetes in adults residing in the cities. In some developing countries, such as those of the Caribbean, urban–rural differences in diabetes prevalence are no longer as pronounced as they were several years ago (Hennis and Fraser 2004, Wilks et al. 2008), and in some developed countries the rates of obesity and diabetes are higher in rural than in urban populations, for example in some parts of the United States such as South Carolina (Patterson et al. 2004).

The Clinical Characteristics of Diabetes in Developing Countries

Some striking features of patients with diabetes in developing countries (see Fig. 24.2), when they are compared with their counterparts in the developed countries, are (1) younger age, (2) lower BMI, and (3) a relatively rapid progression to the diabetic state from IGT (Yajnik 2004a). Indian patients with type 2 diabetes are diagnosed at least 10 years younger than those in Europe, and the age is falling. Earlier manifestation of diabetes means a longer exposure to risk factors and higher risk of developing vascular complications, which reduce life expectancy. Diabetes in the young has serious implications for the productivity and economic development of these populations. In young diabetic women from developing countries there is a risk of dying early, marriage prospects are reduced, chances of marriage breakup are high, there is increased risk of complicated pregnancy, and the resultant children have increased risks of obesity and diabetes (United Nations 2008). A female child of a diabetic mother propagates diabetes to the next generation ("diabetes begets diabetes") (Pettitt et al. 1988). Seventy percent of diabetes in the young in the Pima Indians is contributed by hyperglycemia in pregnancy (Dabelea, Knowler, and Pettitt 2000).

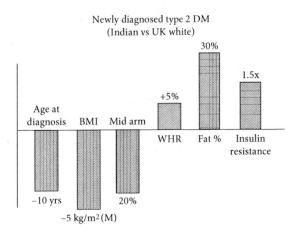

FIGURE 24.2. A comparison of an average type 2 diabetic patient from India with an average white patient from the United Kingdom. The Indian patient is younger, thinner (lower BMI), has a smaller muscle mass (mid-arm circumference), but has higher adiposity (fat percent) and central obesity (waist–hip ratio). The Indian patient is also more insulin resistant

Obesity, Adiposity, and Short Height: The Thin–Fat Syndrome

Many developing populations, especially Asians (Indians, Chinese, and related groups), are prone to diabetes at a BMI lower than the overweight category (set at 25 derived from European data) (WHO Expert Consultation 2004). This higher risk is partly contributed by higher body fat percentage and its more central (truncal and visceral) distribution in these populations. Thus, for a BMI of 25 kg/m², a European man has 18% body fat where an Asian Indian has 28% body fat, and at each BMI the Asians have a higher waist–hip ratio (Deurenberg-Yap et al. 2000). A WHO expert consultation (WHO Expert Consultation 2004) therefore proposed that the public-health action for obesity-related outcomes in Asians should start at a lower BMI and that the desirable BMI for Asians be 23 kg/m². Given the smaller frame of Asians, the IDF has also set the cutpoint for waist circumference at a lower level for this population (for example, 90 cm for Indian men compared with 94 cm for European men) (International Diabetes Federation 2006). It is perhaps more relevant to measure body fat percentage and waist–hip ratio as risk markers for diabetes across populations. One more reason for the higher risk of type 2 diabetes at lower BMI in Asians might be their short stature, which is recognized as an independent risk factor for type 2 diabetes (Asao et al. 2006) and for GDM (Jang et al. 1998). These associations may be ascribable to shorter legs, suggesting a role for impaired growth in early life (Kulkarni et al. 2007).

In addition, hyperglycemia is associated with high plasma triglycerides, low HDL (high-density lipoprotein) cholesterol concentrations, and high blood pressure, characteristics that constitute the so-called *metabolic syndrome*. Many studies in India have shown a high prevalence of metabolic syndrome (approximately 35% at mean age of 40 years in urban Indians) (Misra et al. 2007; Yajnik et al. 2008a). This combination of risk factors could predispose Indians to a rapid progression to diabetes from the intermediate states of IGT and GDM. For example in the Indian Diabetes Prevention Trial, 18% of persons with IGT progressed to diabetes per year (Ramachandran A et al. 2006), compared with 6% of such persons in the Finnish trial (Tuomilehto et al. 2001) and 11% in the American trial (Knowler et al. 2002). Two-thirds of women with GDM in an Indian study were hyperglycemic by 4 years after delivery, which is one of the fastest and highest rates of progression known (Kale et al. 2004).

Increasing Obesity in Adults and Children

Notwithstanding the "thin–fat" characteristic of many developing populations, there is also a progressive increase in obesity in these populations, reflecting the trend across the world (WHO Global Infobase). In China, obesity in men increased from 27.5% to 33.1% between 2002 and 2005, in Indians it rose from 15.0% to 16.8%. In Thailand, 27.9 % of the population is now overweight or obese. The most alarming statistics are for children: 15%–25% of schoolchildren in recent surveys in urban India were overweight (Ramachandran A et al. 2002), a pattern also noted in several developing countries in the Caribbean (Gaskin and Walker 2003; Gaskin et al. 2008). A prospective study in South India found that the rate of overweight in youth aged 5–16 years increased from 4.9% in 2003 to 6.6% in 2005 (Raj et al. 2007). The number of obese children has rapidly increased in China since the introduction of the one-child policy. Obese children usually become obese adults, and obesity in girls may have particularly grave implications for the escalation of the type 2 diabetes epidemic, as they are at higher risk of diabetes in pregnancy, which increases the risk of obesity and diabetes in their offspring.

Pathogenesis of Type 2 Diabetes

Most of the epidemiologic studies in developing countries measure only blood glucose, with insulin measured occasionally. The most commonly reported measurement of insulin resistance is the HOMA (homeostatic model assessment); β-cell function is rarely reported. This could have contributed to the (over)emphasis on insulin resistance as a cause of diabetes in the developing countries.

The risk factors for diabetes can be looked on as those contributing to susceptibility, those acting as precipitating factors, and those accelerating the metabolic deterioration and tissue damage (see Fig. 24.3). Obesity and central obesity precede type 2 diabetes by a long time, and they could be looked on as an intermediate phenotype. However, the mechanisms linking obesity and type 2 diabetes are not entirely clear.

■ Susceptibility to Diabetes

Susceptibility is usually ascribed to genetic factors in a polygenic model, with a strong role for environmental factors in the manifest disease. Genome-wide association studies in Europeans have revealed more than 10 markers, the majority of which affect beta cell function (Frayling 2007). The role of individual genes is likely to be small; the highest risk has been shown for variants in the *TCF7L2* gene (odds ratio 1.35), which has also been shown to be associated with diabetes in developing populations (Chandak et al. 2007). It is not yet clear whether the highly susceptible ethnic groups (who also qualify as developing populations, that is, Pima Indians,

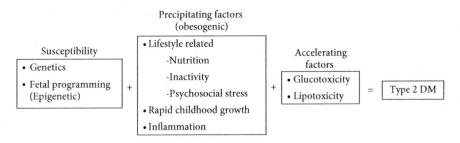

FIGURE 24.3. Risk factors for type 2 diabetes

Hispanics, and South Asian Indians) have a stronger genetic predisposition or if the same susceptibility genes function differently because of environmental influences. For example, the *Pro12Ala* polymorphism in the *PPAR-γ* gene does not protect Indians against type 2 diabetes (Radha et al. 2006), and the *FTO* gene seems to make a variable contribution to obesity and type 2 diabetes in Asians (Sanghera et al. 2008). Altered gene function due to environmental influences may be a key mechanism in the pathogenesis of type 2 diabetes, and the intrauterine period may be particularly important for such an effect (Yajnik 2007).

Hales and Barker made the key observation that low birth weight and thinness at birth (low ponderal index) are risk factors for type 2 diabetes (thrifty phenotype) (Hales and Barker 1992). This focused attention on the importance of intrauterine life as a determinant of later health. The association was confirmed in many other populations, including different ethnic groups in the United States, in the Chinese, in Afro-Caribbeans, and in some but not all studies in India. In Pima Indians the relationship was U-shaped; the contribution of large birth weight presumably reflected maternal diabetes (McCance et al. 1994). In Canadian Indians large birth weight was predictive of diabetes (Dyck, Klomp, and Tan 2001), and in South India diabetes was predicted by shorter length and higher ponderal index (Fall et al. 1998). These studies highlight the importance of intrauterine life and growth in determining risk of future diabetes and also suggest that birth weight may not be the most appropriate indicator of intrauterine exposures.

The link between intrauterine exposures and type 2 diabetes is explained by the concept of fetal programming (Yajnik 2007). A developing system (embryo and fetus) is plastic, that is, capable of taking any of many diverse routes and forms, but the intrauterine environment programs it along certain pathways that help the fetus survive and develop. This is achieved by alterations in structure and function, manifest in growth and body composition, β-cell function, tissue response to hormones, and vascular reactivity. Programming restricts the options for the fetus (predictive adaptive response) (Gluckman and Hanson 2004): if the environment in later life does not match the programming environment, the capabilities of the system may be exceeded and result in disease. The programming stimuli are only beginning to be understood: nutritional factors, metabolic and hormonal milieu, infections, and inflammation all seem to contribute. Given the orchestrated nature of embryonic development, there are windows of opportunity for programming of different systems and functions, and there may be some specificity for certain exposures.

Programming involves altered gene expression rather than a change in DNA sequence. Heritable modifications in the genome not associated with a change in the base sequence are called epigenetic (Robertson 2005). Periconceptional, embryonic, and fetal life are considered the most opportune times for epigenetic manipulation, although it may continue postnatally. Many of these changes are organ specific and contribute to differentiation and development. Methylation of cytosine residues in the CpG dinucleotide regions of DNA and acetylation of lysine residues of the

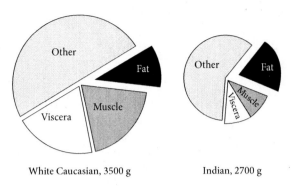

White Caucasian, 3500 g   Indian, 2700 g

FIGURE 24.4. A schematic diagram to compare body composition of Indian and white (UK) newborn babies. The Indian babies are approximately 800 g lighter and have less muscle but higher adiposity than the white babies

histones (responsible for chromatin structure) are two known mechanisms. The importance of methyl group donors in epigenetic programming has been demonstrated in animal models—Agouti mouse (Waterland and Jirtle 2003) and sheep (Sinclair et al. 2007).

For ethical reasons, epigenetic changes are difficult to demonstrate in the human fetus. However, measurements in Indian babies provide some support for possible structural and functional programming. Indian babies are among the smallest in the world: compared with white babies they are 800 g lighter, 4 cm shorter, and 3 ponderal units thinner. However, they have a higher percentage of body fat (adiposity), including higher central fat (abdominal subcutaneous as well as visceral) but smaller lean mass. Indian babies are thus "short-thin–fat" (see Fig. 24.4) (Yajnik et al. 2003). They also have higher concentrations of insulin and leptin in the cord blood but lower concentrations of adiponectin, thus demonstrating higher levels of risk factors for type 2 diabetes from their intrauterine life (Yajnik et al. 2002). Higher circulating homocysteine levels in Indian mothers predicted intrauterine growth restriction (Yajnik et al. 2005), and low maternal vitamin B12 status coupled with normal-to-high folate status predicted higher adiposity and higher insulin resistance in children at age 6 years (Yajnik et al. 2008b). These findings suggest that methyl group metabolism may be important in fetal programming in humans. In addition, they open new possibilities for intervention to prevent adiposity and insulin resistance and therefore prevent diabetes and related disorders.

Postnatal nutrition and growth also influence the risk of diabetes in low-birthweight children. Babies born small but who have grown big in childhood are more adipose, more insulin resistant, and have higher blood pressure and other cardiovascular risk factors (see Fig. 24.5) (Bavdekar et al. 1999). The role of rapid childhood growth in increasing risk of type 2 diabetes was shown in a prospective study in Delhi (Bhargava et al. 2004). Those who developed IGT and diabetes by age 28 years were lighter at birth, had poorer weight gain in the first 2 years of life, but had

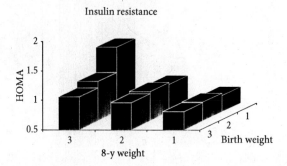

FIGURE 24.5. Mean levels of insulin resistance (HOMA) in 8-year-old children by tertiles of birth weight and 8-year weight. Those born the lightest but grown heaviest are the most insulin resistant. The figure highlights the effect of "rapid transition" in one's lifetime and depicts the effect of a double burden (early life undernutrition and subsequent overnutrition) in an individual

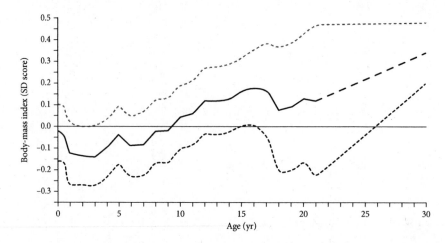

FIGURE 24.6. Mean sex-specific unadjusted SD scores for body-mass index according to age, for subjects in whom impaired glucose tolerance or diabetes developed. Solid line represents the mean SD score and the dash lines represents the 95% confidence intervals

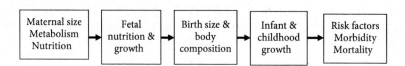

FIGURE 24.7. Current concept of the Developmental Origins of Health and Disease (DOHaD). The figure shows the influence of early life factors (including maternal factors and childhood growth) on the burden of type 2 diabetes and other noncommunicable disease

exaggerated weight gain from early childhood up to adult life compared with those with normal glucose tolerance (see Fig. 24.6). These ideas have led to a change in the nomenclature from "fetal origins" to "developmental origins of health and disease (DOHaD)" (see Fig. 24.7).

■ Complications of Diabetes

Younger age at diagnosis, delay in diagnosis due to poverty and lack of education, and inadequate treatment (due to socioeconomic factors and lack of facilities) contribute to the substantial problem of diabetic complications in developing countries. In African countries acute metabolic complications are still a major cause of death in diabetic patients (McLarty, Kinabo, and Swai 1990). Abnormalities associated with the metabolic syndrome exaggerate the vascular risk. In a population-based cross-sectional study in Chennai (India), 18% of diabetic patients had retinopathy, 6% had peripheral vascular disease, 2% had overt nephropathy, and up to 21% had some evidence of coronary artery disease (Mohan et al. 2007b). In Barbados the annual incidence of lower-extremity amputation is among the highest in the world—396/100,000 diabetic patients (Hennis et al. 2004). Diabetes is one of the leading causes of foot amputation, blindness, renal failure, and cardiovascular disease in many developing countries. The cost of treating these complications is prohibitive, and the necessary technology and expertise are not always available. There is therefore a greater need for basic and translational research in prevention of this disease.

■ Public Health Preventive or Intervention Strategies

Control and Prevention of the Diabetes Epidemic

Secondary and Tertiary Prevention

Given the huge scope and rapid escalation of the diabetes epidemic, all approaches to prevention (primary, secondary, and tertiary) need to be put into action simultaneously. More than 50% of diabetic people remain undiagnosed, and thus one priority is to diagnose as many patients as possible and treat them adequately. This will involve massive education of the public by innovative use of media. Diabetes risk scores individualized for populations could help to diagnose people at high risk (Mohan et al. 2005, 2007a), and use of glucometers and portable machines to measure hemoglobin A1C has facilitated the diagnosis of diabetes in remote areas where laboratory facilities are not available. Education of health workers is important to promote opportunistic screening. Adequate treatment of the newly diagnosed will necessitate the availability of antidiabetic medications in large quantities. Availability of insulin, especially in the African subcontinent, is a big problem, and many children with type 1 diabetes die due to lack of adequate insulin treatment (Beran and Yudkin 2006). Both governmental and nongovernmental agencies (including the pharmaceutical industry) need to bear the responsibility of providing adequate medication at an affordable price. Cost-effective, evidence-based use of drugs and restructuring existing price structures to contain costs, if need be by legislation, may become necessary.

Improved tertiary care to limit the disabilities from diabetic complications is the most expensive aspect of management. It is impossible for poorly funded public health services to meet these needs. Private health care systems in many countries offer this facility but at a considerable cost that is far beyond the reach of large sections of the population. The cost of treating diabetic complications is increasingly unbearable even for the rich countries in the world.

Venkat Narayan and colleagues, who assessed a number of the interventions for feasibility and cost-effectiveness in developing countries (Venkat Narayan et al. 2006), examined cost saving as well as difficulty in reaching the intervention population, technical complexity, capital intensity, and cultural acceptability. The most feasible and cost-effective interventions were (1) moderate glycemic control if the A1C was >9%, (2) blood pressure control if >160/95 mm Hg, and (3) foot care in people at high risk of ulcers.

Primary and Primordial Prevention

The rapidly escalating epidemic of diabetes that is taking place even with the widespread knowledge of its determinants suggests that far more efforts are needed to translate our knowledge into practice. Primary prevention strategy has included manipulation of dietary intake and physical activity to control weight and improve metabolism. The Cuban economic crisis between 1989 and 2000 is of interest in terms of the impact that population-wide interventions may have in developing countries (Franco et al. 2007). During the crisis there was a significant increase in physical activity (30%–67%) and a reduction in BMI (decrease of 1.5 units) with a subsequent reduction in deaths attributable to diabetes by 51%.

Results of recent trials in two developed countries, Finland (Tuomilehto et al. 2001) and the United States (Knowler et al. 2002), and in two developing countries, China (Pan et al. 1997) and India (Ramachandran A et al. 2006), show it is possible to improve glucose metabolism in people with IGT by modification of diet, increased physical activity, and the use of drugs. Although effective in the clinical trial setting, lifestyle modification is difficult to implement in communities. We may have to eventually consider drugs in public health interventions, but there are currently no cost-effective and safe medications as effective as lifestyle changes. The creation of diabetes education programs staffed by health care professionals trained in culturally relevant techniques for diabetes prevention may be one approach to solve this problem. Unfortunately these programs are typically poorly developed and not widely available in developing countries. In Latin America and the Caribbean, for instance, there are a few diabetes education programs, with the Pan American Health Organization (PAHO) Web site (*http://www.paho.org*) listing only 21 educational programs in 19 countries. No information on the efficacy or sustainability of these programs was available to the authors.

Research in novel methods to promote healthy diets, adequate physical activity, and reduction of psychosocial stress is urgently needed. In addition to scientific knowledge, the success of public health interventions depends on careful consideration of proximal determinants, which influence individual and societal behavior. Social, cultural, and political influences assume special importance. In addition, national and international market forces have far-reaching influences (Popkin 2006). The public health solution to the diabetes epidemic will thus involve a complex approach from various sources, including biomedical and social scientists, anthropologists, politicians, and governmental and nongovernmental agencies. In addition to education and empowerment of individuals, the solutions will involve structural changes involving home and neighborhood environments, roads, and public transport systems. Some of these might be achieved only through legislative changes, which are dictated by political will. Adoption of the diabetes resolution by the United Nations in 2006 is an important step in this direction (United Nations 2006).

Diabetes prevention clinical trials have been restricted to those with prediabetes, that is, those with IGT and those who are obese (this is the high-risk approach to prevention), which may divert attention from the real need of improving the health of the "sick societies" (Rose 1985). The trial subjects are usually in their postreproductive years, thus overlooking the benefits of the "life-course" interventions (see Figs. 24.8 and 24.9), including the opportunity to break the intergenerational cycle of diabetes. The changing epidemiology of type 2 diabetes, that is, the increasing affliction of the young and the poor, means that the current model will soon be inadequate. Admittedly, the "early-life" approach needs to be vigorously tested in humans, which is a challenge because it requires special expertise and patience. Such interventions will be necessarily of long duration, which breeds reluctance in the funding and political bodies. However, there can be little disagreement on the need to improve the health of young girls, a universal mandate based on the Millennium Development

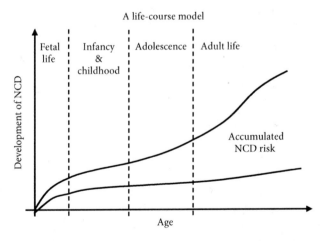

FIGURE 24.8. The World Health Organization's life-course model of noncommunicable disease. The model suggests that noncommunicable diseases have their origins in early life. The risk progressively accumulates throughout the life course, and the disease becomes manifest in later life

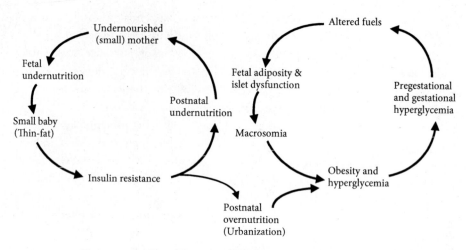

FIGURE 24.9. The interrelationship of two major maternal factors (undernutrition and overnutrition) in fetal programming. An undernourished mother produces a small (thin–fat) insulin-resistant baby. If this baby remains undernourished in postnatal life, the cycle is propagated. If the thin–fat insulin-resistant baby is overnourished it becomes obese and hyperglycemic. An obese and hyperglycemic mother produces a "macrosomic" baby at higher risk of obesity and hyperglycemia. Thus the intergenerational insulin resistance-diabetes cycle is propagated through a girl child. The two aspects of this cycle have been demonstrated in rural and urban India, respectively. Rapid transition shifts the balance from undernutrition to overnutrition and contributes to escalation of the diabetes epidemic. Improving the health of a girl child is of paramount importance in controlling the diabetes epidemic

Goals (United Nations 2000). A recently held UN hearing titled "Women, Diabetes and Development" (April 2008) provided a much-needed synthesis of the special effects that diabetes has on the health of women and on developing societies (United Nations 2008). This should provide an impetus to focus attention on this vital issue. Rapid transition in the developing world creates a special challenge of protecting the fetus from undernutrition ("nutrient-mediated teratogenesis" or thrifty phenotype) as well as inadvertent overnutrition as in obesity and gestational hyperglycemia ("fuel-mediated teratogenesis"). The importance of balanced nutrition and the role of micronutrient nutrition are increasingly apparent, and they call for education of nutritionists and the medical profession to avoid iatrogenic situations, such as may have arisen from overprescription of folic acid in a vitamin B_{12}-deficient population in India (Yajnik et al. 2008b). The current practice of screening for GDM in the third trimester of pregnancy (after a substantial part of fetal programming is over) may not only be inadequate but could also prove harmful to the growing fetus because the dietary restrictions in the mother may create a degree of fetal undernutrition (Jovanovic 2004). This is an important area of research. Again, improving the nutrition and metabolic health of young girls before pregnancy might hold the key.

Parents and caregivers tend to overfeed small babies to achieve normal growth. The growth charts are derived from the well-fed populations, and their use could promote rapid postnatal growth ("centile crossing"), with attendant risk of adiposity and diabetes. This is a priority area for research; there is a need to educate parents and caregivers about the dangers of rapid childhood growth.

In short, the control and prevention of diabetes in developing countries is a mammoth task, and it needs a pragmatic approach based on evidence. The life-course approach and intergenerational health are key concepts, and there is an urgent need to investigate relevant questions in each geographical area. We might have to wait for a few generations to see the "real" decline in incident diabetes.

■ Incidence and Trends of Type 1 Diabetes

The Multinational Project for Childhood Diabetes (DIAMOND) has reported age-adjusted incidence rates for type 1 diabetes (per year, analyzed per 100,000 children aged ≤14 years) from as low as 0.1 in China and Venezuela to as high as 37 in Sardinia and Finland (The DIAMOND Project Group 2006). Asian countries, with the exception of Kuwait, have very low incidence rates of type 1, with 70% having an incidence of <1/100,000 children/year. Among African populations, incidence rates vary between 1 and 9 per 100,000 children per year, whereas in Central America and the West Indies, these range from 2 to 17 per 100,000/year. The global trend for an increasing incidence rate is generally observed in the developing nations, with the exception of Central America and the West Indies.

Quality of Care

Perusal of the literature indicates that the quality of diabetes care is largely suboptimal in the developing world. The factors preventing optimal care include low household income, absence of trained educators, absence of governmental subsidies and support for the treatment of this chronic condition, lack of availability of insulin, and a lack of monitoring reagents and equipment (Alemu et al. 1998; Bassili et al. 2001; Beran and Yudkin 2006; Beran, Yudkin, and De Courten 2005; Elrayah et al. 2005; Ismail et al. 2000). The impact of delivering care in a diabetes center is amply demonstrated by data from Brazil, where patients treated by a multidisciplinary team had more than four times the likelihood of reaching target A1C levels as those being treated by individual endocrinologists (Mourao-Junior et al. 2006).

Complications and Mortality in Patients with Type 1 Diabetes from Developing Countries

The WHO initiated the DIAMOND complications study (DiaComp), which is a multinational, cross-sectional study of complications in type 1 diabetes (Walsh et al. 2005). In patients with a short duration of disease, a significantly higher prevalence of retinopathy was reported from South America and the former socialist economies of Eastern Europe countries than in patients from Northern Europe and the Mediterranean region. A similar trend was observed for microalbuminuria. In patients with disease of long duration the differences between the regions were not marked. Health system performance, as measured by gross national investment per capita, disability-adjusted life expectancy, and purchasing power, showed consistent correlations with complications. Every US$1000 increase in gross national investment per capita was associated with a 19% reduction in prevalence of reported retinopathy, 15% reduction in reported renal disease, and a 45% reduction in reported neuropathy. Data from Tanzania and India, countries not included in the DiaComp project, reaffirm the high rates of vascular complications reported from countries that had been studied as part of the DiaComp project. In Tanzanian patients with a median duration of type 1 diabetes of 3 years microalbuminuria and macroalbuminuria were observed in 12% and 1%, respectively (Lutale et al. 2007). Microproteinuria rates of 55%–73% and macroproteinuria rates of 9.7%–23.7% were reported in a group of Indian patients with type 1 diabetes (Miglani et al. 2004).

Even more disturbing are the mortality data from the developing world, especially from Africa. The life expectancy of a child with type 1 diabetes in rural Mozambique is as low as 7 months (Beran et al. 2005), and in one study only 1% of diabetic children survived 6 years in sub-Saharan Africa (Makame 1992). Other reports from sub-Saharan Africa indicate the estimated life expectancy of children with type 1 disease varies from 1.5 years in rural areas to 3.8 years in the capital, while that in adults varies from 2.9 years in the rural areas to 20 years in the capital city (Yudkin and Beran 2003). A major study from Zimbabwe followed newly diagnosed patients with diabetes and documented an inpatient mortality of 8% and an additional mortality of 41% in a 6-year follow-up, with most deaths being due to infection, hyperglycemic emergencies (ketoacidosis and nonketotic coma), or hypoglycemia (Castle and Wicks 1980). This contrasts with a 40% survival after 40 years in European patients. However, there has been improvement in some parts of Africa, with a study from Ethiopia reporting a 96% 5-year survival (Lester 1992). In contrast to data from Africa, a study from Israel demonstrated a standardized mortality ratio of 2.98 for type 1 patients (the reference population is set at 1.0), which is comparable to the developed economies of Europe (Laron-Kenet et al. 2001). These reports clearly demonstrate that mortality rates in some developing countries, especially parts of sub-Saharan Africa, are very much higher than in the developed world.

■ References

Abegunde DO et al. (2007). The burden and costs of chronic diseases in low-income and middle-income countries. *Lancet* **370**, 1929–38.

Abdulkadri AO, Cunningham-Myrie C, Forrester TF (2009). Economic Burden of diabetes and hypertension in CARICOM states. *Social and Economic Studies* **3 & 4**, 175–197.

Alemu S et al. (1998). Access to diabetes treatment in Northern Ethiopia. *Diabetic Medicine* **15**, 791–4.

Asao K et al. (2006). Short stature and the risk of adiposity, insulin resistance and type 2 diabetes in middle age: the Third National Health and Nutrition Examination Survey (NHANES III), 1988–1994. *Diabetes Care* **29**, 1632–7.

Aschner P (2002). Diabetes trends in Latin America. *Diabetes/Metabolism Research and Reviews* **18** (Suppl. 3), S27–31.

Balasubramanian K et al. (2003). High frequency of type 1B (idiopathic) diabetes in North Indian children with recent-onset diabetes. *Diabetes Care* **26**, 2697.

Barcelo A et al. (2003). The cost of diabetes in Latin America and the Caribbean. *Bulletin of the World Health Organization* **81**, 19–27.

Bassili A et al. (2001). The adequacy of diabetic care for children in a developing country. *Diabetes Research and Clinical Practice* **53**, 187–99.

Bavdekar A et al (1999). Insulin resistance in 8-year-old Indian children, small at birth, big at 8 years, or both? *Diabetes* **48**, 2422–9.

Beran D, Yudkin JS (2006). Diabetes care in sub-Saharan Africa. *Lancet* **368**, 1689–95.

Beran D, Yudkin JS, De Courten M (2005). Access to care for patients with insulin-requiring diabetes in developing countries: case studies of Mozambique and Zambia. *Diabetes Care* **28**, 2136–40.

Bhargava SK et al (2004). Relation of serial changes in childhood body-mass index to impaired glucose tolerance in young adulthood. *New England Journal of Medicine* **350**, 865–75.

Bhatia V et al. (2004). Etiology and outcome of childhood and adolescent diabetes mellitus in North India. *Journal of Pediatric Endocrinology and Metabolism* **17**, 993–9.

Castle WN, Wicks AC (1980). A follow-up of 93 newly diagnosed African diabetics for 6 years. *Diabetologia* **18**, 121–3.

Chandak GR et al. (2007). Common variants in the TCF7L2 gene are strongly associated with type 2 diabetes mellitus in the Indian population. *Diabetologia* **50**, 63–7.

Cunningham-Myrie C, Reid M, Forrester TE (2008). A comparative study of the quality and availability of health information used to facilitate cost burden analysis of diabetes and hypertension in the Caribbean. *West Indian Medical Journal* **57**, 383–92.

Dabelea D, Knowler WC, Pettitt DJ (2000). Effect of diabetes in pregnancy on offspring: follow-up research in the Pima Indians. *Journal of Maternal-Fetal Medicine* **9**, 83–8.

Deurenberg-Yap M et al. (2000). The paradox of low body mass index and high body fat percentage among Chinese, Malays, and Indians in Singapore. *International Journal of Obesity and Related Metabolic Disorders* **24**, 1011–7.

Dyck RF, Klomp H, Tan L (2001). From "thrifty genotype" to "hefty fetal phenotype": the relationship between high birthweight and diabetes in Saskatchewan Registered Indians. *Canadian Journal of Public Health* **92**, 350–4.

Elrayah H et al. (2005). Economic burden on families of childhood type 1 diabetes in urban Sudan. *Diabetes Research and Clinical Practice* **70**, 159–65.

Fall CH et al. (1998). Size at birth, maternal weight and type 2 diabetes in South India. *Diabetic Medicine* **15**, 220–7.

Franco et al. (2007). Impact of energy intake, physical activity, and population-wide weight loss on cardiovascular disease and diabetes mortality in Cuba, 1980–2005. *American Journal of Epidemiology* **166**, 1374–80.

Frayling TM (2007). Genome-wide association studies provide new insights into type 2 diabetes aetiology. *Nature Reviews. Genetics* **8**, 657–62.

Gaede P et al. (2003). Multifactorial intervention and cardiovascular disease in patients with type 2 diabetes. *New England Journal of Medicine* **348**, 383–93.

Gaede P et al. (2008). Effect of a multifactorial intervention on mortality in type 2 diabetes. *New England Journal of Medicine* **358**, 580–91.

Gaskin PS et al. (2008). Misperceptions, inactivity and maternal factors may drive obesity among Barbadian adolescents. *Public Health Nutrition.* **11**, 41–8.

Gaskin PS, Walker SP (2003). Obesity in a cohort of black Jamaican children as estimated by BMI and other measures of obesity. *European Journal of Clinical Nutrition* **57**, 420–6.

Gillies CL et al (2007). Pharmacological and lifestyle interventions to prevent or delay type 2 diabetes in people with impaired glucose tolerance: systematic review and meta-analysis. *British Medical Journal* **334**, 299–302.

Gluckman PD, Hanson MA (2004). Living with the past: evolution, development, and patterns of disease. *Science* **305**, 1733–6.

Gopalan C (1997). Diet related non-communicable diseases in South and South East Asia. In: Shetty PS, McPherson K, eds. *Diet, Nutrition and Chronic Disease: Lessons from a Contrasting World,* pp 10–23. London: John Wiley & Sons.

Goswami R et al. (2001). Islet cell autoimmunity in youth onset diabetes mellitus in Northern India. *Diabetes Research and Clinical Practice* **53**, 47–54.

Hales CN, Barker DJ (1992). Type 2 (non-insulin-dependent) diabetes mellitus: the thrifty phenotype hypothesis. *Diabetologia* **35**, 595–601.

Hennis A et al. (2002). Diabetes in a Caribbean population: epidemiological profile and implications. *International Journal of Epidemiology* **31**, 234–9

Hennis A, Fraser HS (2004). Diabetes in the English speaking Caribbean. *Revista Panamericana de Salud Publica* **15**, 90–3.

Hennis AJ et al. (2004). Explanations for the high risk of diabetes-related amputation in a Caribbean population of black African descent and potential for prevention. *Diabetes Care* **27**, 2636–41.

International Diabetes Federation (2006). *Diabetes Atlas*, 3rd ed. Brussels: IDF.

Ismail IS et al. (2000). Sociodemographic determinants of glycaemic control in young diabetic patients in peninsular Malaysia. *Diabetes Research and Clinical Practice* **47**, 57–69.

Jang HC et al. (1998). Short stature in Korean women: a contribution to the multifactorial predisposition to gestational diabetes mellitus. *Diabetologia* **41**, 778–83.

Jovanovic L (2004). Never say never in medicine: confessions of an old dog. *Diabetes Care* **27**, 610–2.

Kale SD et al. (2004). High risk of diabetes and metabolic syndrome in Indian women with gestational diabetes mellitus. *Diabetic Medicine* **21**, 1257–8.

Kim S, Moon S, Popkin BM (2000). The nutritional transition in South Korea. *American Journal of Clinical Nutrition* **71**, 44–53.

Knowler WC et al. (2002). Reduction in the incidence of type 2 diabetes with lifestyle intervention or metformin. *New England Journal of Medicine* **346**, 393–403.

Ko GT et al. (2002). Prevalence of gestational diabetes mellitus in Hong Kong based on the 1998 WHO criteria. *Diabetic Medicine* **19**, 80.

Kulkarni SR et al (2007). Determinants of incident hyperglycemia 6 years after delivery in young rural Indian mothers: the Pune Maternal Nutrition Study (PMNS). *Diabetes Care* **30**, 2542–7.

Laron-Kenet T et al. (2001). Mortality of patients with childhood onset (0–17 years) type 1 diabetes in Israel: a population-based study. *Diabetologia* **44** (Suppl. 3), B81–6.

Lester FT (1992). Clinical features, complications and mortality in type 1 (insulin-dependent) diabetic patients in Addis Ababa, Ethiopia, 1976–1990. *Quarterly Journal of Medicine* **83**, 389–99.

Lutale JJ et al. (2007). Microalbuminuria among Type 1 and Type 2 diabetic patients of African origin in Dar Es Salaam, Tanzania. *BMC Nephrology* **8**, 2.

Makame M (1992). Childhood diabetes, insulin, and Africa. DERI (Diabetes Epidemiology Research International) Study Group. *Diabetic Medicine* **9**, 571–3.

Martorell R et al. (1998). Obesity in Latin American women and children. *Journal of Nutrition* **128**, 1464–73.

Mather HM, Keen H (1985). The Southall Diabetes Survey: prevalence of known diabetes in Asians and Europeans. *British Medical Journal (Clinical Research ed.)* **291**, 1081–4.

Mbanya C et al. (1999). Standardised comparison of glucose intolerance in West African populations of rural and urban Cameroon, Jamaica, and Caribbean migrants to Britain. *Diabetes Care* **22**, 434–40.

Mbanya JC, Kengne AP, Assah F (2006). Diabetes care in Africa. *Lancet* **368**, 1628–9.

McCance DR et al. (1994). Birth weight and non-insulin dependent diabetes: thrifty genotype, thrifty phenotype, or surviving small baby genotype? *British Medical Journal* **308**, 942–5.

McLarty DG, Kinabo L, Swai AB (1990). Diabetes in tropical Africa: a prospective study, 1981–7. II. Course and prognosis. *British Medical Journal* **300**, 1107–10.

Mennen LI et al. (2001). Habitual diet in four populations of African origin: a descriptive paper on nutrient intakes in rural and urban Cameroon, Jamaica and Caribbean migrants in Britain. *Public Health Nutrition* **4**, 765–72.

Miglani S et al. (2004). Glycaemic control and microvascular complication among patients with youth onset diabetes in India using differing types of insulin and methods of glucose monitoring. *Diabetes Research and Clinical Practice* **65**, 183–5.

Misra A et al. (2007). The metabolic syndrome in South Asians: continuing escalation and possible solutions. *Indian Journal of Medical Research* **125**, 345–54.

Mohan V et al. (2005). A simplified Indian Diabetes Risk Score for screening for undiagnosed diabetic subjects. *Journal of the Association of Physicians of India* **53**, 759–63.

Mohan V et al. (2006). Secular trends in the prevalence of diabetes and impaired glucose tolerance in urban South India—the Chennai Urban Rural Epidemiology Study (CURES-17). *Diabetologia* **49**, 1175–8.

Mohan V et al. (2007a). A diabetes risk score helps identify metabolic syndrome and cardiovascular risk in Indians — the Chennai Urban Rural Epidemiology Study (CURES-38). *Diabetes, Obesity & Metabolism* **9**, 337–43.

Mohan V et al. (2007b). Epidemiology of type 2 diabetes: Indian scenario. *Indian Journal of Medical Research* **125**, 217–30.

Mourao-Junior CA 2nd et al. (2006). Glycemic control in adult type 1 diabetes patients from a Brazilian country city: comparison between a multidisciplinary and a routine endocrinological approach. *Arquivos Brasileiros de Endocrinologia e Metabologia* **50**, 944–50.

Omran AR (1971). The epidemiologic transition: a theory of the epidemiology of population change. *Milbank Memorial Fund Quarterly* **49**, 509–38.

Pan XR et al. (1997). Effects of diet and exercise in preventing NIDDM in people with impaired glucose tolerance. The Da Qing IGT and Diabetes Study. *Diabetes Care* **20**, 537–44.

Patterson PD et al. (2004). Obesity and physical activity in rural America. *Journal of Rural Health* **20**, 151–9.

Pettitt DJ et al. (1988). Congenital susceptibility to NIDDM. Role of intrauterine environment. *Diabetes* **37**, 622–8.

Poon-King T (1968). Prevalence and natural history of diabetes in Trinidad. *Lancet* **1**, 155–60.

Popkin B (2006). Global nutrition dynamics: the world is shifting rapidly toward a diet linked with noncommunicable diseases. *American Journal of Clinical Nutrition* **84**, 289–98

Popkin BM (2004). The nutrition transition: an overview of world patterns of change. *Nutrition Reviews* **62**, S140–3.

Radha V et al. (2006). Role of genetic polymorphism peroxisome proliferator-activated receptor-gamma2 Pro12Ala on ethnic susceptibility to diabetes in South-Asian and Caucasian subjects: evidence for heterogeneity. *Diabetes Care* **29**, 1046–51.

Ragoobirsingh D, Lewis-Fuller E, Morrison EY (1995). The Jamaican Diabetes Survey. A protocol for the Caribbean. *Diabetes Care* **18**, 1277–9.

Raj M et al. (2007). Obesity in Indian children: time trends and relationship with hypertension. *National Medical Journal of India* **20**, 288–93.

Ramachandran A (2005). Epidemiology of diabetes in India: three decades of research. *Journal of the Association of Physicians of India* **53**, 34–8.

Ramachandran A et al. (2001). High prevalence of diabetes and impaired glucose tolerance in India: National Urban Diabetes Survey. *Diabetologia* **44**, 1094–101.

Ramachandran A et al. (2002). Prevalence of overweight in urban Indian adolescent school children. *Diabetes Research and Clinical Practice* **57**, 185–90.

Ramachandran A et al. (2006). The Indian Diabetes Prevention Programme shows that lifestyle modification and metformin prevent type 2 diabetes in Asian Indian subjects with impaired glucose tolerance (IDPP – 1). *Diabetologia* **49**, 289–97.

Ramachandran A et al. (2008). High prevalence of diabetes and cardiovascular risk factors associated with urbanization in India. *Diabetes Care* **31**, 893–98.

Ramachandran P (2008). Changing food consumption patterns in India. *Nutrition Foundation of India Bulletin* **29**, 1–5.

Reddy KS et al. (2005). Responding to the threat of chronic diseases in India. *Lancet* **366**, 1744–9.

Registrar General and Census Commissioner (2006). Population Projections for India and States, Office of the Registrar General and Census Commissioner, New Delhi.

Robertson K (2005). DNA methylation and human disease. *Nature Reviews. Genetics* **6**, 597–610.

Rose G (1985). Sick individuals and sick populations. *International Journal of Epidemiology* **14**, 32–8.

Royle P, Bain L, Waugh N (2005). Systematic reviews of epidemiology in diabetes: finding the evidence. *BMC Medical Research Methodology* **5**, 2.

Sanghera DK et al. (2008). Impact of nine common type 2 diabetes risk polymorphisms in Asian Indian Sikhs: PPARG2 (Pro12Ala), IGF2BP2, TCF7L2 and FTO variants confer significant risk. *BMC Medical Genetics* **9**, 59.

Sawaya AL et al. (1995). Obesity and malnutrition in a Shantytown population in the city of Sao Paulo, Brazil. *Obesity Research* **3**, 107–15.

Seshiah V et al. (2004). Gestational diabetes mellitus in India. *Journal of the Association of Physicians of India* **52**, 707–11.

Seshiah V et al. (2007). Gestational diabetes mellitus manifests in all trimesters of pregnancy. *Diabetes Research and Clinical Practice* **77**, 482–4.

Sinclair KD et al. (2007). DNA methylation, insulin resistance, and blood pressure in offspring determined by maternal periconceptional B vitamin and methionine status. *Proceedings of the National Academy of Sciences of the United States of America* **104**, 19351–6.

Sobngwi E et al. (2001). Diabetes in Africans. Part 1: epidemiology and clinical specificities. *Diabetes and Metabolism* **27**, 628–34.

Sobngwi E et al. (2002). Diabetes in Africans. Part 2. Ketosis-prone atypical diabetes mellitus. *Diabetes Metabolism (Paris)* **22**, 5–12.

The DIAMOND Project Group (2006). Incidence and trends of childhood type 1 diabetes worldwide 1990–1999. *Diabetic Medicine* **23**, 857–66.

Tulloch JA (1961). *The prevalence of diabetes mellitus in Jamaica.* Diabetes 10, 286–8

Tuomilehto J et al (2001). Prevention of type 2 diabetes mellitus by changes in lifestyle among subjects with impaired glucose tolerance. *New England Journal of Medicine* **344**, 1343–50.

UNDP India (1998). Demographic transition in India 1998. Available at: www.undp. org.in/report/preidf. Accessed May 30, 2008.

United Nations (2000). Resolution adopted by the General Assembly 55/2. United Nations Millennium Declaration. Available at http://daccessdds.un.org/doc/UNDOC/GEN/N00/559/51/PDF/N0055951.pdf?OpenElement. Assessed May 30, 2008.

United Nations (2006). Resolution adopted by the General Assembly 61/225. World Diabetes Day. Available at: http://daccessdds.un.org/doc/UNDOC/GEN/N06/507/87/PDF/N0650787.pdf?OpenElement. Assessed May 30, 2008.

United Nations (2008). Diabetes, Women, and Development. Summary of the Meeting, Expert Recommendations for Policy Action, Conclusions and Follow-up Actions. New York: United Nations Headquarters.

Venkat Narayan KM et al. (2006). How should developing countries manage diabetes? *Canadian Medical Association Journal* **175**, 733–6.

Walsh MG et al. (2005). The socioeconomic correlates of global complication prevalence in type 1 diabetes (T1D): a multinational comparison. *Diabetes Research and Clinical Practice* **70**, 143–50.

Waterland RA, Jirtle RA (2003). Transposable elements: targets for early nutritional effects on epigenetic gene regulation. *Molecular Cell Biology* **23**, 5293–300.

WHO Expert Consultation (2004). Appropriate body mass index for Asian populations and its implications for policy and intervention strategies. Lancet **363**, 157–63.

WHO Global Infobase. Advanced Obesity Compare Tool. Available at http://www.who.int/infobase/report.aspx?rid=152. Accessed May 30, 2008.

Wild S et al. (2004). Global prevalence of diabetes: estimates for the year 2000 and estimates for year 2030. *Diabetes Care* **27**, 1047–53.

Wilks R et al. (1999). Diabetes in the Caribbean: results of a population survey from Spanish Town, Jamaica. *Diabetic Medicine* **16**, 875–83.

Wilks R et al. (2008). Jamacia Health and Lifestyle Survey 2007-08 Technical Report. Available at http://www.mona.uwi.edu/reports/health/JHLSII_final_may09.pdf. Accessed May 6, 2010.

Yajnik CS (2004a). Early life origins of insulin resistance and type 2 diabetes in India and other Asian countries. *Journal of Nutrition* **134**, 205–10.

Yajnik CS (2004b). Obesity epidemic in India: intrauterine origin? *Proceedings of the Nutrition Society* **63**, 387–96.

Yajnik CS (2007). Fetal programming of type 2 diabetes. *Diabetes Care* **30**, 2754–5.

Yajnik CS et al. (2002). Adiposity and hyperinsulinemia in Indians are present at birth. *Journal of Clinical Endocrinology and Metabolism* **87**, 5575–80.

Yajnik CS et al. (2003). Neonatal anthropometry: the thin–fat Indian baby. The Pune Maternal Nutrition Study. *International Journal of Obesity and Related Metabolic Disorders* **26**, 173–80.

Yajnik CS et al. (2005). Maternal total homocysteine concentration and neonatal size in India. *Asia Pacific Journal of Clinical Nutrition* **14**, 179–81.

Yajnik CS et al. (2008a). Adiposity, inflammation, insulin resistance and hyperglycaemia in rural and urban Indian men. *Diabetologia* **51**, 39–46

Yajnik CS et al. (2008b). Vitamin B12 and folate concentrations during pregnancy and insulin resistance in the offspring: the Pune Maternal Nutrition Study. *Diabetologia* **51**, 29–38.

Yudkin JS, Beran D (2003). Prognosis of diabetes in the developing world. *Lancet* **362**, 1420–1.

Yusuf S et al. (2001a). Global burden of cardiovascular diseases: part 1: general considerations, the epidemiologic transition, risk factors, and impact of urbanization. *Circulation* **104**, 2746–53.

Yusuf S et al. (2001b). Global burden of cardiovascular diseases: part II: variations in cardiovascular disease by specific ethnic groups and geographic regions and prevention strategies. *Circulation* **104**, 2855–64.

25. The Quality of Diabetes Care and the Prevention and Control of Diabetes in Developing Countries

An Illustration from India

Viswanathan Mohan and Rajendra Pradeepa

■ Main Public Health Messages

- Of the estimated 284.6 million people worldwide in 2010 who have diabetes, approximately 80% reside in developing countries.
- The high prevalence of diabetes in developing countries is attributed to rapid epidemiologic transition that has involved globalization, changes in dietary habits (due to Westernization), decreased physical activity, and fetal undernutrition.
- In general the quality of diabetes care is suboptimal worldwide, particularly in developing nations, where there are numerous barriers to delivering high-quality care. These include financial restrictions, lack of awareness, lack of knowledge about guidelines for care, lack of time for clinicians to spend with patients because of heavy patient loads, and lack of specialty care services.
- Quality of care can be accurately measured using structural, process, and outcome indicators; outcome indicators are the best but are often difficult and expensive to monitor.
- Targeted control of risk factors for diabetes at the population level might reduce the incidence of diabetes (primordial prevention), whereas identification of high-risk groups and effective lifestyle modification in persons with prediabetes can help in primary prevention of diabetes.
- There is a compelling need for broad-based, affordable, and effective community-based preventive programs in both urban and rural areas using lifestyle interventions to prevent diabetes.

- Ultimately, effectively tackling the diabetes epidemic calls for a multisectoral effort involving several departments of the government, nongovernmental organizations, and health care professionals as well as active community participation.

■ Introduction

Developing countries have about 80% of the world's diabetic population. In India the prevalence rates for diabetes in urban areas now approach figures reported for the more affluent migrant Indians living abroad. The epidemic is now shifting to rural areas, where diabetes care is neither available, accessible, nor affordable. This leads to significant morbidity and mortality associated with microvascular and macrovascular complications of diabetes. Luckily, a large body of evidence has shown that effective management and control measures could substantially reduce this burden. An issue of growing concern among diabetes care systems in developing countries is how to combat the current situation and deliver high-quality care while at the same time controlling costs. Unfortunately the quality of diabetes care generally remains suboptimal worldwide. This points to the need to develop and use standard measures of the quality of diabetes care, which will help to track whether diabetes management and control systems are in place in different countries. In addition, urgent preventive strategies should be introduced to reduce the diabetes epidemic, which threatens to overwhelm the economies of developing countries. These strategies should include primary, secondary, and tertiary prevention of diabetes, with a focus on the first two.

This chapter describes the present status of quality of diabetes care and how it can be measured in the context of developing countries. In addition, it assesses the prevention and control activities for diabetes and highlights some successful prevention strategies at the community level in India that can be used as a model for prevention of diabetes in other developing nations.

■ Background/Historical Perspective

Diabetes mellitus has a profound effect on national and individual economies as well as on the health of the individual and the society as a whole. According to the most recent estimates published in the *Diabetes Atlas 2009* by the International Diabetes Federation, of the estimated 284.6 million diabetic individuals in the world in 2010, approximately 80% resided in developing countries (Sicree, Shaw, and Zimmet 2009). This situation is expected to become steadily worse, as the number of individuals with diabetes is predicted to increase to 438.4 million by the year 2030. Unfortunately the largest increases will be seen in the developing countries (Sicree, Shaw, and Zimmet 2009). Moreover in contrast to developed countries, where diabetes predominantly affects older people, in developing nations it affects younger people in the prime of their working lives and thus poses an even greater threat to the economies of these nations.

The epidemic of diabetes will unfortunately be paralleled by a corresponding increase in the prevalence of its complications, both microvascular (retinopathy, nephropathy, and neuropathy) and macrovascular (cardiovascular disease and peripheral vascular disease), which account for much of the premature morbidity associated with this disease and often result in premature mortality. Diabetes and its complications also significantly reduce the quality of life and are responsible for enormous health care costs. Luckily, a large body of evidence has shown that effective management and control measures could substantially reduce this burden. However a marked variability has been documented in preventive and therapeutic approaches, suggesting that the level of diabetes care currently delivered may not be sufficient to bring about the expected health-related gains. According to the World Health Organization (WHO), almost a million people die because of diabetes each year, of whom two-thirds reside in developing countries (World Health Organization 2002). A recent study from India reported that all-cause mortality among persons with diabetes was 18.9 per 1000 person-years (age standardized: 6.3 per 1000 person-years) compared with 5.1 per 1000 person-years (age standardized: 4.4 per 1000 person-years) among persons without diabetes. Over 75% of the deaths among persons with diabetes were due to cardiovascular or renal causes (Mohan et al. 2006a).

Currently India has the largest number of people with diabetes in the world, estimated to be around 50.8 million in 2010, and this figure is projected to dramatically increase to 87 million by 2030 (see Fig. 25.1) (Sicree, Shaw, and Zimmet 2009). In urban areas of India prevalence rates now approach figures reported earlier among affluent migrant Indians living abroad (Mohan et al. 2006b). This change is due to rapid epidemiologic transition involving urbanization and industrialization,

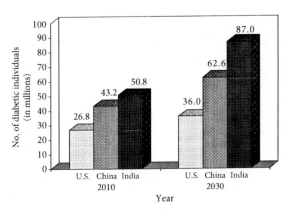

FIGURE 25.1 Estimated number of persons with diabetes in top three countries of the world (Source: Sicree, Shaw, and Zimmet 2009.)

leading to changes in dietary habits that include consumption of an unhealthy diet and sedentary lifestyles, such as decreased physical activity due to the increased use of energy-saving devices. Over the last two decades some of the unique phenotypic features in South Asians collectively called the "Asian Indian Phenotype" or "South Asian Phenotype" have been described (Joshi 2003; Deepa, Sandeep, and Mohan 2006). These include greater insulin resistance, increased central body adiposity despite lower body mass index (BMI), a characteristic dyslipidemia with low high-density lipoprotein cholesterol (HDL-C), increased triglycerides, and excess of small, dense low-density lipoprotein cholesterol (LDL-C), decreased adiponectin, and increased high-sensitivity C-reactive protein levels.

The noncommunicable disease risk factor surveillance recently carried out by the WHO and the Indian Council of Medical Research in six regions of India looked at urban–rural differences in the prevalence of risk factors for these diseases. The study, which developed estimates from self-reports, found that the overall frequency of diabetes was 4.5%. Urban areas had the highest prevalence (7.3%), followed by periurban/slum (3.2%) and rural areas (3.1%) (Mohan et al. 2008). The epidemic is now shifting to rural areas, where diabetes health care services are neither available nor affordable. Unless urgent preventive strategies are introduced, the diabetes epidemic could overwhelm the economies of developing countries such as India, as shown by a 2007 report in *The Economist* ("The Silent Epidemic").

Although effective treatment strategies to prevent or delay diabetes and its associated complications are now available, an issue of growing concern among diabetes care systems in developing countries is how to deliver high-quality care while at the same time controlling costs. If we are to translate science into clinical practice, we must first evaluate the quality of care that is being delivered. Unfortunately the quality of diabetes care generally remains suboptimal worldwide, regardless of a particular country's level of development, health care system, or population characteristics (Alberti, Boudriga, and Nabli 2007; Arday et al. 2002; Reed et al. 2005). This may be attributed to the various barriers to delivery of high-quality care, including financial restrictions and lack of awareness (patient-oriented barriers), lack of knowledge about guidelines and/or lack of time to spend with patients (provider-oriented barriers), and lack of specialty care services and long waiting times for utilization of services (system-oriented barriers). Low family income is one of the barriers to quality diabetes care, as reported in a study by Rayappa and coworkers (Rayappa et al. 1999), where annual family income below 10,000 rupees (approximately US$225) predicted poorer care. Another study, which evaluated the quality of care in known diabetic patients from the middle- and high-income populace of Delhi (Nagpal and Bhartia 2006), concluded that a wide gap exists between practice recommendations and delivery of diabetes care. A similar survey among physicians in Karachi treating the middle- and upper-income population showed inadequacies in physicians' knowledge and in the practice of optimal and acceptable diabetes care, and it recommended physician education as a priority in the developing world (Akhter 2007).

Studies have also shown that awareness and knowledge regarding diabetes among certain Indian subpopulations is very low (Deepa et al. 2005; Nagpal and Bhartia 2006). In addition, there is not enough time for primary care physicians to deliver the services currently recommended for management of chronic diseases, including diabetes (Østbye et al. 2005). Integrating specific features designed to facilitate care for diabetic patients within health care systems may reduce many of these barriers. Diabetes care centers with interdisciplinary team approaches, use of electronic diabetes records, and the use of clinical assistants and diabetes educators might help to ensure better diabetes outcomes (Narayan et al. 2006).

The quality of health care delivery can be assessed by examining several variables: the well-being and quality of life of patients, various clinical and biochemical parameters, and cost of the care delivered. All are important in chronic lifestyle diseases such as diabetes, where care, rather than cure, is the primary end point. Thus it is clear that there is a need for a set of standard measurements to deliver high-quality diabetes care.

■ Measurements of the Quality of Diabetes Care

Assessing the quality of diabetes care is of interest to clinicians, managed care organizations, regulatory agencies, and the public. Hence efforts to measure quality and find ways to improve it have been made by several agencies. Health care providers are now considered to be accountable for the quality of their services. This has resulted in the development of "performance and outcome measures," and a number of organizations have now started to use these measures. Typically, these measures are divided into process and outcome measures, and each measure has its own merits and demerits as discussed below (Donabedian 1980).

Process Measures

Process measures are the most frequently used indicators of quality, and those that have been clearly linked to good outcomes are naturally considered the best. The process indicator focuses on the activity of giving patients care, either directly or indirectly. Patient care functions, including clinical assessments and specific interventions, can be process indicators. Process indicators must be simple, economic, and easy to monitor and interpret. Simplicity suggests that indicators be few in number and readily understandable so that clinicians can focus on a few key targets for improvement. These indicators must also be easy to collect—preferably, built into the process of clinical record keeping—so that the data required are reliably and consistently collected.

Process measures assess whether providers follow predefined procedures for specific types of patients with specific health problems and needs. These procedures, such as treatments, interventions, and prescriptions, are supported by scientific evidence or have only limited scientific support but can be justified by practitioners. Examples of process measures include whether or how often certain diagnostic, preventive, and therapeutic procedures were performed (e.g., the frequency of hemoglobin A1C or microalbuminuria measurements, or eye examination for diabetic retinopathy at a diabetes center). These procedures are incorporated into practice guidelines that set particular standards of care, and they become part of a patient's plan of care. There are many practice guidelines that use process measures. It should be noted that process measures are used to evaluate compliance with guidelines, and outcomes measures (discussed below) are used to evaluate the value of the guidelines.

Certification/Accreditation

Certification/accreditation has been recognized as the gold standard for providing care at the highest level of quality. The process generally evaluates the characteristics of an organization or care provider. An example of this is a hospital or diabetes center applying for certification by the International Organization for Standardization (ISO) 9001 or the Joint Commission International (JCI) of the United States. The ISO 9000 series is an international set of quality standards laid down to bring about uniformity in practices and the documentation of systems in use in an organization. The various benefits of ISO certification in hospitals include standardizing and documenting procedures in various departments; interdepartmental integration and cooperation, which enhances patient satisfaction and services; better time management, which reduces the patient's waiting time; and taking preventive and corrective actions to maintain quality of care (Parvathi, Rema, and Mohan 2000). In addition the JCI is the gold standard for global health care standards for maintaining high levels of patient care and safety (the Joint Commission is the largest accreditor of health care organizations in the United States). Other measures could include accreditation of a laboratory by an organization such as College of American Pathologists (CAP); CAP-accredited laboratories are widely accepted as reference laboratories. Certification of a dietician/nurse as a certified diabetes educator (CDE) is another example of giving a provider a stamp of quality. However, the certification process is usually lengthy and expensive and hence beyond the reach of many institutions/individuals in developing countries.

Implementation of Guidelines for Diabetes Care

Since the publication of the results of the Diabetes Control and Complications Trial (DCCT) and the United Kingdom Prospective Diabetes Study (UKPDS) (Diabetes Control and Complications Trial Research Group 1993; UK Prospective Diabetes Study [UKPDS] Group 1998), there has been considerable interest worldwide in improving the quality of care for diabetic patients. However, trying to apply the results of such clinical trials to real-life situations involves huge challenges. Tight control of diabetes requires frequent testing, more visits to the doctor, and the use of appropriate medications and devices, all of which have tremendous cost implications. Regardless, the results of the DCCT and the UKPDS have led several organizations to formulate guidelines for improving the quality of diabetes care in the United States and United Kingdom. These include the American Diabetes Association (ADA), the National Diabetes Quality Improvement Alliance in the United States, and the National Institute for Clinical Excellence (NICE) in the United Kingdom. The ADA has promulgated evidence-based guidelines for diabetes care that, if met, would have a major impact on reducing the rising burden of diabetic complications (guidelines are available online at http://care.diabetesjournals. org/content/vol30/suppl_1/). The new NICE diabetes guidelines include recommendations to health professionals in the United Kingdom on how to manage the treatment and care of adults and children with type 1 diabetes. The National Diabetes Quality Improvement Alliance, which is a collaborative effort of 13 private and public national organizations, has developed a performance measurement set for improving the quality of diabetes care.

Some of the reasons stated for poor adherence to guidelines are that (1) physicians are unaware of, or do not understand, the rationale behind the guideline and that (2) patients refuse to undergo recommended interventions. Litzelman and Tierney (1996) reported that the failure of physicians to comply with guidelines for preventive care starts from "system" factors, including physicians not being able to recall screening guidelines in the midst of a busy primary care clinic, lack of time to carry out recommended procedures, and a lack of resources.

In developing nations such guidelines may not even be available. In India a set of guidelines for management of type 2 diabetes was developed by the Indian Council of Medical Research with the support of WHO (available online at http:// www.icmr.nic.in/guidelines_diabetes/guide_diabetes.htm).

Recently WHO and the International Diabetes Federation have updated the guidelines for the definition, diagnosis, and classification of diabetes and intermediate hyperglycemia; the new guidelines reflect the evolving body of knowledge of the relationship between blood glucose levels and adverse health outcomes (available online at http://www.idf.org/webdata/docs/WHO_IDF_definition_diag nosis_of_diabetes.pdf). Several other agencies in diabetes-related fields from different parts of the world have come out with similar guidelines that are specific to their part of the world.

Outcome Measures

Outcome measures are undoubtedly the best measures of the quality of care. These need not be final outcomes, however; interim outcome measures, such as glycemic control, are often used. Outcome measures, which are of greater intrinsic interest than process measures, can reflect all aspects of care. Outcome indicators are particularly useful for improving care when they direct caregivers to the processes that contribute to the outcomes. They also help establish priorities by highlighting processes that are particularly troublesome and contribute to poor outcomes. For example, the patient's age, severity of illness, socioeconomic situation, and comorbid conditions all potentially influence clinical outcome. Outcome indicators can be improved if efforts are made to standardize data collection and systems to adjust for case mix are developed and validated.

Over the last decade many efforts have been initiated to assess the quality of diabetes care. In 1997 the Diabetes Quality Improvement Program (DQIP), initiated in the United States, identified "standardized" uniform performance measures for diabetes care that conformed to a national consensus on the assessment of care (Fleming et al. 2001).

These measures retrospectively assess the level of care delivered across the diabetic population using a standardized and systematic approach. The aim of the DQIP was to develop a measurement set that is feasible, reliable, and suitable for uniform application across health care systems, which calls for organizational, financial, and logistical support. The DQIP's recommendations published in 1998 included two sets of measures: an accountability set and a quality-improvement set. The first set of measures, which is evidence based, has received consensus support from the scientific and medical community and has been field-tested. The measures were initially proposed to be used to compare health plans or providers and were chosen to avoid the need to adjust for case mix. The second set of measures, that is, those for quality improvement, was recommended for providing internal information on performance due to concerns about methodology or feasibility. In 2000 a set of patient survey-derived measures (counseling on smoking cessation, self-management, nutritional education, satisfaction, interpersonal skills of the health care team, and functional status) was added after being extensively field-tested (see Table 25.1) (Fleming et al. 2001).

The DQIP has shown that assessing the quality of diabetes care is feasible, at least in the United States. In Asia the Diabcare-Asia project, modeled after a project conducted in Europe several years ago (DIABCARE project), was designed to provide large-scale, yet simple, standardized information about patient characteristics and the care received from 230 diabetes centers in Bangladesh, People's Republic of China, India, Indonesia, Malaysia, Philippines, Singapore, South Korea, Sri Lanka, Taiwan, Thailand, and Vietnam in 1998 (Chuang et al. 2002). The objectives of the project were to describe as well as to investigate the relationship between diabetes control, diabetes management, and complications status in the diabetes centers of each participating country. The data, although subject to referral bias, was at least collected using similar methods and during the same time frame from India, Singapore, and Taiwan. This study showed that 32% to 50% of the diabetic population had poor glycemic control (A1C > 8%), 43% to 67% had high cholesterol (>5.2 mmol/dL), and 47% to 54% had an abnormal level of triglycerides (>1.7 mmol/dL) as depicted in Table 25.2 (Chuang et al. 2001; Lee et al. 2001; Raheja et al. 2001).

In the Diabcare-Asia project the overall mean A1C value measured in a central laboratory among all the diabetic subjects from various countries was 8.6%. The mean A1C values measured centrally in Bangladesh (7.9%), Indonesia (8.1%),

TABLE 25.1 *Set of Measures in the Diabetes Quality Improvement Project*

Accountability Measures* (Quantity Assessment)	Quality Improvement Measures* (Quality Assessment)
Collected from Medical Records or Electronic Data	
Percentage of Diabetic Population Having	Evaluation for
Glycated hemoglobin (A1C) tested annually Poor glycemic control (A1C > 9.5%)	Distribution of A1C levels (<7.0%, 7.0%–7.9%, 8.0%–8.9%, 9.0%–9.9%, ≥10.0%, or undocumented).
Lipid profile test (biennially) Lipids controlled (LDL <130 mg/dL)	Distribution of LDL values (<100, 100–129, 130–159, >159 mg/dL, or undocumented).
Blood pressure controlled (<140/90 mm Hg)	Distribution of BP values (systolic: <140, 140–159, 160–179, 180–200, >200 mm Hg; diastolic: <90, 90–99, 100–119, >119 mm Hg, or undocumented).
Nephropathy assessment High risk (annually) Low risk (biennially)	
Dilated eye examination high risk (annually) Low risk (biennially)	
Foot examination (annually)	
Data from patient survey	
Smoking cessation counseling	Diabetes self-management and nutrition education Interpersonal care

*All measures apply to type 1 and type 2 diabetic patients between 18 and 75 years of age.
LDL, low-density lipoprotein; BP, blood pressure.
Source: Fleming et al. (2001).

Malaysia (8.4%), Korea (8.0%), and Taiwan (8.1%) were significantly lower than the overall mean of 8.6%, whereas those of China (8.8%), India (8.9%), Philippines (8.9%), and Vietnam (8.9%) were significantly higher than the overall mean. The mean central A1C of patients from Sri Lanka and Thailand did not differ significantly from the overall mean (Chuang et al. 2002). In Korea data collected from 1170

TABLE 25.2 *Studies of the Quality of Diabetes Care in Selected Asian Countries—DIABCARE-Asia Project (1998)*

Study Characteristics	Country		
	Singapore* (n = 1697)	India[†] (n = 2269)	Taiwan[‡] (n = 2446)
Type of sites	General hospitals and primary health care centers	Tertiary diabetes care centers	General hospitals and primary health care centers
Total sites (n)	22	26	25
Type 2 diabetes (%)	91.4	90.6	97
Mean age (yrs)	58.1 ± 14.4	54 ± 13	61.6 ± 11.3
Mean duration of diabetes (yrs)	10.1 ± 7.5	10 ± 6.9	10.3 ± 7.3
Level of Care			
Fasting blood sugar (FBS)			
FBS (mmol/L)	9.1 ± 3.1	8.3 ± 3.3	9.0 ± 3.3
FBS >7.8 mmol/L (%)	61	50	59
Glycated hemoglobin (A1C)			
Mean (%)	8.0 ± 1.9	8.9 ± 2.1	8.1 ± 1.6
A1C >2% of normal range (%)	32	50	35
Lipids			
Total cholesterol >5.2 (mmol/L)	67	46	43
Triglycerides >1.7 (mmol/L)	48	54	47

Sources of data: *Lee et al. (2001); [†]Raheja et al. (2001); [‡]Chuang et al. (2001).

diabetic patients from 21 centers (one university hospital and 20 clinics) showed a mean A1C of 7.3% at the hospital and 7.5% at the clinics, and the mean fasting plasma glucose (FPG) levels were 7.0 mmol/L at the hospital and 7.9 mmol/L at the clinics. About 40% of patients had an A1C and an FPG above the normal upper limits (Rhee et al. 2005).

In 2001 the Diabetes Care Excellence Project (DCEP) was set up through the joint efforts of seven diabetes clinics in as many countries (Australia, Austria, Denmark, Germany, India, the Netherlands, and the United States) to document the standards/definitions used at different centers and to assess the feasibility of collecting and comparing data on the quality of diabetes care in real-life settings. The six parameters (glycemic control, lipid profile, hypertension, renal assessment, foot examination, and eye examination) were standardized for all clinics through the specification of quantity and quality measures (disregarding local standards). Patients had to be at least 18 years old, diagnosed as having type 1 or type 2 diabetes, and seen as part of a regular visit in the clinic. The DCEP guidelines are presented in Table 25.3 (Mohan and Hansen, on behalf of the DCEP Group 2001).

Applicability of Measures of Quality to Developing Countries

It is clear from the evidence presented to this point that the quality of diabetes care can now be accurately assessed. However to obtain effective outcomes we must put

TABLE 25.3 *Guidelines for the Diabetes Care Excellence Project*

Parameters	Quality Measures	Quantity Measures
Glycemic control (A1C)	At least one measurement of A1C per year.	$A1C \leq 9.5\%$.
Lipid profile (LDL cholesterol)	At least one biannual measurement of LDL cholesterol (for patients aged 18–75 years).	LDL cholesterol ≤ 130 mg/dL (for patients aged 18–75 years).
Hypertension (blood pressure)	At least one measurement of BP in the past year.	BP < 140/90 mm Hg during the last year.
Renal (microalbuminuria)	One annual screening for microalbuminuria.	—
Foot examination	At least one foot examination in the past year (for patients aged 18–75 years).	—
Eye examination	At least one retinal examination in the past year.	—

LDL, low-density lipoprotein; BP, blood pressure.
Source: Mohan and Hansen (2001).

the measures for measuring quality into practice. Unfortunately, high-quality data on diabetes care are not available for most developing countries.

To make the available medical knowledge and measures of the quality of diabetes care more functional, networking between diabetes centers within the developing countries, preferably in the form of electronic records, can be adopted, as in the case of the Dr. Mohan's Diabetes Specialities Centre (formerly M. V. Diabetes Specialities Centre) model in India, where currently five to six centers in different geographic areas in India are linked through electronic medical records and video conferencing facilities (www.drmohansdiabetes.com). Such networking of clinical databases offers many advantages, such as improved recognition of patterns, interaction with patients, being able to provide tailored health information to patients, and database development based on secondary evidence. Currently, however, not many diabetes centers have electronic databases, and where available, they may not be compatible. Some studies have shown that electronic management systems improve performance outcomes (e.g., carrying out the tests) but not necessarily metabolic outcomes (e.g., better glycemic control, lower blood pressure) (O'Connor et al. 2005).

■ Implications for Health Policy

Diabetes care is different from most other types of medical care in that it is mostly preventive. The prevention of and targeted control of its risk factors could potentially reduce the disease's impact in the developing world. Prevention is classified as primordial, primary, secondary, or tertiary based on the natural history of the disorder (see Fig. 25.2). Primordial prevention involves efforts to prevent the risk factors themselves (e.g., trying to decrease the development of obesity, increase exercise or physical activity, or provide a well-balanced diet) in a community. Primary prevention targets the prevention of diabetes itself by identifying prediabetes through screening programs. Secondary prevention refers to preventing the complications of diabetes by good diabetes control. Tertiary prevention seeks to prevent the worsening of complications to a late stage in those in the early stages of complications; it also involves the offering of rehabilitation measures to those in more advanced stages of the disease.

Primordial Prevention

The clear distinction between primordial and primary prevention lies in the fact that primordial prevention takes place in the community and thus outside the physician-patient relationship and the medical model. But the implementation of primordial prevention in the community raises several unanswered questions: Who would benefit from diabetes prevention? Are such approaches possible at the community level? How will the community respond to such approaches? How should

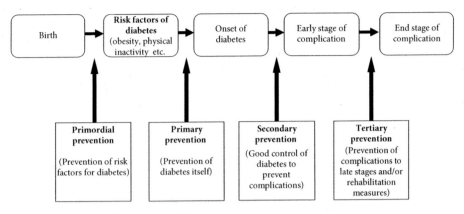

FIGURE 25.2 Levels of prevention of diabetes

results be extrapolated from developed countries to developing countries, where the priorities and approaches may be different?

There are lessons from studies conducted in south India that demonstrate that community-based interventions are not only feasible but are also welcomed by the community (Mohan et al. 2006c). The results of a population-based study, the Chennai Urban Population Study, which involved two residential areas representing the middle- and lower-income groups in Chennai (one of India's largest cities), clearly demonstrated that with affluence, which was invariably associated with decreased physical activity, there was a marked increase in the prevalence rate of diabetes (Mohan et al. 2001; Mohan, Shanthirani, and Deepa 2003). Residents of the area with the higher prevalence of diabetes and greater obesity rate were empowered and motivated to increase physical activity. This led to the residents themselves raising money to build a beautiful park and also to maintain it through a modest annual contribution. A follow-up survey demonstrated that the construction of the park led to a 300% increase in the number of people who exercised in this community (Mohan et al. 2006c). This is a demonstration of the power of community empowerment and has been highlighted in the WHO publication *Preventing Chronic Disease—A Vital Investment* in the section entitled "Improving the built environment in India," where this has been showcased as a model for prevention of noncommunicable diseases in developing countries (World Health Organization Report 2005). Such activities soon spread to other parts of Chennai and finally led to over 200 parks being developed in Chennai through public and governmental efforts. If this model can be replicated, it could lead to prevention not just of type 2 diabetes but of noncommunicable diseases in general.

The U.S. Centers for Disease Control and Prevention (CDC) has reported that screening for undiagnosed diabetes or prediabetes in the general population may be worthwhile, especially for those with risk factors for other chronic diseases, such as hypertension and dyslipidemia (U.S. Centers for Disease Control and Prevention 1998). Along these lines, a massive community-based diabetes prevention program has been initiated in Chennai involving over a million people (Suresh et al. 2005). The Prevention, Awareness, Counseling and Evaluation (PACE) Diabetes Project involves large-scale awareness programs, cost-effective screening for diabetes and prediabetes, and a large community-based diabetes prevention program involving physical activity and yoga. Massive screening camps were undertaken in educational institutions, such as schools and colleges, religious places such as churches, mosques, and temples, in banks, and elsewhere. In addition periodic public awareness campaigns, camps to modify lifestyle and diet, and health exhibitions were organized to empower the community regarding diabetes and its ravages. Furthermore, optimal treatment of diabetes was provided through a network of general practitioners trained in diabetes care. Activities such as the PACE Diabetes Project are expected to have a profound and immediate benefit to the community, as it is a public health initiative aimed at reducing the health, social, and economic burden imposed by diabetes.

It is a paradox that nearly all efforts directed at diabetes in developing countries are currently focused in urban areas, with virtually no prevention or awareness activities in rural areas. In the rural areas activities to control diabetes are a challenge, as awareness levels and accessibility to diabetes care remain woefully inadequate. This inevitably leads to a delay in diagnosis and inadequate management of diabetes and its associated complications. To serve as a model for the 72% of India's population that lives in rural areas and to track the burden of diabetes and make innovative health care available, accessible, and affordable to the rural population of Tamil Nadu (one of India's 28 states), a rural diabetes project has been started by the Madras Diabetes Research Foundation supported by the World Diabetes Foundation in the Chunampet village cluster 110 km (68.4 miles) from Chennai. Innovative real-time "interactive teaching" with empowerment of the community is being conducted with the support of National Agro Foundation, a local nongovernmental organization whose major thrust is increasing farm productivity and training of the youth to improve the living standards of rural poor with income-generating schemes. A mobile van provides diabetes care services using telemedicine facilities for the diagnosis and management of diabetes complications, particularly diabetic retinopathy. The Indian Space Research Organization, Bangalore (one of Southern India's most populous cities), supports this project by providing connectivity to satellites. This project is already improving the diabetes care of rural people who hitherto had no access to diabetes care. The Chunampet model is an example of intersectoral collaboration involving areas of health, agriculture, and the community; this is an excellent model for replication in other parts of India and other developing countries to enhance the economic, social, and health status of rural communities.

Primary Prevention

Evidence from the West suggests that lifestyle changes (primary prevention) could prevent and/or delay the onset of type 2 diabetes in high-risk groups by approximately 58% over 3 to 4 years by changes in lifestyle that involve incorporation of physical activity and appropriate nutrition (Knowler et al. 2002; Tuomilehto et al. 2001). The Indian Diabetes Prevention Programme has also shown that diabetes is preventable by lifestyle modification and to a lesser extent by treatment with metformin. The reduction in the relative risk of diabetes was 28.5% with lifestyle modification, 26.4% with metformin, and 28.2% with lifestyle modification plus metformin when the referent was the control group (Ramachandran et al. 2006). Thus the reduction in relative risk with lifestyle modification was less in the Indian Diabetes Prevention Programme than in the Diabetes Prevention Program in the United States and the Finnish Diabetes Prevention Study (58% in both) (Knowler et al. 2002; Tuomilehto et al. 2001). These successful trials, conducted over the past decade to prevent type 2 diabetes, have used clinic-based approaches targeting high-risk groups. However data on community-/population-based prevention strategies are sparse, and implementation strategies are not well-defined. Moreover, these trials have raised new issues of translating the findings into practice at the community level and in a real-life setting.

One of the major steps in primary prevention is empowering the community by increasing its awareness of diabetes. Very few studies, however, have assessed knowledge levels about diabetes in a community setting within a developing country. In a large study done at Chennai (which is in southern India), we found that 25% of urban residents were not aware of a condition called diabetes, over 88% were unaware that obesity and physical inactivity could predispose to diabetes, and only 25% knew that the most common form of diabetes was preventable (Deepa et al. 2005). Corresponding rural figures would obviously be far worse.

The excess of undiagnosed diabetes in developing countries could be attributed to lack of access to care, lack of awareness (on the part of patient or provider), inertia or inaction of the provider, or something else. Regardless, an estimated 50% of diabetes in urban areas and 60% to 70% of diabetes in rural areas remains undiagnosed. This calls for widespread screening programs for identifying undiagnosed diabetes. Additionally, in developing countries, the prevalence of impaired glucose tolerance is consistently higher than the diabetes prevalence rates (Mohan, Shanthirani, and Deepa 2003; Shera et al. 1999), which substantiates the continuing growth of the diabetes pandemic. There is thus a huge window of opportunity to prevent diabetes itself through specific activities, including effective screening for prediabetes and introducing lifestyle changes at a population level. However performing blood glucose measurements would be expensive and a logistic nightmare, even if funds were available. This calls for cost-effective tools to detect those with undiagnosed diabetes and prediabetes. Ethnicity-specific diabetes risk scores have proved to be a good method for cost-effective screening (Mohan et al. 2005; Ramachandran et al. 2005). It has been shown that a simple Indian Diabetes Risk Score using just four questions and a waist measurement not only identifies undiagnosed diabetes and prediabetes (Mohan et al. 2005) but also helps identify subjects with metabolic syndrome and cardiovascular disease among those with normal glucose tolerance (Mohan et al. 2007). Thus, even those individuals with normal glucose tolerance but a high Indian Diabetes Risk Score should be targeted for prevention of diabetes.

Community-based studies of primary prevention that use lifestyle interventions are essential. In addition, it is mandatory to study the long-term effects of diabetes prevention on rates of heart disease, stroke, and other important outcomes whose risk is increased by diabetes and to find cheaper and more effective ways to prevent such major complications as blindness, kidney failure, and lower-extremity amputation. Thus, there is a compelling need for broad-based, affordable, and effective community-based preventive programs. Such programs can only succeed if there is community empowerment, however. Empowering the community with appropriate information on diabetes and its complications could potentially result in increased knowledge of this widespread disease, which will help individual men and women in taking care of their own, their family's, and their community's health.

Recent research shows a clear link between health, physical activity, and the "built environment" (Berrigan and Troiano 2002). This last term refers to roads, buildings, parks, and other structures that physically define a community. Table 25.4 shows examples of how the urban environment can be reengineered to promote healthy living. It is thus clear that prevention of type 2 diabetes is not a health sector issue alone but instead involves a multisectoral collaboration. This calls for a coherent and well-planned approach, as most developing countries have inadequate funds and resources. Clearly, the leading role for this multisectoral approach to tackling the diabetes burden in developing countries must be played by the ministry of health. However, other governmental departments, including education, social welfare, finance, transport, culture, and sport and youth affairs, in addition to nongovernmental organizations and religious, family, and community welfare organizations, should all work together. Only such a concerted effort would lead to a successful diabetes prevention program as shown in Figure 25.3.

TABLE 25.4 *Redesigning the Urban Environment to Promote Physical Activity*

Environment	How to Redesign
Public utilities	• Construct parks. • Construct walking/cycling lanes. • Provide provisions for sports, fitness, and recreational facilities.
Workplace	• Provide well-lit wide stairs in multistoried buildings in addition to escalators. • Provide spaces for outdoor and indoor games. • Construct gyms.
Schools	• Provide playground facilities and/or indoor stadium.

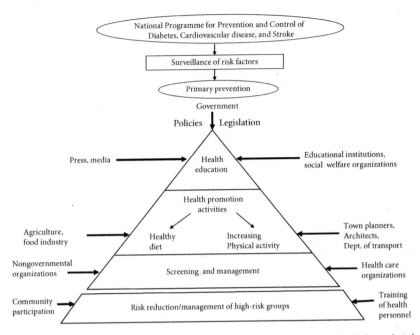

FIGURE 25.3. Multisectoral collaboration—a concerted effort to reduce the diabetes burden in developing countries

■ Areas of Uncertainty or Controversy

Health care in general is a dynamic, growing enterprise; the quality of that enterprise is equally dynamic. Quality in these circumstances remains a major challenge that rests on two basic concepts: appropriate processes of care and patient outcomes or end results of care. Given the substantial public health burden of diabetes, improving care for persons with diabetes should be relevant in the majority of communities and health care systems. They should strive to improve glycemic control, decrease diabetes complications and mortality, and improve quality of life. One area of controversy is concerned with using process versus clinical outcome measures. Much more research may be needed to examine the link between performance on process measures and outcomes of care for diabetic patients.

Another major problem in current diabetes care is the poor translation of knowledge derived from clinical research into routine clinical practice (Berger 1996). Thus, to improve standards and outcomes of diabetes care, efforts in the following areas appear vital: diagnostic procedures and therapeutic management must be evidence based; patients need to become more actively involved in their disease management; and every center/geographic area needs to perform quality assessment based on patient-oriented outcomes.

■ Developments over the Next 5 to 10 Years

Diabetes is likely to remain a huge threat to public health in the years to come. The explosion of the diabetes epidemic in developing regions of the world, combined with the significant morbidity and mortality imposed by its complications, underscores the need for increased focus on prevention and control programs and on developing the necessary resources to tackle this problem. The success of any diabetes prevention and control program ultimately depends on active community participation. However, this will not become a reality unless governments and public health planners use the available evidence-based data to address the challenges of the growing diabetes problem. Luckily, simple interventions that could help prevent diabetes among those at high risk are available and effective. More proactive steps should be taken in developing countries to restructure health policies, with emphasis on prevention of diabetes and improving the quality of diabetes care in those who are already afflicted with the disorder.

■ References

Akhter J (2007). Quality of diabetes care and management of general physicians in Karachi, Pakistan: response to Nagpal and Bhartia. *Diabetes Care* **30** (4), e27.

Alberti H, Boudriga N, Nabli M (2007). "Damm Sokkor": factors associated with the quality of care of patients with diabetes: a study in primary care in Tunisia. *Diabetes Care* **30**, 2013–8.

Arday DR et al. (2002). Variation in diabetes care among states. *Diabetes Care* **25**, 2230–7.

Berger M (1996). To bridge science and patient care in diabetes. *Diabetologia* **39**, 749–57.

Berger M, Mühlhauser I (1999). Diabetes care and patient-oriented outcomes. *JAMA* **281**,1676–8.

Berrigan D, Troiano RP (2002). The association between urban form and physical activity in U.S. adults. *American Journal of Preventive Medicine* **23** (2 Suppl.), 74–9.

Chuang LM et al. (2001). The current state of diabetes management in Taiwan. *Diabetes Research and Clinical Practice* **54** (Suppl. 1), S55–65.

Chuang LM et al. (2002). The status of diabetes control in Asia—a cross-sectional survey of 24,317 patients with diabetes mellitus in 1998. *Diabetic Medicine* **19**, 978–85.

Deepa M et al. (2005). Awareness and knowledge of diabetes in Chennai—the Chennai Urban Rural Epidemiology Study [CURES - 9]. *Journal of the Association of Physicians of India* **53**, 83–7.

Deepa R, Sandeep S, Mohan V (2006). Abdominal obesity, visceral fat and type 2 diabetes— "Asian Indian Phenotype." In: Mohan V, Rao GHR, eds. *Type 2*

Diabetes in South Asians: Epidemiology, Risk Factors and Prevention, pp 138–52. New Delhi: Jaypee Brothers Medical Publishers (P) Ltd.

Diabetes Control and Complications Trial Research Group (1993). The effect of intensive treatment of diabetes on the development and progression of long-term complications in insulin-dependent diabetes mellitus. *New England Journal of Medicine* **329**, 977–86.

Donabedian A (1980). *The definition of quality and approaches to its assessment.* Ann Arbor, MI: Health Administration Press.

Fleming BB et al. (2001). The Diabetes Quality Improvement Project. Moving science into health policy to gain an edge on the diabetes epidemic. *Diabetes Care* **24**, 1815–20.

Joshi SR (2003). Metabolic syndrome—emerging clusters of the Indian Phenotype. *Journal of the Association of Physicians of India* **51**, 445–6.

Knowler WC et al. (2002). Reduction in the incidence of type 2 diabetes with lifestyle intervention or metformin. *New England Journal of Medicine* **346**, 393–403.

Lee WR et al. (2001). A window on the current status of diabetes mellitus in Singapore—the Diabcare-Singapore 1998 study. *Singapore Medical Journal* **42**, 501–7.

Litzelman DK, Tierney WM (1996). Physicians' reasons for failing to comply with computerized preventive care guidelines. *Journal of General Internal Medicine* **11**, 497–9.

Mohan V et al. (2001). Intra-urban differences in the prevalence of the metabolic syndrome in southern India—the Chennai Urban Population Study (CUPS-4). *Diabetic Medicine* **18**, 280–7.

Mohan V et al. (2005). A simplified Indian Diabetes Risk Score for screening for undiagnosed diabetic subjects. *Journal of the Association of Physicians of India* **53**, 759–63.

Mohan V et al. (2006a). Mortality rates due to diabetes in a selected urban south Indian population—the Chennai Urban Population Study (CUPS-16). *Journal of the Association of Physicians of India* **54**, 113–7.

Mohan V et al. (2006b). Secular trends in the prevalence of diabetes and impaired glucose tolerance in urban South India—the Chennai Urban Rural Epidemiology Study (CURES-17). *Diabetologia* **49**, 1175–8.

Mohan V et al. (2006c). Community empowerment—a successful model for prevention of non-communicable diseases in India—the Chennai Urban Population Study (CUPS-17). *Journal of the Association of Physicians of India* **54**, 858–62.

Mohan V et al. (2007). A diabetes risk score helps identify metabolic syndrome and cardiovascular risk in Indians—the Chennai Urban Rural Epidemiology Study (CURES-38). *Diabetes, Obesity & Metabolism* **9**, 337–43.

Mohan V et al. (2008). Urban rural differences in prevalence of self-reported diabetes in India—the WHO–ICMR Indian NCD risk factor surveillance. *Diabetes Research and Clinical Practice* **80**, 159–68.

Mohan V, Hansen JB, on behalf of the DCEP Group (2001). The Diabetes Care Excellence Project (DCEP). *International Diabetes Monitor* **Special issue**, 39–42.

Mohan V, Shanthirani CS, Deepa R (2003). Glucose intolerance (diabetes and IGT) in a selected south Indian population with special reference to family history, obesity and life style factors—the Chennai Urban Population Study (CUPS 14). *Journal of the Association of Physicians of India* **51**, 771–7.

Nagpal J, Bhartia A (2006). Quality of diabetes care in middle- and high-income group populace: the Delhi Diabetes Community (DEDICOM) survey. *Diabetes Care* **29**, 2341–8.

Narayan KM et al. (2006). Diabetes: the pandemic and potential solutions. In: Jamison DT et al., eds. *Disease Control Priorities in Developing Countries*, 2nd ed., pp 591–604. New York: Oxford University Press.

O'Connor PJ et al. (2005). Impact of an electronic medical record on diabetes quality of care. *Annals of Family Medicine* **3**, 300–6.

Østbye T et al. (2005). Is there time for management of patients with chronic diseases in primary care? *Annals of Family Medicine* **3**, 209–14.

Parvathi SJ, Rema M, Mohan V (2000). Role of ISO certification in preventing occupational health hazard in a health sector. *Indian Journal of Occupational and Environmental Medicine* **4**, 149–50.

Raheja BS et al. (2001). DiabCare Asia—India study: diabetes care in India—current status. *Journal of the Association of Physicians of India* **49**, 717–22.

Ramachandran A et al. (2005). Derivation and validation of diabetes risk score for urban Asian Indians. *Diabetes Research and Clinical Practice* **70**, 63–70.

Ramachandran A et al. (2006). The Indian Diabetes Prevention Programme shows that lifestyle modification and metformin prevent type 2 diabetes in Asian Indian subjects with impaired glucose tolerance (IDPP-1). *Diabetologia* **49**, 289–97.

Rayappa PH et al. (1999). The impact of socio-economic factors on diabetes care. *International Journal of Diabetes in Developing Countries* **19**, 7–16.

Reed RL et al. (2005). A controlled before-after trial of structured diabetes care in primary health centres in a newly developed country. *International Journal for Quality in Health Care* **17**, 281–6.

Rhee SY et al. (2005). Diabcare Asia 2001—Korea country report on outcome data and analysis. *Korean Journal of Internal Medicine* **20**, 48–54.

Shera AS et al. (1999). Pakistan National Diabetes Survey: prevalence of glucose intolerance and associated factors in Baluchistan province. *Diabetes Research and Clinical Practice* **44**, 49–58.

Sicree R, Shaw J, Zimmet P (2009). Diabetes and impaired glucose tolerance. In Gan D, ed. *Diabetes Atlas*, 4th ed., pp 1–105. Brussels: International Diabetes Federation.

Suresh S et al. (2005). Large-scale diabetes awareness and prevention in South India. *Diabetes Voice* **50**, 11–4.

The silent epidemic: an economic study of diabetes in developed and developing countries. *A report from the Economist Intelligence Unit.* Available at http://a330.g.akamai.net/7/330/25828/20070613142039/graphics.eiu.com/upload/portal/DIABETES_WEB.pdf. Accessed July 23, 2007.

Tuomilehto J et al. (2001). Prevention of type 2 diabetes mellitus by changes in lifestyle among subjects with impaired glucose tolerance. *New England Journal of Medicine* **344**, 1343–50.

UK Prospective Diabetes Study (UKPDS) Group (1998). Intensive blood-glucose control with sulphonylureas or insulin compared with conventional treatment and risk of complications in patients with type 2 diabetes (UKPDS 33). *Lancet* **352**, 837–53.

U.S. Centers for Disease Control and Prevention (1998). Diabetes Cost-Effectiveness Study Group. The cost-effectiveness of screening for type 2 diabetes. *JAMA* **280**, 1757–63.

World Health Organization (2002). *Global Burden of Disease for the Year 2001 by World Bank Rregion, for Use in Disease Control Priorities in Developing Countries.* 2nd ed. Geneva: World Health Organization.

World Health Organization Report (2005). *Preventing Chronic Disease a Vital Investment. Part Four—Taking Action: Essential Steps for Success, Chapter 1—Planning Step 3—Identify Policy Implementation Steps—"Spotlight. Improving the Built Environment in India,"* p 136. Geneva: World Health Organization.

26. Diabetes Prevention and Control Programs in Developing Countries

Ambady Ramachandran and Chamukuttan Snehalatha

■ Main Public Health Messages

- Diabetes is a major health care burden in both developed and developing countries.
- Primary prevention should be adopted to curb the current epidemic of diabetes.
- There is evidence from well-planned, randomized, controlled prevention programs that primary prevention of type 2 diabetes is possible in developing countries.
- Lifestyle modification and metformin have been shown to be highly effective in reducing incident diabetes in high-risk groups. These interventions are cost saving when taking into account the high cost of care of diabetes and its complications.
- Although targeting high-risk groups has definite benefits, for a widespread, perceivable impact, a population-based, upstream strategy is ideal for preventing diabetes.
- National diabetes control programs have been implemented by the governments of many developed countries. With the help of the American Diabetes Association, the International Diabetes Federation, the World Health Organization, and similar organizations, these national programs have been initiated even in several developing nations.

■ Introduction

Diabetes is a chronic disease that is reaching epidemic proportions in many parts of the world. The International Diabetes Federation estimates that the number of people with diabetes will increase from 194 million in 2003 to 333 million by 2025 (Diabetes Atlas 2006).

■ Background and Historical Perspective

Southeast Asian countries have the highest burden of diabetes. In urban India the prevalence was just 1.2% in 1971, but this rate increased about 900% in three decades to reach 12.1% in 2000 (Ramachandran et al. 2001). Recent data from Asian countries show that the epidemic is no longer solely an urban phenomenon. In countries like India (Ramachandran et al. 2004) and Bangladesh (Abu Sayeed et al. 2003) rural areas experienced an increase of almost 400% in diabetes between 1989 and 2003. The factors associated with the increase were improved socioeconomic, educational, and occupational status and the availability of motorized transport due to the economic transition occurring in rural parts of the countries.

■ Epidemiology

Type 2 diabetes accounts for more than 90% of the diabetic population worldwide. A genetic and environmental interaction is involved in the development of the disease. The genetics of type 2 diabetes are poorly understood, but the environmental factors influencing the expression of the disease are fairly clear. These include overweight, especially central adiposity, physical inactivity, and increased consumption of fats and energy-dense foods, all of which tend to increase insulin resistance. Ethnic group and perinatal factors are also risk factors. Although the genetic factors are not modifiable, sufficient evidence indicates the benefits of modifying the environmental influences, which could reduce the genetic-environmental interaction (Kanaya et al. 2002; Knowler et al. 2002; Pan et al. 1997; Ramachandran et al. 2006; Tuomilehto et al. 2001). Both forms of diabetes, type 1 and type 2, have genetic and environmental etiopathogenic factors. There is insufficient evidence to indicate that type 1 diabetes is preventable, although a few preventive strategies, such as the use of insulin or nicotinamide in high-risk groups and eliminating exposure to bovine protein, have been tested (Akerblom and Knip 1998).

Diabetes causes premature mortality, resulting in 12 to 14 years of life lost (Manuel and Schultz 2004). To reduce adverse impacts, the primary step, undoubtedly, is an optimal treatment that is beneficial in reducing the development of microvascular complications and to a great extent the macrovascular risk as well (Diabetes Control and Complications Trial Research Group 1993; UK Prospective Diabetes Study Group 1998). Early diagnosis and prompt management of hyperglycemia with regular follow-up, patient education, and motivation for adherence to treatment are essential steps to reduce the onslaught of the complications.

■ Public Health Preventive or Intervention Strategies

To avert the epidemic of type 2 diabetes that is spreading globally, the ideal tool is primary prevention, the potential and strategies for which are fairly clear. Whether in developed countries (Knowler et al. 2002; Tuomilehto et al. 2001) or in developing countries (Pan et al. 1997; Ramachandran et al. 2006), the preventive strategies using lifestyle modifications involving healthy food habits and enhanced physical activity are effective. Insulin sensitizers such as metformin (Knowler et al. 2002; Ramachandran et al. 2006) and glitazones (Buchanan et al. 2002; Gerstein et al. 2006) may also have a role. Because lifestyle modification involves behavioral changes, constant motivation is needed for lifelong implementation, and this poses a huge challenge.

Risk Factors

Genetic Risk

The genetic factors for type 2 diabetes are complex and still elusive. However the genetic predisposition is obvious from the heritable nature of the disease. Strong familial aggregation of the disease has been noted in various Asian populations (Ramachandran et al. 2004). Preventive measures should be applied at an early age in boys and girls with a strong family history of diabetes.

Age

The association between the risk factors is strong and complex. Age is probably the strongest unmodifiable risk factor that has a positive influence on modifiable risk factors, such as obesity or excess body fat, particularly visceral adiposity, and activity level. Body weight is strongly related to age, especially between 35 and 65 years (Centers for Disease Control and Prevention 2007). A continued increase in life expectancy and a decline in fertility (and thus a decline in the younger population) are expected to result in faster aging of the global population in the next 50 years. The prevalence of diabetes is known to increase linearly with increasing age. In the developing countries, onset of diabetes occurs at a younger age (45–65 years) than in developed Western regions (≥65 years) (Diabetes Atlas 2003). The DECODA (Diabetes Epidemiology: Collaborative Analysis of Diagnostic Criteria in Asia) study found that the overall effect of age on prevalence of diabetes differed considerably between ethnic groups even after correcting for other confounding factors such as body mass index (BMI) (Qiao et al. 2003). The association between age and diabetes was higher in the Indian and the Maltese populations than in all other populations studied (Europeans, Chinese, and Japanese) (see Fig. 26.1).

Adiposity

Rapid urbanization is producing significant changes in lifestyles not only in urban but even in rural areas (Ramachandran et al. 2008). Risk factors such as obesity and insulin resistance have become more prevalent. The availability of modern devices, including motorized transportation, has reduced the demand for physical work. Obesity also appears to be familial (Davey et al. 2000).

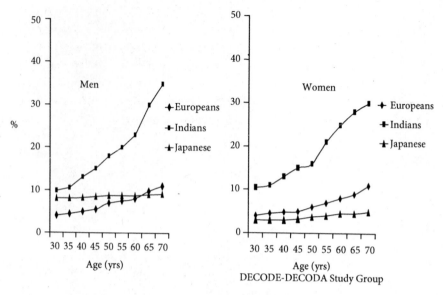

FIGURE 26.1 Age-specific prevalence of diabetes among men and women in different ethnic groups

The adverse effects are manifested even at a young age. In urban southern India, the prevalence of overweight in 2001 was 16% among teenagers and showed a strong association with lack of physical activity and higher socioeconomic status (Ramachandran 2002). Asian countries have a higher prevalence of metabolic syndrome, which is a constellation of cardiovascular risk factors that include hyperglycemia and insulin resistance (Joshi 2003).

The distribution of body fat is a more important determinant for several disorders than the degree of obesity. Asian Indians generally have a lower BMI than many other populations, but among Asian Indians the association of BMI with type 2 diabetes is as strong as in any other population. Asian Indians show a tendency for central adiposity and have a higher percentage of body fat (Banerji et al. 1999; Gallagher et al. 1996; Ramachandran et al. 2004). Insulin resistance is more strongly associated with central adiposity than with BMI.

■ Primary Prevention of Type 2 Diabetes

Definition and Strategies

Primary prevention can be defined as the prevention of a disease by controlling modifiable risk factors through population prevention programs (Rose 1985). The primary prevention of type 2 diabetes, at best, would mean to keep genetically or otherwise susceptible individuals normoglycemic (Tuomilehto 2005). Studies show that in addition to preventing diabetes it helps to improve cardiovascular risk factors as well (Diabetes Prevention Program Research Group 2005; Snehalatha et al. 2008). This requires complementary strategies of (1) preventing the development of modifiable risk factors and (2) preventing those who have the risk factors from developing the disease. Primary prevention programs can be broadly classified as downstream, midstream, or upstream (McKinlay 1975). Downstream programs target individuals having the highest risk of the disease (persons with impaired glucose tolerance [IGT] or impaired fasting glucose [IFG]). Midstream programs target defined populations or communities that have been found to be at increased risk of diabetes (e.g., Pima Indians, Asian Indians). Upstream programs target the whole population and include public policy and environmental interventions intended to increase support for maintaining a healthy lifestyle.

For a perceivable impact, a population approach has to be adopted, which requires participation from the government by investing in programs to prevent noncommunicable diseases.

Downstream Strategies

Downstream programs target the persons with the highest risk. Historically, the major primary prevention studies in diabetes have been downstream programs, as they have selected subjects with IGT, IFG, or women with a history of gestational diabetes.

In developing countries prevention measures are likely to be influenced by the socioeconomic conditions and the structure of the health care system. Currently, no universally validated system exists to identify people at high risk of diabetes.

Identification of High-Risk Subjects

Screening for blood glucose has been used or proposed as the ideal tool to identify individuals with a high risk of developing diabetes or who are symptomatic but have never been diagnosed as having diabetes. Measuring blood glucose is an invasive procedure, and it is costly and time-consuming. Risk of diabetes can be diagnosed with a good sensitivity and high predictive value by models developed using anthropometry, blood glucose, and lipids (Stern et al. 1993) or by using more sophisticated parameters such as proinsulin concentrations (Wareham et al. 1999). The latter methods are not practical because of their high cost and the need for special laboratory tests. Recently, more practical and simple diabetes risk scores have been developed. Assigning points for the noninvasive, nonmodifiable, and modifiable risk factors for diabetes produces a useful risk score. The Cambridge risk score has been shown to predict undiagnosed prevalent diabetes (Park et al. 2002), incident diabetes (Simmons et al. 2007), and all-cause mortality (Spijkerman et al. 2002). Although the main purpose is to identify those who need further investigations by a diagnostic oral glucose tolerance test, such scores also help to identify people at high risk so that preventive action can be taken. Several ethnic-specific risk scores have been published (Glumer et al. 2006); these scores will considerably reduce the cost of screening and can be applied in large numbers even in a primary health care setting. Use of a risk score reduces the need for expensive and cumbersome screening procedures and is therefore economical.

The International Diabetes Federation recommends opportunistic screening by health care personnel (Alberti et al. 2007). The strategy includes the use of a questionnaire to identify people who are at high risk for prediabetes or diabetes to limit the number requiring a diagnostic glucose tolerance test. The criteria included are obesity using gender- and ethnic-specific cut-points for waist circumference, first-degree family history, age (≥45 years in Europids, ≥35 years for other populations), cardiovascular history, including raised blood pressure and/or heart disease, history of gestational diabetes, and use of diabetogenic drugs.

The American Diabetes Association (ADA) recommends an interactive diabetes risk test that helps to categorize people according to their risk levels (ADA Diabetes Risk Test) (Alberti et al. 2007).

Randomized, Controlled, Primary Prevention Studies

Randomized, controlled, primary prevention studies have employed the downstream strategy and selected people with a high risk of developing diabetes, such as those with IGT. Lifestyle modification is the most effective and practical choice and is also cost-effective, especially in the developing countries. Metformin can be used as an alternative if behavioral changes are difficult. This drug is available at an affordable price in countries such as India.

Lifestyle Modification

The Diabetes Prevention Program (DPP) in the United States (Knowler et al. 2002), the Finnish Diabetes Prevention Study (DPS) (Tuomilehto et al. 2001), the Malmo study in Sweden (Erikksson and Lindgarde 1991), the Da Qing study in China (Pan et al. 1997), and the Indian Diabetes Prevention Programme-1 (IDPP-1) (Ramachandran et al. 2006) in India studied the impact of lifestyle modification on the incidence of diabetes in subjects with IGT. What constitutes lifestyle modification may differ in different societies based on social, cultural, economic, and political environments. A comparative analysis of the results is shown in Table 26.1. The DPP and the IDPP-1 also tested metformin as a tool for primary prevention. The Da Qing study and IDPP-1, both from developing countries, involved relatively non-obese and younger participants and differed significantly in the characteristics of their study subjects from the Western studies.

The Da Qing Study

The Da Qing study was one of the earliest primary prevention studies to evaluate the effect of lifestyle modification on the conversion of IGT to diabetes. A very large

TABLE 26.1 *Comparison of the Major Diabetes Prevention Programs in Developing and Developed Countries*

	Da Qing (China)	IDPP (India)	DPP (United States)	DPS (Finland)
Number recruited	577	531	3234	523
Age (years) (mean ± SD)	45.0 (7.0)	45.0 (5.7)	50.6 (10.7)	55.0 (7.0)
BMI (kg/m²) (mean ± SD)	25.8 (3.8)	25.8 (3.5)	34.0 (6.7)	31.2 (4.5)
Waist circumference (cm) (mean ± SD)	—	97.2 ± 13.5	105.1 (14.5)	101.0 (11.0)
Period of follow-up (years)	6	3.0	2.8	3.2
Interventions	Diet, exercise, LSM*, diet + exercise	Met*, LSM* + Met*	LSM*, Met*	LSM*
Cumulative incidence of diabetes in controls	67.7%	55%	11.0/100 person years	23% in 4 years
Relative risk reduction (%)	Diet – 31 Exercise – 46 Both – 42	LSM – 28.5 Met – 26.4 Both – 28.4	LSM – 58 Met – 31	LSM – 58
Dose of metformin	—	500 mg/day	1750 mg/day	—

*LSM, lifestyle modification; Met, metformin.

number of people (110,600) were screened, and 577 were identified with IGT. This subgroup was randomized to the control group or to one of the three treatment groups: diet, exercise, or a combination of the two. A 6-year follow-up showed a cumulative incidence of diabetes of 67.7% in the control group, 43.8% in the diet group, 41.1% in the exercise group, and 46% in the diet-plus-exercise group. The effectiveness of all three treatment modalities was similar after correcting for the baseline confounding variables (adjusted values of 31%, 46%, and 42%, respectively).

Reductions in relative risk were similar in overweight and lean participants. Given the modest weight changes in this study, the major benefits appeared to be due to exercise.

The Indian Diabetes Prevention Programme (IDPP-1)

Epidemiologic data on Asian Indians living in the homeland or in different migrant countries have highlighted the strong tie between a genetic predisposition for diabetes and a low threshold for acquired or environmental risk factors for the disease (Ramachandran et al. 2004). Series of studies by the authors of this chapter have indicated that the rising trend in diabetes is not restricted to urban areas, as it is also observed in rural areas with the rapid pace of social and economic developments (Ramachandran et al. 2008). Urbanization is increasing rapidly, as is the rate of lifestyle-related disorders. The prevalence of IGT and IFG is high, and this large pool of prediabetic men and women could be targeted primarily for prevention of diabetes.

The IDPP-1 was a community-based, randomized controlled study in 531 subjects (421 men and 110 women) who had persistent IGT on two glucose tolerance tests. Their age (mean 45.9 ± 5.7 years) and BMI (25.8 ± 3.5 [weight in kilograms divided by (height in meters)^2] were similar to those of the Chinese cohort but were significantly lower than in the DPP and the DPS. The four arms of the study were (1) control with standard advice, (2) lifestyle modification involving diet and exercise, (3) treatment with metformin, and (4) treatment with lifestyle modification and metformin.

In a median follow-up period of 30 months, a high rate of conversion to diabetes was noted (18.3%/year), probably the highest reported so far. The reductions in relative risk with the various interventions are shown in Table 26.2. Lifestyle modification and metformin were equally effective in reducing the incidence of diabetes, and there were no additional benefits from combining them.

The Japanese Prevention Study

A prevention trial in Japanese men with IGT also showed the benefits of lifestyle modification (Kosaka et al. 2004). Men with IGT were recruited using a health-screening examination and were randomized in a 4:1 ratio to the control group with a standard intervention or to an intensive intervention with diet and exercise. Repeated motivation was given to the study group to maintain lifestyle modification and also to reduce the BMI below 22. The cumulative, 4-year incidence of diabetes was 9.3% in the control group versus 3.0% in the intervention group. The reduction in the risk of diabetes was 67.4% ($p < 0.001$). A linear correlation between incidence of diabetes and BMI was seen. The benefits were not entirely explained by the reduction in weight.

Pharmacologic Interventions

Heneghan and colleagues (Heneghan, Thompson, and Perera 2006), in their editorial in the *British Medical Journal*, brilliantly analyzed the trials of drugs intended

TABLE 26.2 *Relative Risk Reduction with Interventions in IDPP*

Groups	1	2	3	4
	Control	Lifestyle	Metformin	Lifestyle + Metformin
Conversion to DM % (95% CI)	49.6 (41.1–58.1)	35.0 (26.5–43.5)	39.8 (30.3–48.3)	34.7 (26.2–43.2)
Absolute risk reduction %	—	14.4	9.8	14.8
Relative risk	—	0.705	0.803	0.699
p value vs. group 1	—	0.026	0.14	0.023
Cumulative % of remaining free from DM*	35.1	48.5	45.0	56.3
p value vs. group 1	—	0.0134	0.055	0.0354
Number needed to treat to prevent diabetes in 1 person	—	6.9	10.2	6.7

*Comparison of survival experience using Wilcoon (Gehan) statistic. Pairwise comparison, DF1. Median follow-up is 30 months.

Source: Ramachandran et al. (2006).

to achieve primary prevention of diabetes. Metformin reduced the incidence of diabetes by 31% in 2.8 years in the DPP and by 26.4% in the IDPP-1; troglitazone (since withdrawn from the market) was found to be efficacious in both the DPP (Knowler et al. 2002) and the TRIPOD (Troglitazone in Prevention of Diabetes) (Buchanan et al. 2002). In obese subjects orlistat reduced the risk of diabetes in those who had IGT by 37% in relation to placebo (Heymsfield et al. 2000). In the more recently published DREAM (Diabetes Reduction Assessment with Ramipril and Rosiglitazone Medication) trial (Gerstein et al. 2006), rosiglitazone in a daily dose of 8 mg reduced the conversion of IGT and/or IFG to diabetes from 26% with placebo to 11.6% (hazard ratio of 0.40; p <0.001). Ramipril (15 mg daily) did not have any beneficial effect on the risk of diabetes in the DREAM study. Although rosiglitazone was found to be highly effective, the recent concern about its safety (combined with its high cost) might restrict its wide use, especially in the low- and middle-income countries.

The key question is whether the benefits of the drugs are merely due to the glu-cose-lowering property in new-onset diabetes or in people with IGT and IFG. This can only be decided by long-term "washout" studies. The indication from the DPP was that the effectiveness was reduced on withdrawal of the drug (DPP 2003), which is what happened in the washout period in the DREAM study (Gerstein et al. 2006). Metformin's effectiveness depended on age and BMI in the American population; it was almost ineffective in older subjects (>60 years) and those whose BMI was below 30. In the IDPP-1, due to the narrow age range (35–55 years) and lower mean BMI, such variations could not be assessed.

The STOP NIDDM trial was a placebo-controlled study (duration: 3.3 years) with acarbose, an α-glucosidase inhibitor, in 1429 subjects with IGT (Chiasson et al. 2002); the subjects had a mean age of 55 years and a mean BMI of 31. Acarbose was found to be effective in reducing conversion to diabetes, with an absolute reduction in risk of 9.1% and with a 35.8% reduction in relative risk compared with the pla-cebo. In addition a 49% reduction in relative risk of cardiovascular events was noted in the treatment group.

Midstream Strategies

Midstream strategies target defined populations, communities, or groups known to have a high risk of diabetes. Obesity in children and young adults has been recog-nized as a forerunner of obesity-related metabolic disorders in adulthood. In devel-oping countries that are becoming industrialized, levels of physical activity among children are declining. Prolonged hours of television and computer use are contrib-uting to this decline. Use of fat-rich, energy-dense foods is increasing and enhances the rate of obesity or overweight.

A recent study by the authors has shown that there is a high prevalence of cardio-metabolic risk factors even in healthy young children of normal weight in southern India, and there is a clustering of several risk factors (Ramachandran et al. 2007). Among the normal-weight children 64.8% had at least one cardiometabolic abnor-mality. Insulin resistance, increased blood pressure, and dyslipidemia were more com-mon in children who were overweight. Targeting children with overweight and/or abdominal obesity is likely to produce benefits at a young age. In addition adoption of a healthy lifestyle at a young age may help to influence behaviors in adulthood. Studies targeting modification of the behavioral patterns of children have to be planned.

A group in India that can be targeted for midstream projects is the informa-tion technology (IT) professionals. Studies have highlighted a high degree of stress and "burnout" cases among them, causing stress-related disorders such as diabetes, hypertension, and visual and musculoskeletal disorders (Sharma et al. 2006). India has been in the forefront of the IT industry, which employs mostly young people. Most of the IT companies have in-house facilities such as gyms for physical activity, and educating their workers on the importance of lifestyle modification is likely to yield beneficial effects.

Upstream Programs

Upstream programs target the whole population. To be fully effective, primary prevention programs should include all sectors of the society, including those at high risk. The impressive results produced by the implementation of lifestyle modification in all well-executed clinical research settings are definitely impractical, however, even in well-funded health care systems (Heneghan, Thompson, and Perera 2006). Even in the closely monitored clinical trials, the long-term behavioral changes required to achieve the prevention goals seemed difficult to achieve. For example Simmons and co-workers (Simmons et al. 2006) noted that only 20% of the EPIC (European Prospective Investigation into Cancer and Nutrition) participants met three or more of the study's five goals. Their investigation showed that the incidence of diabetes could be reduced in a population-based cohort by the achievement of goals for healthy behavior, the reduction being proportionate to the number of goals achieved. Information on healthy behaviors could be used to identify high-risk groups. The EPIC analysis showed that unhealthy behaviors tend to cluster in particular subgroups (Simmons et al. 2006). Future research should focus on developing low-cost interventions such as increased physical activity and improving nutritional intake among the target populations, which would consist of people with different levels of risk for diabetes. Investments are needed in education, food policies, and physical amenities such as playgrounds and parks to support and encourage the desired changes. Alliances of the government, nongovernmental public interest groups, professional organizations, and individual members of the population can play significant roles in improving a nation's health care awareness and its environment.

National Diabetes Control Programs

Developed Countries

Encouraged by results of the primary prevention programs, many developed countries have initiated major national diabetes control programs for improved diabetes care, primary prevention, and prevention of complications. The Development Program for the Prevention and Care of Diabetes in Finland (DEHKO), which began in 2000, is one of the most comprehensive and well-planned projects (Etu-Seppal 2003). DEHKO comprises three concurrent strategies—a population strategy promoting health care of the entire nation, a high-risk strategy for those at high risk, and a third strategy for early diagnosis of diabetes and management of the newly diagnosed cases. The population strategy focuses on nutritional interventions and improved physical activity to reduce the risk in all age groups. Many other developed nations in Europe, the United States, the United Kingdom, Canada (in the United States through the state-based Diabetes Prevention and Control Programs), and Australia have also included primary prevention of diabetes in their health care agendas (Lefebrve 2005).

Developing Countries

The major burden of diabetes is on the developing countries, which also face serious limitations in health care due to inadequate national economic resources and lack of national health care systems. In recent years considerable public awareness of the seriousness of noncommunicable diseases has been created in several developing countries by the concerted attempts and programs initiated by the International Diabetes Federation, the World Health Organization (WHO), the World Bank, and the World Diabetes Foundation. Local associations of several developing countries, supported and guided by the International Diabetes Federation, WHO, and the World Diabetes Federation, launched the national diabetes control programs. China, India, Bangladesh, Pakistan, Sri Lanka, Costa Rica, El Salvador, Malaysia, African countries, and the Western Pacific regions have all taken major steps in laying down guidelines for effective management of noncommunicable diseases, including diabetes, creating public awareness, and implementing strategies at population levels for the primary and secondary prevention of diabetes, cardiovascular disease, and stroke (Willett et al. 2006). Several nations have also brought forth changes in tobacco legislation that have led to favorable outcomes (Barnoya and Glantz 2004).

Laudable reforms have been undertaken in many developing countries to improve the population's health. Examples include Singapore, which has a Fit and Trim Program for increasing physical activity and healthy diets among schoolchildren; the Republic of Korea, which is building satellite communities around Seoul with ample amenities for physical activity; and Poland, which has removed government subsidies on butter and lard (Willett et al. 2006).

Population studies focusing on the reduction of cardiovascular risk have been successful in some countries. The close association of blood glucose concentrations and cardiovascular disease, with no threshold value, is well known. Therefore, the strategies for reducing risk for cardiovascular disease will also be appropriate for diabetes. The noncommunicable-disease-control program in Mauritius was successful 5 years after implementation in reducing cardiovascular risk factors such as physical inactivity, cigarette smoking, alcohol misuse, hypertension, dyslipidemia, and obesity (Dowse et al. 1995). This was the first project of its kind in a developing country, and it had a high success rate.

Several developed nations have launched similar programs for the reduction of cardiovascular risks (Fortmann et al. 1993). Among the best known was the North Karelia project launched in 1970s in Finland, which had major positive effects on the reduction of cardiovascular risk factors and premature deaths from cardiovascular disease (Puska 1998).

In India, which has the highest number of people with diabetes of any country in the world, a few preliminary steps have been initiated by the government along these lines. Based on the recommendations given by an expert committee, guidelines have been laid down by the Indian Council of Medical Research and the

Government of India for minimum standards of care, prevention, a survey of disease prevalence, and the development of human resources. The Ministry of Health and Family Welfare, Government of India, has launched the pilot phase of the National Programme for Prevention and Control of Diabetes, Cardiovascular Diseases and Stroke (NPDCS 2008). The pilot phase has been undertaken in six districts in six states with a financial outlay of approximately 1.3 million dollars (U.S.).

Under the leadership of the author (A. Ramachandran), a 3-year program was sponsored by the WHO and the World Diabetes Foundation for building national capacity to control diabetes. During the 3-year period of 2005–2007, 3000 physicians and 1100 paramedical persons from rural and semi-urban areas of seven states of India were trained. Workshops of 5 days for physicians and 3 days for paramedicals were conducted on early detection and on the management and preventive aspects of diabetes. The trainees are motivated to improve their practices and also to disseminate the knowledge by means of awareness-raising camps, counseling, and so forth. An independent evaluation of the project's impact showed that the program has been highly effective in improving knowledge and capacity building for diabetes care. Similar programs spanning wider target areas are in progress.

Another project has been designed to enhance the knowledge and skills of Vietnamese nurses and physicians to improve diabetes care (Baumann et al. 2006). Cameroon has also started an initiative to improve health promotion among persons with diabetes by involving a number of strategies, by spreading the messages through schools, churches, and cultural groups and by involving local traditional healers (Tuo-uo-Kpu 2006). The results will throw light on effective strategies applicable to local areas and populations.

■ Economic Issues and Implications

In 2007 the world spent an estimated US$232.0 to US$421.7 billion for diabetes care, and this figure is likely to rise to US$302.5 to US$558.6 billion by 2025 (Diabetes Atlas 2006). The major brunt will be borne by the developing countries. Estimates by WHO are that lost productivity due to diabetes, heart disease, and stroke over the next 10 years will result in lost national income (in billions of international dollars) of 555.7 in China, 303.2 in the Russian Federation, 336.6 in India, 49.2 in Brazil, and 2.5 in Tanzania (Diabetes Atlas 2006).

There are very few studies from developing countries on the economic aspects of diabetes. A study by the authors of this chapter done in 1999 showed the average annual expenditure on diabetes care ranged from US$83 to US$347 among patients who attended a specialty center (Shobhana et al. 2000). As expected, patients who required hospitalization had higher expenditures. Those who attended the government's free clinics had to spend only a small amount (US$9 annually), but it was calculated that an average of US$115 was spent annually per patient by the institution (Shobhana et al. 2000). A more recent study indicated that the expenses had increased further, with an annual average of US$227 spent by the patient on diabetes care (Ramachandran et al. 2007). The more distressing factor was that persons in the lower-income group had to spend nearly one-third of their annual income for diabetes care. There are no data from developing countries on the indirect cost of diabetes care.

■ Economics of the Prevention of Diabetes

A general conclusion drawn from some studies in Western developed countries is that dietary and other lifestyle modifications could prevent most cases of many noncommunicable diseases, including type 2 diabetes, among the high-income populations (Willett et al. 2006). Using modeling methods, Willett and colleagues calculated a range of estimates of the cost-effectiveness of lifestyle interventions, which consisted of dietary modifications (including limiting sodium intake) and enhancing physical activity. The calculations were performed for several regions, including South Asia, other regions of Asia, and sub-Saharan Africa. The cost-effectiveness ratio of reducing cardiovascular diseases ranged from US$25 to US$73 per disability-adjusted life-year (DALY) averted. Depending on the region and the interventions, the interventions could be cost saving. Thus it was inferred that population-wide and community-based interventions appear to be cost-effective modalities.

In the Netherlands, the cost-effectiveness of lifestyle interventions in two community-based programs was computed (Jacobs-van der Bruggen et al. 2007). One new case of diabetes per 20 years was prevented for every 7–30 participants in the health care intervention and for every 300–1500 adults in the community intervention. In the community intervention the cost needed to prevent one case in 20 years was €2000–9000, and for the health care intervention it was €5000 to €21,000. Thus, the former was a more cost-effective intervention. The lifestyle intervention for preventing type 2 diabetes cost US$60 to US$130 per QALY over a lifetime, depending on the region. Because the developing countries have a large population with a high potential of developing diabetes (Diabetes Atlas 2006), such attempts would be highly cost saving (Narayan et al. 2006).

The data have been sparse on the primary prevention of diabetes and its cost-effectiveness in developing countries. Using the IDPP-1 data, relative effectiveness and direct medical costs of interventions were estimated from the perspective of the health care system (Ramachandran et al. 2007). The cost of the screening procedure used to identify one subject with IGT was US$117. The cost-effectiveness of preventing one case of diabetes with lifestyle modification was US$1052. In the IDPP study lifestyle modification was the most cost-effective intervention, followed by metformin. The cost of the intervention was the highest when a combination of lifestyle modification and metformin was used, because both modalities had to be

TABLE 26.3   *Summary of the Total and Incremental Costs of the Interventions of IDPP*

	Control	LSM	Metformin	LSM + Metformin
Total cost of intervention INR ($)	2739 (61)	10,136 (225)	9881 (220)	12,144 (270)
Number needed to prevent 1 case of diabetes (NNT)	—	64	6.9	6.5
Incremental cost (IC) (INR)	—	7397 (164)	7142 (159)	9405 (209)
Cost-effectiveness (CER) IC × NNT (INR)	—	47,341 (1052)	49280 (1095)	61,133 (1359)

implemented, and their combined efficacy was not superior to either of them used separately (see Table 26.3).

. In the Indian context expenditures for health care are borne by either the individual or the family, and thus those with meager earnings tend to neglect health care due to financial constraints. Health insurance plans have not become popular and are currently used mainly by the upper strata of society. The Employees State Insurance plan of India is an integrated security scheme to provide social security to industrial workers and their families in contingencies such as sickness and occupational injury. Proper use is not made of such state insurance plans. In such a scenario, primary prevention of diabetes is the choice to reduce the economic burden on the individual and the society. Preventing diabetes is of enormous value in developing countries because the cost of diabetes care is high.

■ Areas of Uncertainty or Controversy

The clinical trials require intensive input, and they are expensive. The population potentially eligible for lifestyle modification is large in developing countries such as India because such countries have a huge number of people with nondiabetic dysglycemia. Economic and technological insufficiency and the lack of adequately trained personnel such as dietitians and exercise physiologists are great barriers to implementing community-based interventions. Fortunately diabetes education, including self-management, has been found to be highly effective in urban India (Shobhana et al. 1999). Because the cost of patient education is generally low, the intervention may be cost effective. However, the efforts needed to train educators who in turn can practice among rural communities are huge in such a vast country with its diverse social and cultural environment. Involvement of both the governmental and nongovernmental systems and the training of grassroots-level workers are required. By the use of telephone, IT, videos, and programs that make use of folklore, the messages about diabetes can be spread. Input from research in these areas should be tested, and algorithms for follow-up must be developed. The evaluation of impact is not possible in large upstream programs unless trained manpower is made available in all the areas.

■ Implications for Health Policy

In a nutshell, to promote the primary prevention of diabetes we need to improve nutrition and enhance physical activity, both of which will require major behavioral changes in the community. The task is by no means simple. Although metformin has the potential to reduce the risk of conversion of IGT to diabetes, it is not clear whether the effects are long lasting or are only due to the glucose-lowering properties. There are several social, political, economic, and administrative hurdles in developing countries for implementation of major primary prevention programs. Here a lack of adequate financial resources and a lack of trained people pose major hurdles to the implementation of population-based studies. However in several regions attempts have been initiated to implement primary prevention programs with the help of organizations such as the ADA, WHO, and the International Diabetes Federation supported by the World Diabetes Foundation. Both the government and nongovernmental authorities need to be sensitized to the seriousness of the diabetes burden and the possibilities of the primary prevention of diabetes.

■ Developments over the Next 5 to 10 Years

In the next 5 to 10 years more countries are expected to initiate national programs for the control and prevention of diabetes. In general, awareness about diabetes is expected to improve among the general public, which will provide opportunities to implement upstream programs in many developing countries. Results of the ongoing national programs will highlight the cost-effectiveness of the primary prevention of diabetes, an intervention that is more relevant in low-resource countries. It is hoped that policy makers will be sensitized to increase their emphasis on noncommunicable diseases.

■ Acknowledgments

The authors acknowledge the assistance given by Dr. A. Yamuna in organizing the manuscript and the secretarial help of Mrs. Bobby Alex and Mrs. L. Vijaya.

■ References

Abu Sayeed M et al. (2003). Diabetes and impaired fasting glycemia in a rural population of Bangladesh. *Diabetes Care* **26**, 1034–9.

Akerblom HK, Knip M (1998). Putative environmental factors in type 1 diabetes. *Diabetes /Metabolism Reviews* **14**, 31–67.

Alberti KG, Zimmet P, Shaw J (2007). International Diabetes Federation: a consensus on type 2 diabetes prevention. *Diabetic Medicine* **24**, 451–63.

Banerji BA et al. (1999). Body composition, visceral fat, leptin and insulin resistance in Asian Indian men. *Journal of Clinical Endocrinology and Metabolism* **84**, 137–44.

Barnoya J, Glantz S (2004). Association of the California Tobacco Control Program with declines in lung cancer incidence. *Cancer Causes and Control* **15**, 689–95.

Baumann LC et al. (2006). A training program for diabetes care in Vietnam. *Diabetes Educator* **32**, 189–94. Buchanan TA et al. (2002). Preservation of pancreatic B-cell function and prevention of type 2 diabetes by pharmacological treatment of insulin resistance in high-risk Hispanic women. *Diabetes* **51**, 2769–803.

Centers for Disease Control and Prevention (2007). Trend data from the Behavioral Risk Factor Surveillance System. Trend data Rhode Island grouped by age. Available from http://apps.nccd.cdc.gov/brfss/Trends/agechart. asp?qkey=10010&state=RI. Accessed February 23, 2008.

Chiasson JL et al. (2002).The STOP-NIDDM Trial Research Group. Acarbose for prevention of type 2 diabetes mellitus: the STOP-NIDDM randomized trial. *Lancet* **359**, 2072–7.

Davey G et al. (2000). Familial aggregation of central adiposity among southern Indians. *International Journal of Obesity and Related Metabolic Disorders* **24**, 1523–7.

Diabetes Atlas (2003). Second edition, executive summary, pp 11–4. Brussels: International Diabetes Federation.

Diabetes Control and Complications Trial Research Group (1993). The effect of intensive treatment of diabetes on the development and progression of long-term complications in insulin-dependent diabetes mellitus. *New England Journal of Medicine* **329**, 977–86.

Diabetes Prevention Program Research Group (2003). Effects of withdrawal from metformin on the development of diabetes in the diabetes prevention program. *Diabetes Care* **26**, 977–80.

Diabetes Prevention Program Research Group (2005). Impact of intensive lifestyle and metformin therapy on cardiovascular disease risk factors in the Diabetes Prevention Program. *Diabetes Care* **28**, 888–94.

Dowse GK et al. (1995). Changes in population cholesterol concentrations and other cardiovascular risk factor levels after 5 years of the non-communicable disease intervention programme in Mauritius. Mauritius Non-communicable Disease Study Group. *British Medical Journal* **311**, 1255–9.

Eriksson KF, Lindgarde F (1991). Prevention of type 2 (non-insulin-dependent) diabetes mellitus by diet and physical exercise. The 6-year Malmö feasibility study. *Diabetologia* **34**, 891–8.

Etu-Seppal L (2003). DEHKO: Finland moves on primary prevention. *Diabetes Voice* **48**, 1–2.

Fortmann SP et al. (1993). Effect of community health education on plasma cholesterol levels and diet: the Stanford Five-City Project. *American Journal of Epidemiology* **137**, 1039–55.

Gallagher D et al. (1996). How useful is body mass index for comparison of body fatness across age, sex and ethnic groups? *American Journal of Epidemiology* **143**, 228–9.

Gerstein HC et al. (2006). Effect of rosiglitazone on the frequency of diabetes in patients with impaired glucose tolerance or impaired fasting glucose: a randomized controlled trial. *Lancet* **368**, 1096–105.

Glumer C et al. (2006). Risk scores for type 2 diabetes can be applied in some populations but not all. *Diabetes Care* **29**, 410–4.

Heneghan C, Thompson M, Perera R (2006). Prevention of diabetes. Drug trials show promising results, but have limitations. *British Medical Journal* **333**, 764–5.

Heymsfield SV et al. (2000). Effects of weight loss with orlistat on glucose tolerance and progression to type 2 diabetes in obese adults. *Archives of Internal Medicine* **160**, 1321–6.

Jacobs-van der Bruggen MA et al. (2007). Lifestyle interventions are cost-effective in people with different levels of diabetes risk: results from a modeling study. *Diabetes Care* **30**, 128–34.

Joshi SR (2003). Metabolic syndrome-emerging clusters of the Indian phenotype. *Journal of the Association of Physicians of India* **51**, 445–6.

Knowler WC et al. (2002).Reduction in the incidence of type 2 diabetes with lifestyle intervention or metformin. *New England Journal of Medicine* **346**, 393–403.

Kosaka K, Noda M, Kuzuya T (2004). Prevention of type 2 diabetes by lifestyle intervention: a Japanese trial in IGT males. *Diabetes Research and Clinical Practice* **67**, 152–62.

Lefebvre P (2005). Type 2 diabetes mellitus: primary and secondary prevention. The vision of the International Diabetes Federation. In: Ganz M, ed. *Prevention of Type 2 Diabetes*, pp 15–19. West Sussex: John Wiley & Sons, Ltd.

Manuel DG, Schultz SE (2004). Health-related quality of life and health-adjusted life expectancy of people with diabetes in Ontario, Canada, 1996–1997. *Diabetes Care* **27**, 407–14.

McKinlay J (1975). A case for refocusing upstream: the political economy of sickness. In J.Gartley, ed. *Patients, Physicians and Illness: A Sourcebook in Behavioral Science and Health*, pp 9–25. New York: Free Press.

Narayan KMV et al. (2006). Diabetes: the pandemic and potential solutions. In: Jamison DT et al., eds. *Disease Control Priorities in Developing Countries*, 2nd ed., pp 591–603. New York: Oxford University Press.

NPDCS (2008). A new initiative for a healthy nation National programme for prevention and control of diabetes, cardiovascular and stroke (NPDCS). Available at: http://mohfw.nic.in/for%20websitediabetes.htm. Accessed March 11, 2008.

Pan XR et al. (1997). Effects of diet and exercise in preventing NIDDM in people with impaired glucose tolerance: the Da Qing IGT and diabetes study. *Diabetes Care* **20**, 537–44.

Park PJ et al. (2002). The performance of a risk score in predicting undiagnosed hyperglycemia. *Diabetes Care* **25**, 984–8.

Puska P et al. (1998). Changes in premature deaths in Finland: successful long-term prevention of cardiovascular diseases. *Bulletin of the World Health Organization* **76**, 419–25.

Qiao Q et al. (2003). Age-and sex-specific prevalence of diabetes and impaired glucose regulation in 11 Asian cohorts. *Diabetes Care* **26**, 1770–80.

Ramachandran A et al. (2001). High prevalence of diabetes and impaired glucose tolerance in India: National Urban Diabetes Survey. *Diabetologia* **44**, 1094–101.

Ramachandran A et al. (2002). Prevalence of overweight in urban Indian adolescent school children. *Diabetes Research and Clinical Practice* **57**, 185–90.

Ramachandran A, Snehalatha C, Vijay V (2004). Low risk threshold for acquired diabetogenic factors in Asian Indians. *Diabetes Research and Clinical Practice* **65**, 189–95.

Ramachandran A et al (2004). Temporal changes in prevalence of diabetes and impaired glucose tolerance associated with lifestyle transition occurring in the rural population in India. *Diabetologia*. **47**, 860–5.

Ramachandran A et al. (2006). The Indian Diabetes Prevention programme shows that lifestyle modification and metformin prevent type 2 diabetes in Asian Indian subjects with impaired glucose tolerance (IDPP-1). *Diabetologia* **49**, 289–97.

Ramachandran A et al. (2007a). Cost effectiveness of the interventions in the primary prevention of diabetes among Asian Indians: within-trial results of the Indian Diabetes Prevention Programme (IDPP). *Diabetes Care* **30**, 2548–52.

Ramachandran A et al. (2007b). Increasing expenditure on health care incurred by diabetic subjects in a developing country. *Diabetes Care* **30**, 252–6.

Ramachandran A et al. (2007c). Insulin resistance and clustering of cardiometabolic risk factors in urban teenagers in southern India. *Diabetes Care* **30**, 1828–33.

Ramachandran A et al. (2008). High prevalence of diabetes and cardiovascular risk factors associated with urbanization in India. *Diabetes Care* **31**, 893–8.

Rose G (1985). Sick individuals and sick populations. *International Journal of Epidemiology* **14**, 32–8.

Sharma AK, Khera S, Khandekar J (2006). Computer related health problems among information technology professionals in Delhi. *Indian Journal of Community Medicine* **31**, 36–8.

Shobhana R et al. (1999). Patients' adherence to diabetes treatment. *Journal of the Association of Physicians of India* **47**, 1173–5.

Shobhana R et al. (2000). Expenditure on health care incurred by diabetic subjects in a developing country—a study from southern India. *Diabetes Research and Clinical Practice* **48**, 37–42.

Sicree R, Shaw J, Zimmet P (2006). Prevalence and projections. In: Gan D, ed. *Diabetes Atlas*, 3rd ed., pp 16–104. Brussels: International Diabetes Federation.

Sicree R et al. (2006). The economic impacts of diabetes. In: Gan D, ed. *Diabetes Atlas*, 3rd ed., pp 237–65. Brussels: International Diabetes Federation.

Simmons RK et al. (2006). How much might achievement of diabetes prevention behaviour goals reduce the incidence of diabetes if implemented at the population level? *Diabetologia* **49**, 905–11.

Simmons RK et al. (2007). Do simple questions about diet and physical activity help to identify those at risk of type 2 diabetes? *Diabetic Medicine* **24**, 830–5.

Snehalatha C et al. (2008). Beneficial effects of strategies for primary prevention of diabetes on cardiovascular risk factors: results of the Indian Diabetes Prevention Programme. *Diabetes & Vascular Disease Research* **5**, 25–9.

Spijkerman A et al. (2002). What is the risk of mortality for people who are screen positive in a diabetes screening programme but who do not have diabetes on biochemical testing? Diabetes screening programmes from a public health perspective. *Journal of Medical Screening* **9**, 187–90.

Stern MP et al. (1993). Predicting diabetes—moving beyond impaired glucose tolerance. *Diabetes* **42**, 706–14.

Tuomilehto J (2005). A paradigm shift is needed in the primary prevention of type 2 diabetes. In: Ganz M, ed. *Prevention of Type 2 Diabetes*, pp 154–68. West Sussex: John Wiley & Sons.

Tuomilehto J et al. (2001). Prevention of type 2 diabetes mellitus by changes in lifestyle among subjects with impaired glucose tolerance. *New England Journal of Medicine* **344**, 1343–50.

Tuo-uo-Kpu L (2006). Creating awareness on diabetes and its risk factors in the Cite des Palmiers Health District, Douala. 19th IDF World Diabetes Congress 2006. Abstract Book. *Diabetic Medicine* **23** (Special Suppl.).

UK Prospective Diabetes Study Group (1998). Tight blood pressure control and risk of macrovascular and microvascular complications in type 2 diabetes. *British Medical Journal* **317**, 703–13.

Wareham N et al. (1999). Fasting proinsulin concentrations predict the development of type 2 diabetes. *Diabetes Care* **22**, 262–70.

Willett WC et al. (2006). Prevention of chronic disease by means of diet and lifestyle changes. In: Jamison DT et al., eds. *Disease control priorities in developing countries*, 2nd ed., pp 833–50. New York: Oxford University Press.

SECTION 6

EMERGING ISSUES AND SCIENCE IN DIABETES

27. Diabetes in the Young

Actions for the 21st Century

Giuseppina Imperatore, Barbara Linder, and David J. Pettitt

■ Main Public Health Messages

- Diabetes mellitus is one of the most common chronic diseases in children and adolescents.
- The majority of cases of diabetes among youth are type 1.
- Worldwide, the incidence of type 1 diabetes is increasing, especially among young children.
- The incidence of type 1 diabetes varies dramatically around the world.
- Large, long-term intervention studies are needed to identify effective strategies for reducing barriers to diabetes care and improving adherence to treatment and management regimens.
- Since the mid-1990s, type 2 diabetes has become more common among youth.
- The etiology of type 2 diabetes is multifactorial, including environmental, behavioral, and genetic factors.
- The increase in type 2 diabetes is linked to the increase in childhood obesity.
- Children exposed to diabetes in utero appear to develop diabetes at younger ages.
- Small clinical studies give hope that lifestyle modification will increase insulin sensitivity among children at risk for diabetes.
- Schools are natural sites for population-based efforts to prevent type 2 diabetes among children.
- Onset of diabetes in childhood is associated with an increased risk of developing cardiovascular disease in adulthood.
- Children diagnosed with diabetes at age 10 years can expect, on average, about a 19-year reduction in life expectancy.

The findings and conclusions in this paper are those of the authors and do not necessarily represent the official positions of the Centers for Disease Control and Prevention, nor have they been endorsed by the authors cited herein.

- In the United States, higher rates of diabetes-related mortality have been reported among minority children and those of low socioeconomic status.
- The health care delivery system should assure the availability of providers who are competent in caring for type 1 and type 2 patients and are sensitive to the needs of children and adolescents.

■ Introduction

Diabetes mellitus is one of the most common chronic diseases in children and adolescents (National Diabetes Data Group 1995). In this age group the majority of cases are type 1 (SEARCH for Diabetes in Youth Study Group 2006). Worldwide, the incidence of type 1 diabetes is increasing, especially among young children (DIAMOND Project Group 2006). Over the last three decades, however, considerable progress has been made in understanding the pathogenesis and natural history of type 1 disease, thereby increasing our ability to identify those at high risk. And yet we still have no means of preventing or reversing the disease's course. In the last two decades, as a consequence of increasing obesity, type 2 diabetes, once rarely observed in youth, has become much more common, especially among African American, Hispanic, Asian, and Native American youth (SEARCH for Diabetes in Youth Study Group 2006). Although the natural history of early-onset type 2 disease has not been well studied, its prevention in adolescents (as in adults) likely implies the treatment and prevention of obesity. This requires modifying complex behavior patterns that involve the individuals at risk, their families and health care providers, schools, and the community at large.

Well-conducted randomized clinical trials have indicated that the complications of diabetes are preventable. Furthermore, improved pharmacological agents and technologies for insulin administration and glucose monitoring have dramatically changed diabetes management. Unfortunately, not all patients have benefited. In developed countries a large proportion of children and adolescents with diabetes still have elevated levels of risk factors for diabetes complications. And in developing countries children with diabetes may experience premature death because they do not have regular access to insulin and diabetes supplies.

Diabetes care regimens are complex and impose a substantial burden on patients and their families. Success requires comprehensive strategies involving not only the patients, their families, and their health care providers but also the patient's environment. Large, long-term intervention studies are needed to identify effective strategies for reducing barriers to diabetes care and improving adherence; at the same time health policies must assure that children and adolescents with diabetes have access to quality care. Schools, for their part, must offer a supportive environment, including healthy food, a curriculum in physical activity, and personnel trained to manage hypoglycemic or hyperglycemic episodes and assist with insulin administration if needed. The intent should be to establish lifelong healthy behaviors while enhancing the attainment and maintenance of good glycemic control and weight management.

This chapter discusses the epidemiology of type 1 and type 2 diabetes in young people and current etiologic hypotheses. It also highlights the challenges in diabetes classification in youth, and it describes the public health issues of screening, disease outcomes, and potential preventive strategies.

■ Classification of Diabetes in Youth

In the past classification of the two major forms of diabetes in youth was based on clinical characteristics and, in some cases, demographics. Onset before age 15 years and a requirement for insulin soon after diagnosis to control hyperglycemia were criteria used to define type 1. The presence of obesity and/or signs of insulin resistance, membership in a minority racial/ethnic group, and family history have been typically associated with type 2 (American Diabetes Association 2000). However, these criteria may no longer be useful; for example, because early-onset type 2 disease is becoming more common, the age of onset alone is not a definitive criterion. Furthermore the presence of obesity does not necessarily indicate type 2 disease, as individuals with type 1 may also present with obesity (Libman et al. 2003). In 1997 the American Diabetes Association (ADA) and the National Institutes of Health jointly defined type 1 diabetes as a disorder caused by an absolute deficiency of insulin, usually due to autoimmune destruction of the β-cells; type 2 was defined as a disorder resulting from a combination of insulin resistance and progressive β-cell failure (American Diabetes Association 1997). And yet classifying diabetes in youth according to pathophysiology poses numerous challenges. First, specific cutoffs for defining insulin deficiency and insulin resistance are lacking. Fasting C-peptide concentration, a marker of endogenous insulin production, when very low usually indicates type 1 disease, but at the onset of type 1 some individuals may have residual insulin secretion, whereas individuals with long duration of type 2 disease may develop insulin deficiency. Furthermore, glucose toxicity may suppress insulin secretion, and so tests of residual insulin production must be done when the patient is in good metabolic control.

The hallmark of type 1 diabetes is the presence of autoantibodies against the insulin-producing β-cells of the pancreas (diabetes autoantibodies [DAA]) (Wasserfall and Atkinson 2006). The detection of DAA can be used to differentiate between type 1 and type 2, but laboratory methods for measuring DAA are not standardized. In addition DAA titers decline after diagnosis and tend to disappear with longer duration of disease. Therefore DAA titers are less useful for distinguishing between types in persons with diabetes of long duration.

The gold standard for assessing insulin resistance associated with type 2 is the euglycemic hyperinsulinemic clamp, but this procedure is invasive, laborious, and costly. Thus, surrogate markers need to be identified and validated in youth with diabetes. The correct classification of youth-onset diabetes has crucial clinical, prognostic, and public health implications, and the diagnosis may determine the best treatment regimen. In addition, differentiating between type 1 and type 2 may be important because type 2 has become increasingly common in some adolescent populations and is potentially preventable with lifestyle changes. Moreover prevention strategies for type 1 are being tested in large clinical trials (Mahon et al. 2009), and their clinical application would involve correct classification of type. In addition ongoing surveillance of the incidence of childhood and adolescent diabetes requires distinguishing between types to assess temporal trends and the effectiveness of preventive and treatment strategies. An important complicating factor is that the spectrum of diabetes includes phenotypes with characteristics of both types—autoimmunity and insulin resistance (Gale 2006).

■ Epidemiology of Type 1 Diabetes

Prevalence, Incidence, and Trends

Prevalence

The SEARCH for Diabetes in Youth study, a multicenter, population-based study of physician-diagnosed diabetes with onset at age <20 years (SEARCH for Diabetes in Youth Study Group 2006), provides the most recent estimates of type 1 prevalence among U.S. youth. In 2001, in an at-risk population of over 3.4 million youth, the prevalence of type 1 diabetes was 1.54/1000. In the 0- to 9-year age group, the highest prevalence was among non-Hispanic whites, the lowest among American Indians. Type 1 constituted the most common form of diabetes, regardless of race/ethnicity (see Fig. 27.1). In the 10- to 19-year age group, the overall prevalence was 2.3/1000 and was highest in non-Hispanic whites (2.9/1000) and lowest in American Indians (0.5/1000). In this age group type 1 accounted for over 91% of cases among non-Hispanic whites; 74% among Hispanics; 64%, African Americans; 59%, Asians/Pacific Islanders; and 21%, American Indians.

Incidence

Worldwide, diabetes registries have demonstrated that the incidence of type 1 diabetes varies more than 350-fold among countries (DIAMOND Project Group 2006), from 0.1/100,000/year in Venezuela and China to 42/100,000/year in Finland. Variations in incidence are also observed within countries (Muntoni et al. 1997). In the United States incidence varies across racial/ethnic groups. In 2002–2003 in children aged <10 years, the highest incidence (per 100,000 per year) was observed among non-Hispanic whites (23), followed by African Americans (13), Hispanics (12), Asians/Pacific Islanders (6.9), and American Indians (5.2) (see Fig. 27.2) (The

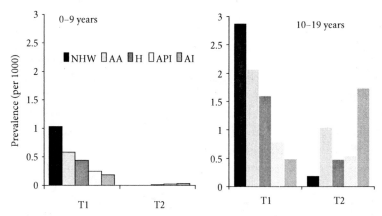

FIGURE 27.1. Prevalence of type 1 and type 2 diabetes per 1000 U.S. youth aged < 20 years in 2001, by age and race/ethnicity. (Source: SEARCH for Diabetes in Youth Study Group 2006.) NHW = Non-Hispanic white; AA = African American; H = Hispanic; API = Asian/Pacific Islander; AI = American Indian; T1 = type 1; T2 = type 2

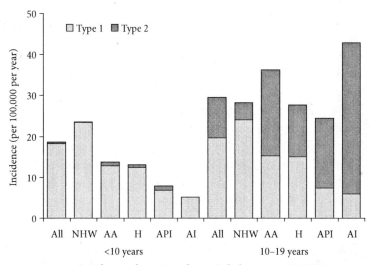

FIGURE 27.2. Incidence of type 1 and type 2 diabetes per 100,000/year among U.S. youth aged <20 years in 2002–2003, by age and race/ethnicity. (Source: writing group for the SEARCH for Diabetes in Youth Study Group 2007.) NHW = Non-Hispanic white; AA = African American; H = Hispanic; API = Asian/Pacific Islander; AI = American Indian

Writing Group for the SEARCH for Diabetes in Youth Study Group 2007). A similar pattern was observed for youth aged 10–19 years (Fig. 27.2). Across all racial/ethnic groups, incidence peaked in the 5–9 and 10–14 age groups and then declined. In all groups among the 0–9-year-olds, type 1 represented the majority of cases. In the 10–19-year-old category, however, the proportion of cases due to type 1 ranged from 85% in non-Hispanic whites to just 14% in American Indians. In the United States every year about 15,000 new cases of type 1 occur in youth aged <20 years (The Writing Group for the SEARCH for Diabetes in Youth Study Group 2007).

Trends

Since the early 1970s, diabetes registries around the world have reported an increase in the incidence of type 1 diabetes. More recently, the World Health Organization-sponsored DIAbetes MONDiale (DIAMOND) project reported an average world-wide annual increase of 2.8% in type 1 incidence (DIAMOND Project Group 2006). The greatest increase was in the 0- to 4-year age group (4.0% per year), followed by those aged 5–9 years (3.0%), with the lowest increase in the 10- to 14-year age group (2.1%). This pattern was primarily seen in European populations. In the United States recent data from Colorado indicated that between 1978–1988 and 2002–2004 in youth aged 0–17 years the average annual increase in incidence of type 1 was 2.7% in non-Hispanic whites and 1.6% in Hispanics (Vehik et al. 2007). As in the DIAMOND project, the highest increase was among children aged 0–4 years.

The increase in incidence of type 1 over such a short period suggests that changes in environmental factors, yet to be identified, are interacting with the genetic background. Among the hypotheses offered is Gale's "spring harvest" (Gale 2005), which suggests an acceleration of the disease's progression in genetically susceptible individuals (thus leading to diagnosis in childhood) rather than an increase in the rate of initiation. Indeed, the observation that the incidence of type 1 has increased in children but decreased in young adults suggests an earlier age of onset rather than a true increase (Pundziute-Lycka et al. 2002; Weets et al. 2002). Some studies have implicated the rapid early growth and increase in childhood obesity seen in most industrialized countries as putative factors for the increased risk of type 1 diabetes (Dahlquist 2005; Hypponen et al. 2000; Knerr et al. 2005). In recent years the proportion of children with type 1 carrying the high-risk HLA (human leukocyte antigen) genotypes has decreased (Fourlanos et al. 2008; Gillespie et al. 2004; Vehik et al. 2008), suggesting that a more hostile environment could increase risk of disease in genetically less susceptible individuals.

Etiopathogenesis and Risk Factors

Although the exact etiology of type 1 diabetes is still unknown, considerable progress has been made in understanding its natural history (Wasserfall and Atkinson 2006). The disease arises from the immune-mediated destruction of the insulin-producing beta cells of the pancreas and is likely initiated and modulated by some environmental factors (Knip et al. 2005) in genetically susceptible individuals, leading ultimately to absolute insulin deficiency.

The preclinical phase is characterized by the presence of DAA and impaired insulin secretion but normal blood glucose levels. As the disease progresses, insulin production declines and hyperglycemia appears (Atkinson 2005). However, the hypothesis that individuals who develop type 1 diabetes are born with definite β-cell mass that is gradually destroyed by the autoimmune process remains to be proven. In addition we still have not identified the environmental factors that can cause or prevent autoimmunity. Moreover, we do not know when β-cell loss starts, at what pace it progresses, and whether genetic or environmental factors can modify its evolution. Finally, we do not know whether, after the onset of frank diabetes, the residual β-cells are able to regenerate. Answering these questions is crucial to ultimately preventing or reversing type 1 disease (Atkinson 2005).

The variation in incidence of type 1 diabetes between racial/ethnic groups and its familial aggregation have been known for a long time, indicating that a genetic susceptibility is involved in the autoimmune process leading to type 1 diabetes. As of today, 12 regions of the genome have been implicated. Of those, genes located in the HLA class II region on chromosome 6 contribute about 50% of the genetic predisposition for type 1 disease (Concannon et al. 2009).

A number of environmental factors are being considered as potential triggers of the autoimmune response and are discussed in chapter 4 of this volume.

■ Epidemiology of Type 2 Diabetes

Prevalence, Incidence, and Trends

Since the mid-1990s, type 2 diabetes has become more common among youth, especially in American Indian, African American, Asian, and Hispanic adolescents. This rise has been reported worldwide and has been reviewed previously (Alberti et al. 2004; Fagot-Campagna et al. 2000; Pinhas-Hamiel and Zeitler 2005). Unfortunately, comparing reports is difficult because of the different case definitions and age ranges used.

The majority of reported studies are from clinics, but before the 1990s it was unusual for pediatric clinics to have patients with type 2 diabetes. By 1999 type 2 represented 8% to 45% of new cases of diabetes in the United States, depending on location (Fagot-Campagna et al. 2000). For example in Cincinnati, Ohio, type 2 rose from less than 4% of all new cases of diabetes before 1992 to 16% of all new cases in children and 33% of new cases in 10- to 19-year-olds in 1994. In Cincinnati the annual incidence (per 100,000) of type 2 in the 10–19 age group increased from 0.7 in 1982 to 7.2 in 1994 (Pinhas-Hamiel et al. 1996). One New York clinic reported a 10-fold increase from 1990 to 2000, with almost 50% of new diabetes cases classified as type 2 in 2000 (Grinstein et al. 2003). In the United States certain ethnic groups, including American Indians, Hispanic Americans, and African Americans, appear to be at highest risk.

In both Japan (Urakami et al. 2006) and Taiwan (Wei et al. 2003) type 2 is the leading cause of childhood diabetes. In Japan urine glucose screening (with confirmation by blood glucose) has been conducted in schools since 1975. Incidence may be underestimated, however, by screening for glycosuria. The annual incidence (per 100,000) of type 2 in Tokyo from 2001 to 2004 was 0.46 in primary school children and 3.66 in junior high school students. Among children aged 6–15 years the overall annual incidence (per 100,000) of type 2 increased from 1.7 in 1974–1980 to 2.7 in 1996–2000, then declined to 1.4 in 2001–2004. This decline, however, was observed mostly among older children (aged 13–15 years), not for younger children (Urakami et al. 2006).

The SEARCH for Diabetes in Youth study has reported population-based incidence (The Writing Group for the SEARCH for Diabetes in Youth Study Group 2007) and prevalence (SEARCH for Diabetes in Youth Study Group 2006) data for U.S. youth aged younger than 20 years. Type 2 was rare in children less than age 10 (see Fig. 27.1). In 2002–2003, annual incidence (per 100,000) in 10- to 19-year-olds was 10 (see Fig. 27.2). Incidence varied by race/ethnicity in this group, ranging from 4 in non-Hispanic whites to 37 in American Indians. Overall, type 2 was more common in minority groups. In the 10–19 group it represented 86.2% of diabetes cases in American Indians, 69.7% in Asians/Pacific Islanders, 57.8% in African Americans, and 46.1% in Hispanics. Prevalence data for 2001 showed a similar racial/ethnic distribution (Fig. 27.1).

Numerous other reports document the high rate of type 2 diabetes among American Indians (Acton et al. 2002; Pavkov et al. 2007) as well as among Canadian (Dean et al. 1998) and Australian (Craig et al. 2007) aboriginal youth. From 1965 to 2003 among the Pima Indians of Arizona, a population at very high risk for type 2 disease, the incidence of type 2 diabetes in youth aged 5–14 years increased almost six times, but it declined in the 25–34 age group (Pavkov et al. 2007). This suggests a shift to a younger age of onset in those at greatest risk.

A yearlong survey of pediatricians (October 2004 to October 2005) was used in England to assess type 2 diabetes among youth aged less than 17 years (Haines et al. 2007). As in other reports from Europe, the annual rate was low (0.53). Incidence rates were higher among minority groups (3.9 and 1.25, respectively, per 100,000 for blacks and South Asians).

In the United States a more definitive picture of temporal trends in type 2 diabetes among youth of all major racial/ethnic groups will be provided by the ongoing SEARCH study (www.searchfordiabetes.org).

Etiopathogenesis and Risk Factors

Although the pathophysiology of type 2 diabetes in the pediatric population has not been well studied, emerging evidence (Druet et al. 2006; Gungor et al. 2005) suggests that the disease is similar to what is typically seen in affected adults, in whom decreased insulin sensitivity and impaired pancreatic beta cell function are hallmarks (Kahn 2003). Initially, insulin resistance occurs that is accompanied by compensatory hyperinsulinemia. Over time, however, there is progressive β-cell failure, resulting in type 2 diabetes.

The etiology of type 2 disease is multifactorial, including environmental, behavioral, and genetic risk factors. Heritability has been demonstrated in adults, and a strong family history is present in most affected children (American Diabetes

Association 2000). The prevailing hypothesis is that environmental factors, such as excessive caloric intake and a sedentary lifestyle, superimposed on a familial phenotype of decreased insulin sensitivity and/or impaired insulin secretion, lead over time to type 2 disease. A genetic predisposition to insulin resistance is thought to partially account for the increased incidence of type 2 diabetes among minorities.

The increase in type 2 disease in children is linked to the increase in childhood obesity in the United States and around the world. Large portions and high-calorie diets coupled with a sedentary lifestyle have led to an epidemic of obesity among youth (Daniels et al. 2005; Huang and Goran 2003). Obesity, superimposed on a high-risk genetic background, is likely the most important contributor to the development of insulin resistance. In children, as in adults, visceral fat appears to be the best predictor of type 2 disease (Lee et al. 2006; Weiss and Caprio 2005).

Youth are diagnosed with type 2 at a mean age of 13.5 years (Gungor et al. 2005). Puberty is associated with transient insulin resistance, thought to be a consequence of increased secretion of growth hormone (Hannon et al. 2006). Pubertal youth who have risk factors for type 2 diabetes may be unable to undergo a normal puberty-related compensatory increase in insulin secretion, leading to the development of diabetes. Other clinical characteristics that may indicate insulin resistance include acanthosis nigricans in boys or girls and polycystic ovary syndrome in girls. Generally girls are at greater risk (American Diabetes Association 2000; Pinhas-Hamiel et al. 1996; Scott et al. 1997).

In Utero Exposure to Maternal Diabetes as a Risk Factor for Type 2 Diabetes

Since the 1970s several human studies have found striking long-term effects of the diabetic uterine environment on growth and development, including higher rates of obesity (Pettitt et al. 1983, 1987; Silverman et al. 1993), impaired glucose tolerance (Clausen et al. 2008; Silverman et al. 1995), and type 2 diabetes (Pettitt et al. 1988) as well as diagnosis of diabetes at a younger age (Pettitt et al. 2008; Stride et al. 2002). Obesity associated with this intrauterine exposure is well described among the Pima Indians (Dabelea and Pettitt 2001; Pettitt et al. 1983, 1987, 1991) and among the racially mixed population from the Chicago Diabetes in Pregnancy Center (Silverman, Landsberg, and Metzger 1993). By age 15 to 19, severe obesity (≥140% of standard) was found among 58% of Pima children who were exposed to diabetes *in utero*, compared with only 17% of those whose mothers did not have diabetes (Pettitt et al. 1983). Higher rates of type 2 diabetes have also been described among offspring of Pima women with this kind of diabetes (Dabelea et al. 2001; Pettitt et al. 1988, 1991). By age 20 to 24, Pima children exposed to diabetes in utero were much more likely to have type 2 diabetes (45%) than were those whose mothers developed diabetes after they delivered (8.6%) (Pettitt et al. 1988).

Similar findings have been described in other populations (Silverman et al. 1995) and among whites from Denmark (Clausen et al. 2008). Evidence that these findings are not simply genetic or familial associations is provided by the sibling studies in the Pima Indians (Dabelea et al. 2000) and by carefully conducted studies in experimental animals (Aerts and Van Assche 2006; Gauguier et al. 1994). Offspring exposed to diabetes in utero appear to develop diabetes at younger ages. Among subjects with maturity-onset diabetes of the young due to mutations in the HNF1-α (MODY3) that they inherited from their mothers, those born after their mothers were already hyperglycemic developed their disease at a significantly younger age (15.3 years) than those whose mothers were euglycemic at pregnancy (27.5 years) (Stride et al. 2002). Similarly, individuals with type 2 diabetes in the SEARCH for Diabetes in Youth Study developed diabetes an average of 1.7 years earlier if they were exposed to diabetes in utero than if their mothers developed diabetes after they were born (Pettitt et al. 2008). In both of these studies paternal diabetes was not a risk factor for an earlier diagnosis. Thus the diabetic pregnancy and its effect on the offspring represent a trans-generational vicious cycle (Dabelea et al. 2001), with female offspring of diabetic women more likely to have diabetic pregnancies themselves (Pettitt et al. 1991).

In Utero Exposure to Undernutrition as a Risk Factor for Type 2 Diabetes

In 1992 Barker and Hales proposed the thrifty phenotype hypothesis, which postulates that exposure to undernutrition during fetal life and infancy produces physiological and structural changes that later in life predispose the affected person to type 2 diabetes (Hales and Barker 1992). In support of this hypothesis a recent meta-analysis of 32 populations showed an inverse association between birth weight and risk of type 2 diabetes (Whincup et al. 2008). The overall reduction of type 2 diabetes for a 1-kg increase in birth weight was about 20%. However a positive relationship between birth weight and type 2 disease was observed in two American Indian populations in which there was a very high prevalence of both maternal diabetes and young-onset type 2 diabetes as well as in a population of predominantly young adults of European origins. This pattern suggests that in individuals who develop type 2 diabetes at a younger age, high birth weight, which is usually a result of exposure to maternal diabetes, may play a more predominant role. This hypothesis, however, needs to be confirmed in large longitudinal studies that include individuals of diverse racial and ethnic background.

■ Primary Prevention

Primary Prevention of Type 1 Diabetes

Since the 1980s a number of randomized clinical trials have tested the use of agents to induce immunosuppression or immunological tolerance or to prevent the initiation of the autoimmune process in high-risk individuals (Sherr et al. 2008). In the

European Nicotinamide Diabetes Intervention Trial, individuals treated with nicotinamide, which prevents autoimmunity in animal models, progressed to diabetes at a rate similar to that for controls (28% vs. 30%). The Diabetes Prevention Trial Type 1 tested whether the use of parenteral or oral insulin would induce immunological tolerance and prevent the onset of type 1 diabetes in first- or second-degree relatives of type 1 patients. Individuals with positive DAA and an estimated 5-year risk of developing diabetes of at least 50% were randomly assigned to treatment with parenteral insulin or to close observation. Those with a 5-year diabetes risk of 25%–50% were randomly assigned to either daily oral insulin or placebo. Both approaches failed to prevent or delay overt diabetes. However, a post hoc analysis suggested some beneficial effect of oral insulin in individuals with very high DAA titers. Type 1 Diabetes TrialNet (http://www2.diabetestrialnet.org) is currently testing the use of oral insulin to prevent type 1 in a much larger cohort. Finally, in a population-based sample of high-risk children in Finland, intranasal insulin failed to induce immunotolerance and to retard progression to diabetes (Nanto-Salonen et al. 2008).

A number of prevention studies have focused on dietary factors operating in early life. Based on epidemiologic evidence that dietary intake of omega-3 fatty acids is associated with reduced risk of autoimmunity in children at increased risk for type 1 diabetes (Norris et al. 2007), TrialNet is testing whether supplementing the diet of mothers or infants with docosahexaenoic acid (DHA), an omega-3 fatty acid usually contained in fish, prevents type 1 disease in high-risk individuals.

The Trial to Reduce IDDM in the Genetically at Risk (2007), a multicenter international study, is assessing whether the use of casein hydrolysate formula (as compared with conventional cow's milk-based formula) decreases the incidence of type 1 diabetes in children with high-risk HLA genotypes who have first-degree relatives with type 1.

Primary Prevention of Type 2 Diabetes

The primary prevention of type 2 diabetes essentially means the treatment or prevention of obesity. There is clear evidence (Knowler et al. 2002; Li et al. 2008; Lindstrom et al. 2006) that lifestyle modification in adults can prevent or delay the onset of type 2 disease, but studies are lacking in children. Nevertheless, as in adults, obesity is the most important modifiable risk factor for type 2 diabetes in youth. Since 1980 the prevalence of obesity has doubled for children and tripled in the adolescent age range (Ogden et al. 2002, 2006; Troiano and Flegal 1998). The obesity epidemic in children has been linked to increased consumption of sugared beverages and fast foods, increased screen time, and reduced physical activity—all modifiable targets (Johnson-Taylor and Everhart 2006). Although no large-scale studies have demonstrated prevention in children, small clinical studies have demonstrated that lifestyle modification aimed at promoting weight loss and decreasing sedentary activity is associated with improvements in insulin sensitivity (Carrel et al. 2005; Ritenbaugh et al. 2003; Rosenbaum et al. 2007; Savoye et al. 2007). In addition, exercise improves insulin sensitivity, independent of changes in weight (McMurray et al. 2000). One school-based study in Mexican American fourth-graders demonstrated a lower mean fasting glucose (within the normal range) in the intervention schools than in the control schools (Trevino et al. 2004), and a recent program in Philadelphia elementary schools lowered the prevalence of overweight (Foster et al. 2008).

Prevention of diabetes in children will require the modification of complex behavior patterns. Treating and preventing obesity is challenging and must involve the individual, the family, health care providers, and the community, including schools (Daniels et al. 2005; Dietz 2001; Ebbeling et al. 2002; Epstein et al. 1998). Education programs alone are not adequate; successful interventions must include behavior modification.

Individualized, formal treatment in the medical setting may be required for children who are already obese and should include age-specific goals for physical activity and nutrition. Studies also show that limiting sedentary activity, such as watching television or using a computer, leads to increased physical activity and weight loss (Epstein et al. 2008; Robinson 1999). In addition, a focus on eliminating sugared beverages can lead to weight loss (Ebbeling et al. 2006). Lifestyle interventions are most likely to succeed when there is family involvement in the behavior modification process (Epstein et al. 1990; Golan and Crow 2004; Wrotniak et al. 2004). Peer pressure is particularly important in the population at highest risk for type 2 diabetes—adolescents—and thus focusing on social norms and self-efficacy skills may need to be given primacy.

Schools are a natural choice for population-based efforts, as children spend almost half of their waking hours there and are essentially a captive audience. Schools provide one to two meals daily and offer an excellent environment for physical education and the teaching of healthy behaviors. They can promote healthy eating by changing offerings from the cafeteria and vending machines. Physical education focused on fun activities that promote moderate–vigorous physical activity should be provided in all years. Numerous school-based studies have been conducted; although some have reduced body mass index (BMI) or body fat, many have not had an appreciable effect on weight (Doak 2006; Sharma 2006; Story 1999; Summerbell et al. 2005). Further research is needed to define the successful components of a school-based obesity prevention program and to translate such efforts into practice.

Primary prevention should also be aimed at promoting maternal health during pregnancy, as gestational diabetes in the mother (Dabelea et al. 2000) and low birth weight (Hales 2001; Jones 2007) are associated with the development of obesity and type 2 diabetes in the offspring. Attempts to prevent the long-term effects of the diabetic pregnancy must start early and continue throughout the offspring's life. Although randomized controlled trials to demonstrate the effectiveness of controlling diabetes during pregnancy have not been conducted and would raise serious ethical objections, data demonstrating a high correlation between maternal glucose levels during pregnancy and outcomes both at birth (Metzger et al. 2008; Pettitt et al. 1980) and during childhood (Clausen et al. 2008; Pettitt et al. 1991) suggest that normalizing glucose during pregnancy should be beneficial in the long term. Some studies also suggest that breast-feeding may help prevent obesity later in childhood and subsequent type 2 diabetes (Owen et al. 2006).

Unfortunately, although changes that lead to weight loss may prevent type 2 diabetes, weight loss is often difficult to maintain. Studies in adults demonstrate that several drugs used to treat type 2 diabetes—metformin (Knowler et al. 2002), acarbose (Chiasson et al. 2002), and rosiglitazone (DREAM Trial Investigators 2006)—also prevent or delay the onset of the disorder. Comparable studies have not been done in children. The U.S. Food and Drug Administration has not approved these drugs for the prevention of type 2 diabetes, but there are several drugs approved for treating obesity (Padwal and Majumdar 2006; Yanovski 2002).

■ Diabetes Complications in Youth

Acute Complications: Incidence, Trends, Risk Factors, and Prevention Strategies

In children and adolescents with diabetes, acute complications are more common than chronic complications and, at this age, carry a greater risk of morbidity and mortality (Dahlquist and Kallen 2005; Patterson et al. 2007). Acute complications include diabetic ketoacidosis (DKA), hyperosmolar nonketotic syndrome, and hypoglycemia.

Diabetic Ketoacidosis

If untreated, DKA, which is a serious acute complication of childhood diabetes caused by insulin deficiency, can lead to coma and even death. In population-based studies mortality rates in children with DKA have ranged from ~0.15% to 0.3%. The majority of these deaths are due to cerebral edema. DKA may be the initial clinical presentation of both type 1 and type 2 diabetes (Rewers et al. 2008) or can occur in individuals with an established diagnosis.

In 2006 among U.S. youth aged 0–17 years, about 64% of hospital discharges with diabetes as the first-listed diagnosis were due to DKA (CDC National Diabetes Surveillance System, available at http://www.cdc.gov/diabetes/statistics/hosp/kidtable1.htm). The SEARCH study reported that at the onset of diabetes one out of four youth presented with DKA, and 93% of the children with DKA were hospitalized (Rewers et al. 2008). DKA was more common in children aged <5 years than in those aged 15–19 years (38% versus 14%), but rates did not differ significantly by gender or race/ethnicity. In Europe the frequency of DKA in newly diagnosed type 1 diabetes ranged from 26% in Germany to 67% in Romania (Levy-Marchal, Patterson, and Green 2001). The youngest children, youth of families with limited resources, and those who are uninsured or underinsured are more likely to present at the onset of diabetes with DKA (Maniatis et al. 2005; Rewers et al. 2008; Rosenbauer, Icks, and Giani 2002). Limited data are available on temporal trends of DKA at initial presentation. In Finland the frequency of DKA at the initial presentation of type 1 diabetes decreased from 29.5% in 1982–1991 to 18.9% in 1992–2001 (Hekkala, Knip, and Vejola 2007). In contrast, frequency has not decreased in Australia (Bui et al. 2002).

Rapid recognition of classical symptoms of diabetes such as polydypsia, polyuria, polyphagia, and weight loss will help reducing the occurrence of DKA. Fortunately, interventions aimed at increasing awareness among parents, school personnel, and health care providers have demonstrated a dramatic impact in its prevalence at initial presentation of diabetes. In Italy, for example, an intensive community-based awareness campaign reduced the prevalence of DKA at diagnosis of type 1 diabetes from 83% to 13% (Vanelli et al. 1999). Improvements in health care access, especially for those at the low end of the socioeconomic spectrum, are also necessary for reducing the prevalence of DKA at diabetes presentation.

The risk of DKA in youth with established type 1 diabetes varies from 1 to 12 per 100 patients per year. In a U.S. cohort of children aged <19 years with type 1 diabetes the overall incidence of DKA was 8 per 100 patient-years, but it reached 12 per 100 patient-years in adolescent girls, suggesting they are particularly vulnerable (Rewers et al. 2002). Similar rates have been reported in the United Kingdom (7.1 per 100 patient-years) (Smith et al. 1998) and in Australia (12 per 100 patient-years) (Thomsett 1999). In contrast, a Swedish study found that, in children on an intensive-treatment regimen, only 1.5 per 100 patient-years experienced DKA (Nordfeldt et al. 1999).

Limited data are available on secular trends in DKA among youth with established diabetes. In the province of Ontario, Canada, rates of DKA hospitalizations among children aged <19 years remained relatively stable in the period 1991–1999 (Curtis et al. 2002). Similar trends have been found in the Netherlands (Hirasing et al. 1996).

Hypoglycemia

Hypoglycemia, the most common acute complication of diabetes, may range from a very mild lowering of blood glucose levels with minimal or no symptoms to severe hypoglycemia resulting in very low glucose levels, nerve damage, coma, and death if not treated.

Estimates of incidence vary because different glucose levels have been used to define cases. In Colorado, the overall incidence of severe hypoglycemia was 19 per 100 patient-years and decreased significantly with age in girls (per 100 patient-years it was 24 in those aged <7 years, 19 in those 7–12, and 14 in those aged 13) but not in boys (23 per 100 patient-years in those aged <7 years; 22, aged 7–12; and 20, ≥13). Non-Hispanic white ethnicity, longer duration of diabetes, the presence of psychiatric disorders, and underinsurance predicted severe hypoglycemia (Rewers et al. 2002).

The incidence of severe hypoglycemia at a diabetes center in Western Australia was 7.8 per 100 patient-years in 1992, but it was 16.6 per 100 patient-years in 2002, corresponding to a significant decrease in glycosylated hemoglobin (A1C). With newer insulin analog therapy and more experience with intensive diabetes management, the incidence of hypoglycemia stabilized. Thus, the age- and gender-adjusted incidence rate increased significantly by 18% per year from 1992 to 1998 but remained stable thereafter. Of those who experienced severe hypoglycemia, 47% had one episode; 21%, two; and 32%, three or more (Bulsara et al. 2004). Severe hypoglycemia was more common in younger children, individuals with lower A1C levels, those with longer diabetes duration, and children of low social class; it was less common in children on insulin pumps. Data from a tertiary diabetes care center showed that in children with type 1 diabetes during 2002–2003 the rate of severe hypoglycemia was lower than that observed during 1997–1998 (18.5 per 100 patient-years vs. 47.1 per 100 patient-years), and glycemic control was improved in the later period (Svoren et al. 2007).

Despite recent pharmacological and technological advances in diabetes management (Nordfeldt et al. 2003; Shalitin and Phillip 2007), obtaining as close to normal glucose levels as possible while avoiding hypoglycemia still presents substantial challenges. Clearly, improved technologies for predicting and preventing severe hypoglycemia are needed. Fortunately the use of case managers supplemented by psychoeducational modules seems to significantly reduce the incidence of severe hypoglycemia (Svoren et al. 2003).

Hyperglycemic Hyperosmolar Nonketotic Syndrome

Hyperglycemic hyperosmolar nonketotic syndrome (HHNS) is a rare but serious complication of diabetes that is associated with a risk of death close to 45%. HHNS is characterized by severe hyperglycemia (usually over 600 mg/dL), a marked increase in serum osmolality (>330 mOsm/L), and mild ketoacidosis. This complication occurs most commonly in obese adolescents with type 2 disease and presents with signs of severe dehydration and depressed mental status. So far, 29 cases have been described, with the majority involving African American males. Underlying infections, undiagnosed diabetes, diabetes mismanagement, and substance abuse are associated with HHNS (Pinhas-Hamiel and Zeitler 2007).

Chronic Complications: Incidence, Prevalence, Trends, Risk Factors, and Prevention Strategies

Retinopathy

In young people with diabetes, retinopathy is usually asymptomatic, but it is a predictor of proliferative retinopathy and, if untreated, of future vision loss. Very limited population-based data exist for children and adolescents, especially nonwhite youth. In youth with type 1 diabetes, the prevalence of retinopathy ranges from 10% to 45% (Kernell et al. 1997; Kullberg et al. 2002; Mohsin et al. 2005; Olsen et al. 2004). The Diabetes Incidence Study in Sweden (DISS), a nationwide population-based prospective study of adolescents and young adults aged 15–34 years, found that after 10 years of diabetes, retinopathy was present in 39% of patients, but only 1.8% had proliferative retinopathy (Nordwall et al. 2004). In Norway 89% of type 1 patients diagnosed before age 15 in 1973–1982 developed diabetic retinopathy after 25 years of disease, while 11% developed proliferative retinopathy (Skrivarhaug et al. 2006). More recent studies in Europe and Australia have indicated a favorable trend in the occurrence of severe retinopathy (Hovind et al. 2003; Mohsin et al. 2005). In contrast the U.S. Pittsburgh Epidemiology of Diabetes Complications (EDC) study did not detect a significant decline in cumulative incidence of proliferative retinopathy (Pambianco et al. 2006).

Data for retinopathy in youth with type 2 diabetes are scarce. Of note, however, among 178 Pima Indians diagnosed with type 2 before age 20, 45% had diabetic retinopathy by age 30 (Pavkov et al. 2006). In Japanese individuals with onset before age 30, the incidence of background retinopathy was 48 per 1000 person-years after an average of 6 years of diabetes; among those with background retinopathy the incidence of proliferative retinopathy was 58 per 1000 person-years (Yokoyama et al. 2000).

Limited data indicate that youth with type 2, despite a short duration of diabetes, have a greater prevalence of severe retinopathy than those with type 1 (Henricsson et al. 2003). Risk factors identified for the onset and progression of retinopathy include poor glucose control, high blood pressure, albuminuria, hyperlipidemia, smoking, duration of diabetes, and pregnancy. In the DCCT (Diabetes Control and Complications Trial), adolescents (aged 13–17 years) in the intensive-treatment group with no retinopathy at study entry had a 53% decreased risk of retinopathy; those with retinopathy at entry had a 70% reduced risk of retinopathy progression (The Diabetes Control and Complications Trial Research Group 1993). These benefits persisted after the end of the study, clearly demonstrating that in adolescents, tight glucose control should be reached as early as possible after the onset of type 1 disease. It is unknown whether this is also true for type 2 youth. Regardless, current guidelines for youth with diabetes recommend maintaining glucose concentrations at as close to normal values as possible as a measure to prevent the onset and progression of diabetic retinopathy (Silverstein et al. 2005).

Nephropathy

Diabetic kidney disease, or nephropathy, is diagnosed by measuring albumin levels in the urine; microalbuminuria is the early marker of diabetic renal disease. High levels of urinary protein (macroalbuminuria) appear after 15–25 years of diabetes (Harvey et al. 2001; Hovind et al. 2003; Skrivarhaug et al. 2006) and signal a decline in renal function leading to end-stage renal disease (ESRD), a relatively common cause of death among persons with type 1 diabetes.

A recent longitudinal study of children and adolescents with type 1 found an incidence of persistent microalbuminuria of 4.6 per 1000 patient-years (Stone et al. 2006). In the EURODIAB cohort of type 1 patients (mean age 33 years, mean duration 19 years), prevalence was 22% for microalbuminuria and 7.8% for macroalbuminuria (Mattock et al. 2001). Data for 27,805 children, adolescents, and adults with type 1 diabetes from 262 diabetes centers in Germany and Austria revealed that after 40 years of diabetes about a quarter had microalbuminuria, but only 9.4% had developed macroalbuminuria or ESRD (Raile et al. 2007).

Downward trends in the incidence of nephropathy have been reported in Europe. In Denmark in patients with type 1 diabetes the cumulative incidence of nephropathy was significantly lower in those diagnosed in 1979–1984 (13.7%) than in patients diagnosed in 1965–1969 (31.1%) (Hovind et al. 2003). Similar findings have been reported by the Linköping Diabetes Complications Study. In the United States, however, the Pittsburgh EDC study reported no significant difference in the cumulative incidence of nephropathy after 25 years of type 1 diabetes between patients diagnosed in 1965–1969 and those diagnosed in 1975–1980 (Pambianco et al. 2006).

Data on prevalence, incidence, and trends for nephropathy among youth with type 2 disease are limited. In the Pima Indians 57% of individuals who developed type 2 before age 20 had developed nephropathy by age 30 (Krakoff et al. 2003), and early-onset type 2 conferred a higher risk of developing ESRD and of dying by middle age (Pavkov et al. 2006).

As in retinopathy, nephropathy seems to be more frequent in young-onset type 2 disease than in comparable cases of type 1 (Eppens et al. 2006; Maahs et al. 2007; Svensson et al. 2003; Yokoyama et al. 2000). This finding warrants further research to identify the factors that confer the elevated risk of nephropathy associated with early-onset type 2.

Modifiable risk factors for diabetic nephropathy include poor glucose control, hypertension, hyperlipidemia, and smoking. Both the DCCT and the UKPDS (United Kingdom Prospective Diabetes Study) have unquestionably demonstrated the role played by glucose control. The adolescent subgroup enrolled in the intensive-treatment group of the DCCT showed a 10% reduction (primary prevention cohort) and 55% reduction (secondary prevention cohort) in the risk of microalbuminuria compared with the conventionally treated group. These effects persisted well beyond the period of intensive glucose control (White et al. 2001).

Although in children with type 1 diabetes it is unclear whether hypertension is the cause or the result of nephropathy (Schultz et al. 2001), the current ADA guidelines recommend treating microalbuminuria with an angiotensin-converting enzyme (ACE) inhibitor even if blood pressure is not elevated (Silverstein et al. 2005).

Neuropathy

Symptomatic neuropathy is rare in children and adolescents with type 1 diabetes (Hyllienmark, Brismar, and Ludvigsson 1995), but subclinical involvement of the peripheral nervous system is common in this group. Among 80 children and adolescents with type 1 disease with a mean long-term A1C of 8.4% after 13 years of diabetes, subclinical neuropathy, ascertained by nerve conduction, was present in 59% (Nordwall et al. 2006). In the EURODIAB cohort, the incidence of neuropathy was 23.5% over 7 years of follow-up and a mean diabetes duration of 15 years (Tesfaye et al. 2005); prevalence was 46% in Eastern Europe but 25% in northwestern Europe (Toeller et al. 1999). The DiaComp study, a multinational cross-sectional study of complications in type 1 diabetes with onset before age 15 years, reported a remarkable geographic variation in prevalence, ranging from less than 1% in Italy to 59% in Puerto Rico (Walsh et al. 2004). These differences, after controlling for glucose control and hypertension, were partly explained by health care system and socioeconomic factors (Walsh et al. 2005).

Longer duration of diabetes and poor glucose control are the major risk factors for neuropathy (Vinik et al. 2000). The DCCT found that intensive glucose control reduced the risk of developing clinical neuropathy by 60%–69% (The Diabetes Control and Complications Trial Research Group 1995) and that this benefit extends well beyond the end of intensive treatment (Martin et al. 2006).

No data are available on the prevalence or incidence of neuropathy in youth with type 2 diabetes. However, limited data indicate that, despite a short disease duration, individuals with type 2 disease have a prevalence of peripheral and autonomic neuropathy similar to that seen in type 1 (Eppens et al. 2006).

Cardiovascular Diseases

Cardiovascular diseases (CVD), the leading cause of mortality and morbidity in diabetic adults (Gregg et al. 2007; Krolewski 1987; Orchard et al. 2003; Skrivarhaug et al. 2006; Soedamah-Muthu et al. 2004), are uncommon in children and adolescents with diabetes. However, increased thickness of the carotid artery intima and impaired endothelium function, both markers of early atherosclerosis, have been described in the young (Donaghue et al. 1997). Childhood-onset diabetes is associated with an increased risk of developing CVD early in adulthood (Laing et al. 2003; Larsen et al. 2002). The Pittsburgh EDC study reported an annual incidence rate of coronary artery disease of approximately 1% among persons with type 1 diabetes aged 28–38 years (Pambianco et al. 2006); a similar incidence rate was found in the EURODIAB cohort (Soedamah-Muthu et al. 2004).

Data on CVD in youth with type 2 disease are scarce. A study of 20 patients with mean age of 15.5 years and mean duration of diabetes of 1.7 years showed increased arterial stiffness compared with obese and healthy-weight controls (Gungor et al. 2005). The SEARCH study found that type 2 disease, compared with type 1, was associated with increased arterial stiffness (Wadwa et al. 2010). Future research is needed to determine if this increase represents an early sign of future progression to CVD.

The role of hyperglycemia in the development of macrovascular diseases is less clear than it is for microvascular complications. The DCCT/EDIC (Epidemiology of Diabetes Interventions and Complications) study has reported that intensive glucose control in type 1 patients resulted in a 42% reduction of any CVD event and a 57% reduction in major CVD events compared with the conventional treatment group (Nathan et al. 2005). A recent meta-analysis of randomized controlled trials comparing interventions to improve glycemic control with conventional treatment in type 1 and type 2 diabetes found that improved glycemic control substantially reduced cardiac and peripheral vascular events in type 1, whereas in type 2 the effect was more modest and limited to peripheral vascular disease and stroke (Stettler et al. 2006). This suggests that hyperglycemia's role in the development of CVD may differ between type 1 and type 2 patients. Recently, the UKPDS showed that, in adults, intensive treatment of hyperglycemia soon after the diagnosis of type 2 disease resulted in significant decreases in the incidence of myocardial infarction and in all-cause mortality (Holman et al. 2008), suggesting that early intensive glucose control may protect these patients from developing CVD. Whether this is also true for type 2 youth remains to be established.

Other risk factors for the initiation and progression of atherosclerosis, which is typically associated with type 2 disease, include dyslipidemia, hypertension, endothelial dysfunction, and increased platelet activity and coagulability (Beckman, Creager, and Libby 2002). In children with type 1 diabetes, despite normal levels of LDL (low-density lipoprotein) cholesterol, elevated LDL oxidation has been observed, which may lead to accelerated atherogenesis (Nishimura et al. 2001). In the SEARCH study, 35% of type 2 participants had elevated apoB (apolipoprotein B > 100 mg/dL), 36% had dense LDL, and 23% had elevated LDL cholesterol (>130 mg/dL). In contrast, among those with type 1, only 10% had elevated apoB; 8%, dense LDL; and 11%, elevated LDL cholesterol. However, the prevalence of these lipid abnormalities increased substantially with poor glycemic control in both groups (Albers et al. 2008). These results stress the importance of good glucose control in youth with diabetes.

Mortality

Children diagnosed with diabetes at age 10 years experience, on average, a 19-year reduction in life expectancy (Narayan et al. 2003). Among youth the majority of diabetes-related deaths are due to acute complications such as DKA and hypoglycemia. The EURODIAB study reported that individuals diagnosed before the age of 15 years experienced an average doubling of their risk of death (versus their national mortality rates). The standardized mortality ratio ranged from 1.6 in the 0- to 4-year age group to 2.2 in the 10–14 age group (Patterson et al. 2007). EURODIAB also detected differences across countries. For example in Iceland the risk of death did not differ between persons with and without diabetes, whereas in Bulgaria, diabetic children had almost five times the risk of mortality as Bulgarian children as a whole. Differences in diabetes incidence rates and in socioeconomic status did not seem to explain these discrepancies.

In the United States higher rates of diabetes-related mortality have been reported among minority children and those of low socioeconomic status (Centers for Disease Control and Prevention 2007). In 2003–2004 the diabetes death rate for black youth was 2.5 per 1 million, almost three times that of white youth (0.9 per 1 million). Moreover the diabetes death rate in black youth significantly increased after 1998, while in white youth this rate did not change significantly during 1994–2004. Nationwide children living in counties with higher unemployment rates have been found to have higher diabetes mortality, increasing by 2.5% per 1% increase in the unemployment rate (DiLiberti and Lorenz 2001).

Very limited mortality data exist for youth with type 2 diabetes. A study from Sweden, however, reported a mortality ratio of 2.9 in such patients aged 15–34 years for 1983–1999 (Waernbaum et al. 2006).

■ Quality of Care in the Young: Where are the Gaps?

Despite the development of national consensus guidelines for the management of childhood diabetes (Hanas et al. 2006; Silverstein et al. 2005), numerous observational studies have revealed wide discrepancies in the control of diabetes and risk factors for complications in youth (Bell et al. 2009; Craig et al. 2007; Dabelea et al. 2009; Lawrence et al. 2009; Liu et al. 2009; Mayer-Davis et al. 2009).

The ADA currently recommends age-specific targets for glucose control: an A1C of 7.5% for adolescents aged 13–18 years, <8% for those aged 6–12 years, and A1C of 7.5%–8.5% for children less than 6 years old (Silverstein et al. 2005). Unfortunately, data suggest that youth do not generally attain these levels. In the United States among participants in the SEARCH study, the proportion of youth with poor glucose control was high, especially in those aged ≥15 years or from ethnic/racial minority groups (Bell et al. 2009; Dabelea et al. 2009; Lawrence et al. 2009; Liu et al. 2009; Mayer-Davis et al. 2009). In this age group, 50% of African American, 36% of Hispanic, and 22% of non-Hispanic white youth with type 1 diabetes had an A1C ≥9.5% (Bell et al. 2009; Lawrence et al. 2009; Mayer-Davis et al. 2009).

Data for 2005 from 21 pediatric diabetes centers in 17 countries in Europe, Japan, and North America revealed that among adolescents aged 11–18 years the mean A1C was 8.2% (de Beaufort et al. 2007). Of concern is the finding that no significant changes in mean A1C occurred between 1998 and 2005 (mean A1C = 8.6% and 8.7%, respectively, in 1998 and 2005). During 1994–2004 in Germany in a large cohort of patients with type 1 diabetes, mean A1C was 8.5% in adolescents (12–16 years) and 8.6% in young adults (17–26 years) (Schwab et al. 2006). More than 60% of the patients had an A1C >7.5%. A nationwide Scottish study of children aged

0–15 years with type 1 reported a mean A1C of 9.1%. Adolescents (aged 10–15 years) had significantly worse glycemic control (mean A1C 9.5%) than younger children (Scottish Study Group for the Care of the Young Diabetic 2001). The survey also detected significant variation in A1C levels across centers: in only 3 out of 18 centers did at least half of the patients have an A1C <8.5%. From these data it emerges that, despite the technological and therapeutic progress in diabetes management, glucose control in children is still suboptimal. Reaching good glycemic control is greatly influenced by the level of support that youth receive from their parents and siblings, peers, their school, the health care system, and the community at large (Hains et al. 2007, 2008). It is, therefore, critical to identify barriers that prevent a large proportion of youth with diabetes from achieving the desirable level of glycemic control.

In addition to glucose control treatment of cardiovascular risk factors is an essential part of diabetes management. The American Heart Association and the ADA state that in children and youth with diabetes (both type 1 and type 2), optimal lipid concentrations are <100 mg/dL for LDL cholesterol, >35 mg/dL for HDL (high-density lipoprotein) cholesterol, and <150 mg/dL for triglycerides (American Diabetes Association 2003; Williams et al. 2002). The ADA also recommends lipid screening at diagnosis of type 1 disease in children older than 2 years if they have other CVD risk factors or at age 12 if they do not. If the lipid profile is normal, testing for lipids should be repeated every 5 years. In youth with type 2 disease lipid screening should be performed at diagnosis and, if normal, repeated every 2 years (Silverstein et al. 2005). If lipid abnormalities are identified, initial treatment should focus on aggressive management of diet, exercise, and glycemic control. If these modalities prove inadequate, pharmacological therapy should be considered.

The SEARCH study recently reported a high prevalence of lipid abnormalities in a large population-based sample of youth with diabetes (Kershnar et al. 2006). About half of the participants had an LDL cholesterol concentration above the desirable level of 100 mg/dL. Among children aged >10 years, 24% of those with type 2 and 15% of those with type 1 had an LDL cholesterol concentration >130 mg/dL; 3% of those with type 1 and 9% of those with type 2 had an LDL cholesterol concentration >160 mg/dL. Yet the use of lipid-lowering drugs was very rare (Kershnar et al. 2006). Similarly in Germany and Austria among over 27,000 patients with type 1 disease who were aged 0–26 years, the prevalence of dyslipidemia was very high (29% in those aged 12–16 years and 34% in those aged 17–26), but less than 1% of the patients received lipid-lowering therapy (Schwab et al. 2006).

In adults, hypertension is a risk factor for the development of both microvascular and macrovascular complications. The ADA recommends that, as in adults, children with diabetes have their blood pressure measured at every physical examination. Blood pressure levels between the 90th and 95th percentile for age, gender, and height should be treated with diet and exercise, and levels above the 95th with pharmacological treatment (Silverstein et al. 2005). In a large sample of U.S. youth with diabetes, the prevalence of hypertension was 16% in children aged 3–9 years and 30% in those aged 10–19. The highest prevalence (73%) was among those with type 2 disease (Rodriguez et al. 2006). This suggests that implementation of the guidelines is suboptimal.

Unhealthy dietary habits in children and adolescents with diabetes, in addition to compromising healthy growth and development, can increase the risk of acute and chronic complications. The ADA recommends that youth with diabetes consume a diet rich in fruits and vegetables, whole grains, low-fat dairy, and lean protein (Franz et al. 2004). United States data on dietary practices of youth with type 1 or type 2 disease showed that only one in five met recommendations for intake of fruits, vegetables, and grains; only 6.5% met the recommendations for consumption of saturated fat, and none met the guidelines for whole-grain consumption (Mayer-Davis et al. 2006). These findings are consistent with those of a case-control study comparing dietary intake among adolescents between those with type 1 diabetes and those without diabetes (Helgeson et al. 2006).

■ Implications for Health Policy

Policies that empower youth to take control of managing their diabetes, that provide these youth with opportunities for diabetes education, and that assure an environment that promotes a healthy lifestyle could facilitate the prevention or delay of major complications and reduce the burden of disease in this population.

Diabetes management requires the coordination of mealtimes and intake, physical activities, monitoring of blood glucose, and drug administration. Family involvement is essential and, when supported by a multidisciplinary health care team, has been demonstrated to improve glucose control (Laffel et al. 2003; Wysocki et al. 2007). Psychological treatments, especially those involving the whole family, may also improve diabetes outcomes (Winkley et al. 2006). A family-centered approach and consideration of behavioral interventions may be particularly important during adolescence, when youth are facing peer pressure to conform and are seeking to establish independence from their parents.

The health care delivery system should assure the availability of providers who are competent in caring for type 1 and type 2 patients and are sensitive to the needs of children and adolescents. This recommendation should not be limited to secondary and tertiary care centers, as youth with type 2 disease are likely to be diagnosed and treated at primary care facilities. The transition from adolescence into adulthood can be difficult, and diabetes control can deteriorate (Fleming, Carter, and Gillibrand 2002; Kipps et al. 2002; Tsamasiros and Bartsocas 2002). Having the adolescent patient see both pediatric and adult providers during this transition may be helpful (Kollipara and Kaufman 2008). In addition policy makers should assure that young adults with diabetes are not denied health care coverage after becoming ineligible for coverage under their parents' insurance.

School nurses and other personnel are an essential component of the diabetes management team, and thus school personnel should receive training on diabetes and its management. The U.S. National Diabetes Education Program (NDEP) has produced a school guide on diabetes management for school nurses and other personnel (available at http://ndep.nih.gov/diabetes/pubs/catalog.htm#PubSchoolPer), but there is an urgent need to reach a consensus on policies to increase physical activity and enhance access to healthy food in school settings and to facilitate diabetes self-management behaviors there. The collaboration of advocates and policy makers, health care providers, the public health community, industry, and the education sector would enhance this process.

Not surprisingly, a lack of health insurance can negatively affect the course of diabetes, increase rates of hospital admission, and prolong stays at the hospital (Keenan, Foster, and Bratton 2002; Todd et al. 2006). Lack of insurance is usually associated with lower socioeconomic status and is more common in minority groups. Policies to provide quality health care coverage for all children and to assure reimbursement for insulin administration and glucose-monitoring devices that are appropriate for youth are needed.

■ Economic Issues and Implications

Even though diabetes is one of the most common chronic diseases in children and adolescents, data on the disease's economic burden relative to this age group remain limited (Icks, Holl, and Giani 2007). And yet such data are crucial for assessing the health care costs of the disease and evaluating the economic efficiency of diabetes prevention and control programs in this population.

Data from an administrative database using insurance claims for more than 3 million persons in the United States indicated that, in 2002, among children aged 0–18 years, medical costs for diabetes were over US$5000 per patient; outpatient care constituted the largest proportion of these costs (Zhang and Imai 2007). The cost of diabetes supplies alone was $384 per patient. In Sweden medical care expenditures for children with diabetes were about eight times more than those for their nondiabetic counterparts (Wirehn et al. 2008). These estimates are comparable to those obtained from adult populations (Ettaro et al. 2004). In Germany inpatient care accounts for about a quarter of the total cost of diabetes expenditures among insulin-treated youth (Icks et al. 2004). Not surprisingly youth with diabetes are more likely to be hospitalized than nondiabetic youth (Icks et al. 2001). In Germany the costs for hospitalization after the onset of diabetes were estimated at US$506 per person-year (in 1997 prices), totaling US$12.4 million for the diabetic population aged 1–19 years, which represented the majority of the total costs associated with pediatric diabetes in the country (Icks et al. 2001). More than half of hospitalizations were for diabetes education or metabolic control; 17% were due to DKA or severe hypoglycemia. In light of increasing health care costs, strategies aimed at reducing hospitalization rates are warranted.

There are very limited data on the indirect costs of diabetes in youth, and essentially no data for direct and indirect costs for youth with type 2 disease. There is also a lack of data on the health care costs due to diabetes complications in children with type 1 or type 2 diabetes.

■ Screening for Diabetes: Who, Where, Why?

Any successful screening program must satisfy several criteria: the condition must be common and serious; it should have a prolonged latency period; the screening test should be sensitive and specific; an adequate intervention strategy for patients detected by screening should be available; and screening should be cost effective.

Type 1

Currently, screening for type 1 diabetes is not recommended because no preventive intervention is available. Even so, there is considerable discussion about whether population screening for identifying children at high risk for this disease should be implemented. Screening costs can be substantial, ranging from US$245 per child if only individuals at elevated genetic risk are periodically screened for autoimmune markers to US$733 if the entire child population is periodically tested for these markers (Hahl et al. 1998). It is unclear who should bear the costs of the screening, who should perform it, and how often it should be done. In addition, for a person to know that she or he is at risk for type 1 diabetes may create apprehension and adversely affect quality of life, access to health care and life insurance, and future opportunities for employment. The lack of effective preventive strategies poses an additional ethical concern. Until screening becomes more appropriate, increased education of the general population, especially health care providers and school personnel, on the signs and symptoms of hyperglycemia may be an effective way to increase the early recognition of new-onset diabetes, thus preventing DKA with its significant morbidity (Vanelli et al. 1999).

Type 2

Screening for type 2 diabetes can identify youth with prediabetes (American Diabetes Association 2000), a group that may benefit from prevention programs, as well as those who already have type 2 disease. The definitive demonstration that type 2 diabetes can be prevented in adults with prediabetes has provided a compelling argument for screening of high-risk youth.

Early diagnosis of type 2 diabetes and the prompt institution of treatment may provide opportunities to preserve β-cell function, although studies addressing this question have not been conducted. Early diagnosis also allows identification and treatment of comorbidities, such as hypertension and dyslipidemia, which contribute to the long-term morbidity and mortality of type 2 diabetes.

Another rationale for screening is that type 2 disease may remain asymptomatic for long periods of time. One adult in three with type 2 diabetes is undiagnosed (Cowie et al. 2006), and many adults with the disease are diagnosed only after they present with a complaint related to one of its long-term microvascular or macrovascular complications (Harris and Eastman 2000). Presumably, identification of individuals early in the disease will allow treatment to normalize blood glucose values and thus prevent long-term complications. Although it has been established that normalization of blood glucose prevents complications (The Diabetes Control and Complications Trial Research Group 1993), studies have not addressed whether early diagnosis through screening also results in improved outcomes. Regardless, evidence has emerged recently that adolescents with type 2 diabetes already have a significant prevalence of microvascular complications (Eppens et al. 2006) as well as risk factors for macrovascular complications (Rodriguez et al. 2006), suggesting that aggressive early intervention in youth may be warranted.

Unlike the case in adults, among youth, population-based screening has not revealed a significant prevalence of undiagnosed type 2 diabetes (Baranowski et al. 2006; Dolan et al. 2005). However, data from both population-based screening (Baranowski et al. 2006; Dolan et al. 2005) and clinic settings (Goran et al. 2004; Sinha et al. 2002) demonstrate that the prevalence of prediabetes is high. Therefore targeted screening of high-risk individuals may be justified. In children targeted screening for prediabetes and type 2 disease has been supported, despite a lack of research in this area, because the disorder meets many of the public health criteria for screening (American Diabetes Association 2000): it is common and serious; there is a prolonged latency period; screening is sensitive and specific; and treatment is available.

The ADA and the American Academy of Pediatrics (American Diabetes Association 2000) have recommended screening of obese children (BMI >85th percentile for age and sex) who have two or more of the following risk factors: (1) family history of diabetes in a first- or second-degree relative, (2) high-risk race/ethnicity (American Indian, African American, Hispanic American, Asian/Pacific Islander), or (3) signs of insulin resistance (acanthosis nigricans, hypertension, dyslipidemia, polycystic ovary syndrome). Screening should begin at age 10 years (or at puberty) and be repeated every 2 years. Screening can be done with either a fasting blood glucose or a 2-hour oral glucose tolerance test (OGTT). The ADA recommends the fasting blood glucose because of its convenience.

Which screening test is best remains a controversial issue in adults as well as in children. Whereas the ADA recommends fasting blood glucose, the World Health Organization (WHO) recommends an OGTT (Alberti and Zimmet 1998). The two organizations also disagree about the definition of impaired fasting glucose ($\geq$100 mg/dL per the ADA vs. $\geq$110 mg/dL by the WHO standard). Data in children indicate that, as in adults, many children diagnosed with type 2 diabetes based on an abnormal OGTT would have been missed with a fasting glucose (Invitti et al. 2003; Libman and Arslanian 2007; Sinha et al. 2002). Although individuals with either impaired fasting glucose (IFG) or impaired glucose tolerance (IGT) may be at risk for the development of diabetes and/or CVD, these two groups are not interchangeable (Unwin et al. 2002). Further research is needed to better understand the different pathophysiologies of IFG and IGT and the implications for screening.

The use of an A1C value to screen for diabetes is controversial, but is currently recommended by the ADA (International Expert Committee 2009). Large trials have not been performed to establish appropriate cutoff values, and issues with standardization and the need for population-specific cutoffs need to be considered. Nevertheless, the A1C measure is an attractive tool because it does not require fasting and can, therefore, be done "on the spot" during a medical visit. Recent studies support its usefulness as a screening tool (Peters et al. 1996; Rohlfing et al. 2000). At the very least, the A1C value may be a useful tool to determine which individuals need further follow-up and diagnostic testing.

Further research is needed to establish the most accurate and cost-effective approaches to screening in youth.

■ Developments over the Next 5 to 10 Years

Management of Type 1 Diabetes: How to Assure Access?

The introduction of insulin analogs, the use of continuous subcutaneous insulin infusion, improved devices for self-monitoring of blood glucose, better behavioral and educational programs, and enhanced communication technologies have dramatically changed diabetes management (Nordfeldt et al. 2003; Shalitin et al. 2007). In the near future it is conceivable that a system able to sense glucose levels and deliver insulin accordingly, the so-called "artificial pancreas," will be available (Steil and Rebrin 2005). Islet transplantation, today limited to patients who have undergone kidney transplant or have frequent episodes of hypoglycemia, might be offered as a cure for type 1 diabetes (Merani and Shapiro 2006). And yet, despite these rapid improvements, a large proportion of youth with diabetes, especially those from families with reduced means, have poor glycemic control or inadequate control of other risk factors for diabetes complications. Moreover, a large proportion of individuals with type 1 diabetes, particularly in developing countries, still lack regular access to insulin and diabetes supplies (International Diabetes Federation, available at http://www.eatlas.idf.org/Insulin_and_diabetes_supplies).

Clearly, there is a gap between the scientific and technological progress achieved and its implementation. To reduce this gap international efforts are needed to assure that children and adolescents around the world do not suffer premature death and disability because their diabetes is mismanaged and that they all benefit from the new technologies. Policies aimed at improving access to care and reducing costs are imperative and will require the collaboration of governments, health care systems, patient and health care provider organizations, industry, and community leaders.

Identification of Strategies for the Prevention or Reversal of Type 1 Diabetes

The prevention of type 1 diabetes can not be separated from the identification of environmental agents involved in the autoimmune process. Although a variety of factors have been investigated, including viral infections, dietary factors during infancy, and vitamin D deficiency (Knip et al. 2005), there is as yet no clear evidence that any of these factors are causative.

The Environmental Determinants of Diabetes in the Youth (TEDDY 2007), a multicenter, multinational, epidemiologic study conducted in six clinical centers in the United States and Europe, is enrolling high-risk newborns to identify infectious agents and dietary or other environmental factors that are associated with an increased risk of autoimmunity and type 1 diabetes. Identification of such factors will lead to a better understanding of type 1's pathogenesis and eventually to its prevention.

Identification of Strategies for the Prevention of Obesity and Type 2 Diabetes

With increases in risk factors such as obesity and inactivity among children and adolescents, the prevalence of early-onset type 2 diabetes and its complications will increase (Lee 2008). In high-risk adults lifestyle interventions reduce the incidence of this disease (Knowler et al. 2002; Li et al. 2008; Lindstrom et al. 2006), and these interventions are cost effective (Herman et al. 2005). Whether this is true for youth is still uncertain. Although the pathophysiology of type 2 diabetes in youth is characterized by the same metabolic abnormalities as in adults, the progression to β-cell failure appears to be more rapid in youth (Gungor and Arslanian 2004).

Most important, the development and implementation of effective, sustainable interventions for the prevention of type 2 diabetes in youth requires interaction among a variety of sectors of the society, including public health and medical communities, local and national governments, industry, media, transportation, urban planners, and educators. Engaging these disparate groups in working toward a common goal may represent the greatest challenge.

■ References

Acton KJ et al. (2002). Trends in diabetes prevalence among American Indian and Alaska Native children, adolescents, and young adults. *American Journal of Public Health* **92**, 1485–90.

Aerts L, Van Assche FA (2006). Animal evidence for the transgenerational development of diabetes mellitus. *International Journal of Biochemistry & Cell Biology* **38**, 894–903.

Albers JJ et al. (2008). Prevalence and determinants of elevated apolipoprotein B and dense low-density lipoprotein in youths with type 1 and type 2 diabetes. *Journal of Clinical Endocrinology and Metabolism* **93**, 735–42.

Alberti G et al. (2004). Type 2 diabetes in the young: the evolving epidemic: the International Diabetes Federation Consensus Workshop. *Diabetes Care* **27**, 1798–811.

Alberti KG, Zimmet PZ (1998). Definition, diagnosis and classification of diabetes mellitus and its complications. Part 1: diagnosis and classification of diabetes mellitus provisional report of a WHO consultation. *Diabetic Medicine* **15**, 539–53.

American Diabetes Association (1997). Report of the Expert Committee on the Diagnosis and Classification of Diabetes Mellitus. *Diabetes Care* **20**, 1183–97.

American Diabetes Association (2000). Type 2 diabetes in children and adolescents. American Diabetes Association. *Diabetes Care* **23**, 381–9.

American Diabetes Association (2007). Diabetes care in the school and day care setting. *Diabetes Care* **30** (Suppl. 1), S66–73.

Atkinson MA (2005). ADA Outstanding Scientific Achievement Lecture 2004. Thirty years of investigating the autoimmune basis for type 1 diabetes: why can't we prevent or reverse this disease? *Diabetes* **54**, 1253–63.

Baranowski T et al. (2006). Presence of diabetes risk factors in a large U.S. eighth-grade cohort. *Diabetes Care* **29**, 212–7.

Beckman JA, Creager, MA, Libby P (2002). Diabetes and atherosclerosis: epidemiology, pathophysiology, and management. *JAMA* **287**, 2570–81.

Bell RA et al. (2009). Diabetes in Non-Hispanic white youth: Prevalence, incidence, and clinical characteristics: the SEARCH for Diabetes in Youth Study. *Diabetes Care* **32** (Suppl. 2), S102–11.

Bui TP et al. (2002). Trends in diabetic ketoacidosis in childhood and adolescence: a 15-yr experience. *Pediatric Diabetes* **3**, 82–8.

Bulsara MK et al. (2004). The impact of a decade of changing treatment on rates of severe hypoglycemia in a population-based cohort of children with type 1 diabetes. *Diabetes Care* **27**, 2293–8.

Carrel AL et al. (2005). Improvement of fitness, body composition, and insulin sensitivity in overweight children in a school-based exercise program: a random-ized, controlled study. *Archives of Pediatrics & Adolescent Medicine* **159**, 963–8.

Centers for Disease Control and Prevention (2007). Racial disparities in diabetes mortality among persons aged 1–19 years--United States, 1979–2004. *Morbidity and Mortality Weekly Report* **56**, 1184–7.

Chiasson J et al. (2002). Acarbose for prevention of type 2 diabetes mellitus: the STOP-NIDDM randomised trial. *Lancet* **359**, 2072–7.

Clausen TD et al. (2008). High prevalence of type 2 diabetes and pre-diabetes in adult offspring of women with gestational diabetes mellitus or type 1 diabetes: the role of intrauterine hyperglycemia. *Diabetes Care* **31**, 340–6.

Concannon P et al. (2009). Genetics of type 1A diabetes. *New England Journal of Medicine* **360**, 1646–54

Cowie CC et al. (2006). Prevalence of diabetes and impaired fasting glucose in adults in the U.S. population: National Health and Nutrition Examination Survey 1999–2002. *Diabetes Care* **29**, 1263–8.

Craig ME et al. (2007a). Type 2 diabetes in indigenous and non-indigenous children and adolescents in New South Wales. *Medical Journal of Australia* **186**, 497–9.

Craig ME et al. (2007b). Diabetes care, glycemic control, and complications in children with type 1 diabetes from Asia and the Western Pacific Region. *Journal of Diabetes Complications* **21**, 280–7.

Curtis JR et al. (2002). Recent trends in hospitalization for diabetic ketoacidosis in Ontario children. *Diabetes Care* **25**, 1591–6.

Dabelea D et al. (2000). Intrauterine exposure to diabetes conveys risks for type 2 diabetes and obesity: a study of discordant sibships. *Diabetes* **49**, 2208–11.

Dabelea D, Pettitt DJ (2001). Intrauterine diabetic environment confers risks for type 2 diabetes mellitus and obesity in the offspring, in addition to genetic susceptibility. *Journal of Pediatric Endocrinology & Metabolism* **14**, 1085–91.

Dabelea D et al. (2009). Diabetes in Navajo Youth: Prevalence, incidence, and clinical characteristics: the SEARCH for Diabetes in Youth Study. *Diabetes Care* **32** (Suppl. 2) S141–7.

Dahlquist G, Kallen B (2005). Mortality in childhood-onset type 1 diabetes: a population-based study. *Diabetes Care* **28**, 2384–7.

Dahlquist G (2005). Can we slow the rising incidence of childhood-onset autoimmune diabetes? The overload hypothesis. *Diabetologia* **49**, 20–4.

Daniels SR et al. (2005). Overweight in children and adolescents: pathophysiology, consequences, prevention, and treatment. *Circulation* **111**, 1999–2012.

de Beaufort CE et al. (2007). Continuing stability of center differences in pediatric diabetes care: do advances in diabetes treatment improve outcome? The Hvidoere Study Group on Childhood Diabetes. *Diabetes Care* **30**, 2245–50.

Dean HJ et al. (1998). Screening for type-2 diabetes in aboriginal children in northern Canada. *Lancet* **352**, 1523–4.

Delamater AM et al. (1999). Risk for metabolic control problems in minority youth with diabetes. *Diabetes Care* **22**, 700–5.

DIAMOND Project Group (2006). Incidence and trends of childhood type 1 diabetes worldwide 1990–1999. *Diabetic Medicine* **23**, 857–66.

Dietz WH (2001). The obesity epidemic in young children. Reduce television viewing and promote playing. *British Medical Journal* **322**, 313–4.

DiLiberti JH, Lorenz RA (2001). Long-term trends in childhood diabetes mortality: 1968–1998. *Diabetes Care* **24**, 1348–52.

Doak CM (2006). The prevention of overweight and obesity in children and adolescents: a review of interventions and programmes. *Obesity Reviews* **7**, 111–36.

Dolan LM et al. (2005). Frequency of abnormal carbohydrate metabolism and diabetes in a population-based screening of adolescents. *Journal of Pediatrics* **146**, 751–8.

Donaghue KC et al. (1997). The effect of prepubertal diabetes duration on diabetes. Microvascular complications in early and late adolescence. *Diabetes Care* **20**, 77–80.

DREAM (Diabetes REduction Assessment with ramipril and rosiglitazone Medication) Trial Investigators et al. (2006). Effect of rosiglitazone on the frequency of diabetes in patients with impaired glucose tolerance or impaired fasting glucose: a randomised controlled trial. *Lancet* **368**, 1096–105.

Druet C et al. (2006). Characterization of insulin secretion and resistance in type 2 diabetes of adolescents. *Journal of Clinical Endocrinology and Metabolism* **91**, 401–4.

Ebbeling CB, Pawlak DB, Ludwig DS (2002). Childhood obesity: public-health crisis, common sense cure. *Lancet* **360**, 473–82.

Ebbeling CB et al. (2006). Effects of decreasing sugar-sweetened beverage consumption on body weight in adolescents: a randomized, controlled pilot study. *Pediatrics* **117**, 673–80.

Eppens MC et al. (2006). Prevalence of diabetes complications in adolescents with type 2 compared with type 1 diabetes. *Diabetes Care* **29**, 1300–6.

Epstein LH et al. (1990). Ten-year follow-up of behavioral, family-based treatment for obese children. *JAMA* **264**, 2519–23.

Epstein LH et al. (1998). Treatment of pediatric obesity. *Pediatrics* **101**, 554–70.

Epstein LH et al. (2008). A randomized trial of the effects of reducing television viewing and computer use on body mass index in young children. *Archives of Pediatrics & Adolescent Medicine* **162**, 239–45.

Ettaro L et al. (2004). Cost-of-illness studies in diabetes mellitus. *Pharmacoeconomics* **22**, 149–64.

Fagot-Campagna A et al. (2000). Type 2 diabetes among North adolescents: an epidemiologic health perspective. *Journal of Pediatrics* **136**, 664–72.

Fleming E, Carter B, Gillibrand W (2002). The transition of adolescents with diabetes from the children's health care service into the adult health care service: a review of the literature. *Journal of Clinical Nursing* **11**, 560–7.

Foster GD et al. (2008). A policy-based school intervention to prevent overweight and obesity. *Pediatrics* **121**, e794–802.

Fourlanos S et al. (2008). The rising incidence of type 1 diabetes is accounted for by cases with lower-risk human leukocyte antigen genotypes. *Diabetes Care* **31**, 1546–9.

Franz MJ et al. (2004). Nutrition principles and recommendations in diabetes. *Diabetes Care* **27** (Suppl. 1), S36–46.

Gale E (2005). Spring harvest? Reflections on the rise of type 1 diabetes. *Diabetologia* **48**, 2445–50.

Gale E (2006). Declassifying diabetes. *Diabetologia* **49**, 1989–95.

Gauguier D et al. (1994). Higher maternal than paternal inheritance of diabetes in GK rats. *Diabetes* **43**, 220–4.

Gillespie KM et al. (2004). The rising incidence of childhood type 1 diabetes and reduced contribution of high-risk HLA haplotypes. *Lancet* **364**, 1699–700.

Golan M, Crow S (2004). Targeting parents exclusively in the treatment of childhood obesity: long-term results. *Obesity Research* **12**, 357–61.

Goran MI et al. (2004). Impaired glucose tolerance and reduced beta-cell function in overweight Latino children with a positive family history for type 2 diabetes. *Journal of Clinical Endocrinology and Metabolism* **89,** 207–12.

Gregg EW et al. (2007). Mortality trends in men and women with diabetes, 1971 to 2000. *Annals of Internal Medicine* **147**, 149–55.

Grinstein G et al. (2003). Presentation and 5-year follow-up of type 2 diabetes mellitus in African-American and Caribbean-Hispanic adolescents. *Hormone Research* **60**, 121–6.

Gungor N, Arslanian S (2004). Progressive beta cell failure in type 2 diabetes mellitus of youth. *Journal of Pediatrics* **144**, 656–9.

Gungor N et al. (2005). Type 2 diabetes mellitus in youth: the complete picture to date. *Pediatric Clinics of North America* **52**, 1579–609.

Hahl J et al. (1998). Costs of predicting IDDM. *Diabetologia* **41**, 79–85.

Haines L et al. (2007). Rising incidence of type 2 diabetes in children in the U.K. *Diabetes Care* **30**, 1097–101.

Hains AA et al. (2009). Attributions of teacher reactions to diabetes self-care behaviors. *Journal of Pediatric Psychology* **34**, 97–107.

Hains AA et al. (2007). Attributions of adolescents with type 1 diabetes related to performing diabetes care around friends and peers: the moderating role of friend support. *Journal of Pediatric Psychology* **32**, 561–70.

Hales CN (2001). The thrifty phenotype hypothesis. *British Medical Bulletin* **60**, 5–20.

Hales CN, Barker DJP (1992). Type 2 (non-insulin dependent) diabetes mellitus; the thrifty phenotype hypothesis. *Diabetologia* **35**, 595–601.

Hanas R et al. (2006). ISPAD Clinical Practice Consensus Guidelines 2006–2007. *PediatricDiabetes* **7**, 341–2.

Hannon TS, Janosky J, Arslanian SA (2006). Longitudinal study of physiologic insulin resistance and metabolic changes of puberty. *Pediatric Research* **60**, 759–63.

Hanberger L et al. (2008). A1C in children and adolescents with diabetes in relation to certain clinical parameters: the Swedish Childhood Diabetes Registry SWEDIABKIDS. Diabetes Care **31**, 927–9.

Harris MI, Eastman RC (2000). Early detection of undiagnosed diabetes mellitus: a US perspective. *Diabetes/Metabolism Research and Reviews* **16**, 230–6.

Harvey JN et al. (2001). Population-based survey and analysis of trends in the prevalence of diabetic nephropathy in type 1 diabetes. *Diabetic Medicine* **18**, 998–1002.

Hekkala A, Knip M, Veijola R (2007). Ketoacidosis at diagnosis of type 1 diabetes in children in northern Finland: temporal changes over 20 years. *Diabetes Care* **30**, 861–6.

Helgeson VS et al. (2006). Diet of adolescents with and without diabetes: trading candy for potato chips? *Diabetes Care* **29**, 982–7.

Henricsson M et al. (2003). The incidence of retinopathy 10 years after diagnosis in young adult people with diabetes: results from the nationwide population-based Diabetes Incidence Study in Sweden (DISS). *Diabetes Care* **26**, 349–54.

Herman WH et al. (2005). The cost-effectiveness of lifestyle modification or metformin in preventing type 2 diabetes in adults with impaired glucose tolerance. *Annals of Internal Medicine* **142**, 323–32.

Hirasing RA et al. (1996). Trends in hospital admissions among children aged 0–19 years with type I diabetes in The Netherlands. *Diabetes Care* **19**, 431–4.

Holman RR et al. (2008). Long–term follow–up after tight control of blood pressure in type 2 diabetes. *New England Journal of Medicine* **359**, 1565–76.

Hovind P et al. (2003). Decreasing incidence of severe diabetic microangiopathy in type 1 diabetes. *Diabetes Care* **26**, 1258–64.

Huang TT, Goran MI (2003). Prevention of type 2 diabetes in young people: a theoretical perspective. *PediatricDiabetes* **4**, 38–56.

Hyllienmark L, Brismar T, Ludvigsson J (1995). Subclinical nerve dysfunction in children and adolescents with IDDM. *Diabetologia* **38**, 685–692.

Hypponen E et al. (2000). Obesity, increased linear growth, and risk of type 1 diabetes in children. *Diabetes Care* **23**, 1755–60.

Icks A, Holl RW, Giani G (2007). Economics in pediatric type 1 diabetes—results from recently published studies. *Experimental and Clinical Endocrinology & Diabetes* **115**, 448–54.

Icks A et al. (2004). Direct costs of care in Germany for children and adolescents with diabetes mellitus in the early course after onset. *Journal of Pediatrics, Endocrinology and Metabolism* **17**, 1551–9.

Icks A et al. (2001). Hospitalization among diabetic children and adolescents and the general population in Germany. German Working Group for Pediatric Diabetology. *Diabetes Care* **24**, 435–40.

International Expert Committee (2009). International Expert Committee report on the role of the A1C assay in the diagnosis of diabetes. *Diabetes Care* **32**, 1327–34.

Invitti C et al. (2003). Prevalence and concomitants of glucose intolerance in European obese children and adolescents. *Diabetes Care* **26**, 118–24.

Johnson-Taylor WL, Everhart JE (2006). Modifiable environmental and behavioral determinants of overweight among children and adolescents: report of a work-shop. *Obesity (Silver Spring)* **14**, 929–66.

Jones RH (2007). Intra-uterine origins of type 2 diabetes. *Archives of Physiology and Biochemistry* **113**, 25–9.

Kahn SE (2003). The relative contributions of insulin resistance and beta-cell dysfunction to the pathophysiology of Type 2 diabetes. *Diabetologia* **46**, 3–19.

Karnik SK et al. (2007). Menin controls growth of pancreatic beta–cells in pregnant mice and promotes gestational diabetes mellitus. *Science* **318**, 806–9.

Keenan HT, Foster CM, Bratton SL (2002). Social factors associated with prolonged hospitalization among diabetic children. *Pediatrics* **109**, 40–4.

Kernell A et al. (1997). Prevalence of diabetic retinopathy in children and adolescents with IDDM. A population-based multicentre study. *Diabetologia* **40**, 307–10.

Kershnar AK et al. (2006). Lipid abnormalities are prevalent in youth with type 1 and type 2 diabetes: the SEARCH for Diabetes in Youth Study. *Journal of Pediatrics* **149**, 314–9.

Kipps S et al. (2002). Current methods of transfer of young people with Type 1 diabetes to adult services. *Diabetic Medicine* **19**, 649–54.

Knerr I et al. (2005). The accelerator hypothesis: relationship between weight, height, body mass index and age at diagnosis in a large cohort of 9,248 German and Austrian children with type 1 diabetes mellitus. *Diabetologia* **48**, 2501–4.

Knip M et al. (2005). Environmental triggers and determinants of type 1 diabetes. *Diabetes* **54** (Suppl. 2), S125–36.

Knowler WC et al. (2002). Reduction in the incidence of type 2 diabetes with lifestyle intervention or metformin. *New England Journal of Medicine* **346**, 393–403.

Kollipara S, Kaufman FR (2008). Transition of diabetes care from pediatrics to adulthood. *School Nurse News* **25**, 27–9.

Krakoff J et al. (2003). Incidence of retinopathy and nephropathy in youth-onset compared with adult-onset Type 2 diabetes. *Diabetes Care* **26**,76–81.

Krolewski AS (1987). Magnitude and determinants of coronary artery disease in juvenile-onset, insulin-dependent diabetes mellitus. *American Journal of Cardiology* **59**, 750–5.

Kullberg CE et al. (2002). Prevalence of retinopathy differs with age at onset of diabetes in a population of patients with Type 1 diabetes. *Diabetic Medicine* **19**, 924–31.

Laffel LM et al. (2003). Impact of ambulatory, family-focused teamwork intervention on glycemic control in youth with type 1 diabetes. *Journal of Pediatrics* **142**, 409–16.

Laing SP et al. (2003). Mortality from heart disease in a cohort of 23,000 patients with insulin-treated diabetes. *Diabetologia* **46**, 760–5.

Larsen JB et al. (2002). Silent coronary atheromatosis in type 1 diabetic patients and its relation to long-term glycemic control. *Diabetes* **51**, 2637–41.

Lawrence JM et al. (2009). Diabetes in Hispanic American youth: prevalence, incidence, demographics, and clinical characteristics: the SEARCH for Diabetes in Youth Study. *Diabetes Care* 2009 **32** (Suppl 2), S123–S132.

Lee JM (2008). Why young adults hold the key to assessing the obesity epidemic in children. *Archives of Pediatrics and Adolescent Medicine* **162**, 682–7.

Lee JM et al. (2006). An epidemiologic profile of children with diabetes in the U.S. *Diabetes Care* **29**, 420–1.

Levy-Marchal C, Patterson CC, Green A (2001). Geographical variation of presentation at diagnosis of Type I diabetes in children: the EURODIAB Study. *Diabetologia* **44**, B75–80.

Li G et al. (2008). The long-term effect of lifestyle interventions to prevent diabetes in the China Da Qing Diabetes Prevention Study: a 20-year follow-up study. *Lancet* **371**, 1783–9.

Libman IM, Arslanian SA (2007). Prevention and treatment of type 2 diabetes in youth. *Hormone Research* **67**, 22–34.

Libman IM et al. (2003). Changing prevalence of overweight children and adolescents at onset of insulin-treated diabetes. *Diabetes Care* **26**, 2871–5.

Lindstrom J et al. (2006). Sustained reduction in the incidence of type 2 diabetes by lifestyle intervention: follow-up of the Finnish Diabetes Prevention Study. *Lancet* **368**, 1673–9.

Liu LL et al. (2009). Type 1 and type 2 diabetes in Asian and Pacific Islander U.S. Youth: The SEARCH for Diabetes in Youth Study. *Diabetes Care* **32** (Suppl. 2), S133–40.

Maahs DM et al. (2007). Higher prevalence of elevated albumin excretion in youth with type 2 than type 1 diabetes: the SEARCH for Diabetes in Youth Study. *Diabetes Care* **30**, 2593–8.

Mahon JL et al. (2009). The TrialNet Natural History Study of the Development of Type 1 Diabetes: objectives, design, and initial results. *Pediatric Diabetes* **10**, 97–104.

Maniatis AK et al. (2005). Increased incidence and severity of diabetic ketoacidosis among uninsured children with newly diagnosed type 1 diabetes mellitus. *Pediatric Diabetes* **6**, 79–83.

Martin CL et al. (2006). Neuropathy among the Diabetes Control and Complications Trial cohort 8 years after trial completion. *Diabetes Care* **29**, 340–4.

Mattock MB et al. (2001). Plasma lipids and urinary albumin excretion rate in Type 1 diabetes mellitus: the EURODIAB IDDM Complications Study. *Diabetic Medicine* **18**, 59–67.

Mayer-Davis EJ et al. (2006). Dietary intake among youth with diabetes: the SEARCH for Diabetes in Youth Study. *Journal of the American Dietetic Association* **106**, 689–97.

Mayer-Davis EJ et al. (2009). Diabetes in African American Youth: Prevalence, incidence, and clinical characteristics: the SEARCH for Diabetes in Youth Study. *Diabetes Care* **32** (Suppl. 2), S112–22.

McMurray RG et al. (2000). The influence of physical activity, socioeconomic status, and ethnicity on the weight status of adolescents. *Obesity Research* **8**, 130–9.

Merani S, Shapiro AM (2006). Current status of pancreatic islet transplantation. *Clinical Science (London)* **110**, 611–25.

Metzger BE et al. (2008). Hyperglycemia and adverse pregnancy outcomes. *New England Journal of Medicine* **358**, 1991–2002.

Mohsin F et al. (2005). Discordant trends in microvascular complications in adolescents with type 1 diabetes from 1990 to 2002. *Diabetes Care* **28**, 1974–80.

Muntoni S et al. (1997). Incidence of insulin-dependent diabetes mellitus among Sardinian heritage children born in Lazio region, Italy. *Lancet* **349**, 160–2.

Nanto-Salonen K et al. (2008). Nasal insulin to prevent type 1 diabetes in children with HLA genotypes and autoantibodies conferring increased risk of disease: a double-blind, randomised controlled trial. *Lancet* **372**, 1746–55.

Narayan KM et al. (2003). Lifetime risk for diabetes mellitus in the United States. *JAMA* **290**, 1884–90.

Nathan DM et al. (2005). Intensive diabetes treatment and cardiovascular disease in patients with type 1 diabetes. *New England Journal of Medicine* **353**, 2643–53.

National Diabetes Data Group, eds. (1995). *Diabetes in America*, 2nd ed. Bethesda, MD: National Institutes of Health/National Institute of Diabetes and Digestive and Kidney Diseases. NIH Publication No. **95**–1468.

Nishimura R et al. (2001). Mortality trends in type 1 diabetes. The Allegheny County (Pennsylvania) Registry 1965–1999. *Diabetes Care* **24**, 823–7.

Nordfeldt SL et al. (1999). Adverse events in intensively treated children and adolescents with type 1 diabetes. *Acta Pediatrica* **88**, 1184–93.

Nordfeldt S et al. (2003). Prevention of severe hypoglycaemia in type I diabetes: a randomised controlled population study. *Archives of Disease in Childhood*, **88**, 240–5.

Nordwall M et al. (2004). Declining incidence of severe retinopathy and persisting decrease of nephropathy in an unselected population of Type 1 diabetes—the Linkoping Diabetes Complications Study. *Diabetologia* **47**, 1266–72.

Nordwall M et al. (2006). Early diabetic complications in a population of young patients with type 1 diabetes mellitus despite intensive treatment. *Journal of Pediatric Endocrinology* **19**, 45–54.

Norris JM et al. (2007). Omega-3 polyunsaturated fatty acid intake and islet autoimmunity in children at increased risk for type 1 diabetes. *JAMA* **298**, 1420–8.

Ogden CL et al. (2002). Prevalence and trends in overweight among US children and adolescents, 1999–2000. *JAMA* **288**, 1728–32.

Ogden CL et al. (2006). Prevalence of overweight and obesity in the United States, 1999–2004. *JAMA* **295**, 1549–55.

Olsen BS et al. (2004). The significance of the prepubertal diabetes duration for the development of retinopathy and nephropathy in patients with type 1 diabetes. *Journal of Diabetes and Its Complications* **18**, 160–4.

Orchard TJ et al. (2003). Insulin resistance-related factors, but not glycemia, predict coronary artery disease in type 1 diabetes: 10-year follow-up data from the Pittsburgh Epidemiology of Diabetes Complications study. *Diabetes Care* **26**, 1374–9.

Owen CG et al. (2006). Does breastfeeding influence risk of type 2 diabetes in later life? A quantitative analysis of published evidence. *American Journal of Clinical Nutrition* **84**, 1043–54.

Padwal R, Majumdar S (2006). Metabolic risk factors, drugs, and obesity. *New England Journal of Medicine* **354**, 974–5.

Pambianco G et al. (2006). The 30-year natural history of type 1 diabetes complications: the Pittsburgh Epidemiology of Diabetes Complications Study experience. *Diabetes* **55**, 1463–9.

Patterson CC et al. (2007). Early mortality in EURODIAB population–based cohorts of type 1 diabetes diagnosed in childhood since 1989. *Diabetologia* **50**, 2439–42.

Pavkov ME et al. (2006). Effect of youth-onset type 2 diabetes mellitus on incidence of end-stage renal disease and mortality in young and middle-aged Pima Indians. *JAMA* **296**, 421–6.

Pavkov ME et al. (2007). Changing patterns of type 2 diabetes incidence among Pima Indians. *Diabetes Care* **30**, 1758–63.

Peters AL et al. (1996). A clinical approach for the diagnosis of diabetes mellitus: an analysis using glycosylated hemoglobin levels. Meta-analysis Research Group on the Diagnosis of Diabetes Using Glycated Hemoglobin Levels. *JAMA* **276**, 1246–52.

Pettitt DJ et al. (1988). Congenital susceptibility to NIDDM. Role of intrauterine environment. *Diabetes* **37**, 622–8.

Pettitt DJ et al. (1983). Excessive obesity in offspring of Pima Indian women with diabetes during pregnancy. *New England Journal of Medicine* **308**, 242–5.

Pettitt DJ et al. (1991). Abnormal glucose tolerance during pregnancy in Pima Indian women. Long-term effects on offspring. *Diabetes* **40** (Suppl. 2), 126–30.

Pettitt DJ et al. (1980). Gestational diabetes: infant and maternal complications of pregnancy in relation to third-trimester glucose tolerance in the Pima Indians. *Diabetes Care* **3**, 458–64.

Pettitt DJ et al. (1987). Obesity in offspring of diabetic Pima Indian women despite normal birth weight. *Diabetes Care* **10**, 76–80.

Pettitt DJ et al. (2008). Association between maternal diabetes in utero and age at offspring's diagnosis of type 2 diabetes. *Diabetes Care* **31**, 2126–30.

Pinhas-Hamiel O et al. (1996). Increased incidence of non-insulin-dependent diabetes mellitus among adolescents. *Journal of Pediatrics* **128**, 608–15.

Pinhas–Hamiel O, Zeitler P (2005). The global spread of type 2 diabetes mellitus in children and adolescents. *Journal of Pediatrics* **146**, 693–700.

Pinhas–Hamiel O, Zeitler P (2007). Acute and chronic complications of type 2 diabetes mellitus in children and adolescents. *Lancet* **369**, 1823–31.

Pundziute–Lycka A. et al. (2002). The incidence of type I diabetes has not increased but shifted to a younger age at diagnosis in the 0–34 years group in Sweden 1983–1998. *Diabetologia* **45**, 783–91.

Raile K et al. (2007). Diabetic nephropathy in 27,805 Children, adolescents, and adults with type 1 diabetes: effect of diabetes duration, A1C, hypertension, dyslipidemia, diabetes onset, and sex. *Diabetes Care* **30**, 2523–8.

Rewers A et al. (2002). Predictors of acute complications in children with type 1 diabetes. *JAMA* **287**, 2511–8.

Rewers A et al. (2008). Presence of diabetic ketoacidosis at diagnosis of diabetes mellitus in youth: the Search for Diabetes in Youth Study. *Pediatrics* **121**, e1258–66.

Ritenbaugh C et al. (2003). A lifestyle intervention improves plasma insulin levels among Native American high school youth. *Preventive Medicine* **36**, 309–19.

Robinson TN (1999). Reducing children's television viewing to prevent obesity: a randomized controlled trial. *JAMA* **282**, 1561–7.

Rodriguez BL et al. (2006). Prevalence of cardiovascular disease risk factors in U.S. children and adolescents with diabetes: the SEARCH for diabetes in youth study. *Diabetes Care* **29**, 1891–6.

Rohlfing CL et al. (2000). Use of GHb (HbA1c) in screening for undiagnosed diabetes in the U.S. population. *Diabetes Care* **23**, 187–191.

Rosenbauer J, Icks A, Giani G (2002). Clinical characteristics and predictors of severe ketoacidosis at onset of type 1 diabetes mellitus in children in a North

Rhine–Westphalian region, Germany. *Journal of Pediatric Endocrinology* **15**, 1137–45.

Rosenbaum M et al. (2007). School–based intervention acutely improves insulin sensitivity and decreases inflammatory markers and body fatness in junior high school students. *Journal of Clinical Endocrinology and Metabolism* **92**, 504–8.

Savoye M et al. (2007). Effects of a weight management program on body composition and metabolic parameters in overweight children: a randomized controlled trial. *JAMA* **297**, 2697–704.

Schultz CJ et al. (2001). Blood pressure does not rise before the onset of microalbuminuria in children followed from diagnosis of type 1 diabetes. Oxford Regional Prospective Study Group. *Diabetes Care* **24**, 555–60.

Schwab KO et al. (2006). Spectrum and prevalence of atherogenic risk factors in 27,358 children, adolescents, and young adults with type 1 diabetes: cross-sectional data from the German diabetes documentation and quality management system (DPV). *Diabetes Care* **29**, 218–25.

Scott CR et al. (1997). Characteristics of youth–onset noninsulin–dependent diabetes mellitus and insulin–dependent diabetes mellitus at diagnosis. *Pediatrics* **100**, 84–91.

Scottish Study Group for the Care of the Young Diabetic (2001). Factors influencing glycemic control in young people with type 1 diabetes in Scotland: a population-based study (DIABAUD2). *Diabetes Care* **24**, 239–44.

SEARCH for Diabetes in Youth Study Group (2006). The burden of diabetes mellitus among US youth: prevalence estimates from the SEARCH for Diabetes in Youth Study. *Pediatrics* **118**, 1510–8.

Shalitin S, Phillip M (2007). The role of new technologies in treating children and adolescents with type 1 diabetes mellitus. *PediatricDiabetes* **8** (Suppl. 6), 72–9.

Sharma M (2006). School–based interventions for childhood and adolescent obesity. *Obesity Reviews* **7**, 261–269.

Sherr J et al. (2008). Prevention of type 1 diabetes: the time has come. *Nature Clinical Practice. Endocrinology & Metabolism* **4**, 334–43.

Silverman BL, Landsberg L, Metzger BE (1993). Fetal hyperinsulinism in offspring of diabetic mothers. Association with the subsequent development of childhood obesity. *Annals of the New York Academy of Sciences* **699**, 36–45.

Silverman BL et al. (1995). Impaired glucose tolerance in adolescent offspring of diabetic mothers. Relationship to fetal hyperinsulinism. *Diabetes Care* **18**, 611–7.

Silverstein J et al. (2005). Care of children and adolescents with type 1 diabetes: a statement of the American Diabetes Association. *Diabetes Care* **28**, 186–212.

Sinha R et al. (2002). Prevalence of impaired glucose tolerance among children and adolescents with marked obesity. *New England Journal of Medicine* **346**, 802–10.

Skrivarhaug T (2006). Long–term mortality in a nationwide cohort of childhood-onset type 1 diabetic patients in Norway. *Diabetologia* **49**, 298–305.

Skrivarhaug T et al. (2006). Low risk of overt nephropathy after 24 yr of childhood-onset type 1 diabetes mellitus (T1DM) in Norway. *Pediatric Diabetes* **7**, 239–46.

Smith CP et al. (1998). Ketoacidosis occurring in newly diagnosed and established diabetic children. *Acta Pediatrica* **87**, 537–41.

Soedamah–Muthu SS et al. (2004). Risk factors for coronary heart disease in type 1 diabetic patients in Europe: the EURODIAB Prospective Complications Study. *Diabetes Care* **27**, 530–7.

Steil GM, Rebrin K (2005). Closed-loop insulin delivery—what lies between where we are and where we are going? *Expert Opinion on Drug Delivery* **2**, 353–62.

Steinberger J, Daniels SR (2003). Obesity, insulin resistance, diabetes, and cardiovascular risk in children: an American Heart Association scientific statement from the Atherosclerosis, Hypertension, and Obesity in the Young Committee (Council on Cardiovascular Disease in the Young) and the Diabetes Committee (Council on Nutrition, Physical Activity, and Metabolism). *Circulation* **107**, 1448–53.

Stettler C et al. (2006). Glycemic control and macrovascular disease in types 1 and 2 diabetes mellitus: meta–analysis of randomized trials. *American Heart Journal* **152**, 27–38.

Stone ML et al. (2006). Natural history and risk factors for microalbuminuria in adolescents with type 1 diabetes: a longitudinal study. *Diabetes Care* **29**, 2072–7.

Story M (1999). School–based approaches for preventing and treating obesity. *International Journal of Obesity* **23** (Suppl. 2), S43–51.

Stride A et al. (2002). Intrauterine hyperglycemia is associated with an earlier diagnosis of diabetes in HNF–1alpha gene mutation carriers. *Diabetes Care* **25**, 2287–91.

Summerbell CD et al. (2005). Interventions for preventing obesity in children. *Cochrane Database of Systematic Reviews* **3**, CD001871.

Svensson M et al. (2003). Signs of nephropathy may occur early in young adults with diabetes despite modern diabetes management: results from the nationwide population-based Diabetes Incidence Study in Sweden (DISS). *Diabetes Care* **26**, 2903–9.

Svoren BM et al. (2003). Reducing acute adverse outcomes in youths with type 1 diabetes: a randomized, controlled trial. *Pediatrics* **112**, 914–22.

Svoren BM et al. (2007). Temporal trends in the treatment of pediatric type 1 diabetes and impact on acute outcomes. *Journal of Pediatrics* **150**, 279–85.

Tesfaye S et al. (2005). Vascular risk factors and diabetic neuropathy. *New England Journal of Medicine* **352**, 341–50.

The Diabetes Control and Complications Trial Research Group (1993). The effect of intensive treatment of diabetes on the development and progression of long–term complications in insulin–dependent diabetes mellitus. *New England Journal of Medicine* **329**, 977–86.

The Diabetes Control and Complications Trial Research Group (1995). The effect of intensive diabetes therapy on the development and progression of neuropathy. *Annals of Internal Medicine* **122**, 561–8.

The Writing Group for the SEARCH for Diabetes in Youth Study Group (2007). Incidence of diabetes in youth in the United States. *JAMA* **297**, 2716–24.

The S. T. O. P. (2006). Presence of diabetes risk factors in a large U.S. eighth-grade cohort. *Diabetes Care* **29**, 212–7.

The Environmental Determinants of Diabetes in the Young (TEDDY) study: study design (2007). *Pediatric Diabetes* **8**, 286–98.

TRIGR Study Group (2007). Study design of the Trial to Reduce IDDM in the Genetically at Risk (TRIGR). *Pediatric Diabetes* **8**, 117–37.

Thomsett M (1999). How well are we doing? Metabolic control in patients with diabetes. *Journal of Paediatrics and Child Health* **35**, 479–82.

Todd J et al. (2006). Increased rates of morbidity, mortality, and charges for hospitalized children with public or no health insurance as compared with children with private insurance in Colorado and the United States. *Pediatrics* **118**, 577–85.

Toeller M et al. (1999). Prevalence of chronic complications, metabolic control and nutritional intake in type 1 diabetes: comparison between different European regions. EURODIAB Complications Study group. *Hormone and Metabolic Research* **31**, 680–5.

Trevino RP et al. (2004). Impact of the Bienestar school–based diabetes mellitus prevention program on fasting capillary glucose levels: a randomized controlled trial. *Archives of Pediatrics & Adolescent Medicine* **158**, 911–7.

Troiano RP, Flegal KM (1998). Overweight children and adolescents: description, epidemiology, and demographics. *Pediatrics* **101**, 497–504.

Tsamasiros J, Bartsocas CS (2002). Transition of the adolescent from the children's to the adults' diabetes clinic. *Journal of Pediatric Endocrinology & Metabolism* **15**, 363–7.

Tunstall–Pedoe H et al. (1994). Myocardial infarction and coronary deaths in the World Health Organization MONICA Project. Registration procedures, event rates, and case-fatality rates in 38 populations from 21 countries in four continents. *Circulation* **90**, 583–612.

Unwin N et al. (2002). Impaired glucose tolerance and impaired fasting glycaemia: the current status on definition and intervention. *Diabetic Medicine* **19**, 708–23.

Urakami T, Owada M, Kitagawa T (2006). Recent trend toward decrease in the incidence of childhood type 2 diabetes in Tokyo. *Diabetes Care* **29**, 2176–7.

Vanelli M et al. (1999). Effectiveness of a prevention program for diabetic ketoacidosis in children. An 8–year study in schools and private practices. *Diabetes Care* **22**, 7–9.

Vehik K et al. (2007). Increasing incidence of type 1 diabetes in 0- to 17-year-old Colorado youth. *Diabetes Care* **30**, 503–9.

Vehik K et al. (2008). Trends in high-risk HLA susceptibility genes among Colorado youth with type 1 diabetes. *Diabetes Care* **31**, 1392–6.

Vinik AI et al. (2000). Diabetic neuropathies. *Diabetologia* **43**, 957–73.Wadwa RP et al. (2010).Measures of arterial stiffness in youth with type 1 and type 2 diabetes: the SEARCH for diabetes in youth study. *Diabetes Care* **33**, 881–6.

Waernbaum I et al. (2006). Excess mortality in incident cases of diabetes mellitus aged 15 to 34 years at diagnosis: a population-based study (DISS) in Sweden. *Diabetologia* **49**, 653–9.

Walsh MG et al. (2004). A multinational comparison of complications assessment in type 1 diabetes: the DiaMond substudy of complications (DiaComp) level 2. *Diabetes Care* **27**, 1610–7.

Walsh MG et al. (2005). The socioeconomic correlates of global complication prevalence in type 1 diabetes (T1D): a multinational comparison. *Diabetes Research and Clinical Practice* **70**, 143–50.

Wasserfall CH, Atkinson MA (2006). Autoantibody markers for the diagnosis and prediction of type 1 diabetes. *Autoimmunity Reviews* **55**, 424–8.

Weets I et al. (2002). The incidence of type 1 diabetes in the age group 0–39 years has not increased in Antwerp (Belgium) between 1989 and 2000: evidence for earlier disease manifestation. *Diabetes Care* **25**, 840–6.

Wei JN et al. (2003). National surveillance for type 2 diabetes mellitus in Taiwanese children. *JAMA* **290**, 1345–50.

Weiss R, Caprio S (2005). The metabolic consequences of childhood obesity. *Best Practice & Research. Clinical Endocrinology & Metabolism* **19**, 405–19.

White NH et al. (2001). Beneficial effects of intensive therapy of diabetes during adolescence: outcomes after the conclusion of the Diabetes Control and Complications Trial (DCCT). *Journal of Pediatrics* **139**, 804–12.

Williams CL et al. (2002). Cardiovascular health in childhood: a statement for health professionals from the Committee on Atherosclerosis, Hypertension, and Obesity in the Young (AHOY) of the Council on Cardiovascular Disease in the Young, American Heart Association. *Circulation* **106**, 143–60.

Winkley K et al. (2006). Psychological interventions to improve glycaemic control in patients with type 1 diabetes: systematic review and meta-analysis of randomised controlled trials. *British Medical Journal* **333**, 65.

Wirehn AB et al. (2008). Age-specific direct healthcare costs attributable to diabetes in a Swedish population: a register-based analysis. *Diabetic Medicine* **25**, 732–7.

Whincup PH et al. (2008). Birth weight and risk of type 2 diabetes: a systematic review. *JAMA* **300**, 2886–97.

Wrotniak BH et al. (2004). Parent weight change as a predictor of child weight change in family-based behavioral obesity treatment. *Archives of Pediatrics & Adolescent Medicine* **158**, 342–7.

Wysocki T et al. (2007). Randomized trial of behavioral family systems therapy for diabetes: maintenance of effects on diabetes outcomes in adolescents. *Diabetes Care* **30**, 555–60.

Yanovski SZ (2002). Obesity. *New England Journal of Medicine* **346**, 591–602.

Yokoyama H et al. (2000). Higher incidence of diabetic nephropathy in type 2 than in type 1 diabetes in early–onset diabetes in Japan. *Kidney International* **58**, 302–11.

Zhang P, Iami K (2007). The relationship between age and healthcare expenditure among persons with diabetes mellitus. *Expert Opinion Pharmacotherapy* **8**, 49–57.

28. PUBLIC HEALTH GENOMICS OF TYPE 1 DIABETES, TYPE 2 DIABETES, AND DIABETIC COMPLICATIONS

Robert L. Hanson, Robert G. Nelson, and William C. Knowler

■ Main Public Health Messages

- Recent population-based twin studies have suggested that the genetic component of type 1 diabetes is larger than previously thought.
- Polymorphisms in the major histocompatibility complex (MHC) locus strongly influence the risk of type 1 diabetes.
- Of variants identified outside the MHC region, those in the insulin gene probably have the strongest effects on risk of type 1 diabetes.
- Identification of individuals with high-risk MHC class II haplotypes could theoretically identify about 95% of individuals who would develop type 1 diabetes by age 20 years. This measure has very low specificity, however.
- A potential strategy for identifying individuals at high risk for type 1 diabetes is to initiate genetic screening in newborns and follow those with high-risk genotypes for development of islet cell autoimmunity and possibly for signs of deficient insulin secretion.
- At present there is no effective treatment for those identified as at high risk for type 1 diabetes, and thus, genetic screening programs do not have a strong public health rationale.
- Having a mother with type 2 diabetes is more risky than having a father with type 2 in terms of development of the disease in offspring.
- Exposure of the child to a diabetic intrauterine environment is a strong risk factor for subsequent obesity and type 2 diabetes.
- The concordance rate for type 2 diabetes is higher for monozygotic twins than for twins who are dizygotic.
- A large number of variants associated with risk of type 2 diabetes have been recently identified. However, these associations involve modest effects.

- Although there are effective preventive strategies for type 2 diabetes, the presently identified susceptibility genes do not provide predictive abilities strong enough to warrant genetic screening.

■ Introduction

The term "genomics" generally refers to the study of an organism's entire genome and how the genome acts, often in concert with environmental factors, to influence the organism's phenotype. This field of study has grown in recent years as the basic genome sequence has become known for an increasing number of organisms, including humans. Technological advances in methods for genotyping have led to an enhanced ability to survey polymorphic DNA sequences on a genomic basis. With respect to human diseases, such as diabetes mellitus, these genomic tools are increasingly being used to map genes that influence susceptibility to disease. The present chapter reviews these efforts from a public health perspective for studies of type 1 and type 2 diabetes. To facilitate the understanding of these studies, we first review the epidemiologic approaches applied to human genetics.

■ Genetic Epidemiologic Methods

Familial Aggregation

Traditionally investigators have assessed the extent to which a disease aggregates in families to quantify the potential influence of genetic factors. These assessments can be accomplished by classical epidemiologic designs (e.g., case-control or cohort studies), and they do not require genotyping any markers. Familial aggregation can be quantified, for example, by the odds ratio (OR) that compares the prevalence of disease among individuals who have a family history of the disease with those who do not have such a history. Thus, the OR may represent the odds of having the disease if a specified relative (e.g., a sibling) is affected divided by the odds if that relative is unaffected. As such, the OR reflects the influence of familial, potentially genetic, factors on the occurrence of the disease.

Heritability (h^2) is another measure of familial aggregation, widely used by geneticists, that quantifies the potential influence of genetic factors more explicitly. As used in the study of quantitative traits, it is the proportion of trait variance attributable to additive genetic effects and is estimated from the correlation for a given trait among pairs of relatives as a function of their genetic similarity. Heritability can also be calculated for dichotomous traits (e.g., presence of diabetes) if one assumes that affection status is reflective of an underlying continuous liability distribution.

Twin Studies

Studies of twins offer a powerful way to estimate heritability. Because monozygotic twins have their entire genome in common, whereas dizygotic twins share on average half of their genes, the extent to which the correlation in liability among monozygotic twin pairs (r_{mz}) exceeds that among dizygotic twin pairs (r_{dz}) provides an estimate of the heritability $[h^2 = 2^*(r_{mz} - r_{dz})]$. The appeal of twin studies rests, in part, on the ability to assess the role of shared environmental factors in contributing to familial aggregation, thereby providing an estimate of h^2 that, in contrast to that provided by studies of other types of relatives, is robust to confounding by a shared environment. However, ability to assess shared environmental factors rests on the assumption that these factors are shared equally between monozygotic and dizygotic twins, and so heritability estimates can still be confounded if this assumption is violated. For example if risk of diabetes is conferred by placental or behavioral factors that are shared to a greater degree among monozygotic than among dizygotic twins, the heritability could be overestimated.

Although twin studies and other studies of familial aggregation may establish the potential importance of genetic factors, they do not estimate the number of genes involved or how they influence traits. And although there are various techniques, such as segregation analysis, that can make such estimates from the pattern of inheritance in families, more conclusive evidence and identification of the specific genetic elements involved requires examination of variation in DNA.

Linkage Studies

Linkage studies examine the co-transmission of disease status, or other traits, with marker alleles within families. For complex diseases, such as diabetes, nonparametric allele-sharing methods, which do not require specification of the mode of inheritance, are most commonly employed. Linkage studies can be performed for specific candidate genes to evaluate their role in disease susceptibility or on a genome-wide basis to identify potentially novel susceptibility loci. The evidence for linkage is often given in terms of the logarithm of the odds (LOD) score. Because most polymorphisms in the genome are not likely a priori to be linked to a disease susceptibility locus, stringent statistical criteria are generally considered necessary before linkage is declared statistically significant (Lander and Kruglyak 1995; Morton 1998). Traditionally an LOD score >3 (which corresponds to $p < 0.0001$) has been taken to indicate "significant" linkage, and an LOD score in the range of 2.0–3.0 is taken as "suggestive." Linkage studies rely on recent recombination events to identify the loci of interest, and therefore, the resolution of this method is generally low, particularly for a complex disease such as diabetes where obligate recombination events can not be identified with confidence. A linkage peak is typically localized to an interval of ~20 centiMorgans (cM), which may contain hundreds of genes; therefore, other methods are required to identify the polymorphisms that confer susceptibility.

Association Studies

Association studies examine the co-occurrence of specific marker alleles with disease status; for example, they may examine whether a particular allele is more common in diabetic than in nondiabetic individuals. These studies do not require family data and may employ familiar epidemiologic techniques, such as case-control designs. For an association study, all individuals in a sample are potentially informative, in contrast to a linkage study, in which only individuals with a parent who is heterozygous at the risk locus are informative. Thus, association studies can be much more powerful than linkage studies, provided the risk associated with a locus is captured by a single functional polymorphism and that a marker that is highly concordant (that is, in strong linkage disequilibrium) with this polymorphism is genotyped. Because linkage disequilibrium reflects historical recombination (rather than recent recombination), association studies typically have finer resolution than linkage studies, but as a consequence they require a larger number of markers to reliably capture the relevant haplotypic information. Traditionally association studies have been used for candidate genes and for fine-mapping linkage peaks, but recent advances in genotyping technology that allow for typing hundreds of thousands of markers simultaneously have made genome-wide association studies feasible. Such studies have been powerful tools for identifying susceptibility genes for type 1 and type 2 diabetes.

"Population stratification," which refers to any process that leads to a population being composed of different genetic subpopulations, is a potential confounder in association studies. If a population contains two or more subpopulations at different risk for the disease, association can be detected with any allele that differs in frequency between the subpopulations, regardless of whether the allele is tightly linked to a functional polymorphism. For example, the Gm system of human immunoglobulin G contains several haplotypes, and one of these, $Gm^{3;5,13,14}$, is inversely associated with type 2 diabetes in American Indians ($p < 0.0001$); however, $Gm^{3;5,13,14}$ is also a marker of European admixture, and there is no association with diabetes once there is control for the degree of European heritage ($p = 0.30$) (Knowler et al. 1988). Thus ethnic admixture, or any other form of population stratification, is an important potential confounder in genetic studies, and a number of techniques have been developed to control for it.

Family-based association designs are an important tool for controlling for population stratification; a variety of designs have been developed to test for association within families (Abecasis, Cardon, and Cookson 2000; Lake, Blacker, and Laird 2000; Martin et al. 2000; Spielman, McGinnis, and Ewens 1993). These designs share the common feature that they test whether a specific allele(s) is transmitted more commonly (or more often than expected by chance) to affected family members than to unaffected family members. Because these tests also assess co-transmission between disease and marker, they can be considered tests of both linkage and association. As such, within-family association tests are generally less powerful than conventional association tests, but they are robust to detection of "spurious" associations due to population stratification.

Measures of Public Health Importance

The population attributable fraction (PAF) is probably the most widely used epidemiologic measure of the public health impact of a given exposure on the occurrence of a disease, such as diabetes. The PAF is the proportion by which disease incidence could be reduced if all of the exposed individuals had the same risk as the unexposed. For a genetic polymorphism, the "exposure" represents the high-risk genotype or genotypes. The PAF can be calculated for a specific allele, and it is often used to describe the potential importance of a given polymorphism in causing disease in a population. Although genetic risk factors are generally considered unmodifiable in that appropriate interventions do not attempt to eliminate the "exposure," it is possible that the difference in risk among genotypes can be eliminated by environmental manipulation, such as medicine or lifestyle modification. The existence of such interventions suggests that treatment could abolish the excess risk associated with the polymorphism.

A feature of the PAF that is often not appreciated is that its calculation assumes that the risk associated with exposure is determined from incidence data. For a diallelic locus, for example, with three possible genotypes, the formula is:

$$PAF = 1 - 1/(P_{LL} + P_{LH}HR_{LH} + P_{HH}HR_{HH})$$

Here, P_{LL}, P_{LH}, and P_{HH} represent, respectively, the proportions of the population homozygous for the low-risk genotype and heterozygous and homozygous for the high-risk genotype, and HR_{LH} and HR_{HH} represent the hazard rate ratios for the heterozygotes and high-risk homozygotes relative to the low-risk homozygotes. When the data are taken from a case-control study, the ORs (OR_{LH}, OR_{HH}) are substituted for the hazard rate ratios. If the cases are incident cases and controls are drawn from the population at risk, then the OR is a valid estimate of the hazard rate ratio, but few genetic studies have had this design; often they have used prevalent cases and placed additional selection criteria on controls. As an example, Figure 28.1 shows the PAF calculated from an incidence study and from a case-control study using prevalent cases for a hypothetical common polymorphism in relation to the cumulative incidence of disease. The estimate from the prevalence study approximates nicely that from the incidence study when the cumulative incidence is low, but it diverges when the cumulative incidence is high. Because type 2 diabetes, in particular, is common in many populations, and because many genetic mapping studies are designed to sample cases and controls to maximize power, rather than for representativeness of the population, estimates of PAF derived from such studies should be treated with caution.

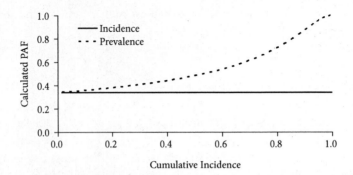

FIGURE 28.1. PAF (population-attributable fraction) calculated for a hypothetical marker with allele frequency = 0.29 for the high-risk allele and a hazard ratio of 1.8 per copy of the risk allele, as a function of the cumulative incidence of the disease. PAF is calculated for an incidence study (i.e., assuming the hazard ratios are accurately estimated) and for a case-control study based on prevalent cases (assuming the prevalence odds ratio approximates the hazard ratio). The odds ratios in the prevalence study are calculated from the cumulative incidence in each genotype, given the known hazard ratios, whereas the total cumulative incidence is taken as a weighted average of the genotype-specific values (assuming Hardy-Weinberg equilibrium)

Locus-specific heritability is another measure of the importance of a particular polymorphism in determining susceptibility to a disease. This measure represents the proportion of the population variance in susceptibility to the disease of interest that is potentially explained by a given polymorphism (or polymorphisms). In contrast to measures such as the allelic OR, which reflect the strength of association between a genetic variant and disease, both PAF and locus-specific h^2 depend on the frequency of the polymorphism in addition to the strength of association. However, they account for the frequency in different ways and thus can give different impressions about the importance of the variant in question. It is important to consider this issue in the interpretation of these numbers. For example the Pro12Ala amino acid substitution in the $PPARG$ gene (a target for thiazolidinediones) has been reproducibly associated with type 2 diabetes in many studies with an OR of ~1.15 per copy of the proline allele (Altshuler et al. 2000). Because this allele has a high frequency (~0.93 in most European populations), this corresponds to a PAF of ~23%, but if the prevalence of diabetes is 10%, the locus-specific h^2 is only ~0.1%. Because the OR is modest, the extent to which the polymorphism causes individuals to bear something other than the average risk in the population is small, despite the fact that the risk allele is common, and this is reflected in the low locus-specific h^2. However, if an intervention was available to eliminate the increased risk associated with the proline allele, the incidence of diabetes in the population could be reduced by about 20%, because the risk allele is very common. (Clearly, for very rare but highly protective alleles, the PAF could be very high while h^2 could be vanishingly small.) Thus, which measure is appropriate depends on which aspect of disease one wishes to consider—the h^2 is probably more appropriate if one seeks to explain variation in disease risk in the population, whereas the PAF is more appropriate if one is considering a targeted intervention.

Type 1 Diabetes

Heritability and the MHC Locus

Classical twin studies showed a very high concordance rate (nearly 100%) for late-onset diabetes among monozygotic twin pairs and a lower concordance rate (~50%) for younger-onset diabetes (Tattersall and Pyke 1972). This finding has been interpreted as suggesting that genetic factors are very important in conferring risk for type 2 diabetes, whereas they are less important, but still significant, for type 1 diabetes. These early twin studies, however, were not population based, and classification of diabetes was not well developed. More recent population-based twin studies have suggested that the genetic component of type 1 diabetes is larger than previously appreciated (whereas that for type 2 diabetes may be smaller, as described later in this chapter).

These studies were conducted with population-based twin registries in Scandinavia (Table 28.1) (Hyttinen et al. 2003; Kaprio et al. 1992; Kyvik, Green, and Beck-Nielsen 1995). A summary estimate of heritability of type 1 diabetes over all these studies is 0.86 (95% confidence interval [CI] 0.77–0.95). The variable age at onset of type 1 diabetes complicates the estimates of heritability, and studies have generally attempted to account for this by using a model that assumes a genetic influence on ultimate susceptibility rather than on age of onset. The estimates are further limited by relatively small samples and the studies' restricted geographic range; nonetheless, these data suggest that variability in susceptibility to type 1 diabetes is determined, in large part, by genetic factors.

Polymorphisms in the major histocompatibility complex (MHC, also called human leukocyte antigen or HLA) locus strongly influence risk of type 1 diabetes, as they do for other autoimmune diseases (Rotter and Landau 1984; Thomson et al. 1984). The effect of the MHC locus is powerful, and this effect has been repeatedly replicated in both linkage and association studies (Concannon et al. 2005; Nejentsev et al. 2007; Thomson 1984). Many alleles associated with type 1 diabetes have been identified in the MHC region; because this region is highly polymorphic and has a high degree of linkage disequilibrium, it has been difficult to identify which polymorphisms are functionally related to diabetes susceptibility. The MHC class II loci have the strongest associations with disease (Todd, Bell, and McDevitt 1987). In most populations the serologic DR3,DQ2 and DR4,DQ8 haplotypes are strongly associated with diabetes, and individuals who are heterozygous for these two haplotypes have the highest risk. In white populations more than 90% of individuals with type 1 diabetes have at least one of these haplotypes, compared with fewer than 40%

TABLE 28.1   *Twin Studies Comparing Concordance Rates for Monozygotic and Dizygotic Twins for Type 1 and Type 2 Diabetes*

Study	Monozygotic Concordance	Dizygotic Concordance	h^2 (SE)
Type 1 diabetes			
Denmark	0.38	0.06	0.72 (0.21)
Finland (older cohort)	0.13	0.03	0.76 (0.11)
Finland (younger cohort)	0.27	0.04	0.88 (0.05)
Summary			**0.86 (0.05)**
Type 2 diabetes			
Denmark	0.33	0.23	0.26 (0.30)
Finland	0.20	0.09	0.39 (0.12)
Japan	0.87	0.43	0.54 (0.13)
USA	0.41	0.10	0.68 (0.23)
Summary			**0.47 (0.08)**

Studies were conducted by ascertainment of co-twins of an affected proband. The concordance rate is the proportion of pairs in which both twins were affected. Summary estimates of heritability (h^2) were made as a weighted average of the estimates for the individual studies, with the inverse of the variance as the weight. There was no significant heterogeneity in heritability estimates for either type 1 ($p = 0.57$) or type 2 ($p = 0.56$) diabetes. SE, standard error.

of individuals without diabetes (Devendra, Liu, and Eisenbarth 2004; Thomson 1984). Naturally, there must be other MHC haplotypes that are underrepresented among people with type 1 diabetes compared with the general population, and DR15,DQ6 is a major such "protective" haplotype (Devendra, Liu, and Eisenbarth 2004). In some populations heterozygotes for other haplotypes at the DR locus are at high risk, such as DR3/DR9 in Chinese and African Americans (Dorman and Bunker 2000). Molecular studies suggest that a number of haplotypes in the class II regions are associated with greatly increased risk (particularly DRB1*0301-DQA1-0501-DQB1*0201 and DRB1*04-DQA1-0301-DQB1*0302), although there are many subtypes that can be ordered according to the degree of risk (Cucca et al. 2001). Moreover there are additional MHC class I variants, primarily in the A and B loci, that appear to contribute to risk of type 1 diabetes even when the analysis is conditioned on the DR/DQ variants, and there may be additional loci in the MHC region that contribute as well (Eike et al. 2009; Nejentsev et al. 2007). Among class I alleles, the HLA-A*24 and HLA-B*39 alleles are associated with the highest risk (Nejentsev et al. 2007).

Susceptibility Variants Outside the MHC Region

A number of other variants outside the MHC region are reproducibly associated with type 1 diabetes (see Table 28.2). Variants in the insulin gene (INS) probably have the strongest effects of those identified to date outside the MHC region (Bennett et al. 1995; Spielman, McGinnis, and Ewens 1993). The diabetes-associated variants consist of variable-number tandem-repeat polymorphisms located approximately 596 base pairs upstream of INS. Depending on the number of repeats, there are two common classes of alleles: those in class I are short (26–63 repeats) and associated with increased risk, and class III alleles are long (140–210 repeats) and associated with lower risk (the intermediate-length class II alleles are at low frequency). More recently studies of biologic and positional candidates have identified several other variants with reproducible associations with type 1 diabetes. These include variants in or near the lymphoid protein tyrosine phosphatase non-receptor 22 [PTPN22] (Bottini et al. 2004; Onengut-Gumuscu et al. 2004), the interleukin-2 receptor-α [IL2RA] (Lowe et al. 2007), and cytotoxic t-lymphocyte antigen 4 [CLTA4] (Nisticò et al. 1996).

Very recently genome-wide association studies with follow-up replication studies have identified several additional variants in the interferon-induced helicase 1 [IFIH1], the C-type lectin domain family 16-A [CLEC16A], the phosphotyrosine protein phosphatase non-receptor 2 [PTPN2], as well as two regions on chromosome 12 that are not clearly associated with specific genes (Smyth et al. 2006; Todd et al. 2007), and several other genes (Concannon et al. 2008; Cooper et al. 2008; Grant et al. 2009). These variants, particularly the ones identified in genome-wide association studies, generally have much weaker effects than those identified earlier, with OR s 1.1–1.3 per copy of the susceptibility allele. As the values in Table 28.2 demonstrate, the PAF values are not additive across loci, but they do show the importance of the MHC class II and INS variants. The h^2 estimates demonstrate that the MHC region is the major contributor to variation in susceptibility to type 1 diabetes. In fact because there are multiple susceptibility alleles in this region, the allele-specific estimate shown in Table 28.2 underestimates the influence of this locus. Analyses of haplotype sharing in relatives suggest that the MHC locus accounts for 40%–50% of the total heritability in liability to type 1 diabetes (Concannon et al. 2005; Rotter and Landaw 1984).

■ Public Health Implications

For optimal application in population screening, genetic tests should be highly predictive, be acceptable to the population, and identify a condition amenable to treatment. Identification of individuals with high-risk MHC class II haplotypes is very sensitive and could theoretically identify ~95% of individuals who would develop type 1 diabetes by age 20 years (Skyler 2007). However the specificity remains low,

TABLE 28.2 *Gene Regions with Variants Reproducibly Associated with Type 1 Diabetes*

Chromosome	Gene/Region	Variation	Risk Allele	Frequency	Odds Ratio	PAF	h^2
1	PTPN22	rs2476601	A	0.14	1.98	0.23	0.012
2	INS	VNTR	Class I	0.63	2.80	0.78	0.048
2	IFIH1	rs1990760	T	0.61	1.17	0.18	0.001
2	CTLA4	rs3087243	T	0.46	1.18	0.15	0.001
6	MHC Class I	A&B	Multiple (HLA-B*39)	0.01	3.55	0.05	0.004
6	MHC Class II	DR & DQ	Multiple DR3, DR4		7.20, 10.8		
		rs3129934	T	0.25	6.90	0.84	0.134
6	BACH2	rs11755527	G	0.44	1.14	0.11	0.001
10	IL2RA	ss52580101	A	0.11	1.59	0.12	0.005
10	PRKCQ	rs947474	A	0.84	1.15	0.21	0.001
12	ERBB3	rs2292239	C	0.70	1.28	0.30	0.003
12	C12orf30	rs17696736	A	0.65	1.22	0.23	0.002
15	CTSH	rs3825932	C	0.68	1.16	0.19	0.001
16	CLEC16A	rs12708716	A	0.71	1.23	0.26	0.002
18	PTPN2	rs2542151	A	0.81	1.30	0.35	0.002
21	UBASH3A	rs887864	T	0.37	1.10	0.07	0.001
22	C1QTNF6	rs229541	C	0.60	1.13	0.14	0.001

In some cases multiple SNPs (single nucleotide polymorphisms) in linkage disequilibrium are associated, and the one with the strongest association is listed. Where possible, the odds ratio is taken from Todd et al. (2007), as this study has the largest sample. The odds ratio is generally listed per copy of the risk allele (except for MHC [major histocompatibility complex] haplotypes DR3, DR4, and HLA-B*39, where it is given for carriers versus noncarriers). There are multiple risk alleles at both MHC loci; the strongest alleles are listed here; these include the strongest associations among the serologic DR3 and DR4 haplotypes. For comparability with other markers and calculation of PAF (population attributable fraction) and h^2 (heritability), the SNP in the MHC II region with the strongest association is also shown. The odds ratio for the class I HLA-B*39 allele is calculated conditional on the MHC class II effects. PAF and h^2 are calculated for a population of European origin, as most of the published data are relevant to such a population. PAF is calculated under the assumption of a multiplicative model from the odds ratio; h^2 is calculated under the assumption of a multiplicative model by iterative solution of the equations in Hanson et al. (2006), assuming a disease prevalence of 0.003. Allele frequencies are taken from European HapMap (International HapMap Consortium 2007) frequencies if available.

as <5% of individuals with these high-risk haplotypes will develop the disease by age 20 years. Thus screening would result in a large number of "false positives." Development of persistent islet cell autoimmunity in individuals with high-risk MHC haplotypes is associated with a high risk of progression to type 1 diabetes, particularly if there is also evidence from metabolic testing of impaired insulin secretion (DPT1 2002; DPT1 2005). Thus one potential strategy to identify individuals at high risk of type 1 diabetes is to initiate genetic screening in newborns and to follow those with high-risk genotypes for development of islet autoimmunity (and potentially for signs of deficient insulin secretion). Intervention to prevent diabetes could then be initiated in those who developed a high-risk profile. Pilot studies to assess the feasibility of such programs in the United States and Finland suggest that the programs are well accepted (Kupila et al. 2001; Rewers et al. 1996). However at present there is no effective preventive treatment for the high-risk individuals, and thus there is no strong public health rationale for initiating programs in genetic screening.

■ Type 2 Diabetes

Familial Aggregation

Type 2 diabetes has long been recognized as having a familial occurrence, and thus a positive family history is a strong risk factor for the disease. Offspring of an affected mother have a modestly higher risk of the disease than offspring of an affected father (Karter et al. 1999). This difference could, in part, reflect mitochondrial inheritance, or it could suggest the sharing of environmental factors between mother and child (perhaps due to child-rearing practices); alternatively it may reflect exposure of the child to a diabetic intrauterine environment, which occurs when the mother has hyperglycemia during pregnancy. The latter is a strong risk factor for subsequent obesity and type 2 diabetes in the child and represents a nongenetic mechanism of familial transmission (Pettitt et al. 1988). In populations where many women of childbearing age have diabetes, this form of familial transmission is an important public health problem. In the Pima Indians, among whom the prevalence of type 2 diabetes is high at young ages, the overall incidence of diabetes has remained largely constant in recent years, but the incidence of type 2 diabetes in childhood has increased, largely due to exposure to a diabetic intrauterine environment (Dabelea et al. 1998; Pavkov et al. 2007).

Among pairs of Pima siblings discordant for exposure to the intrauterine environment the sibling born after onset of maternal diabetes was at higher risk of the disease than the one born before maternal diabetes developed (OR 3.7, 95% CI 1.3–11.3), despite the presumably similar genetic risk (Dabelea et al. 2000). In Pima sibling pairs under age 45 years, diabetes was found to be familial in that the risk was higher if the co-sib had diabetes than if he or she did not (OR 2.8, 95% CI 2.3–3.3).

This familial risk was largely unmodified if both siblings were exposed to a diabetic intrauterine environment (OR 2.6, 95% CI 1.2–5.4) or if the mother was tested and found not to have diabetes after the birth of both siblings (OR 2.9, 95% CI 2.3–3.9), or if the siblings were of unknown or discordant exposure status (OR 2.7, 95% CI 2.2–3.3). These findings suggest that both intrauterine and other familial, presumably genetic, factors have an important influence on risk of type 2 diabetes in this population.

Several twin studies have compared monozygotic with dizygotic twins to assess the role of genetic factors in risk for type 2 diabetes (Table 28.1) (Kaprio et al. 1992; Mastuda and Kuzuya 1994; Newman et al. 1987; Poulsen et al. 1999). These studies have uniformly demonstrated a higher concordance rate for type 2 diabetes among monozygotic than among dizygotic twins, although the extent of the difference has been variable. A summary estimate of heritability across all four studies suggests that 47% of the variation in liability to type 2 diabetes is explained by genetic factors. This estimate, although strongly suggestive of a substantial genetic contribution to the pathogenesis of type 2 diabetes, is subject to the limitations of twin studies discussed above; variable age of onset is particularly a problem for studies of type 2 diabetes.

Candidate Gene and Linkage Studies

A large number of candidate gene studies have been conducted for type 2 diabetes, by both linkage and association methods. Many of these studies have identified variants with nominally significant linkage or association, but few of them have achieved the stringent levels of statistical significance advocated by many authorities to ensure low levels of type I error (the error of declaring a difference when in truth there is not one). Consequently most of the findings have not been replicated consistently across studies. However, two such variants showed consistent association with type 2 diabetes across populations in multiple studies. As discussed above a Pro12Ala variant in the peroxisome proliferator-activated receptor-γ gene (PPARG) has a modest but reproducibly consistent association with type 2 diabetes (Altshuler et al. 2000). Similarly, a glutamine-lysine polymorphism in codon 23 of the potassium inwardly rectifying subfamily J-11 (KCNJ11) gene (which is part of the sulfonylurea receptor complex) has a modest but consistent association with type 2 diabetes across multiple populations (Gloyn et al. 2003). The lysine allele is associated with a higher prevalence of diabetes, with an OR of 1.14 (the modest OR is typical of most widely replicated variants for type 2 diabetes). More recently association mapping targeted at several candidate genes for type 2 diabetes identified single nucleotide polymorphisms (SNPs) in the wolframin gene (WFS1) that are reproducibly associated with diabetes across several populations (Sandhu et al. 2007). Variants in TCF2 (also known as HNF1B, which also causes maturity-onset diabetes in youth, a monogenic form of diabetes) were similarly identified in candidate gene studies and confirmed in a genome-wide association study (Gudmondsson et al. 2007).

A large number of genome-wide linkage studies have been conducted in an attempt to identify susceptibility loci for type 2 diabetes. In contrast with type 1 diabetes, however, there are no loci with consistently strong statistical evidence for linkage; most loci have been detected with evidence that is suggestive of linkage but not definitive. Even so, there are several regions identified as linked to type 2 diabetes across numerous populations, most notably on chromosome 1q and chromosome 20q (Ghosh et al. 2000; McCarthy 2003; Zouali et al. 1997). Efforts to finely map these regions by genotyping a dense map of SNPs have not revealed clear evidence of particular variants that explain the linkage signals, although variants in HNF4A may play some role in the chromosome 20 region (Silander et al. 2004). It is possible that common variants, which confer susceptibility to type 2 diabetes but which were not captured by the association markers, exist in these regions or that the linkage results were spurious. It is also likely, however, that there are multiple susceptibility variants, some of which may be rare, which are not amenable to detection by association studies.

Another region linked to type 2 diabetes in several populations is on chromosome 10q. Fine-mapping studies in this region in an Icelandic population identified variants in the transcription factor 7-like 2 gene (TCF7L2) that were strongly associated with type 2 diabetes (Grant et al. 2006). These associations have been widely replicated in numerous other populations; rs7903146 is the SNP that appears most consistently associated, with a summary OR of 1.46 (95% CI 1.42–1.51) per copy of the high-risk T allele (Cauchi et al. 2007). In terms of the OR this represents the strongest effect of any polymorphism yet identified for type 2 diabetes. However, the effect does not appear to be similar in all populations. Among Pima Indians, for example, the OR is only 1.04 (95% CI 0.82–1.32), and this is significantly lower than the global OR of 1.46 (Guo et al. 2007). The basis for this heterogeneity remains unexplained, although there does appear to be some interaction with obesity.

Genome-wide Association Studies

The recent technological developments that have made genome-wide association studies feasible have resulted in a large number of variants that have been reproducibly associated with type 2 diabetes, although most of the effect sizes have been extremely modest. Several large studies in European populations initially identified six regions, in addition to TCF7L2, in which SNPs were consistently associated with type 2 diabetes (see Table 28.3) (DGI 2007; Scott et al. 2007; Sladek et al. 2007; Steinthorsdottir et al. 2007; Zeggini et al. 2007). Among the hundreds of thousands of SNPs tested, those with the lowest *p* values in any given study did not generally replicate in other studies. However, a few of the SNPs were associated across several studies, and these SNPs were generally replicated in several large population studies. By combining the data from several genome-wide association studies, additional SNPs were subsequently identified that were also replicated in other populations (Zeggini et al. 2008). Whereas most of these studies were conducted in

TABLE 28.3 *Gene Regions with Variants Reproducibly Associated with Type 2 Diabetes*

Chromosome	Gene/Region	Variant	Risk Allele	Frequency	Odds Ratio	PAF	h^2
1	NOTCH2	rs10923931	T	0.12	1.13	0.03	0.001
2	THADA	rs7578597	T	0.92	1.15	0.23	0.001
3	PPARG	rs1801282	C	0.93	1.15	0.23	0.001
3	ADAMST9	rs4607103	C	0.80	1.09	0.13	0.001
3	IGF2BP2	rs4402960	T	0.29	1.14	0.08	0.002
4	WFS1	rs10010131	G	0.73	1.11	0.14	0.001
6	CDKAL1	rs7754840	C	0.31	1.14	0.08	0.002
7	JAZF1	rs864745	T	0.52	1.10	0.10	0.001
8	SLC30A8	rs13266634	C	0.75	1.14	0.18	0.002
9	CDKN2A/B	rs10811661	T	0.79	1.21	0.26	0.003
10	CDC123	rs12778790	G	0.48	1.11	0.10	0.002
10	HHEX	rs1111875	C	0.56	1.13	0.13	0.002
10	TCF7L2	rs7903146	T	0.25	1.46	0.20	0.014
11	KCNQ1	rs2237892	C	0.93	1.40	0.47	0.004
11	KCNJ11	rs5219	T	0.29	1.14	0.08	0.002
12	TSPAN8	rs7961581	C	0.23	1.09	0.04	0.001
16	FTO	rs8050136	A	0.45	1.17	0.14	0.003
17	TCF2	rs4430796	G	0.53	1.10	0.10	0.001

In some cases multiple SNPs (single nucleotide polymorphisms) in linkage disequilibrium are associated, and the one with the strongest association is listed. The odds ratio is listed per copy of the risk allele and is taken from Zeggini et al. (2008) or a weighted sum of studies included in Zeggini et al. (2008) and other genome-wide association studies. PAF (population attributable fraction) and h^2 (heritability) are calculated for a population of European origin, as most of the published data are relevant to such a population. PAF is calculated under the assumption of a multiplicative model from the odds ratio; h^2 is calculated under the assumption of a multiplicative model by iterative solution of the equations in Hanson et al. (2006), assuming a disease prevalence of 0.10. Allele frequencies are taken from European HapMap (International HapMap Consortium 2007) frequencies if available.

populations of European origin, recent genome-wide association studies conducted in Asians identified additional SNPs in the potassium voltage-gated channel KQT-like subfamily-1 (KCNQ1) gene that were well replicated in Asians and Europeans (Unoki et al. 2008; Yasuda et al. 2008). These SNPs were not initially identified in the European studies because the risk allele is extremely common (frequency of 0.93) in

Europeans, and thus the power to detect an association is low (the allele frequency is 0.61 in East Asians).

Thus the total number of genes with reproducibly associated variants for type 2 diabetes is approximately 18 currently, although there are several other variants with evidence that is only slightly weaker than for these. For many variants the more common allele is associated with increased risk, and thus the PAF is often fairly high despite the modest ORs. However the variance in liability explained by most of these variants is considerably below 1%, except for TCF7L2, where it is 1.4%. If these are representative of the variants that influence susceptibility to type 2 diabetes, many more must be discovered to account for the heritability of the disease. The mechanisms by which these variants influence risk for type 2 diabetes is currently unknown; in fact, it is generally not clear that the variants themselves are causal. However several variants are associated with diminished insulin secretion in nondiabetic individuals, and this finding suggests that some of the genetic mechanisms involved result in insulin secretory dysfunction (Grant et al. 2006; Grarup et al. 2007; Yasuda et al. 2008).

■ Public Health Implications

Several studies have analyzed the known type 2 diabetes susceptibility variants in an attempt to derive risk scores that may help to stratify individuals into those with the highest and lowest risk (Lango et al. 2008; van Hoek et al. 2008). Conceivably, a cost-effective strategy would be the delivery of a preventive intervention to those at the highest risk. The utility of the risk scores depends in part on how effective the available treatments are in preventing type 2 diabetes. In individuals with impaired glucose tolerance, for example, there are effective preventive treatments for type 2 diabetes (DPP 2002; Tuomilehto et al. 2001). At present the most effective approach appears to be lifestyle intervention with a diet-and-exercise program designed to produce weight loss. Several medicines, including metformin, thiazolidinediones, and acarbose, are also effective. Analyses of individuals who participated in the Diabetes Prevention Program suggest that for most variants the carriers of risk alleles respond at least as well to lifestyle treatment as do those who do not carry the alleles (Florez et al. 2006; Moore et al. 2008). The results are most striking for TCF7L2 (see Fig. 28.2); the hazard ratio for those homozygous for the high-risk T allele at rs7903146 was 1.81 in the placebo group relative to those homozygous for the C allele. Among individuals who received the lifestyle intervention, the incidence of diabetes was decreased, and homozygotes for the T allele received proportionately greater benefit, such that the hazard ratio was only 1.15. Nonetheless, individuals with the low-risk CC genotype still had a substantial incidence of diabetes and derived benefit from the intervention; in fact individuals with the CC genotype constituted a much larger proportion of the cases than did those with the TT genotype. Thus an intervention targeted at only those with the high-risk genotype

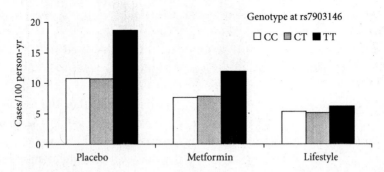

FIGURE 28.2. Incidence rates in the diabetes prevention program by intervention group and genotype at the rs7903146 polymorphism in TCF7L2. Numbers of individuals by genotype are 1747 for CC, 1454 for CT, and 336 for TT. (Data are from Florez et al. 2006.)

would leave out a substantial number of individuals for whom diabetes could be prevented by intervention.

The utility of genetic screening for diabetes prevention also depends on how well the genetic tests predict the development of diabetes. Because the variance in susceptibility explained by the established type 2 diabetes-associated variants is small, even in the aggregate, the ability of these variants to discriminate between individuals at high and low risk is marginal. Furthermore the existing variants appear to add minimally to available clinical information about obesity, age, and glucose intolerance in the prediction of diabetes (van Hoek et al. 2008). Although future genetic research may identify other variants that will help to increase prediction, at present there is little public health justification for screening for genetic variants associated with the risk of type 2 diabetes.

With the exception of KCNQ1 most of the susceptibility variants identified to date have been found in populations of European origin. Although in many cases these variants are associated with type 2 diabetes in non-European populations as well, identification of the strongest genetic predictors in these populations will require population-specific studies.

■ Complications of Diabetes

Microvascular complications (such as retinopathy, nephropathy, and neuropathy) are strongly associated with diabetes and may have a genetic basis. Although macrovascular complications, such as ischemic heart disease, are somewhat more common in individuals with diabetes than in those without diabetes, they are less specific to diabetes and will not be reviewed here. Familial aggregation of diabetic nephropathy has been observed in numerous populations (Pettitt et al. 1990; Seaquist et al. 1989). The occurrence of any degree of retinopathy appears to be less heritable, but more severe forms of the disease do appear to be familial (Hallman et al. 2005; Looker et al. 2007). There have been numerous candidate gene studies for both complications, but few consistent associations have been identified. A potential exception is the carnosinase-1 gene (CNDP1). The region on chromosome 18 containing this gene was identified as linked to nephropathy in a genome-wide linkage study (Vardarli et al. 2002), and subsequent fine-mapping identified a microsatellite repeat (5-Leu) that appeared to be associated with lower risk of nephropathy (Janssen et al. 2005). This finding has been replicated in one study (Freedman et al. 2007), but insufficient evidence is available at present to determine whether it will be widely reproducible. Similarly, variants in the unc-13 homolog B gene (UNC13B) have shown some evidence for association with nephropathy in individuals with type 1 diabetes, but further replication studies are needed (Tregouet et al. 2008).

■ Future Directions in Genomic Medicine and Public Health

Recent years have seen substantial progress in elucidating the genetic factors involved in both type 1 and type 2 diabetes. Genome-wide association studies, in particular, have proven to be a powerful tool for identifying genetic variants that may influence susceptibility to disease. In the near future it is likely that these studies, which may include large-scale genomic sequencing, will identify additional risk variants. As large-scale genotyping is likely to become less expensive in the near future, it may be possible to incorporate genetic information into public health programs, such as genetic screening for diabetes prevention. With the ability to genotype large numbers of variants simultaneously, it may not be necessary to map the susceptibility genes to engage in prediction of risk. With a multivariable score derived from a large number of markers, enough information may be present in the genomic profile to overcome statistical "noise" associated with false-positive signals. For type 1 diabetes a primary challenge is the identification of effective preventive therapies, even if prediction can be improved. For type 2 diabetes effective preventive therapies are feasible, although they still require improvement, and developing effective genetic prediction tools remains challenging. For diabetic complications future studies will need to identify genetic variants that influence risk and their potential response to preventive therapies. Although progress has been made in understanding the genetics of diabetes, much work remains to translate genomic information into public health practice.

■ References

Abecasis GR, Cardon LR, Cookson WO (2000). A general test of association for quantitative traits in nuclear families. *American Journal of Human Genetics* **66**, 279–92.

Altshuler D et al. (2000). The common PPARγ Pro12Ala polymorphism is associated with decreased risk of type 2 diabetes. *Nature Genetics* **26**, 76–80.

Bennett ST et al. (1995). Susceptibility to human type 1 diabetes at *IDDM2* is determined by tandem repeat variation at the insulin gene minisatellite locus. *Nature Genetics* **9**, 284–92.

Bottini N et al. (2004). A functional variant of lymphoid tyrosine phosphatase is associated with type I diabetes. *Nature Genetics* **36**, 337–8.

Cauchi S et al. (2007). *TCF7L2* is reproducibly associated with type 2 diabetes in various ethnic groups: a global meta-analysis. *Journal of Molecular Medicine* **85**, 777–82.

Concannon P et al (2005). Type 1 diabetes: evidence for susceptibility loci from four genome-wide linkage scans in 1,435 multiplex families. *Diabetes* **54**, 2995–3001.

Concannon P et al. (2008). A human type 1 diabetes susceptibility locus maps to chromosome 21q22.3. *Diabetes* **57**, 2858–61.

Cooper JD et al. (2008). Meta-analysis of genome-wide association study data identifies additional type 2 diabetes risk loci. *Nature Genetics* **40**, 1399–401.

Cucca F et al. (2001). A correlation between the relative predisposition of MHC class II alleles to type 1 diabetes and the structure of their proteins. *Human Molecular Genetics* **10**, 2025–37.

Dabelea D et al. (1998). Increasing prevalence of type II diabetes in American Indian children. *Diabetologia* **41**, 904–10.

Dabelea D et al. (2000). Intrauterine exposure to diabetes conveys risks for type 2 diabetes and obesity: a study of discordant sibships. *Diabetes* **49**, 2208–11.

Devendra D, Liu E, Eisenbarth GS (2004). Type 1 diabetes: recent developments. *British Medical Journal* **328**, 750–4.

Diabetes Genetics Initiative (DGI) (2007). Genome-wide association analysis identifies loci for type 2 diabetes and triglyceride levels. *Science* **316**, 1331–6.

Diabetes Prevention Program (DPP) Research Group (2002). Reduction in the incidence of type 2 diabetes with lifestyle intervention or metformin. *New England Journal of Medicine* **346**, 393–403.

Diabetes Prevention Trial—Type 1 (DPT1) Study Group (2002). Effects of insulin in relatives of patients with type 1 diabetes mellitus. *New England Journal of Medicine* **346**, 1685–91.

Diabetes Prevention Trial—Type 1 (DPT1) Study Group (2005). Effects of oral insulin in relatives of patients with type 1 diabetes: The Diabetes Prevention Trial—Type 1. *Diabetes Care* **28**, 1068–76.

Dorman JS, Bunker CH (2000). *HLA-DQ* locus of the human leukocyte antigen complex and type 2 diabetes mellitus: a HuGe review. *Epidemiologic Reviews* **22**, 218–27.

Eike MC et al. (2009). Conditional analyses on the T1DGC MHC data set: novel associations with type 1 diabetes around *HLA-G* and confirmation of *HLA-B*. *Genes & Immunity* **10**, 56–67.

Florez JC et al. (2006). *TCF7L2* polymorphisms and progression to diabetes in the Diabetes Prevention Program. *New England Journal of Medicine* **355**, 241–50.

Freedman BI et al. (2007). A leucine repeat in the carnosinase gene *CNDP1* is associated with diabetic end-stage renal disease in European Americans. *Nephrology, Dialysis, Transplantation* **22**, 1131–5.

Ghosh S et al. (2000). The Finland-United States Investigation of Non-insulin-dependent Diabetes Mellitus Genetics (FUSION) study I: an autosomal genome scan for genes that predispose to type 2 diabetes. *American Journal of Human Genetics* **67**, 1174–85.

Gloyn AL et al. (2003). Large-scale association studies of variants in genes encoding the pancreatic β-cell K_{ATP} channel subunits Kir6.2 (*KCNJ11*) and SUR1 (*ABCC8*) confirm that the *KNCJ11* E23K variant is associated with type 2 diabetes. *Diabetes* **52**, 568–72.

Grant SF et al. (2006). Variant of transcription factor 7-like 2 (*TCF7L2*) gene confers risk of type 2 diabetes. *Nature Genetics* **38**, 320–3.

Grant SF et al. (2009). Follow-up analysis of genome-wide association data identifies novel risk loci for type 1 diabetes. *Diabetes* **58**, 290–5.

Grarup N et al. (2007). Studies of association of variants near the *HHEX, CDKN2A/B,* and *IGF2BP2* genes with type 2 diabetes and impaired insulin release in 10,705 Danish subjects: validation and extension of genome-wide association studies. *Diabetes* **56**, 3105–11.

Gudmondsson J et al. (2007). Two variants on chromosome 17 confer prostate cancer risk and the one in *TCF2* protects against type 2 diabetes. *Nature Genetics* **8**, 977–83.

Guo T et al. (2007). TCF7L2 is not a major susceptibility gene for diabetes in Pima Indians: analysis of 3,501 individuals. *Diabetes* **56**, 3082–8.

Hallman DM et al. (2005). Familial aggregation of severity of diabetic retinopathy in Mexican Americans from Starr County, Texas. *Diabetes Care* **28**, 1163–8.

Hanson RL et al. (2006). Design and analysis of genetic association studies to finely map a locus identified by linkage analysis: sample size and power calculations. *Annals of Human Genetics* **70**, 332–49.

Hyttinen V et al. (2003). Genetic liability of type 1 diabetes and the onset age among 22,650 young Finnish twin pairs: a nationwide follow-up study. *Diabetes* **52**, 1052–5.

International HapMap Consortium (2007). A second generation human haplotype map of over 3.1 million SNPs. *Nature* **449**, 851–61.

Janssen B et al. (2005). Carnosine as a protective factor in diabetic nephropathy: association with a leucine repeat of the carnosinase gene *CNDP1*. *Diabetes* **54**, 2320–7.

Kaprio J et al. (1992). Concordance for type 1 (insulin-dependent) and type 2 (non-insulin-dependent) diabetes mellitus in a population-based cohort of twins in Finland. *Diabetologia* **35**, 1060–7.

Karter AJ et al. (1999). Excess maternal transmission of type 2 diabetes: the Northern California Kaiser Permanente Diabetes Registry. *Diabetes Care* **22**, 938–43.

Knowler WC et al.(1988). $Gm^{3;5,13,14}$ and type 2 diabetes mellitus: an association in American Indians with genetic admixture. *American Journal of Human Genetics* **43**, 520–6.

Kupila A et al. (2001). Feasibility of genetic and immunological prediction of type I diabetes in a population-based birth cohort. *Diabetologia* **44**, 290–7.

Kyvik KO, Green A, Beck-Nielsen H (1995). Concordance rates of insulin dependent diabetes mellitus: a population based study in Danish twins. *British Medical Journal* **311**, 913–7.

Lake SL, Blacker D, Laird NM (2000). Family-based test of association in the presence of linkage. *American Journal of Human Genetics* **67**, 1515–25.

Lander E, Kruglyak L (1995). Genetic dissection of complex traits: guidelines for interpreting and reporting linkage results. *Nature Genetics* **11**, 241–7.

Lango H et al. (2008). Assessing the combined impact of 18 common genetic variants of modest effect sizes on type 2 diabetes risk. *Diabetes* **57**, 3129–35.

Looker HC et al. (2007). Genome-wide linkage analyses to identify loci for diabetic retinopathy. *Diabetes* **56**, 1160–6.

Lowe CE et al. (2007). Large scale genetic fine mapping and genotype-phenotype associations implicate polymorphism in the *IL2RA* region in type 1 diabetes. *Nature Genetics* **39**, 1074–82.

Martin ER et al. (2000). A test for linkage and association in general pedigrees: the pedigree disequilibrium test. *American Journal of Human Genetics* **67**, 146–54.

Matsuda A, Kuzuya T (1994). Diabetic twins in Japan. *Diabetes Research and Clinical Practice* **24** (Suppl.), S63–7.

McCarthy MI (2003). Growing evidence for diabetes susceptibility genes from genome scan data. *Current Diabetes Reports* **3**, 159–67.

Moore AF et al. (2008). Extension of type 2 diabetes genome-wide association scan results in the Diabetes Prevention Program. *Diabetes* **57**, 2503–10.

Morton NE (1998). Significance levels in complex inheritance. *American Journal of Human Genetics* **62**, 690–7.

Nejentsev S et al. (2007). Localization of type 1 diabetes susceptibility to the MHC class I genes *HLA-B* and *HLA-A*. *Nature* **450**, 887–92.

Newman B et al. (1987). Concordance for type 2 (non-insulin-dependent) diabetes mellitus in male twins. *Diabetologia* **30**, 763–8.

Nisticò L et al. (1996). The *CTLA-4* gene region of chromosome 2q33 is linked to, and associated with, type 1 diabetes. *Human Molecular Genetics* **5**, 1075–80.

Onengut-Gumuscu S et al. (2004). A functional polymorphism (1858C/T) in the *PTPN22* gene is linked and associated with type I diabetes in multiplex families. *Genes and Immunity* **5**, 678–80.

Pavkov ME et al. (2007). Changing patterns of type 2 diabetes incidence among Pima Indians. *Diabetes Care* **30**, 1758–63.

Pettitt DJ et al. (1988). Congenital susceptibility to NIDDM: role of intrauterine environment. *Diabetes* **37**, 622–8.

Pettitt DJ et al. (1990). Familial predisposition to renal disease in two generations of Pima Indians with type 2 (non-insulin-dependent) diabetes mellitus. *Diabetologia* **33**, 438–43.

Poulsen P et al. (1999). Heritability of type II (non-insulin-dependent) diabetes mellitus and abnormal glucose tolerance—a population-based twin study. *Diabetologia* **42**, 139–45.

Rewers M et al. (1996). Newborn screening for HLA markers associated with IDDM: Daisy Autoimmunity Study in the Young (DAISY). *Diabetologia* **39**, 807–12.

Rotter JI, Landaw EM (1984). Measuring the genetic contribution of a single locus to a multilocus disease. *Clinical Genetics* **26**, 529–42.

Sandhu MS et al. (2007). Common variants in *WFS1* confer risk of type 2 diabetes. *Nature Genetics* **39**, 951–3.

Scott LJ et al. (2007). A genome-wide association study of type 2 diabetes in Finns detects multiple susceptibility variants. *Science* **316**, 1341–5.

Seaquist ER et al. (1989). Familial clustering of diabetic kidney disease: evidence for genetic susceptibility to diabetic nephropathy. *New England Journal of Medicine* **320**, 905–6.

Silander K et al. (2004). Genetic variation near the hepatocyte nuclear factor-4α gene predicts susceptibility to type 2 diabetes. *Diabetes* **53**, 1141–9.

Skyler JS (2007). Prediction and prevention of type 1 diabetes: progress, problems and prospects. *Clinical Pharmacology & Therapeutics* **81**, 768–71.

Sladek R et al. (2007). A genome-wide association study identifies novel risk loci for type 2 diabetes. *Nature* **445**, 881–5.

Smyth DJ et al. (2006). A genome-wide association study of nonsynonymous SNPs identifies a type 1 diabetes locus in the interferon-induced helicase (*IFIH1*) region. *Nature Genetics* **38**, 617–9.

Spielman RS, McGinnis RE, Ewens WJ (1993). Transmission test for linkage disequilibrium: the insulin gene region and insulin-dependent diabetes mellitus (IDDM). *American Journal of Human Genetics* **59**, 983–9.

Steinthorsdottir V et al. (2007). A variant in *CDKAL1* influences insulin response and risk of type 2 diabetes. *Nature Genetics* **39**, 770–5.

Tattersall RB, Pyke DA (1972). Diabetes in identical twins. *Lancet* **300**, 1120–5.

Thomson G (1984). HLA DR antigens and susceptibility to insulin-dependent diabetes mellitus. *American Journal of Human Genetics* **36**, 1309–17.

Todd JA, Bell JI, McDevitt HO (1987). HLA-DQ$_\beta$ gene contributes to susceptibility and resistance to insulin-dependent diabetes mellitus. *Nature* **329**, 599–604.

Todd JA et al. (2007). Robust associations of four new chromosome regions from genome-wide analyses of type 1 diabetes. *Nature Genetics* **39**, 857–64.

Tregouet DA et al (2008). G/T substitution in intron 1 of the *UNC13B* gene is associated with increased risk of nephropathy in patients with type 1 diabetes. *Diabetes* **57**, 2843–50.

Tuomilehto J et al. (2001). Prevention of type 2 diabetes mellitus by changes in lifestyle among subjects with impaired glucose tolerance. *New England Journal of Medicine* **344**, 1343–50.

Unoki H et al. (2008). SNPs in *KCNQ1* are associated with susceptibility to type 2 diabetes in East Asian and European populations. *Nature Genetics* **40**, 1098–102.

Van Hoek M et al. (2008) Predicting type 2 diabetes based on polymorphisms from genome-wide association studies: a population-based study. *Diabetes* **57**, 3122–8.

Vardarli I et al (2002). Gene for susceptibility to diabetic nephropathy in type 2 diabetes maps to 18q22.3-23. *Kidney International* **62**, 2176–83.

Yasuda K et al. (2008). Variants in *KCNQ1* are associated with susceptibility to type 2 diabetes mellitus. *Nature Genetics* **40**, 1092–7.

Zeggini E et al. (2007). Replication of genome-wide association signals in UK samples reveals risk loci for type 2 diabetes. *Science* **316**, 1336–40.

Zeggini E et al. (2008). Meta-analysis of genome-wide association data and large-scale replication identifies additional susceptibility loci for type 2 diabetes mellitus. *Nature Genetics* **40**, 638–45.

Zouali H et al. (1997). A susceptibility locus for early-onset non-insulin dependent (type 2) diabetes mellitus map to chromosome 20q, proximal to the phosphoenopyruvate carboxykinase gene. *Human Molecular Genetics* **6**, 1401–8.

29. Promising Technological Frontiers in Monitoring and Treatment

David C. Klonoff

■ Main Public Health Messages

- For monitoring diabetes control, self-monitoring of blood glucose is the established technology, continuous glucose monitoring the emerging technology, and the artificial pancreas the technology of the future.
- More information on blood glucose leads to improved outcomes.
- Self-monitoring of blood glucose improves control in type 1 and type 2 diabetes.
- Information from self-monitoring of blood glucose educates, motivates, and protects patients.
- Continuous glucose monitoring provides maximal information for making treatment decisions.
- Information from continuous glucose monitoring can be analyzed retrospectively and also acted on in real time.
- Continuous glucose monitoring improves mean glycemia and decreases glycemic variability.
- The safety, efficacy, and economic impact of closed-loop control systems are currently unknown.
- Telemonitoring permits real-time case management in response to multiple types of measurements.
- Telemonitoring is at an early stage of development and is potentially both effective and cost-effective.
- Insurance coverage for patients and reimbursement of health care providers for device management are major nontechnical barriers to the adoption of new diabetes technologies.

■ Introduction

The current technology for self-monitoring of blood glucose (SMBG) levels has been well established since the 1980s. This practice is beneficial to patients with diabetes from both a clinical and an economic standpoint. Knowledge of their blood glucose levels can allow patients to select appropriate doses of insulin to regulate these levels. Continuous glucose monitoring will be the next widely adopted method for glucose monitoring. This practice has been used since the turn of the 21st century, but only in limited cases thus far. The information provided by this technology can permit significantly more adjustments in insulin dosing and other therapies than spot testing from SMBG can provide. The next generation of technology that will permit adjustment of insulin dosage and with automatic control is closed-loop control. This technology, which is not yet commercially available, will revolutionize diabetes management. Such an approach, also known as the artificial pancreas, is currently being developed. An artificial pancreas will link continuous blood glucose measurement with automatically controlled insulin delivery, using nonliving components made of silicon, plastic, and metal. This chapter analyzes the technology, benefits, economic aspects, problems, and controversies associated with SMBG, continuous glucose monitoring, and the artificial pancreas as well as telemonitoring technology for diabetes management.

■ Background/Historical Perspective

Self-Monitoring of Blood Glucose

SMBG provides significant benefits to patients with diabetes. It improves control in type 1 patients and in insulin-treated type 2 patients. Arguably, it also improves control in type 2 patients who are receiving oral agents or dietary therapy only. SMBG is a tool for preventing severe hypoglycemia in any patient with diabetes. For this tool to improve control in diabetes, however, the patient must know how to respond to the measured blood glucose values.

Benefits

The four principal benefits of SMBG are to (1) treat high or low blood glucose levels by adjusting therapy to achieve the targeted hemoglobin A1C level; (2) protect the patient by allowing immediate confirmation of hypoglycemia or hyperglycemia; (3) educate the patient about the effects of diet, exercise, and other factors on glycemia; and (4) motivate healthy behavior.

In type 1 diabetes and in insulin-treated type 2 diabetes many studies have demonstrated that the frequency of SMBG is correlated with improved control (Levine et al. 2001). Although increased frequency of testing is correlated with decreased A1C levels, above about six to seven tests per day the improvement in control levels off.

Whether patients with type 2 disease who are not treated with insulin benefit from SMBG is a controversial issue. Two recent meta-analyses of randomized controlled trials of SMBG as a component of non-insulin therapy came to similar conclusions about the beneficial effect on A1C of this practice. They found a statistically significant decrease of approximately 0.4% with this practice in comparison with nonmonitoring controls, which was calculated to reduce the risk of microvascular complications by 14% (Sarol 2005; Welschen et al. 2005). The ROSSO nonrandomized study of SMBG in 3268 type 2 patients is the only study that has quantified hard endpoints rather than measuring A1C as a surrogate endpoint for the risk of diabetic complications. ROSSO reported that SMBG was associated with decreased diabetes-related morbidity and all-cause mortality in the entire study population as well as in a subgroup of patients who were not receiving insulin therapy (Martin et al. 2006).

Several factors have limited the demonstration of benefits of SMBG in type 2 populations, including: (1) inadequately specific instructions from health care providers about how to adjust therapy in response to glucose levels; (2) the absence of a consensus on the optimal frequency and timing of testing; (3) a dearth of postprandial blood glucose testing, which would have yielded unexpectedly (to the patient) high glucose values that would have led to behavior modification; and (4) the cost, pain, and inconvenience of frequent testing. Any improvements in these factors will probably increase the benefit of SMBG in this population. Furthermore many reported study protocols assessing the performance of SMBG in type 2 subjects have failed to instruct SMBG users what to do with the information and have not included specific dietary, exercise, or medication interventions in response to hyperglycemic readings (Klonoff et al. 2008).

Optimal Frequency

A problem with advising patients to increase their frequency of SMBG is the lack of a consensus on how frequently they should test and at what time relative to meals. A global consensus conference to address this issue was convened in 2004 (Bergenstal and Gavin 2005). The panel's findings were reported in 2005, and they are summarized in Table 29.1.

Economic Aspects

An economic analysis of providing SMBG in Germany in type 2 diabetes patients who were not receiving insulin assumed a decrease in mean A1C of 0.39%. The benefit attained was 1 month of added life per patient at a cost of approximately $40,000 per life-year gained. The total savings for monitoring seven times per week over 10 years was equal to 6% of the insurance-covered direct costs for diabetes. In a comparison with the costs of other interventions that are considered appropriate, SMBG was concluded to be cost-effective (Neeser, Erny-Albrecht, and Weber 2006).

TABLE 29.1   *Recommendations for Frequency of Self-Monitoring of Blood Glucose According to the Global Consensus Panel on Glucose Monitoring*

Regimen Frequency of Self-Monitoring

Insulin therapy (multiple daily injections or insulin pump) ≥3–4×/day

Patients above target on other regimens (orals and/or daily insulin) ≥2×/day

Patients at target on oral agents or daily insulin ≥1×/day + 1 profile/week

Patients at target on oral agents plus daily insulin ≥1×/day + frequent profiles

Patients on nonpharmacologic therapy ≥1 profile/week

A profile is defined as a premeal and a postmeal glucose test.
Source: Bergenstal, Gavin, and Global Consensus Conference on Glucose Monitoring Panel (2005).

Problems and Controversies

The accuracy of SMBG may be surprisingly poor in some circumstances, and errors may exceed 10%–20%. Patients rarely follow all of the manufacturer's recommendations for proper testing, such as washing their hands, storing strips in the original container, disposing of expired strips, applying blood properly to the strips, inserting strips properly into meters, cleaning the meters weekly, checking the strips and control solution for expiration, and comparing control values with the control range. When the patient does not calibrate the meter with the calibration code printed on the strip bottle, the reading might be inaccurate. In that case, if inaccurate glucose readings are being delivered by the monitor, the risk of insulin misdosing will be significantly greater than when patients correctly code their meters themselves or else use automatically coded meters (Raine et al. 2007). Many clinical chemists are advocating the establishment of external quality analysis programs for glucose meters to assess their performance after they are approved for use and marketed.

Alternate-site blood glucose testing is useful for patients who wish to avoid the pain, waste of blood, and trauma to the fingertips of finger-stick blood glucose testing. The forearm and palm are good sites for sampling blood glucose when the patient wants a break from fingertip trauma. Alternate-site testing should be avoided when (1) the blood glucose level is rising or falling rapidly; (2) the blood glucose level is very low; (3) the patient has eaten within the past 2 hours; and (4) a continuous glucose monitor is being calibrated with capillary blood glucose values.

Other Candidate Analytes for Home Monitoring

A1C is an intracellular analyte found within red blood cells. Blood levels of this glycated hemoglobin molecule reflect control over a period of 2 to 3 months; correspondingly, A1C is the best indicator of glycemic control over the past 2 to 3 months. Two devices are approved by the Food and Drug Administration (FDA) for self-monitoring of A1C. The Micromat II device (BioRad, Hercules, California) was the first to be approved, but the product is intended primarily for use by health care professionals. The A1cNow+ device (Metrika, Sunnyvale, California), the second to be approved, is intended for use by patients at home or by health care professionals. The A1cNow+ device comes with a set of 10 test cartridges that are to be used with one disposable monitor. The A1cNow+ replaced the A1cNow, which used a monitor that was disposed of after each test. An organization with links to governmental regulatory agencies, the National Glycohemoglobin Standardization Program (NGSP), evaluates every laboratory and home test for A1C, sets accuracy standards, and certifies which methods meet its standards. Currently both self-testing monitors for A1C are certified by the NGSP (Bode et al. 2007).

The glycation gap, which is based on fructosamine measurement, and the hemoglobin glycation index (HGI), which is based on mean blood glucose level, are two indices of A1C adjusted for glycemia measured by other means. The glycation gap is the difference between measured blood A1C and the A1C predicted from serum fructosamine testing based on a population regression equation of A1C on fructosamine. The HGI is the difference between measured blood A1C and the A1C predicted from the mean blood glucose level (calculated from SMBG tests) based on a population regression equation of A1C on mean blood glucose levels.

These two gaps could be thought of as an individual's inherent tendency to glycate proteins. This tendency could affect basement membrane proteins and cause microvascular disease, or it could affect hemoglobin molecules and produce a measure of mean glycemia (Cohen et al. 2006). Whether biological variation in glycation is in fact an independent risk factor for diabetic microvascular complications that is distinct from that attributable to mean blood glucose or fructosamine levels is controversial.

A marker for determining the average degree of glycemic control over the past few days or weeks would allow assessment of mean glycemia in patients who are undergoing rapid rises or declines in that measure. An A1C test changes too slowly to reflect such rapid change. The term fructosamine refers to a family of glycated serum proteins that is comprised mostly of albumin, a small amount of globulins, and a very small amount of other serum proteins. No product currently exists for home monitoring of serum fructosamine. Several portable assays are under development for measuring glycated albumin to assess control during periods of rapidly changing glucose levels. Two major obstacles to adoption of glycated albumin testing in the home and laboratory are the following: (1) the technical challenge of calibrating this test to mean glycemia; and (2) the extensive amount of education that will be necessary to convince health care providers to use this test when they already may be comfortable using A1C as a marker of mean glycemia.

Home lactate monitors are used in the athletic community to determine the lactate threshold that reflects peak performance. The clinical significance of monitoring blood lactate in patients with diabetes is unknown. The rise in blood glucose after eating might be expected to be accompanied by a rise in blood lactate in states of inadequate perfusion. Home-testing kits for blood ketone and cholesterol as well as urine microalbumin are also available.

Continuous Glucose Monitoring

Continuous glucose monitors, which give both retrospective and real-time information, provide important information that is not detectable even with frequent SMBG, such as otherwise unrecognized periods of preprandial hypoglycemia, postprandial hyperglycemia, and glycemic variability. The real-time monitors sound an alarm when the glucose level is above or below preset boundaries or when it is time for calibration against a finger-stick measurement. Their data can be downloaded into a computer for analysis at a later time.

Technology

Nine continuous glucose monitors have been approved by the FDA for use in the United States or carry CE (Conformite Europeene) marking for use in Europe; they are listed in Table 29.2 (Bode et al. 2004; Deiss et al. 2006; Feldman et al. 2003; Garg and Jovanovic 2006; Garg, Schwartz, and Edelman 2004; Gross et al. 2000; Maran et al. 2002; Medtronic n.d.; Potts, Tamada, and Tierney 2002). Currently, outside of a research setting, most continuous glucose monitoring in the United States is performed with the Guardian REAL Time System, the Seven, or the Freestyle Navigator. Several continuous blood glucose monitors for hospital use are under

TABLE 29.2 *Continuous Glucose Monitoring Systems*

- Continuous Glucose Monitoring System Gold (CGMS Gold) (Medtronic Diabetes, Northridge, CA) (Gross et al. 2000)
- GlucoWatch G2 Biographer (Cygnus, Inc., Redwood City, CA) (Potts, Tamada, and Tierney 2002)
- Guardian Telemetered Glucose Monitoring System (TGMS) (Medtronic Diabetes, Northridge, CA) (Bode et al. 2004)
- Guardian RT (Medtronic Diabetes, Northridge, CA) (Deiss et al. 2006)
- Guardian REAL TIME (Medtronic Diabetes, Northridge, CA) (Mastrototaro and Lee 2009)
- GlucoDay-S (A. Menarini Diagnostics, Florence, Italy) (Maran et al. 2002)
- STS Short Term Sensor (Dexcom, San Diego, CA) (Garg, Schwartz, and Edelman 2004)
- Seven (Dexcom, San Diego, CA) (Garg and Jovanovic 2006)
- FreeStyle Guardian (Abbott Diabetes Care, Alameda, CA) (Feldman et al. 2003)

All devices have been approved for marketing in the United States except for GlucoDay-S, which is available only in Europe.

development. The GlucoWatch has been withdrawn from the market. The earlier-generation versions of current products are rarely used in clinical practice.

The first continuous glucose monitor to be approved by the FDA was the CGMS; the second generation of this product is the CGMS Gold. For the past few years many users of this product (including the author of this chapter) have omitted the word "Gold" when they have referred to this product. The CGMS measures interstitial fluid glucose continuously with a sensor that is inserted subcutaneously into the abdominal wall. The device contains an enzyme that catalyzes glucose, which creates an electronic current. The current is (1) measured by the sensor, (2) stored in a monitor that is attached to the sensor by a wire and worn on the hip like a pager, and (3) converted by the monitor into a glucose value that equals the blood glucose value. The device must be calibrated four times per day with an SMBG level that is entered into the monitor. This device calculates and stores a reading every 5 minutes over a 72-hour period, which is the approved life of the sensor. After the sensor has been in place for 72 hours, it is removed. The monitor is then plugged into a docking station, which transfers the stored calculated data into a computer. The CGMS provides only retrospective data, which means that the glucose values are presented only after the sensor has been removed. The caregiver and patient can then study the data later and plan modified behavior or insulin dosing based on measured patterns of glycemia. In 2008 an offshoot of the CGMS, known as the iPro Recorder, was approved. This device is a wireless version of the CGMS Gold with a compact transmitter (the Minilink) linking the sensor and the monitor.

The Guardian RT device contains the same sensor as the CGMS Gold, but this device provides continuous glucose data readings every 5 minutes in real time, and it also stores data for retrospective analysis. The Guardian RT transmits data by way of a large transmitter taped to the body to a handheld device, which reveals to the patient the current glucose value.

The Guardian REAL Time System, approved in 2007, contains most of the features of the Guardian RT, but it uses a small olive-sized "Minilink" wireless transmitter to send data from the sensor to the portable monitor. The Guardian REAL Time System can also transmit real-time glucose data into a dedicated insulin pump. The combination monitor-pump product is known as the Paradigm REAL Time System (Lee et al. 2007).

The STS family of continuous sensors, like the CGMS family, uses a subcutaneous wire that is inserted into the skin and left in place to measure and transmit glucose levels in real time. The first-generation product, the STS, which was approved for 3 days of measurements, has been supplanted by the second-generation product, the Seven, which was approved in 2007 for 7 days of use. These devices transmit data to a hand-held glucose monitor.

The Freestyle Navigator monitor uses a needle sensor, like the Guardian REAL TIME and the Seven. This device, which was approved in 2008, is the most recent continuous sensor on the market in the United States. This monitor is approved for up to 5 days of use. The device transmits glucose readings every minute to a handheld monitor that displays directional arrows to indicate which way the glucose level is heading and how quickly.

In terms of future products in the United States, the GlucoDay-S uses microdialysis to (1) rinse interstitial fluid by passing crystalloid fluid through the skin, (2) measure the glucose content of this fluid, and (3) store the dialysate for eventual disposal. The measured glucose concentration is converted by a proprietary formula to a blood glucose level. This device is also available only in Europe. Additional microdialysis products for continuous glucose monitoring from Europe will likely be introduced in the next few years. The GlucoWatch, which removed interstitial fluid from the skin through a method using an electric current, known as reverse electrophoresis, is no longer on the market and will likely not be reintroduced because of poor accuracy and frequent skin irritation.

A noninvasive method for measuring glucose would involve applying light to the body and measuring the interaction with glucose. No such product is currently approved. The main barriers to developing this technology are the small signal from glucose relative to other biological molecules in the body and the difficulty separating the glucose signal from other biological molecules and metabolites of glucose with similar optical properties. Many companies have tried to develop such a product but have gone bankrupt without succeeding.

Performance

A continuous glucose monitor provides both point information and trend data. Currently available continuous monitors are less accurate than blood glucose monitors, however. Mean absolute differences between continuously measured data points and reference blood glucose values have been reported to be in the range of 13%–21%. Home blood glucose monitors tested under similar conditions are usually reported to have mean absolute differences of no more than 5%–10%. On the other hand the trend information provided by continuous monitors permits prediction of future glucose levels. This information can be particularly useful in real-time monitors by predicting impending hypoglycemia when the blood glucose level is at the low end of the normal range and the trend is downward.

The accuracy of continuous glucose monitors is generally less in the hypoglycemic range than in the euglycemic and hyperglycemic ranges. This disparity is unfortunate because the greatest need for continuous glucose data is to prevent or react to incipient hypoglycemia.

Clinical and Laboratory Standards Institute, the largest developer of standards in the United States, and Diabetes Technology Society, together developed "Performance Metrics for Continuous Interstitial Glucose Monitoring; Approved Guideline (POCT05-A)" in 2008. This guideline provides recommendations for methods for determining analytical and clinical metrics of continuous interstitial glucose monitors (Clinical and Laboratory Standards Institute 2008).

The performance of a continuous glucose monitor is most often described mathematically using error grid analysis. This analysis system was developed to classify measurement errors according to their clinical importance rather than by their mathematical magnitude. Because continuous glucose monitors present information on trends as well as point data, it is logical to express their performance in a way that incorporates their accuracy in providing both types of information. Error grid analysis can be applied simultaneously to point measurements and to trend measurements for every data point that is generated by a continuous glucose monitor, and the performance can be expressed as a blended rating (Kovatchev et al. 2004).

Another function of a continuous glucose monitor is to sound an alarm for impending hypoglycemia. Because of inherent inaccuracy problems with existing monitors, the user must accept a tradeoff between sensitivity and specificity when deciding at which glucose level a hypoglycemic alarm should sound. This problem is analogous to using a smoke detector that can be tuned up to report any smoke within hundreds of yards of the monitor, which will result in false alarms in the interests of sensitivity, or could be tuned down to respond only to thick nearby smoke, which will result in delayed warnings or even missed warnings in the interests of specificity. A manufacturer of a continuous glucose monitor can determine an optimal point for maximizing both sensitivity and specificity by applying a receiver operator curve analysis of the sensitivity and specificity of event detection at various alarm thresholds. Regulatory considerations might mandate that patients be notified by way of alarms at specific predetermined levels of hypoglycemia and hyperglycemia. At these mandated threshold levels for sounding an alarm a device might not be detecting such events with an optimal combination of sensitivity and specificity given the performance of its sensor.

Several mathematical tools have been proposed to express mathematically the degree of glycemic variability and burden of high and low glycemic extremes that can be recognized by continuous glucose monitoring. Such formulas are needed because of recent evidence that glycemic variability may represent an independent risk factor for increasing oxidative stress and the release of proinflammatory cytokines, which can lead to diabetic complications.

Outcomes

Ten randomized controlled studies of continuous glucose monitoring technologies have been conducted. The endpoint in eight studies was the A1C level as a surrogate marker for morbidity and mortality related to diabetes; in the other two it was the time spent hypoglycemic or hyperglycemic. Five studies evaluated the CGMS, two the GlucoWatch, one the Guardian REAL TIME, one the STS, and one the Seven. The use of continuous glucose monitoring was associated with improved A1C levels in three of five CGMS studies, in one of the two GlucoWatch studies, and in the single Guardian REAL TIME study (Deiss et al. 2006; Klonoff 2005), and it was associated with decreased time spent in extreme glycemic levels in the STS and Seven studies (Garg and Jovanovic 2006; Garg, Schwartz, and Edelman 2004).

The Continuous Glucose Sensor Human Clinical Trial, a 1-year multicenter, randomized controlled study of real-time continuous glucose monitors in the management of type 1 diabetes that was organized by the Juvenile Diabetes Research Foundation, began in December 2006. This was the largest study ever conducted on the performance of continuous glucose monitoring. The Guardian RT, the STS, and the FreeStyle Navigator were all tested: 322 adults and children with a glycated hemoglobin level of 7.0% to 10.0%, who were already receiving intensive therapy for type 1 diabetes, were randomized either to a group with continuous glucose monitoring or to a control group performing home monitoring with a blood glucose meter. The subjects were stratified into three cohorts according to age. The primary outcome was the change in the glycated hemoglobin level at 26 weeks. A significant difference among subjects 25 years of age or older favored continuous monitoring. This cohort's mean difference in change was −0.53%, but there was no statistically significant difference between groups in the 15 to 24 years of age cohort or the 8 to 14 years of age cohort (JDRF Continuous Glucose Monitoring Study Group 2008).

Based on an empirical finding in some studies that use of the CGMS can lower A1C by 0.3%, this outcome has been estimated to represent approximately one-sixth of the reduction of complications attained by the DCCT (Diabetes Control and Complications Trial). An analysis of the benefits from the DCCT multiplied by one-sixth concluded that use of the CGMS per the protocols used in the studies reviewed could possibly provide 1 additional year of life, of sight, of the absence of end-stage renal disease, and of the absence of amputation. An economic analysis of the benefits of using the GlucoWatch by a medical economics expert employed by the product's manufacturer found that using the GlucoWatch in a simulated population of children and adolescents with type 1 diabetes, if employed for the life of the cohort, would delay the first serious diabetes complication by 4.1 years. Treating 18 subjects would prevent one case of blindness and 1.4 cases of renal failure. The intervention would cost $91,059/year of life, $61,326/quality-adjusted year of life (QALY), and $9930/year free of a major complication. If the GlucoWatch ceased to be effective after age 17, the cost per QALY gained would increase to $103,178 (Eastman, Leptien, and Chase 2003). In general, interventions costing over $100,000 per QALY gained are considered expensive, and those under $50,000 per QALY gained are considered reasonable.

Problems

The accuracy of currently available continuous glucose monitors is insufficient for any of them to have received FDA approval for a primary indication. This means that if a continuous glucose monitor demonstrates an extreme glucose value that might require action, the patient must check a blood glucose level with a standard blood glucose monitor and act only on that result. When patients wearing real-time continuous glucose monitors will no longer be required to carry a standard blood glucose monitor, the continuous glucose monitors will increase in popularity.

Reimbursement

Many insurers have been reluctant to reimburse patients for the use of continuous glucose monitoring equipment and extremely reluctant to reimburse physicians for the time spent on explaining, inserting, and removing these monitors and interpreting the data obtained. These insurers claim that the evidence supporting the use of this technology is inadequate. Additional robust research that demonstrates the clinical and economic benefits of this technology under defined conditions will be needed in order to unlock reimbursement for this technology. After additional outcomes data have been collected, the next step for overcoming the reimbursement barrier will probably be development of evidence-based clinical guidelines.

Closed-Loop Control (Artificial Pancreas)

An artificial pancreas is defined as a device or system of integrated devices containing only synthetic materials that substitutes for an endocrine pancreas by sensing the blood glucose level, determining the amount of insulin needed, and then delivering the appropriate amount of insulin (Klonoff 2007). The four components of an artificial pancreas are listed in Table 29.3. The use of such a system to manage diabetes can result in physiologic glycemic levels without finger-stick blood glucose measurements, insulin injections, or hypoglycemic events. In spite of difficult problems that remain to be solved, recent engineering advances have produced individual components that can be combined into closed-loop systems as well as several investigational closed-loop systems that have actually controlled blood glucose under defined conditions without human input. No artificial pancreas is currently available commercially, but components that could go into an artificial pancreas are now coming onto the market. At this time multiple versions of entire systems are under investigation in humans, animals, and in computerized models.

Technical Problems

The creation of an artificial pancreas will require solutions to significant technical, economic, and political problems. The technical problems related to efficacy include

TABLE 29.3   *The Four Components of an Artificial Pancreas*

- Automatic glucose monitor
- Automatic insulin delivery system
- Algorithm to link glucose levels with insulin delivery
- Transmitters and receivers to link all components

how to create (1) a very accurate continuous glucose sensor with little lag time between fluctuations in blood glucose and measured glucose levels; (2) a method for delivering insulin physiologically; (3) an effective controller for providing appropriate amounts of insulin to maintain glycemia within a physiological range; and (4) a multicomponent system using wireless communication that is not subject to electromagnetic interference from surrounding radiofrequency-emitting equipment. The full costs, specific benefits, and ratio of costs to benefits of closed-loop control are all currently unknown. Finally, if an artificial pancreas can be created, this device will undergo extremely rigorous scrutiny from such political sectors as (1) regulatory agencies (concerned with safety), (2) insurance companies (concerned with efficacy), and (3) the legal system (concerned with liability). Any instances of device failure could result in crippling regulations, denials of coverage, or lawsuits against the manufacturer alleging product liability.

An implanted continuous glucose sensor may malfunction for many reasons, including (1) calibration drift, (2) a lag between concentrations of arterial blood glucose and interstitial fluid glucose during rapid fluctuations, (3) sensor fouling, (4) rejection and fibrosis, and (5) local inflammatory complications.

An implanted or external insulin reservoir that comprises part of an artificial pancreas might develop many problems, depending on the delivery site, including (1) the absence of physiological nonglucose stimuli that trigger insulin release; (2) nonphysiological delivery of infused insulin into the systemic circulation rather than to the portal circulation and the liver; (3) insulin denaturation within the reservoir; (4) local complications from controlled insulin delivery; and (5) surgical and anesthestic risks of implantation and explanation.

Almost all controllers currently under development have similar problems. These devices lack (1) adequate models to predict insulin requirements in a large variety of situations; (2) programming for bidirectional control (a basic principle of control theory), in that they respond to hyperglycemia with insulin delivery but not to hypoglycemia with any counterregulatory substance that will raise the blood glucose level; and (3) effective solutions for responding to glycemic spikes, because they cannot distinguish noise (no prandial insulin bolus is needed) from a mealtime rise (a prandial insulin bolus is needed).

When an artificial pancreas is developed, outcomes data will be required for this tool to become widely adopted. The developers and users of this technology will need to demonstrate safety, effectiveness, and cost-effectiveness for this technology to become widely adopted and reimbursed.

The use of glucagon infusion to overcome excess insulin therapy would be an attractive feature of an artificial pancreas from the physiological standpoint. The availability of glucagon would permit tighter control of hyperglycemia with less risk of "overshoot hypoglycemia." The disadvantages from an engineering standpoint are the complexity of building two separate infusion systems and the possibility of glucagon denaturation within the pump. Animal data from a single laboratory using glucagon in addition to insulin for closed-loop control is promising.

Controversies

The first artificial pancreas systems will probably control basal insulin delivery automatically and require manual programming of insulin at mealtimes. The optimal times for use of such a system may be overnight, during activities known to be associated with glycemic variability, or throughout the entire day.

The FDA has assembled an Artificial Pancreas Working Group to address issues of glucose-sensing hardware, software control, and insulin dosing. Clinical trials of closed-loop systems will initially take place in a hospital setting and eventually move to the home setting.

Telemonitoring

Physiological data in diabetes will increasingly be transmitted, responded to, and archived by telemonitoring technologies. More frequent and more accurate glucose monitoring leads to improved glucose control and better clinical outcomes by allowing insulin to be delivered in optimal quantities at optimal times. Recent engineering advances are leading to improved intermittent testing of blood glucose and the advent of continuous measurements of glucose levels. In the next couple of decades, systems will likely be developed to analyze continuous glucose values, calculate necessary insulin dosages, and deliver appropriate amounts of insulin automatically and without painful needlesticks. Management of diabetes will eventually include telemonitoring and case management by telemedicine in response to wirelessly transmitted data about glucose levels and other physiologic measurements.

Telemonitoring, also known as biotelemetry, combines timely transmission of monitored data with remote interpretation of the data in order to rapidly respond to changes in health status. Patients with diabetes currently generate a large amount of data from SMBG, with two tests per day equaling 730 data points annually. These patients will soon be generating even more data from increasing use of continuous glucose monitors, many of which measure glucose levels up to every 5 minutes, which generates 288 new data points every day. To provide optimal and timely telemedicine care, health care providers need systems for recognizing and responding rapidly to deviations from expected values and also for archiving the thousands of self-monitored data points per patient per year that are increasingly being generated.

Technology

Telemonitoring involves transmission of chemical, electronic, mechanical, video, or audio data. The data can be transmitted through a telephone modem, personal digital assistant, computer, or cell phone to a central repository where it is stored and in some cases automatically analyzed. The data may be transmitted automatically from the monitor directly into the transmitter, or it may be manually entered by the patient. A summary of the data or a computer-generated analysis of the data can be returned to the patient by an automated phone call, a text message on the cell phone, an e-mail message, or a posting onto a secure patient-specific Web site. The frequency of data transmission may be either monthly or daily if the patient must make a manual connection from the monitor to the transmitter, or else automatically in real time if the monitor also contains a transmitter. In selected situations, a case manager might mail, fax, or even personally phone the patient with new directions, depending on the situation's urgency.

Data that have been transmitted in diabetes telemonitoring programs include blood glucose levels, insulin dosages, blood pressure, weight, skin temperature, retinal photographs, and lifestyle events such as eating and exercise. The trend toward less costly global positioning technology will soon enable telemonitoring devices to also automatically report a patient's location at all times.

Outcomes

An improvement in A1C levels or a decreased frequency of diabetic complications has been shown in some but not all studies of telemonitoring. The study populations, methods, and endpoints in reported telemedicine studies in the literature are very different, but telemonitoring programs have mostly been well accepted by patients because they provide empowerment and save travel time. In 2000, Columbia University and the State University of New York (SUNY) Upstate Medical University received a $28 million grant from the U.S. government for a multicenter telemedicine program for underserved rural and inner-city residents with diabetes (Starren et al. 2002). This is the largest telemedicine effort ever funded by the U.S. government. Each patient receives a home telephone unit consisting of four components that are listed in Table 29.4. The program, which is called Informatics for Diabetes Education and Telemedicine (IDEATel), will serve as a test bed for the national use of Internet technology to increase access to health care, and it will be a model to develop more effective treatments for other diseases.

Economic Aspects

For health care providers a telemonitoring program may require additional time for data review and case management in some programs, but it can also save time by

TABLE 29.4   *The Four Functions of the Informatics for Diabetes Education and Telemedicine (IDEATel) Home Telemedicine Unit*

- Synchronous videoconferencing over standard telephone lines
- Electronic transmission for self-monitored glucose and blood pressure readings
- Secure Web-based messaging and clinical data review
- Access to Web-based educational materials

Source: Starren et al. (2002).

decreasing face-to-face contact with patients. A very limited amount of economic data (that includes many assumptions) about small telemonitoring programs indicates that they can be cost saving. Telemonitoring technology is intended to allow managed care organizations to maintain their quality of service while reducing costs associated with serving people with chronic illnesses. Telemedicine care may turn out to be especially cost saving in a capitated reimbursement model.

Problems

Adoption of telemonitoring programs is currently hampered by the limited amount of data about the efficacy and economics of large telemedicine programs. Health care providers must be convinced that these programs will not create an increased workload that is not reimbursed by payers.

■ Implications for Health Policy

Technology is increasingly becoming an important part of the monitoring and treatment of people with diabetes. SMBG, continuous glucose monitoring, closed-loop control, and telemonitoring are evolving technologies that will empower patients to control their glycemia better and experience better outcomes. The insurance coverage of patients and reimbursement of health care providers for device management are major nontechnical barriers to adoption of new diabetes technologies. Well-designed clinical trials will be needed to justify the use and reimbursement of each new device. The challenge for the developers of new technology is to create products that clearly are both effective and cost-effective.

■ Areas of Uncertainty or Controversy

Numerous controversies within the area of diabetes technology are likely to be debated over the next few years. Among the expected controversies are the following eight issues: (1) What are the benefits of SMBG in type 2 diabetes? (2) What is the benefit of continuous glucose monitoring? (3) How significant is glycemic variability as an independent risk factor for complications in diabetes? (4) What type of performance data related to the accuracy of hypoglycemic and hyperglycemic alarms should be collected in clinical trials of continuous glucose monitors? (5) What is the best method for randomizing subjects into user and nonuser cohorts in unblinded clinical trials of diabetes devices to avoid contamination of the nonusers with the information and attitudes of investigators who have seen subjects benefit from use of the technologies? (6) How must the first closed-loop system perform to be adopted by the diabetes community? (7) Can telemedicine for diabetes be made sufficiently beneficial to justify the additional equipment and personnel costs that are necessary for this type of intervention? (8) Which technologies will be useful for management of hospitalized patients, and what will be the goal of treatment?

■ Developments over the Next 5 to 10 Years

Based on current trends in diabetes technology, three predictions are in order: First, within the next 5 to 10 years, a closed-loop artificial pancreas system will appear on the market. This device will likely require some manual control at various times, such as at mealtime. Second, within the next 10 years, improved optics and data-processing technology will lead to the development of an optical noninvasive glucose monitor. Third, new monitoring technologies of currently recognized physiological processes as well as yet-unrecognized physiological processes will be combined with improved wireless transmission technologies to create sophisticated continuous automatic remote displays of patient health that will contain globally calculated real-time health scores. Maintaining the privacy of such remotely monitored and electronically stored data will become an increasing challenge. In conclusion, the number of novel products using new technology will increase, as will the responsibility to use this technology wisely.

■ References

Bergenstal RM, Gavin JR 3rd; Global Consensus Conference on Glucose Monitoring Panel (2005). The role of self-monitoring of blood glucose in the care of people with diabetes: report of a global consensus conference. *American Journal of Medicine* **118** (Suppl. 9A), 1S–6S.

Bode B et al. (2004). Alarms based on real-time sensor glucose values alert patients to hypo- and hyperglycemia: the guardian continuous monitoring system. *Diabetes Technology & Therapeutics* **6**, 105–13.

Bode B et al. (2007). Advances in hemoglobin A1c point of care technology. *Journal of Diabetes Science and Technology* **1**, 405–11.

Cohen RM et al. (2006). Evidence for independent heritability of the glycation gap (glycosylation gap) fraction of HbA1c in nondiabetic twins. *Diabetes Care* **29**, 1739–43.

Clinical and Laboratory Standards Institute (2008). Performance metrics for continuous interstitial glucose monitoring; approved guideline. POCT05-A (28)33. http://www.clsi.org/source/orders/free/POCT05-A.pdf.

Deiss D et al. (2006). Improved glycemic control in poorly controlled patients with type 1 diabetes using real-time continuous glucose monitoring. *Diabetes Care* **29**, 2730–2.

Eastman RC, Leptien AD, Chase HP (2003). Cost-effectiveness of use of the GlucoWatch Biographer in children and adolescents with type 1 diabetes: a preliminary analysis based on a randomized controlled trial. *Pediatric Diabetes* **4**, 82–6.

Feldman B et al. (2003). A continuous glucose sensor based on wired enzyme technology—results from a 3-day trial in patients with type 1 diabetes. *Diabetes Technology & Therapeutics* **5**, 769–79.

Garg S, Jovanovic L (2006). Relationship of fasting and hourly blood glucose levels to HbA1c values: safety, accuracy, and improvements in glucose profiles obtained using a 7-day continuous glucose sensor. *Diabetes Care* **29**, 2644–9.

Garg SK, Schwartz S, Edelman SV (2004). Improved glucose excursions using an implantable real-time continuous glucose sensor in adults with type 1 diabetes. *Diabetes Care* **27**, 734–8.

Gross TM et al. (2000). Performance evaluation of the MiniMed continuous glucose monitoring system during patient home use. *Diabetes Technology & Therapeutics* **2**, 49–56.

Juvenile Diabetes Research Foundation Continuous Glucose Monitoring Study Group et al. (2008). Continuous glucose monitoring and intensive treatment of type 1 diabetes. *New England Journal of Medicine* **359**, 1464–76.

Klonoff DC (2005). Continuous glucose monitoring: roadmap for 21st century diabetes therapy. *Diabetes Care* **28**, 1231–9.

Klonoff DC (2007). The artificial pancreas: how sweet engineering will solve bitter problems. *Journal of Diabetes Science and Technology* **1**, 72–81.

Klonoff DC et al. (2008). Consensus report of the Coalition for Clinical Research—Self-Monitoring of Blood Glucose. *Journal of Diabetes Science and Technology* **2**, 1030–53.

Kovatchev BP et al. (2004). Evaluating the accuracy of continuous glucose-monitoring sensors: continuous glucose-error grid analysis illustrated by TheraSense Freestyle Navigator data. *Diabetes Care* **27**, 1922–8.

Lee S et al. (2007). Combined insulin pump therapy with real-time continuous glucose monitoring significantly improves glycemic control compared to multiple daily injection therapy in pump naive patients with type 1 diabetes; single center pilot study experience. *Journal of Diabetes Science and Technology* **1**, 400–4.

Levine BS et al. (2001). Predictors of glycemic control and short-term adverse outcomes in youth with type 1 diabetes. *Journal of Pediatrics* **139**, 197–203.

Maran A et al. (2002). Continuous subcutaneous glucose monitoring in diabetic patients: a multicenter analysis. *Diabetes Care* **25**, 347–52.

Martin S et al. (2006). Self-monitoring of blood glucose in type 2 diabetes and long-term outcome: an epidemiological cohort study. *Diabetologia* **49**(2):271–8. Epub 2005 Dec 17.

Mastrototaro J, Lee S (2009). The integrated MiniMed Paradigm REAL-Time insulin pump and glucose monitoring system: implications for improved patient outcomes. *Diabetes Technology & Therapeutics* **1**, S37–43.

Neeser K, Erny-Albrecht KM, Weber C (2006). Cost-effectiveness of self-monitoring of blood glucose in type 2 diabetic patients not receiving insulin. *Diabetes Care* **29**, 480.

Potts RO, Tamada JA, Tierney MJ (2002). Glucose monitoring by reverse
    iontophoresis. *Diabetes/Metabolism Research and Reviews* **18** (Suppl. 1), S49–53.
Raine CH III et al. (2007). Significant insulin dose errors may occur if blood
    glucose results are obtained from miscoded meters. *Journal of Diabetes Science
    and Technology* **1**, 205-19.
Sarol JN Jr (2005). Self-monitoring of blood glucose as part of a multi-component
    therapy among non-insulin requiring type 2 diabetes patients: a meta-analysis
    (1966–2004). *Current Medical Research and Opinion* **21**, 173–84.
Starren J et al. (2002). Columbia University's Informatics for Diabetes Education
    and Telemedicine (IDEATel) project: technical implementation. *Journal of the
    American Medical Informatics Association* **9**, 25–36.
Welschen LM et al. (2005). Self-monitoring of blood glucose in patients with type 2
    diabetes who are not using insulin: a systematic review. *Diabetes Care* **28**, 1510–7.

30. TRANSLATION RESEARCH AND MAJOR ONGOING CLINICAL TRIALS

Evan M. Benjamin

■ Main Public Health Messages

- Several efficacious treatments reduce the morbidity and mortality of people with diabetes, but the consistent application of these interventions into practice continues to be a challenge for translation research.
- The quality of diabetes care in the United States remains suboptimal.
- Translation research focuses on assessing the value of treatments and on how treatments can be implemented and sustained in real-world settings.
- Phase Two translation research, which seeks to understand how advances can be adopted in community-based and often uncontrolled conditions, has received little attention in diabetes.
- Some of the important questions in translational research cannot be addressed in randomized trials.
- Planning the research question and selecting the specific outcome measures are key steps in performing effective translation research.
- Through community-based participatory research, issues related to lifestyle, diet, physical activity, and cultural preferences might be explored.
- Clinical guidelines for professionals as part of a multifaceted intervention have had some success in improving diabetes care.
- Interventions targeting patients have been moderately successful in improving diabetes outcomes.
- Structured case management, including clinical practice guidelines, reminders, patient education, and ongoing clinician-patient interaction, can improve the quality of diabetes care.
- A number of translation trials have already had an impact on the treatment of diabetes and its complications as well as on the prevalence of diabetes.

■ Introduction

Diabetes is a chronic disease that imposes huge public health and economic burdens despite the availability of known efficacious treatments. Diabetes is the leading cause of new cases of blindness among working-age adults and of end-stage renal disease and amputation among the general population. People with diabetes have two to four times the risk of cardiovascular disease as those without diabetes. Over the past several years high-quality evidence has supported the efficacy of several treatments to reduce morbidity and mortality in people with diabetes. Interventions such as improving glycemic control, blood pressure, and lipid control; smoking cessation; and early detection and management of retinopathy and nephropathy appear not only successful but also highly cost-effective. The consistent application of these interventions into practice remains the challenge of translation research.

Translation research is applied research for health care and policy that strives to study how to translate available knowledge and make it useful for reducing the burden of diabetes (Narayan et al. 2004). Although both basic and clinical research have provided treatments for diabetes care, the quality of such care continues to remain suboptimal (McGlynn et al. 2003; Saaddine et al. 2002, 2006). Translation research explores the reasons why efficacious treatments have not reduced the burden of diabetes and evaluates potential solutions. Although proven treatments and research studies that document the efficacy of treatments are widely available, we continue to observe inadequate implementation of such treatments. To mitigate and reduce the burden of a disease, research must not only focus on the efficacy of a treatment but also illuminate how such treatment can be translated into clinical practice at a population level.

Translation research may be considered an extension of effectiveness research, but it also takes on other components of health services research, public health, and community medicine. Figure 30.1 shows translation research in the context of other types of research and public health assessments.

■ Background/Historical Perspective

Translation research is oriented toward understanding solutions to real-world health care delivery problems. As opposed to basic science, which helps to characterize the scientific root of the problem, or epidemiologic research, which aims to characterize the extent of the problem, translation research is interested in the implementation of known treatments and how they can be generalized across populations to reach most people who can benefit from the treatment. Translation research focuses on assessing the effectiveness of treatments and on how treatments can be implemented and sustained in real-world settings. This research may focus on clinical microsystems as well as on health policy to accelerate the translation of efficacious treatments into practice.

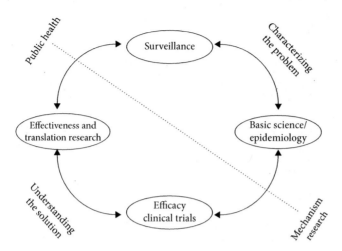

FIGURE 30.1. Translation research in context

Phase One translation research looks at ways in which we can apply basic scientific discoveries to human health under controlled conditions, such as in clinical research. Phase Two translation research seeks to understand how discoveries that are effective in improving human health can be adopted in community-based and often uncontrolled conditions.

In 1974, the Diabetes Mellitus Research in Education Act (Public Law 93-354) initiated a program to guide the federal government's approach to diabetes research in the future. The Act provided that:

1. the National Institutes of Health establish Diabetes Research and Training Centers (DRTCs);
2. the Centers for Disease Control (CDC, now the Centers for Disease Control and Prevention) support diabetes control programs within departments of public health throughout the states; and that
3. the Diabetes Mellitus Interagency Coordinating Committee be formed to help coordinate the diabetes-related activities of federal agencies.

One of the specific aims of the DRTCs was to "translate the advances in the field of diabetes research with least delay and to improve care . . . in the setting of model care administration and through outreach programs in the regional community." This principal charge reflects both Phase One and Phase Two translation research as defined above.

The principal aim of the Diabetes Mellitus Research in Education Act notwithstanding, Phase Two translation research has received little attention in diabetes. Although there continues to be new research conducted on basic and clinical science and on efficacy, we continue to be challenged to identify ways of translating research into community-based practice that will decrease society's burden of diabetes (Hiss 2001).

It has often been assumed that Phase One translation research would be adequate to improve the health of a community and that widespread adoption of science as a result of Phase One research would occur through word of mouth, the medical literature, and national/regional scientific meetings.

Although the activities in developing and disseminating information described above are useful, they are not sufficient to adopt new science into community practice. Publications and meetings do help to produce awareness that new treatments exist, and yet this awareness does not adequately address true implementation issues at the community level that must be understood to convert new science into real-world applications (Hiss 2001).

Translation research fits into the context of research on effectiveness and efficacy and of public health assessments as shown in Figure 30.1 (Greenfield et al. 1994). Efficacy trials attempt to understand mechanisms and to test associations of intervention under ideal conditions. In contrast, effectiveness research uses both observational and experimental designs to test associations and interventions in real-world, but usually controlled, settings. Effectiveness research is concerned with both patient outcomes and outcomes at the level of the health care system. This kind of research may look at outcomes in quality of care, quality of life, patient satisfaction, and resource utilization as well as such classic outcomes as mortality. Translation research is considered an extension of effectiveness research, as it tries to understand how efficacious treatments can be applied in real-world, uncontrolled populations. Specifically, translation research looks at the sustainability of applying treatments over time as well as their generalizability to populations. It takes effectiveness research to a public health level by attempting to understand how optimal health care can be created for as many people as possible. This research attempts to evaluate systems of care as well as health policies that could be created to accelerate the translation of research into practice. The current challenge of effectiveness research is that it fails to penetrate community-based practice and continues to look at the application of efficacious treatments only in controlled circumstances. The laboratory for translation research is the community, and the research subjects are highly varied, uncontrolled members of that community (Garfield et al. 2003).

■ Design for Diabetes Translation Research

Diabetes is a multifactorial disease with a complex biology and etiology. The life-long nature and chronicity of the disease, the numerous challenges in treating and managing it, and the complex relationships among patients, their community, and the health care system make delivering high-quality care with the most efficacious treatment a daunting assignment. We do know that we have the ability to apply currently available efficacious treatments to reduce the burden of diabetes, but we must learn how to make evidence and efficacious treatments part of clinical and public health practice.

At this point, the planning and selection of outcome measures to be used in diabetes translation research and the design for such research continue to evolve. Beginning with studies aimed at documenting quality of care using a variety of measures, translation research has evolved toward better and more standard characterization of quality of care and a better understanding of barriers to improving quality of care. Numerous small studies have tested simple patient-, provider-, and system-level interventions to improve care. Some of the more advanced studies have included multicenter investigations using a common protocol and the testing of specific models of care. Other studies have documented the practicality of system-wide redesign and its effect on diabetes care.

Planning the research question and selecting the specific outcome measures are key steps in performing effective translation research. The goal is to create a research design that will maximize generalizability and minimize bias in the research study. Because the barriers to effective translation are complex, any intervention to study translation must be designed to study the impact of complex and multidisciplinary interventions targeted to improve practice.

The outcomes to be evaluated in translation research include not only traditional measures of effectiveness (quality of care, quality of life, etc.) but also the impact on the community and on health disparities. In designing the research question and defining the variables to be assessed, translation research should incorporate an evaluation of an intervention to improve the overall health of a community that includes all members of that community.

Rigorous evaluation does not always require randomized trials. Although a randomized trial is often an effective design in clinical research, its use in translation research is limited by the complex nature of patients and the community in which they live. Because of the barriers to the delivery of health care, some of the important questions in translation research cannot be addressed in randomized trials. The design of diabetes translation research may need to involve more complicated nonrandomized trials that are either quasi-randomized trials with clustering or perhaps observational studies and interrupted time series with controls at a second site or a second time. Some researchers have proposed that before-and-after studies that include concurrent control groups have their place in translation research and can provide robust results (Eccles et al. 2003; Glasziou et al. 2007).

When trying to translate research into practice, one of the best approaches is to look at redesigning the system with the idea of offering care that is patient centered; often the solution is to offer multiple interventions in our health care system simultaneously. Because these changes are numerous and the barriers complex, the design of translation research needs also to be multifactorial. The focus of the research, whether at the patient, provider, or system level, needs to be reflected in the design of translation research.

■ Community-Based Research and Systems of Care

One example of translation research is community-based participatory research (O'Toole et al. 2003). One barrier to translating evidence into practice is that patients in a variety of settings need individualized recommendations specific to their health literacy, cultural orientation, and goals; community-based participatory research brings together patients, families, members of the community, health care providers, and researchers to craft specific interventions to overcome barriers in communities. Real-world circumstances in which patients live in communities and receive care in local practice settings and interact with family and community members in their day-to-day lives are the basis for community-based participatory research (Israel et al. 1998). This type of research allows translational researchers to evaluate how well a change in health policy or clinical systems could penetrate a community.

Issues related to lifestyle, diet, physical activity, and cultural preferences that intersect with the health care delivery system are at the core of translation research and can be explored with community-based research. Diabetes treatment requires community-wide efforts not only to prevent diabetes but also to improve diet and exercise as part of fundamental efforts in treatment and prevention. The dissemination of information and the promotion of appropriate lifestyle changes and treatments need to happen at the community level for the health care system to be successful at decreasing the burden of diabetes. Working at the community level empowers patients and community stakeholders with a level of control to improve health care in their community.

Community-based research is challenged by the need to balance an idealized, controlled research environment with the demands of real-world communities. Communities may want a customized approach to improving a particular health problem, but this request needs to be balanced by the need for evaluation and sharing of information so that the intervention is more generalizable to other communities (O'Toole et al. 2003).

The current health care system is much better designed for the management of acute diseases than it is for managing chronic disorders. As promoted in the Chronic Care Model (Wagner, Austin, and Von Korff 1996), a new system of care and newer ways of thinking are needed to tackle chronic, complex diseases such as diabetes. Translation research must incorporate the principles of complex systems and must be designed to understand the system as a whole. To perform diabetes translation research means to understand that new systems must be created and tested to translate the results of efficacy and effectiveness trials into clinical care. As a result, translation research needs to be multidisciplinary and incorporate concepts from change management and performance improvement as well as the disciplines of economics, health services research, and human factors research. The Institute of Medicine's landmark report, *Crossing the Quality Chasm* (Institute of Medicine 2001), calls for a rethinking of the health care delivery system to achieve breakthroughs in effectiveness, safety, patient centeredness, and efficiency.

■ Dissemination of the Findings of Research

Translation research gives us the opportunity to disseminate the findings of research in efficacy and effectiveness. In this sense translation research becomes not only the application to a real-world community setting but also includes dissemination research to help spread change. Years ago most research was designed to study questions of efficacy and was not designed to disseminate information into the community (Bero et al. 1998). Similarly our current research system is designed to reward researchers for funding and for publications and not for dissemination. Translation research is an additional opportunity not only to disseminate actively but also to test the best way in which that dissemination can occur.

■ Gaps in Diabetes Care

The numerous barriers to care at the level of the provider, the patient, and the system help to explain the suboptimal state of diabetes care in the United States. At the provider level, forgetfulness and time constraints (Chin, Zhang, and Merrell 1998; McFarlane et al. 2002; McVea et al. 1996), a perception of the patient as nonadherent (Chin et al. 1998; Dalewitz, Khan, and Hershey 2000; Jacques and Jones 1993), and inadequate knowledge on the part of providers (Bernard et al. 1999; Drass et al. 1998) may act as barriers. In addition, one study found that primary care providers perceived diabetes as requiring more resources and being more difficult to treat than other chronic diseases, such as hypertension (Larme and Pugh 1998). Diabetes is often accompanied by numerous comorbid conditions, whose demands for treatment compete with the need for diabetes treatment (Konen, Curtis, and Summerson 1996). At the level of patients, an incomplete understanding of the gravity of diabetes, little motivation toward prevention, insufficient time, lack of social and economic resources, and poor health literacy are barriers (Bernard et al. 1999; Drass et al. 1998; Hiss 1996, 2001; Larme and Pugh 1998). At the level of the health care system, the status of diabetes as a chronic disease constitutes a potential barrier in a system that is better designed for acute care (Etzwiler 1997; Hiss 2001; Wagner 1998). In addition our current health care system often lacks information systems to identify patients, track their status, and prompt providers about ongoing needs in preventive care and treatment. The use of reminders or other tools to overcome forgetfulness as well as time constraints and competing demands has not been common in practice (Adelman and Harris 1999; Dickey and Kamerow 1996; Helseth et al. 1999).

Overall, the level of implementation of diabetes care in the United States remains suboptimal. The National Diabetes Quality Report Card reported that annual eye exams were performed in only 60% of patients with diabetes, lipid profiles were performed in only 76%, and adequate control of blood pressure was achieved in just one-third (McFarlane et al. 2002; Saaddine 2002). Although care has improved over the past few years, recent studies still show significant opportunities to translate effective treatments into daily practice, with 20% of patients still with poor glycemic control as defined by a hemoglobin A1C > 9%. Other data from the National Health and Nutrition Examination Survey over time has shown consistent suboptimal care, with only 40% of patients achieving a target A1C level of <7% (Saaddine et al. 2006).

Several efficacious strategies to prevent or delay the complications of diabetes have emerged during the past decade, including controlling blood pressure, lipids, and hyperglycemia; early detection and treatment of diabetic retinopathy, nephropathy, and foot disease; therapy with aspirin; the use of angiotensin-converting enzyme or ACE inhibitors; and the employment of influenza and pneumococcal vaccination (Narayan et al. 2000). Although many of these treatments are relatively cost-effective, their implementation has been far from optimal.

■ Public Health Preventive or Intervention Strategies

Interventions to Overcome Barriers to Diabetes Translation

The challenge of providing effective diabetes care has, thus far, defied a simple solution. Small regional studies have tested numerous provider-, system-, or patient-level interventions to improve care in both primary care and community settings. Although these interventions have had some documented success, further research is clearly needed to understand how to more effectively translate efficacious treatments into practice. Translation research needs to be conducted to understand the long-term impact of interventions at the patient, provider, and system levels on health outcomes, quality of life, and cost of care.

Providers

Successful translation research has often included health care providers as subjects, which is appropriate because these professionals need to know how to incorporate the latest research into their clinical practice. In addition they need to feel empowered by believing they have a role in improving the quality of care they provide. They must also feel that the care they offer has the highest scientific validity. Unfortunately translation research interventions that have included an educational component for providers have been only moderately successful at improving adherence to process measures. Interventions to educate providers, however, have usually been part of a more complex intervention that also focuses on systems of care and on the organization of practices, covering such areas as continuous quality improvement (CQI), performance feedback, manual and electronic reminder systems, and consensus development of local guidelines (Benjamin, Schneider, and Hinchey 1999; Lobach and Hammond 1997; Mazze et al. 1994). Clinical practice guidelines have been used in many settings (Davis and Taylor-Vaisey 1997; Feder et al. 1995). Most guidelines focus on stepped intensification programs to improve glycemic control and on the use of a reminder checklist to improve adherence to screening and other processes of care. Unfortunately guidelines alone have been only minimally effective in improving care (Grol 2001), as have consensus recommendations disseminated through mass mechanisms such as societies (e.g., the American Diabetes Association) or at health system levels (Lomas 1991). When included as part of a multifaceted strategy, however, clinical guidelines have been associated with more success (Anderson and Lexchin 1996; Wensing, van der Weijden, and Grol 1998). Having health care providers take an active part in modifying and adopting national guidelines has also helped them to feel empowered to lead the translation of research into practice (Benjamin et al. 1999; Feder et al. 1995). One study looked at the effect of combining educational meetings and materials for providers with patient education (Pieber et al. 1995); A1C values, blood pressure, and blood pressure control improved in the intervention group, but other studies have shown no benefit of combined provider and patient education (Kinmonth et al. 1998).

Systems

When guidelines have been used in managed and primary care settings, systems interventions using CQI techniques focused on provider education and feedback and on agreed-upon goals have often been employed (Fox and Mahoney 1998; O'Connor et al. 1996; Sidorov et al. 2000; Sperl-Hillen et al. 2000). The use of guidelines to educate providers combined with a performance feedback approach such as CQI has been successful in numerous small settings (Friedman et al. 1998; Mazze et al. 1994; Rith-Najarian et al. 1998). The use of computerized reminder systems for providers or such systems combined with performance feedback programs can improve outcomes for patients with diabetes (Integrated Care Evaluation Team 1994; Nilasena and Lincoln 1995; Sperl-Hillen et al. 2000). Patient tracking systems or other reminder systems to improve regular follow-up have also reduced no-show rates and improved rates of processes of care such as retinal examinations (Aubert et al. 1998; Halbert et al. 1999; Peters and Davidson 1998).

The evidence that electronic medical records can enhance adherence to quality measures has been mixed. In a study that evaluated an electronic medical record system to facilitate communication between team members and consultants, the intervention group carried out more processes of care, including measurement of A1C and lipid levels (Branger et al. 1999). Elsewhere, use of an electronic medical record system to remind physicians to order tests was effective when linked to multidisciplinary QI efforts (Ornstein et al. 1998). A more recent study (Keating et al. 2004) found associations with higher quality of care (as defined by four process measures and two outcome measures) among practices that received diabetes performance report cards and in practices that routinely enrolled patients in active disease management programs.

Another approach to improve systems was attempted using the Breakthrough Series collaborative model pioneered by the Institute for Healthcare Improvement in Cambridge, Massachusetts (Kilo 1998). A state-level application of the Breakthrough Series model attempted to rapidly test numerous changes in the design of delivery systems to improve care based on the Chronic Care Model. The collaboration was able to demonstrate improvement in processes as well as outcomes for patients with diabetes (Daniel et al. 2004).

Finally, a recent meta-regression analysis of the effects of QI strategies for type 2 diabetes on glycemic control (Shojania et al. 2006) revealed that most QI strategies for diabetes produce only modest improvements in glycemic control. Use of case management programs was associated with the largest reductions in A1C values in a comparison with several other QI strategies, including patient reminders, patient education, electronic patient registries, audit and feedback, CQI, and reminders to the clinician. The smaller impact of these other QI strategies has been evaluated in relatively few trials, and therefore the impact of these strategies cannot be fully determined.

Patients

Interventions targeting patients have been modestly successful in improving diabetes outcomes (Anderson et al. 1995; Greenfield et al. 1988), and the addition of patient-oriented interventions to system-based interventions has also been shown to lead to improvements in both process and outcome measures (Litzelman et al. 1993). One study found improved glycemic control when nurses called patients monthly to educate them and remind them of their medical regimen and to reinforce upcoming appointments (Weinberger et al. 1995).

Education in self-management, including skill building, has helped improve glycemic control and the abilities of patients to cope with chronic disease. Specific teaching programs have shown improvements in quality of life, glycemic control, and adherence to screening recommendations (Glasgow et al. 1992, 1997; Gruesser et al. 1993; Vinicor et al. 1987).

The recent TRIAD (Translating Research Into Action for Diabetes) study compared reminders to physicians with the addition of performance feedback and structured case management. It concluded that structured case management, which included clinical practice guidelines, reminders, patient education, and ongoing clinician-patient interaction, was associated with the best improvement in the quality of care (Mangione et al. 2006). These findings reinforce an earlier meta-analysis which found that case management in which a nurse or pharmacist could interact more with patients and make independent medication changes was associated with improvements in quality of care, including glycemic control (Keating et al. 2004).

Future Research

The translation research studies reviewed in this chapter have laid the foundation for understanding interventions that will help improve the quality of diabetes care and translate efficacious interventions into practice. Further translation trials need to be conducted that include ways to tease out the impact of professional roles for case managers; the impact of reminder systems, feedback systems, and provider and patient education programs; and the role of information technology. Future research should also include detailed economic evaluations as well as an evaluation of the changes in quality of life for patients with diabetes. Implementation of specific QI strategies and translation efforts needs to be fully evaluated from the patient, provider, and system perspectives.

Improving outcomes such as glycemic and blood pressure control is more challenging than improving processes of care, such as obtaining an annual blood test. Processes can often be improved readily in the microenvironment, but to improve outcomes, such as glycemic control, requires identification of a high-risk patient and then the implementation of targeted interventions to improve the desired outcome. To achieve the improvement of outcomes rather than just processes will require more research efforts to understand the impact of education, case management, and patient participation, all within the context of the community and health care system. Future research to understand the roles of physician practice patterns, decision support tools, and local micro-systems is needed.

Clinical Trials

A number of important translational trials currently in progress have already had an impact on the treatment of diabetes and its complications as well as on the prevention of diabetes. These trials represent both Phase One translation research, in which basic science discoveries are being applied to human health under controlled circumstances, and Phase Two translation research, in which knowledge of effectiveness is applied to human health through health delivery, policy, or other interventions in often uncontrolled circumstances.

Tables 30.1 and 30.2 summarize some of the important ongoing clinical trials as of August 2007 (http://clinicaltrials.gov/). The trials are selected and organized based on their type and the type of translation being evaluated. Current prevention trials (see Table 30.1) listed are evaluating both the scientific efficacy and the sustainability of interventions in prevention. Phase One translation prevention studies are assessing the impact of medications to prevent diabetes—oral and injectable insulin for type 1 diabetes and rosiglitazone and metformin for type 2. Phase Two translation prevention studies are evaluating the sustainability of lifestyle modifications and

TABLE 30.1   Clinical Trials for the Prevention of Diabetes

Study Title	Purpose	Design	Outcome Measures	Start Time	End Time
Phase One Translation Trials					
Oral Insulin for Prevention of Diabetes in Relatives at Risk for Type I Diabetes	To determine whether the oral administration of insulin will prevent or delay the development of type 1 diabetes in relatives of patients with type 1 diabetes who are positive for insulin autoantibodies.	Randomized, double-blind, placebo-controlled efficacy study.	The development of type 1 diabetes.	Feb 2007	7–8 years
LANCET Trial: Trial of Long Acting Insulin Injected to Reduce C-Reactive Protein (CRP) in Patients with Type 2 Diabetes	To determine whether Lantus, a long-acting insulin, either alone or in combination with metformin is effective in reducing CRP in adults with type 2 diabetes.	Phase 4—randomized open-label efficacy study enrolling 800 patients.	The percentage reduction in CRP in patients with type 2 diabetes.	Aug. 2006	Expected April 2008
CANOE: A Lifestyle and Combination Medication Therapy Diabetes Prevention Study	To determine whether individuals with impaired glucose tolerance can be prevented from progressing to diabetes with a healthy-living lifestyle intervention with and without a combination of rosiglitazone and metformin.	Phase 3—randomized, double-blind, placebo-controlled efficacy study enrolling 200 patients.	Development of diabetes secondary outcome measures, including changes in lipids, CRP, and insulin levels.	June 2004	Expected Nov. 2009

Phase Two Translation Trials

Diabetes Prevention Program Outcomes Study (DPPOS)	To determine the impact of intensive lifestyle modification on the risk of developing diabetes. To determine whether risk reduction can be sustained up to 10 years and what impact it has on diabetes-related complications.	Phase 4—prevention trial enrolling 200 patients who will be followed for 10 years.	The development of diabetes and determining whether the delay or prevention of diabetes will translate into decreases in other diabetes end-stage organ complications.	Sept. 2002	2012
Type 2 Diabetes Primary Prevention for At-Risk Girls	Evaluate two approaches to prevent obesity and type 2 diabetes in young girls at risk: nutrition education program or after-school dance classes.	Phase 2 and 3 randomized single-blind efficacy study enrolling 240 patients who will be followed for 2 years.	Weight, onset of type 2 diabetes.	April 2003	2006
ATTEMPT: Assessment of the Treatment Effect in Metabolic Syndrome without Perceptible Diabetes	To assess the use of guidelines in training of physicians to help improve the control of the metabolic syndrome.	Phase 4—pre/post study design examining 2500 patients.	Cardiovascular risk assessment.	Feb. 2005	Jan. 2009
Feasibility of a Patterned Approach to Prevent Diabetes	To attempt to translate the Diabetes Prevention Program findings into a sustainable public health scale.	Phase 2—randomized, factorial-assigned safety and efficacy study enrolling 216 patients.	Weight loss, total cost of the program, and cost-effectiveness of the program. Secondary measures will include self-report of physical activity.	March 2006	July 2007

TABLE 30.2 *Clinical Trials for the Treatment of Diabetes*

Study Title	Purpose	Design	Outcome Measures	Start Time	End Time
Phase One Translation Trials					
An Evaluation of Exenatide and Rosiglitazone in Subjects with Type 2 Diabetes	To evaluate the metabolic effects of adding Exenatide and rosiglitazone or both to an existing regimen of metformin in subjects with inadequate glycemic control.	Phase 3—treatment-randomized open-label efficacy study enrolling 140 subjects to be followed for 20 weeks each.	Glycemic control.	Oct. 2005	2008
Clinical Trial Assessing the Impact of the Availability of Inhaled Insulin on Glucose Control	To assess the impact on glucose control from inhaled insulin on patients with type 2 diabetes who are not well controlled on two or more oral antidiabetic agents.	Phase 3—treatment-randomized open-label efficacy study enrolling 1,100 individuals to be followed for 1 year each.	Glycemic control.	April 2005	2008
Rosiglitazone vs. Sulfonylurea on Progression of Atherosclerosis in Patients with Heart Disease and Type 2 Diabetes (APPROACH)	To test the safety and effectiveness of rosiglitazone against sulfonylurea. To reduce or slow the development of atherosclerosis.	Phase 3—randomized double-blind, active-control safety and efficacy study enrolling 600 patients.	The progression of arthrosclerosis as measured by intravascular ultrasound.	Jan. 2005	2008
Rosiglitazone to Reverse Metabolic Defects in Diabetes	To examine whether rosiglitazone can safely and effectively reverse the early markers of type 2 diabetes and delay onset of the disease in people with prediabetes.	Phase 2—intervention treatment study enrolling 70 patients with either impaired glucose tolerance or diabetes to be followed for 3 months each.	Metabolic syndrome markers and development of diabetes.	Oct. 2004	2007

Study	Description	Design	Primary Outcome	Start	End
Low-Carbohydrate Diet Compared to Calorie- and Fat-restricted Diet in Patients with Obesity and Type 2 Diabetes	To test whether a low-carbohydrate diet not specifically restricted in calories compared to a low-fat calorie-restricted diet over 2 years will cause greater reduction in body weight in patients with obesity and type 2 diabetes.	Phase 3—treatment-randomized open-label safety efficacy study enrolling 156 patients.	A reduction in body weight. Additional outcome will be effects on serum lipid concentrations.	Sept. 2004	Dec. 2007
Coronary Artery Revascularization in Diabetes Study (VA Cards)	To compare percutaneous coronary stenting (PCI) with drug-eluting stents to coronary bypass surgery for angiographically significant coronary artery disease in patients with diabetes.	Phase 4—randomized uncontrolled parallel-assignment efficacy study enrolling 790 patients.	Time to either death or nonfatal myocardial infarction.	July 2006	June 2010
ASCEND: A study of Cardiovascular Events in Diabetes	To determine whether 100 mg of daily aspirin vs. placebo and/or supplementation with 1 g daily omega-3 fatty acids or placebo prevents serious vascular events in patients with diabetes who are not known to have arterial disease.	Phase 4—prevention-randomized, double-blind, placebo-controlled safety efficacy study enrolling 10,000 patients.	Major cardiovascular events, death.	March 2005	2010

(continued)

TABLE 30.2 (continued)

Study Title	Purpose	Design	Outcome Measures	Start Time	End Time
RECORD Study: Rosiglitazone Evaluated for Cardiac Outcomes and Regulation of Glycemia and Diabetes Studies	To understand the impact rosiglitazone has on cardiac complications in patients with diabetes.	Randomized open-label trial in patients treated with rosiglitazone as add-on therapy to either metformin or sulfonylurea. Study will enroll 4400 patients.	Cardiovascular death and hospitalization for cardio-vascular disease, myocardial infarction, or heart failure.	2001	2008
Phase Two Translation Trials					
The DYNAMIC Study: Diabetes Nurse, Case Management, and Motivational Interviewing for Change	To evaluate the impact of a combination of nurse case management and enhanced behavioral change counseling on glycemic control, blood pressure, and lipid control in patients with type 2 diabetes.	Three-year randomized control trial. A total of 820 patients will be enrolled and followed for 3 years.	Glycemic, lipid, and blood pressure control.	Sept. 2006	2009
Treatment-Improving Insulin Therapy with Enhanced Care Management	To test a nurse care management program in supporting patients' self-care and adherence to insulin treatment regimens.	Phase 3—randomized open-label efficacy study enrolling 324 patients who will be followed for 12 months.	Glycemic control as measured by A1C.	Feb. 2007	Feb. 2010

ENHANCE Study: *Enhancing Adherence in Type 2 Diabetes*	To test a behavioral intervention based on social cognitive theory to improve adherence to regimens in three different groups of people with diabetes. 1. Those with well-controlled blood glucose and no concurrent renal insufficiency. 2. Those with less-well-controlled glucose and no chronic renal insufficiency. 3. Those with chronic renal insufficiency regardless of glucose control.	Phase 3 educational counseling, randomized efficacy study enrolling 288 patients.		May 2004	Dec. 2008
ADDITION Study: *Intensive Treatment and Complication Prevention in Screen-detected Type 2 Diabetes*	To identify best models to screen patients to identify undiagnosed diabetes and to study the effects of routine care compared with an intensive protocol where blood glucose, blood lipids, blood pressure, aspirin, and lifestyle modification are combined in a specific multi-intensive treatment strategy.	Phase 4—randomized open-label safety efficacy study enrolling 3000 patients.	Cardiovascular mortality and morbidity, including myocardial infarction, stroke, revascularization procedures, and amputations.	Jan. 2001	July 2009

(continued)

TABLE 30.2 (*continued*)

Study Title	Purpose	Design	Outcome Measures	Start Time	End Time
COACH: Community Outreach in Cardiovascular Health	To test the effectiveness of a nurse practitioner, community health worker, and physician team in the management of risk factors for heart disease in patients with diabetes.	Phase 4—randomized, active-control, parallel trial enrolling 500 patients.	Measurement of intermediate outcomes of lipids, blood pressure, and glycemic control.	July 2006	Sept. 2009
CHAMPP: Community Partnership to Examine Racial and Ethnic differences in Health Care for Hypertension and Diabetes	To attempt to identify factors that contribute to racial and ethnic differences in hypertension and diabetes care among minority patients seen at community health centers.	Observational study of health care as well as focus groups of patients with hypertension and diabetes. Study is enrolling 1200 patients.	To identify barriers to high-quality health care delivery among African American and Hispanic patients.	Oct. 2006	2008

| DQIP-DCMP: Diabetes Quality Improvement Program and Diabetes Case Management Program | To test whether nationally agreed upon performance measures can be used to accelerate the translation of research into practice to improve diabetes care. To evaluate the impact of a diabetes nurse case management program on improving adherence to performance measures. | Pre/post evaluation enrolling 20,000 patients. | Intermediate outcomes of glycemic, lipid, and blood pressure control. | April 2007 | April 2008 |
| *Can Group Visits Improve Outcome of Veterans with Diabetes?* | To evaluate the effect of group medical clinics on blood sugar, blood pressure, and the cost of diabetes care. | Phase 3—randomized, single-blind, parallel, assigned-efficacy study enrolling 280 patients. | Glycemic and blood pressure control. | June 2006 | Jan. 2008 |

education to prevent diabetes in real-world settings as well as assessing the training of providers in reducing the patient's cardiovascular risk.

The current treatment trials (Table 30.2) listed are evaluating the efficacy of new treatments as well as interventions involving the health care delivery system that could improve the health of people with diabetes. Phase One translation treatment studies are assessing the impact of new treatments on glycemic control, lipid control, blood pressure, and weight as well as long-term outcomes. Numerous Food and Drug Administration phase 3 drug trials of the new class of DPP-4 inhibitors (inhibitors of dipeptidyl peptidase 4), including drugs such as Exanatide, Vilvagliptin, and SYR-322, are currently under way. Other trials are evaluating the impact of rosiglitazone on reversing cardiovascular defects. Inhaled insulin, aspirin, omega-3 fatty acids, and specific diets are also being evaluated in patients with diabetes. Phase Two translation treatment studies are evaluating whether nurse case management programs alone or in combination with other team members can improve self-care and outcomes in patients with diabetes. Other Phase Two translation trials are assessing whether behavioral interventions as well as group clinics and protocols can improve adherence to diabetes self-management.

These trials and others will continue to help us understand not only the efficacy of interventions and prevention but also the best ways in which we can use them to improve the health of a community. Ongoing trials need to be conducted to further evaluate the health care delivery system and to accelerate the movement of known research into practice.

■ References

Adelman AM, Harris R (1999). Improving performance in a primary care office. *Clinical Diabetes* **16**, 154–60.

Anderson GM, Lexchin J (1996). Strategies for improving prescribing practice. *Canadian Medical Association Journal* **154**, 1013–7.

Anderson RM et al. (1995). Patient empowerment. Results of a randomized controlled trial. *Diabetes Care* **18**, 943–9.

Aubert RE et al (1998). Nurse case management to improve glycemic control in diabetic patients in a health maintenance organization. A randomized controlled trial. *Annals of Internal Medicine* **129**, 605–12.

Benjamin EM, Schneider MS, Hinchey KT (1999). Implementing practice guidelines for diabetes care using problem-based learning. A prospective controlled trial using firm systems. *Diabetes Care* **22**, 1672–8.

Bernard AM et al. (1999). What do internal medicine residents need to enhance their diabetes care? *Diabetes Care* **22**, 661–6.

Bero LA et al. (1998). Closing the gap between research and practice: an overview of systematic reviews of interventions to promote the implementation of research findings. The Cochrane Effective Practice and Organization of Care Review Group. *British Medical Journal* **317**, 465–8.

Branger PJ et al. (1999). Shared care for diabetes supporting communication between primary and secondary care. *International Journal of Medical Informatics* **53**, 133–42.

Chin MH, Zhang JX, Merrell K (1998). Diabetes in the African-American Medicare population. Morbidity, quality of care, and resource utilization. *Diabetes Care* **21**, 1090–5.

Dalewitz J, Khan N, Hershey CO (2000). Barriers to control of blood glucose in diabetes mellitus. *American Journal of Medical Quality* **15**, 16–25.

Daniel DM et al. (2004). A state level application of the Chronic Illness Breakthrough Series. *Joint Commission Journal on Quality and Safety* **30**, 103–8, 57.

Davis DA, Taylor-Vaisey A (1997). Translating guidelines into practice. A systematic review of theoretic concepts, practical experience and research evidence in the adoption of clinical practice guidelines. *Canadian Medical Association Journal* **157**, 408–16.

Dickey LL, Kamerow DB (1996). Primary care physicians' use of office resources in the provision of preventive care. *Archives of Family Medicine* **5**, 399–404.

Drass J et al. (1998). Diabetes care for Medicare beneficiaries. Attitudes and behaviors of primary care physicians. *Diabetes Care* **21**, 1282–7.

Eccles M et al. (2003). Research designs for studies evaluating the effectiveness of change and improvement strategies. *Quality & Safety in Health Care* **12**, 47–52.

Etzwiler DD (1997). Chronic care: a need in search of a system. *Diabetes Educator* **23**, 569–73.

Feder G et al. (1995). Do clinical guidelines introduced with practice based education improve care of asthmatic and diabetic patients? A randomized controlled trial in general practices in east London. *British Medical Journal* **311**, 1473–8.

Fox CH, Mahoney MC (1998). Improving diabetes preventive care in a family practice residency program: a case study in continuous quality improvement. *Family Medicine* **30**, 441–5.

Friedman NM et al. (1998). Management of diabetes mellitus in the Lovelace Health Systems' EPISODES OF CARE program. *Effective Clinical Practice* **1**, 5–11.

Garfield SA et al. (2003). Considerations for diabetes translational research in real-world settings. *Diabetes Care* **26**, 2670–4.

Glasgow RE et al. (1992). Improving self-care among older patients with type II diabetes: the "Sixty Something…" Study. *Patient Education and Counseling* **19**, 61–74.

Glasgow RE et al. (1997). Long-term effects and costs of brief behavioral dietary intervention for patients with diabetes delivered from the medical office. *Patient Education and Counseling* **32**, 175–84.

Glasziou P et al. (2007). When are randomized trials unnecessary? *British Medical Journal* **334**, 349–51.

Greenfield S et al. (1988). Patients' participation in medical care: effects on blood sugar control and quality of life in diabetes. *Journal of General Internal Medicine* **3**, 448–57.

Greenfield S et al. (1994). The uses of outcomes research for medical effectiveness, quality of care, and reimbursement in type 2 diabetes. *Diabetes Care* **17** (Suppl. 1), 32–9.

Grol R (2001). Successes and failures in the implementation of evidence-based guidelines for clinical practice. *Medical Care* **39**, II46–54.

Gruesser M et al. (1993). Evaluation of a structured treatment and teaching program for non-insulin-treated type II diabetic outpatients in Germany after the nationwide introduction of reimbursement policy for physicians. *Diabetes Care* **16**, 1268–75.

Halbert PJ et al. (1999). Effect of multiple patient reminders in improving diabetic retinopathy screening. A randomized trial. *Diabetes Care* **22**, 752–5.

Helseth LD et al. (1999). Primary care physicians' perceptions of diabetes management. A balancing act. *Journal of Family Practice* **48**, 37–42.

Hiss RG (1996). Barriers to care in non-insulin-dependent diabetes mellitus. The Michigan experience. *Annals of Internal Medicine* **124**, 146–8.

Hiss RG (2001). The concept of diabetes translation: addressing barriers to widespread adoption of new science into clinical care. *Diabetes Care* **24**, 1293–6.

Institute of Medicine (2001). *Crossing the Quality Chasm*. Washington, DC: National Academy Press.

Integrated Care Evaluation Team (1994). Integrated care for diabetes; clinical, psychosocial, and economic evaluation. *British Medical Journal* **308**, 1208–12.

Israel BA et al (1998). Review of community-based research: assessing partnership approaches to improve public health. *Annual Review in Public Health* **19**, 173–202.

Jacques CH, Jones RI (1993). Problems encountered by primary care physicians in the care of patients with diabetes. *Archives of Family Medicine* **2**, 739–41.

Keating NL et al. (2004). The influence of physicians' practice management strategies and financial arrangements on quality of care among patients with diabetes. *Medical Care* **42**, 829–39.

Kilo CM (1998). A frame work for collaborative improvement: lessons from the Institute for Healthcare Improvement's Breakthrough Series. *Quality Management in Health Care* **6**, 29–36.

Kinmonth AL et al. (1998). Randomised controlled trial of patient centred care of diabetes in general practice: impact on current wellbeing and future disease risk. The Diabetes Care from Diagnosis Research Team. *British Medical Journal* **317**, 1202–8.

Konen JC, Curtis LG, Summerson JH (1996). Symptoms and complications of adult diabetic patients in a family practice. *Archives of Family Medicine* **124**, 146–8.

Larme AC, Pugh JA (1998). Attitudes of primary care providers toward diabetes: barriers to guideline implementation. *Diabetes Care* **21**, 1391–6.

Litzelman DK et al. (1993). Reduction of lower extremity clinical abnormalities in patients with non-insulin-dependent diabetes mellitus. A randomized, controlled trial. *Annals of Internal Medicine* **119**, 36–41.

Lobach DF, Hammond WE (1997). Computerized decision support based on a clinical practice guideline improves compliance with care standards. *American Journal of Medicine* **102**, 89–98.

Lomas J (1991). Words without action? The production, dissemination, and impact of consensus recommendations. *Annual Review of Public Health* **12**, 41–65.

Mangione CM et al. (2006). The association between quality of care and the intensity of diabetes disease management programs. *Annals of Internal Medicine* **145**, 107–16.

Mazze RS et al. (1994). Staged diabetes management. Toward an integrated model of diabetes care. *Diabetes Care* **17** (Suppl. 1), 56–66.

McFarlane SI et al. (2002). Control of cardiovascular risk factors in patients with diabetes and hypertension at urban academic medical centers. *Diabetes Care* **25**, 718–23.

McGlynn EA et al. (2003). The quality of health care delivered to adults in the United States. *New England Journal of Medicine* **348**, 2635–45.

McVea K et al. (1996). An ounce of prevention? Evaluation of the "Put Prevention into Practice" program. *Journal of Family Practice* **43**, 361–9.

Narayan KM et al. (2000). Translation research for chronic disease: the case of diabetes. *Diabetes Care* **23**, 1794–8.

Narayan KM et al. (2004). Diabetes translation research: where are we and where do we want to be? *Annals of Internal Medicine* **140**, 958–63.

Nilasena DS, Lincoln MJ (1995). A computer-generated reminder system improves physician compliance with diabetes preventive care guidelines. *Proceedings of the Annual Symposium on Computer Applications in Medical Care* New Orleans, LA, 640–5.

O'Connor PJ et al. (1996). Continuous quality improvement can improve glycemic control for HMO patients with diabetes. *Archives of Family Medicine* **5**, 502–6.

Ornstein SM et al. (1998). Electronic medical records as tools for quality improvement in ambulatory practice: theory and a care study. *Topics in Health Information Management* **19**, 35–43.

O'Toole TP et al. (2003). Community-based participatory research: opportunities, challenges and the need for a common language. *Journal of General Internal Medicine* **18**, 592–4.

Peters AL, Davidson MB (1998). Application of a diabetes managed care program. The feasibility of using nurses and a computer system to provide effective care. *Diabetes Care* **21**, 1037–43.

Pieber TR et al. (1995). Evaluation of a structured teaching and treatment programme for type 2 diabetes in general practice in a rural area of Austria. *Diabetic Medicine* **12**, 349–54.

Rith-Najarian S et al. (1998). Reducing lower-extremity amputations due to diabetes. Application of the staged diabetes management approach in a primary care setting. *Journal of Family Practice* **47**, 127–32.

Saaddine JB et al. (2002). A diabetes report card for the United States: quality of care in the 1990's. *Annals of Internal Medicine* **136**, 565–74.

Saaddine JB et al. (2006). Improvements in diabetes processes of care and intermediate outcomes: United States, 1988–2002. *Annals of Internal Medicine* **144**, 465–74.

Shojania KG et al. (2006). Effects of quality improvement strategies for type 2 diabetes on glycemic control. *JAMA* **296**, 427–40.

Sidorov J et al. (2000). Barriers to control of blood glucose in diabetes mellitus. *American Journal of Managed Care* **6**, 1217–26.

Sperl-Hillen J et al. (2000). Improving diabetes care in a large health care system: an enhanced primary care approach. *Joint Commission Journal of Quality Improvement* **26**, 615–22.

Vinicor F et al. (1987). DIABEDS: a randomized trial of the effects of physician and / or patient education on diabetes patient outcomes. *Journal of Chronic Diseases* **40**, 345–56.

Wagner EH (1998). Chronic disease management: what will it take to improve care for chronic illness? *Effective Clinical Practice* **1**, 2–4.

Wagner EH, Austin BT, Von Korff M (1996). Organizing care for patients with chronic illness. *Milbank Quarterly* **74**, 511–44.

Weinberger M et al. (1995). A nurse-coordinated intervention for primary care patients with non-insulin-dependent diabetes mellitus: impact on glycemic control and health-related quality of life. *Journal of General Internal Medicine* **10**, 59–66.

Wensing M, van der Weijden T, Grol R (1998). Implementing guidelines and innovations in general practice: which interventions are effective? *British Journal of General Practice* **48**, 991–7.

31. PUBLIC HEALTH DECISION MAKING AND RISK PERCEPTION

Julie S. Downs, Wändi Bruine de Bruin, Baruch Fischhoff, and Elizabeth A. Walker

■ Main Public Health Messages

- Decision science provides a systematic approach to characterizing people's decisions and behaviors. A *normative analysis* of optimal decision making is compared to *descriptive research* about how people actually make decisions, to reveal gaps between the two that should be targeted by *prescriptive interventions.*
- There has been little work to date applying decision science to the primary prevention of diabetes or to management of the disease to prevent its complications. However, decision science provides basic tenets, general methods, and empirical results on related problems that can inform our understanding of decisions relevant to avoiding and managing diabetes.
- Decision science research has shown promise in improving decisions and changing behavior in a variety of other health and nonhealth risks.
- Risk perception is an important predictor of disease-prevention behavior, but its role must be understood in the context of other cognitively mediated factors such as individuals' values, emotions, social pressures, and resources.
- Future research may benefit from employing decision science concepts, theoretical constructs, and methods to develop high-quality interventions subject to rigorous empirical evaluations.

■ Introduction

Seminal studies have found that the risk of diabetes complications can be significantly reduced with improved metabolic control, for both type 1 (DCCT 1993) and type 2 diabetes (UKPDS 1998). Many of the behaviors that are important for primary prevention of type 2 diabetes (e.g., healthy eating, physical activity) can also help to control diabetes and reduce the risk of complications for those with the disease. One successful study that focused on lifestyle changes found an average 58% reduction in risk, from an average weight loss of 5.6 kg (Knowler et al. 2002). A successful medical intervention reduced risks by 31% through consistent use of the biguanide metformin, which affects gluconeogenesis, also as part of the Diabetes Prevention Program (DPP) (Crandall et al. 2008; Knowler et al. 2002). Metformin's effects were most promising among participants whose body mass index (BMI, defined as weight in kilograms divided by squared height in meters) was above 35 and who were younger than 60 years of age (Knowler et al. 2002).

These impressive intervention effects depend on the choices of individuals, who must understand their risks and the opportunities for risk reduction, then adhere to often demanding regimes, whether lifestyle changes or consistent medication. The noteworthy success of the DPP must owe something to the intensity of the intervention, helping individuals to make and maintain these choices. The resulting cost is a major reason why it has not been adopted as widely as it might. Those costs include places to exercise and coaches to give motivation and guidance regarding nutrition and exercise. Few health insurance plans cover services that require such intensive, individualized treatments. Even if the resources were available, the logistics of providing individual services are often a challenge.

These programs could be more effective to the extent that individuals can make and adhere to their decisions by themselves, without the need for such extensive intervention resources. Although intervention developers have worked hard to facilitate individuals' diabetes-related decisions, they have done so without the potential benefit of basic research in the psychology of decision making, a burgeoning field over the last 50 years, which has just begun to extend itself to chronic health problems. Fisher and his colleagues (2002) called for taking advantage of decision science research. Here, we provide an introduction designed to make the field more accessible to diabetes researchers and practitioners. We hope, in effect, to help diabetes professionals see into the "black box" of individual decision making by presenting theory, results, and methods from decision science (Fischhoff 1999, 2005, 2009).

Decision science provides a theoretical framework for understanding decisions. It begins with *normative analysis*, applying the tools of decision theory to identify the optimal choices for specific decisions by considering the values and capabilities of the individuals making them. ("Normative," in decision science terminology, refers to how people should make decisions in order to achieve the best possible outcomes, rather than to following the social norms familiar to psychologists and sociologists.) The next step is *descriptive research* examining how people actually make choices, in terms comparable to the normative analysis, so that, ultimately, opportunities to help people can be identified. Finally, *prescriptive interventions* can be designed to help people make better choices by closing the gap between the normative ideal and the descriptive reality, as illustrated in Figure 31.1. Such interventions provide essential feedback to the normative and descriptive research by showing how well they have illuminated the problem.

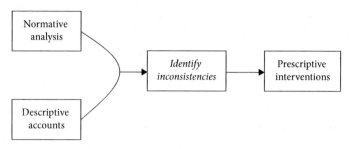

FIGURE 31.1. Decision science structures problems into normative, descriptive, and prescriptive perspectives

Because it begins by normatively characterizing decisions in analytical terms, the decision science perspective looks at behavior through a cognitive lens. It accommodates noncognitive processes such as affect, cultural factors, and socioeconomic factors through their effects on cognitive processes. For example affective processes can affect cognition by signaling which possible outcomes or processes are most relevant, making judgments more (or less) optimistic and affecting task involvement (Slovic et al. 2007). Analogously, general feelings of self-efficacy (or internal locus of control) may predispose people to spend more cognitive effort, in the expectation that this effort will result in better decisions and outcomes. Cultural factors (e.g., social norms) may also affect cognition by shaping the importance that people assign to different outcomes and altering the process of communicating and learning about decisions. Socioeconomic factors can affect cognition by shaping people's perceptions of the options that they are contemplating and of the resources that they have at their disposal to implement decisions effectively.

Because so many chronic diseases are preventable or manageable through behavioral changes, decision science could provide a valuable resource for understanding and improving health decisions and the outcomes that follow them. With its combination of empirical and analytical methods, decision science provides broadly applicable approaches to help people make health decisions in ways that are informed by both medical and social science. It is especially helpful for decisions made in the face of uncertainty whether individuals make them on their own or in consultation with health care providers.

■ Background/Historical Perspective

Decision science begins by creating a normative account of how a "rational" individual would make a decision to achieve the best possible outcome, given available scientific knowledge. This normative step entails integrating scientific expertise from the key disciplines relevant to the decision. Asking experts to summarize their knowledge in a formal model ensures that researchers take a structured, disciplined look at the decision. Normative analyses seek to identify the choice having the highest expected value (or expected utility, in the language of decision theory) for decision makers, in terms of the outcomes that matter most to them. Decision science, unlike most public health perspectives, is neutral regarding how sound those values are. As such it recognizes that the optimal decision might be different, for example, for a person who prefers longer life than for one who prefers richer quality of life. It also recognizes that people may make normatively correct choices in pursuit of goals that public health or other authorities might reject. When that happens, interventions would gain more traction by trying to change people's values rather than their decision-making process. The focus on *expected* values reflects the fact that chance plays a role in many important decisions. As a result, even the best decision-making process will not always lead to the most preferred outcome—just the best chances.

To emphasize a point that is sometimes confused: decision science does not assume that people are actually rational in this formal sense. Rather, the normative analysis forces researchers to specify the decisions that people face before venturing to design programs for them, offer them advice, or explain behaviors revealed in descriptive studies. A normative analysis assumes that decision makers have (1) stable, well-articulated preferences, so that they know what they want, no matter how options are presented to them; (2) coherent beliefs that they can apply consistently to their decisions; and (3) the cognitive capacity and skills needed to combine those assessments of values and facts in order to choose wisely. But descriptive research has documented ways in which the assumptions underlying normative decision analyses often do not hold. For example, people's preferences may be inconsistent, affected by irrelevant variations in how options are described (Tversky and Kahneman 1981), such as preferring ground beef more if it is described as 80% lean rather than as 20% fat. The inferences that people draw from their beliefs may be affected by context effects, such as the "anchoring" biases induced by the presence of irrelevant numerical cues (Tversky and Kahneman 1974). Individuals' cognitive capabilities are sufficiently limited to impair their mental mathematics or cause paralysis (or chaos), if they do try to attend to everything. Even when they execute these mental operations well, people may be misinformed about their values (i.e., what should be important to them) or about their world (i.e., what will follow from their choices).

Many theoretical accounts of individuals' imperfect decision-making processes are cast in terms of their reliance on simplification strategies (called *heuristics*, see Box 31.1) that can lead to reasonable choices but can also induce bias. One example is "satisficing," a heuristic that leads decision makers to consider options only until they find one that passes critical thresholds (e.g., any sandwich that is healthy, tasty, and inexpensive enough, but that may not provide the best combination of healthiness, tastiness, and value). Satisficing makes decision making manageable, but imperfect, in the sense of not always leading to the best possible outcome—only to decisions that are "good enough" (Simon 1956).

Embedding descriptive research in normative analysis allows researchers to ask the critical question of how important heuristic-induced biases are. Some

---

BOX 31.1 *Heuristics in Risk Perception*

People often rely on heuristics to make judgments when they lack statistical evidence. For example, reliance on the *availability heuristic* means judging the probability of events by the ease with which examples come to mind. Although often valid, relying on availability can lead to overestimating the probability of events that are particularly vivid or receive disproportionate media attention. Conversely, it can lead to an underestimating of events that are prevalent but do not make the news, such as diabetes. For example, people think that homicide is a more common cause of death than diabetes, even though about twice as many people actually die from diabetes.

Another heuristic, described by Tversky and Koehler's support theory, compares the arguments that support the occurrence and non-occurrence of an event. When people use this heuristic, an event will seem less likely the more explicitly they consider alternatives, bringing to mind reasons for it not happening. Similarly, an event will seem more likely if broken down into its constituent parts, each of which will stimulate thinking of reasons why it will happen. Thus, diabetes will seem less likely if people think about it as a single disease than if they think about it as a condition possibly leading to blindness, amputation, and its other dire complications. Similarly, the perceived probability of being able to manage the disease will increase if people with diabetes see all the things that they can do to improve their situation.

---

decisions are sensitive to small biases, whereas others are resilient. Recognizing such differential sensitivity makes decision scientists reluctant to make sweeping generalizations about human competence, instead of helping them to focus on those problems that matter most, as obstacles to effective decision making. In the case of health decisions, research has often found that people have a fairly accurate understanding of the *relative* size of many of the risks they face. Moreover, those who see a risk as larger are more likely to protect against it (Brewer et al. 2007). When asked precise questions about personal risks, even adolescents can produce probability judgments with good construct validity (e.g., predictions for obtaining a high school diploma are negatively correlated with self-reported risks for dropping out) and good predictive validity (e.g., 15- to 16-year-olds who give higher probabilities of becoming a parent by age 20 are more likely to have that happen; Bruine de Bruin et al. 2007).

From a decision science perspective, interventions should focus on the critical gaps between the normative ideal and the descriptive reality. Closing those gaps requires an understanding of individuals' psychology, so that better ways of thinking can be made intuitively meaningful. Thus in order to prevent and manage chronic diseases such as type 2 diabetes, people need to know the risks they face and the probabilities for reducing them by adopting various lifestyle changes such as diet and exercise. They cannot wait until they are certain about having a disease, by which time it is too late for prevention. Nor can they wait for firm promises that interventions will succeed for them—assurances that medical science cannot provide. The fact that so many people do not adopt those measures suggests that messages may not be reaching the most important audiences or may not be providing relevant information in ways that motivate and facilitate action.

Perceptions of Chronic Disease Risks

The objective risks of chronic diseases are well documented. In 2006 an estimated 24.9% of Americans had cardiovascular disease (CVD), 23.4% had high blood pressure, 25.9% of adults had prediabetes, and 10.7% had diabetes, with type 2 diabetes accounting for over 90% of all diabetes cases (CDC 2007). The lifetime risk for CVD is one in two for women at age 40 and two in three for men at that age, directly accounting for 37% of all deaths and as a contributing cause for an additional 21% of deaths. Cancers account for 23% of all deaths. Although diabetes accounts for fewer deaths directly, it is one of the strongest risk factors for CVD, giving it an indirect role in many more deaths (Thom et al. 2006)

People typically rank their perceived risks in line with these objective risks. For example Jia and her colleagues found that a sample of ethnic minority adults correctly listed heart disease as the most common of 10 medical conditions, with diabetes ranked second by men and third by women, closely followed by breast, prostate, cervical, and colorectal cancer (Jia et al. 2004). These judgments roughly reflect experts' rankings of these risks, with physicians ranking diabetes as less of a risk than heart disease, high blood pressure, arthritis, or cancer and more of a risk than asthma, kidney failure, AIDS, or blindness (Walker et al. 2003).

Although generally accurate in a relative sense, lay people's risk judgments are often inaccurate in an absolute sense (Slovic 2001). For instance Jia and her colleagues (2004) found that liver cancer's lifetime risk of 0.1%–0.5% was estimated at 18%, lung cancer's 7% risk was estimated at 20%, and cervical cancer's 2%–3% risk was estimated at 21%. In contrast the risk of diabetes was overestimated by a much smaller degree: the real risk of 15% was estimated at 25%. This difference is consistent with people's tendency to amplify perceptions of risks that they dread, such as cancer or HIV (Slovic 2001). By contrast diabetes may not be as dreaded and may evoke less strong perceptions of risk, because it is ubiquitous but not seen as catastrophic. As a result, it may not receive the attention it deserves.

Although consistent with the body of decision science research, the ideas expressed above are mere speculations. Studies have not systematically examined peoples' existing mental models of diabetes or how they can be changed to better serve diabetes-related decisions. Decision-making heuristics are abstract rules whose operation in specific settings has not been studied directly in the context of diabetes. For example, although the availability of bad health outcomes should increase the perceived risks of diabetes, we do not know which events individuals tend to observe and associate with diabetes and how those perceptions affect their decisions. Individuals typically display an *optimistic bias*, judging their own risks as less than those of otherwise comparable individuals in situations where they can imagine asserting some control (Weinstein 1987), meaning that judgments of population risks (as in Jia et al. 2004) do not capture individual risks. However we do not know what people view as the factors contributing to diabetes risk, nor whether they think that they can control them. Conducting these studies could both direct interventions and provide baseline estimates of decision-making processes that are being shaped.

Eliciting Risk Perceptions

Evaluating individuals' risk perceptions requires knowing their actual personal risk, in terms of the chances of the risky outcomes happening to them. However investigators rarely have outcome information about their research participants except in intensive prospective studies. The desire to get around that methodological challenge has prompted studies to ask people either to estimate population risks or to compare their personal risk to the population average, which is likely to be skewed by optimistic bias. As people gain personal experience with a risky event, whether through their own choices or involuntary exposure, their estimates of personal risk tend to decline much more than their population estimates. A plausible mechanism is the illusion of control, whereby people exaggerate the effectiveness of the measures that they take (or imagine that they will take) to control risks (Langer 1975). Familiarity with an event increases the opportunities to learn (or imagine) ways in which it might be controlled through personal actions. In addition individuals' personal actions (and commitments to act) are more salient to them than are others' actions (and commitments), making them feel as though they are doing particularly well at taking advantage of the risk-reduction opportunities that they have discovered. If substantiated in the context of diabetes, unwarranted feeling of personal control would be a likely target for intervention. Understanding the fine structure of individuals' beliefs would be essential to conveying this sobering message in a way that was convincing without being discouraging—so that individuals acquire a feeling of self-efficacy for what they could be doing and escape the complacency of what may not really be helping much.

From a methodological perspective, distinguishing between personal and population risk is one of the many details that need to be considered when designing and interpreting studies eliciting risk judgments (Fischhoff 1994, 2009). Another is eliciting enough background information about the individual to assess the construct validity of that individual's beliefs. Even when one cannot assess the absolute accuracy of risk judgments, one may be able to tell whether individuals are sensitive to the factors that increase and decrease their risk. For example, people with a family history of a disease often develop a sense of vulnerability related to medically established risk factors (Walter et al. 2004). This pattern of results is consistent with the psychological account sketched above: proximity to family members with a disease makes that risk available to people, leading them to feel more vulnerable, perhaps enough to overcome the optimistic bias. Such sensitivity to risk factors can lead to positive behaviors, as people who perceive more risk are more likely to take subsequent protective behaviors (Brewer et al. 2007). That sensitivity might create a temptation for educators to exaggerate risks so as to encourage such behaviors. But such exaggeration risks making claims that lose recipients' trust as a result of being inconsistent with their observations of the world. At the extreme, overly high risk perceptions can even elicit a fatalistic attitude that there is nothing one can do to reduce one's risk, which tends to lead to inertia, undermining the perceived efficacy of preventive health behaviors (Caban and Walker 2006). These complex patterns of responses speak to the need for detailed descriptions of risk beliefs before interventions are developed, with the hope to move target individuals or groups closer to the normative ideal.

Another important class of potentially relevant covariates of individuals' risk judgments includes the beliefs of these individuals regarding socially normative behavior in their social group. In addition to setting values for what is proper behavior, socially normative behavior can send signals regarding the soundness of decisions. For example people seem to gain weight in response to weight gain among those with whom they (implicitly) compare their own weight, suggesting that they look for social cues about the health impact of obesity as well as its social acceptability (Christakis and Fowler 2007; see Box 31.2). The success of anti-smoking regulations in changing smoking behavior has had a similarly recursive effect, whereby observing less smoking among others further reduces smoking (Brownson et al. 2006). Prescriptive interventions will be most effective if the strategies and the responses that they promote can capitalize on both aspects of social norms, the information and the values that they convey. Indeed reducing exaggerated perceptions of others' alcohol use has had some success in reducing unhealthy drinking behaviors, especially when the comparisons involve groups with which individuals most identify. The importance of personally relevant norms to these processes suggests that mass media campaigns will have less effect unless they evoke such meaningful comparison groups. For example the widely disseminated advertisement "Friends don't let friends drive drunk" might or might not be processed as "Your friends don't let their friends drive drunk." When people have accurate perceptions of their friends' behavior, telling them what is typical of others in general has little effect (Lewis and Neighbors 2006). If anything, the recurrent evocation of problem behavior could backfire. For example media campaigns regarding the ubiquity of obesity may, ironically, contribute to the perception that being overweight is socially normative.

Risk Perceptions for Intervention

The complexity of the beliefs revealed in these examples carries a message for the complexity of the interventions needed to create sustained change. Some prescriptive

---

BOX 31.2   *Decision Processes by Which Norms May Affect Behavior*

Social norms may affect decisions by changing values or perceptions. For example, obesity may spread within social networks by changing perceptions of how socially acceptable one's weight is and of how much of a health problem it appears to be. In the absence of social factors, gaining 20 pounds may be cause for concern about both appearance and health risks and thus an impetus for a change in behavior, as depicted in this simple diagram:

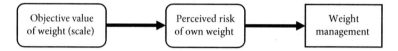

However, if others are also putting on 20 pounds, that might seem like an acceptable change. Conversely, if others in one's social circle maintain a healthy weight or even lose weight, then that may seem like the right thing to do, in terms of both style and health. Thus, social comparison may affect behavior through perceptions and not just through motivation.

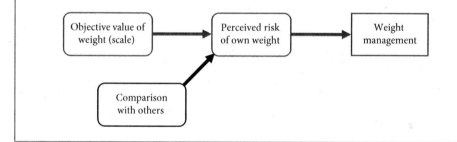

---

interventions provide only summary statistics regarding risks, expecting individuals to fill in the picture by themselves, as far as providing the reasons why those assertions are true. Some decision aids seek to help people understand uncertain medical choices by showing users the probabilities associated with the possible outcomes of their choices. Given the vagaries of qualitative risk judgments, it is essential that patients be given such information quantitatively from an authoritative source. However summary statistics may not stand on their own and provide patients with full enough mental models for them to feel comfortable making fateful choices. Research that evaluates decision aids has found that such aids often improve patient knowledge and increase patients' participation in the decision-making process, especially with more complex and intensive decisions. However, there is much less evidence showing that such aids improve patients' decisions, satisfaction, or health outcomes (O'Connor et al. 1999).

Risk calculators are pervading public health outreach efforts, and their use is likely to increase given how well they lend themselves to the Internet. The American Diabetes Association (www.diabetes.org) has two online calculators to help individuals assess their personal diabetes risks. The Diabetes Risk Test assesses the user's risk of developing type 2 diabetes, with prediabetes as an interim step. Diabetes PHD, which has been shown to have clinical value for screening (Engelgau, Narayan, and Herman 2000), assesses users' risk of developing diabetes complications conditioned on personal health decisions (e.g., whether they smoke) and clinical indicators (e.g., metabolic control, blood pressure, cholesterol). The Diabetes PHD calculator allows the individual to choose a behavior change, such as losing weight or quitting smoking, then to see its effect on his or her future risk of diabetes complications. Based on decision science research, both calculators have the advantage of providing some context (e.g., risk factors) for their summary statistics. They might have more of a chance of improving decisions and behaviors if they provided a mechanistic understanding about how these factors worked so that users would understand why, say, blood pressure mattered, in addition to their detailed advice on how to reduce risk factors.

■ Public Health Strategies

Prescriptive interventions designed to close the gaps might be directed at the individual, family, work-site, community, environmental, and regulatory levels (see Box 31.3). The National Diabetes Education Program (www.ndep.nih.gov), a

---

BOX 31.3   *Environmental Interventions*

Some interventions aim to change behavior not by influencing individuals' beliefs and values but by changing the environment within which they make decisions based on those perspectives. For example, physical activity has been found to increase when people have better access to exercise facilities, when planning makes communities more walkable, and when students have physical education classes in schools. Behavior can also be improved by removing bad options, such as by making unhealthy food less available. Economic incentives could include subsidizing public transportation or healthy foods. Although theoretically attractive, such interventions should take advantage of the most promising strategies and require evaluation to ensure success. Their design would benefit from the normative approach of decision science, first characterizing the decisions that individuals face and then those that they could face with feasible changes in their environment. That normative research requires descriptive empirical studies of what people value, what they see as possible, and how they respond to changes.

collaboration of governmental and nongovernmental agencies, aims to span these strata in development and dissemination of culturally appropriate, coordinated programs for at-risk individuals, health care providers, and health systems managers. Although decision science has not been actively used in this work, it offers a natural complement to NDEP's programs. Once a decision has been identified as critical to an individual's diabetes risk, decision science has tools for producing normative analyses of how that decision should be made (given the goals of the individual making it), understanding how the decision is made, and how to close the gap between the normative ideal and the descriptive reality. The generality of decision science means that it can be applied to a wide variety of decisions—and that it depends vitally on collaboration with subject-matter experts and practitioners.

Decision science has informed other interventions, including the development of clinical decision aids (e.g., Garg et al. 2005) and the evaluation of patient involvement in clinical decisions (e.g., Say et al. 2006). The decision science methodology most directly relevant to developing messages to improve people's understanding of the processes creating and controlling risks is the mental models approach (Morgan et al. 2001). Like other decision science approaches, it starts with a normative analysis. In this case the form of the analysis is an *influence diagram* summarizing the factors creating and controlling a risk. It reduces the science deemed relevant to predicting decision outcomes to those facts most worth knowing. Such analyses are informed by both medical research, which provides the facts, and psychological research, which assesses individuals' priorities (determining which outcomes to predict).

This analysis also provides a framework for descriptive research analyzing people's beliefs in terms of how well they understand the facts most critical to their choices. Those mental models are elicited by open-ended interviews, structured around the normative analysis, which is also used as a coding scheme for the beliefs raised in the interviews. The precision of the model typically allows highly reliable coding, often revealing misconceptions that researchers might not otherwise have considered had they merely developed a knowledge test without first gathering these qualitative insights. Structured surveys can be used to assess the prevalence and inter-relationships of the beliefs (including misconceptions) found most central to understanding. These structured surveys are domain-specific tests, with formal models structuring their item selection and open-ended interviews informing their question wording, to use terms familiar to the target audience.

For example, in an early application Bostrom and her colleagues used the mental models approach to investigate people's understanding of the detection and remediation of radon in the home. They found that although people generally knew that radon posed a risk, many did not appreciate the feasibility of addressing the problem, which undermined their motivation to test lest they find a problem that could not be fixed (Bostrom et al. 1992). The normative analysis identified facts such as the risks and remediation effectiveness as vital to effective decision making. The descriptive analysis not only showed these gaps, but revealed the intuitive theories that supported them and that would have to be addressed in any attempt to improve understanding. Notably, many individuals had learned that radioactive substances *can* cause permanent contamination, a fact that is often true but not with radon, whose decay products have short half-lives. As a result, very small amounts of radon can release a lot of energy and pose a great danger. However once the influx is stopped, the problem is over, with no further contamination. That message is easy enough to convey once the misunderstanding has been identified.

As a second example, in a project on adolescents' sexual decisions, Downs and her colleagues (2004) found that adolescent girls do not see opportunities to exert control over having sex in the face of pressure from would-be partners. In this case the descriptive research revealed lack of awareness of the decision options that the adolescent girls could evaluate in terms of how well they met their circumstances and values. In effect, the normative-descriptive comparison revealed the ultimate gap, of girls not even seeing that they could make a choice and potentially control the situation. As a result, the initial focus of the intervention, an interactive video, was to make decision points salient. Having accomplished this, the intervention engaged young women in cognitive role playing, devising and practicing options for managing the stages in a sexual encounter. For women who believe that they have a choice, information about sexually transmitted infections (STIs) matters. The intervention presented information about STIs in ways that built on the young women's intuitive mental models. Descriptive research found that young women tended to generalize their thinking about STIs from their knowledge about AIDS. As a result a valuable place to start explaining STIs was by distinguishing between those caused by bacteria and viruses, two basic biology concepts that were accessible. This simple organizing device helped teens to understand how, for example, treatment options differ for bacterial infections (which can generally be cured by antibiotics) and viral ones (which may be treated but not cured, hence tend to recur or become chronic). The intervention also emphasized (and graphically illustrated) the difficulty of diagnosing many STIs (especially those in asymptomatic males). The intervention based on closing these gaps between the normative and descriptive accounts of decisions succeeded in changing behavior and preventing acquisition of disease (Downs et al. 2004).

As seen in Table 31.1, projects using the mental models approach span a wide range of health behaviors. All follow the same research strategy: characterize the decisions facing people, understand their current beliefs, and then close the most critical gaps. Although applicable to diabetes-related decisions, the methodology has rarely been used in this domain. Rather, most interventions have focused on changing the attitudes and perceived social norms expressed in decisions that individuals are presumed to make (Munro et al. 2007). Most such interventions use models of health behavior focused on these constructs, such as the Health Belief Model, the Theory of Planned Behavior, Protection Motivation Theory, or the Transtheoretical Model (Weinstein 1993). Because the models use a common set of constructs for all decisions, their application to any specific decision requires researchers and practitioners to make choices in adapting the general constructs. For example, an

TABLE 31.1   *Sample Findings from Mental Models Studies of Risk*

Topic	Sample Finding
Childhood vaccination	Parents who lack a conceptual understanding of how vaccines stimulate immune response are less equipped to assess rumors that vaccines were unsafe.
Avian flu	Experts see a need to focus on nonpharmaceutical interventions such as hand washing and using masks and gloves because pharmaceutical interventions would likely be insufficient.
HIV/AIDS	Adolescents understand most key concepts about HIV risk, but they hold key misconceptions that are typically ignored in educational programs.
Fraudulent e-mail	Better conceptual understanding of the computer and Internet environment reduces vulnerability to fraudulent e-mail attacks, but increases in the perceived severity of consequences do not.
Terrorism	Responses to communication materials on risk are unintentionally affected by the fear evoked by these communications.

For more information the reader should consult sds.hss.cmu.edu/risk.

intervention promoting change in individuals' perceptions of subjective norms, beliefs, and attitudes about diabetes would require dedicated research on the specific diabetes-related norms, beliefs, and attitudes that ought to be changed. Decision science provides a systematic approach to that research following the path described above, creating a normative model of the specific domain, then conducting descriptive research to reveal how people think about the concepts in that model.

Although there have been many diabetes behavioral interventions based on health behavior models (e.g., Jones et al. 2003, using the Transtheoretical Model), the opportunity for cross-fertilization with decision science has thus far been missed. Likewise the familiar health behavior models have played scant roles in decision science research since Dawes and Corrigan (1974) established that models that express very different psychological processes can have similar predictive success, leaving researchers with little ability to distinguish among them. Rather, decision science research has focused on domain-specific decisions with multiple possible behaviors. This focus also avoids the limitation of focusing on intentions rather than behavior or clinical outcomes. A meta-analysis has found that behavior changes less than intentions predict (Webb and Sheeran 2006). Unlike the traditional models, which look at intentions to perform a single, focal act (e.g., exercise), decision science examines multiple possible outcomes (e.g., exercising and not exercising). This may be particularly pertinent to the preventive or self-management behaviors related to type 2 diabetes. Other decision options are implicitly available, when individuals focus their attention on them. However, they may not receive the same evaluation as when they are examined explicitly (Beyth-Marom et al. 1993; Fischhoff 1996).

■ Implications for Health Policy

Public policies are often based on program designers' intuition about what people need to know and what they already know, presuming that there is no need for formal analysis and empirical research. Often the resultant programs are not subjected to empirical evaluation, forcing adopters to rely on their face validity (Hill et al. 2007). When informational programs are evaluated but show little success, it is hard to know whether the problem is that information will not work or whether the specific intervention, without systematic formative research, has not worked (Seymour et al. 2004). In addition to guiding the design of such intervention, decision science can guide the forensic analysis of why an informational intervention has not worked. Was it the wrong information, telling people things that they already knew, or failing to address the barriers to action? Was the information insufficient or presented in ways that frustrated recipients' attempts to integrate it with their existing mental models? Did the message ask people to do the impossible, such as withstanding strong social pressure to act in unhealthy ways or providing no viable alternative actions? When information misses the target, for any of these reasons, the failures may undermine the decision-making processes essential to behavioral change. It can also undermine faith in the individuals who were failed by the intervention but who may be held responsible for their lack of improvement.

From this perspective interventions may benefit from addressing individuals' psychology and circumstances in a coordinated way. The successful Diabetes Prevention Program did so by providing not only individual counseling but also opportunities to practice lifestyle changes. Its widespread implementation may be hampered by being embedded in a society without strong social norms for healthier lifestyles. Unfortunately interventions directed at social norms face uncertain prospects. Social norms are notoriously difficult to manipulate without sustained, intensive, multifaceted programs. Moreover, diet-related interventions face the challenge that eating is so basic a drive that demand can be effectively inelastic, whatever is done to try to reduce consumption.

Although not decision scientists themselves, Hill and his colleagues (2007) have proposed interventions that look at food choice as a decision and then try to change how these choices present themselves. For example they suggest that work sites encourage healthier behaviors, perhaps by making stairs more visible and legitimating the hitherto uncommon choice of walking where appropriate, pointing to dress codes as an analogous form of informal norm setting. They suggest that schools grade lunchroom choices, then provide students (and parents) with diet report cards. A full analysis of such incremental changes would ask whether they can scale up to create overall changes, much in the way that those concerned with environmental changes consider whether tactical decisions (e.g., recycling, compact fluorescent light bulbs) can make enough of a difference or represent a distraction from strategic change (Gardner and Stern 2008).

Thus the success of interventions depends on their integration of tactical and strategic measures. From a tactical perspective designers need to understand how individuals make the many small choices that they face. For example when they consider whether to take the stairs or the elevator, what comes into their minds, what social pressures do they experience, and what other costs are incurred (e.g., getting sweaty, risking injury)? Those decisions can be studied with the usual decision science methods. That is, researchers can first conduct normative analyses of how the choices affect outcomes that individuals value. They can then conduct descriptive studies focused on how individuals perceive the expected outcomes following different choices. By comparing the normative and descriptive results, they can develop interventions directed at either psychology (e.g., perceptions of the costs and benefits of lifestyle changes) or circumstances (e.g., social and economic barriers to healthy diet). That research may reveal that seemingly attractive behaviors are actually unattractive in certain circumstances or even infeasible. For example employees who could use the stairs may worry about appearing to judge companions who may be disabled or less fit; hence they decide to avoid awkwardness by using the elevator. Only by understanding the complex structure of such seemingly simple choices is it possible to create interventions that meet individuals' multiple goals.

Once a suite of suitable tactics has been identified, organizations can consider strategies for incorporating them into programs with mutually reinforcing elements. For example firms or schools can adopt goals that relieve individuals of the burden of pressuring others to change. Incentives might be provided in the form of financial rewards or group recognition. The strategic analysis would also consider ways in which the organization provides disincentives for change (e.g., cafeteria food prices, health insurance programs). Sound behavioral science can help to design programs that have a chance of working with real people facing real constraints and to evaluate programs in a scientifically sound way. Implementing unrealistic programs not only wastes the resources invested in them, but it incurs the opportunity costs of leaving the problem unaddressed and the direct costs of alienating those who are asked to do the impossible—change their behavior in ways whose logic they cannot see or whose acts they cannot implement. When research shows that behavioral change requires alterations in individuals' physical and social environments, strong leadership may be needed in addition to strong science.

One class of structural change that is consistent with a decision science perspective involves pay-for-performance programs, whereby health care providers receive incentives for good health outcomes in their patients. Here, too, proper execution requires integrating tactical and strategic levels, looking at the information, incentives, and options provided to both those whose behavior should be changed and those rewarded for making those changes happen. For example management must provide rewards and facilities for preventive services. Assessing impacts may require technology to track clinical information (e.g., medications, test results, physician notes) or incentives for providers (e.g., external audits, public recognition) within privacy constraints (Casalino et al. 2003). To date few empirical studies have evaluated pay-for-performance approaches for the prevention or treatment of chronic diseases.

■ Economic Issues and Implications

There has been much more research on the cost-effectiveness of medical interventions than of behavioral ones. Because behavioral interventions are more difficult to standardize, they differ more in their implementation than do medical interventions, making it harder to calculate the cost-effectiveness of a "type" of behavioral intervention. With complex interventions, it is hard to determine the cost-effectiveness of specific program elements, which cannot be separated from those of the overall package (Chodosh et al. 2005).

A noteworthy exception is the DPP, in which costs were carefully evaluated for both lifestyle modification (healthy eating and physical activity) and pharmaceutical intervention (metformin), compared with placebo (Herman et al. 2005). Both interventions prevented or delayed the development of type 2 diabetes, with the lifestyle intervention being almost twice as effective as metformin (Knowler et al. 2002). The lifestyle intervention was also more cost-effective, in terms of both medical and nonmedical costs (e.g., absenteeism), and covered all age groups and body weights. In contrast, the metformin intervention was ineffective for those with a BMI less than 35 and for older individuals (Herman et al. 2005). The lifestyle intervention was beneficial for all groups, although its cost was not fully recouped in reduced medical costs.

Without rigorously collected evaluation data from multiple prevention programs, we have only the most basic guidelines for estimating cost-effectiveness (see Box 31.4). Communications are inexpensive, compared to pharmacological and counseling interventions, and thus may have an advantage in enhancing cost-effectiveness. Decision science offers inexpensive ways to develop the form and content of communications targeting specific decisions as faced by specific audiences. Whether decision science can provide effective (and cost-effective) communications is an open question. The choice of communication channel (e.g., Internet, affinity groups, family members) is, of course, critical to ensuring that messages providing useful, comprehensible information arrive from credible sources.

BOX 31.4 *Calculating Cost-Effectiveness*

To conduct the meta-analyses needed to estimate cost-effectiveness across classes of prevention programs, there must be enough published studies reporting both cost and effectiveness data, a standard rarely met for behavioral interventions. For example, despite the many efforts to prevent smoking among adolescents, there are only enough studies to provide a weak signal supporting their cost-effectiveness. Probably the most studied topic for behavioral intervention is HIV prevention. A meta-analysis of different kinds of HIV prevention interventions found two predictors of cost-effectiveness: the prevalence of the disease in the target population, which affects the number of potential targets of an intervention, and the cost of the intervention.

■ Areas of Uncertainty or Controversy

There is broad agreement that economic and health behavior models do not describe precisely how people make many decisions, even when such models predict that behavior. Simple linear models can often provide such good predictions, in the hands of investigators attuned to the kinds of things that matter to people (Dawes and Corrigan 1974). However understanding the psychological processes responsible for the behavior requires other, complementary research, like the decision science approaches described here. Those approaches begin with normative analyses that facilitate a hard look at the nature and difficulty of the decisions that individuals face. Thus decision science recognizes both the value and the limits of economic and health behavior models.

Given its focus on the intellectual demands of decision making, decision science has naturally focused on cognitive processes. Over the past decade or so it has increasingly accommodated affective processes, examining how they influence cognitive processes (sometimes sharpening them, sometimes distorting them) and how aware people are of those effects. For example there is growing understanding of why people fail to predict how "hot" emotions will lead them to evaluate decisions differently from how they think about the decisions in a "cold" state (Loewenstein 1996).

The social cognitive models that have guided most behavioral interventions have long been subject to lively controversy over their theoretical foundations and relative effectiveness, and to the extent that comparisons are possible, no model has emerged as a clear winner (Weinstein 2007). However evaluations do find that interventions using any of these models tend to be more effective than interventions using none. This pattern may reflect the fact that each model serves as a checklist, ensuring that the researchers consider the basic issues that can matter, including both cognitive factors (e.g., risk perception) and social-normative ones (e.g., comparison of others' behavior and values). If the different models use correlated measures, they should predict outcomes similarly well, even if they embody different theoretical formulations of how health behaviors are chosen. As a result,

the effectiveness of any intervention will depend primarily on how well it is implemented, a function of the skill of the investigators, the quality of their relationships
with practitioners and subjects, and the resources available. That implementation
should be facilitated by the decision science practices of engaging in a structured
analysis of the content domain, comparing that normative analysis to a descriptive
account of actual understanding and providing missing knowledge in a comprehensible form.

A decision science approach could also help to take full advantage of new
technologies for diabetes self-management. Many new devices, such as those providing for continuous blood glucose monitoring, generate large amounts of data.
Unless individuals can cope with that information stream, the technologies may not
achieve their potential. They could even undermine individuals' health if providers
assume that patients are better informed than they actually are and then withdraw
the informational support they would otherwise provide.

■ Developments over the Next 5 to 10 Years

Decision science continues to expand its focus on the role of emotion in decision
making, distinguishing the roles of specific emotions. For example although
an earlier view assumed that positive and negative emotions have opposite
effects, recent research finds that happiness and anger both encourage optimistic assessments, pushing people toward action (Lerner and Keltner 2000).
As we learn more about the effects of different emotions and contexts, we will
deepen our understanding of the effects of emotions and individuals' ability to
manage them when making choices. Applied to health behaviors, this research
could help people to stay the course with planned behavioral changes, despite
fluctuating feelings.

The growing field of behavioral economics applies the principles of decision science to design programs that manipulate incentive structures in order to
alter behaviors. Such manipulation is, of course, the stock-in-trade of marketing.
However, it can also be applied to inducing people to do things that are in their
own best interests but that they do not pursue on their own. These failures may
have environmental causes (e.g., missing critical data, lacking needed resources)
and individual ones (e.g., inability to focus, a lack of self-discipline). The incentives
to change behavior could be financial or beneficial in terms of time and convenience
(Sunstein and Thaler 2003; Thaler and Sunstein 2008). For example the increased
convenience of calorie-dense, low-cost snack foods contributes to the increase in
obesity rates. People might benefit from being rewarded for resisting that temptation or having healthier choices subsidized.

Finally, within the realm of cognitive processes, there is growing research
interest in how individuals understand not just summary estimates of risks and
benefits but also the quality of the evidence underlying them. For example before

committing to an intervention, one could reasonably want to know whether its promise of effectiveness reflected one person's claim or a consensus of leading opinions (just as clinicians would want to see a comprehensive meta-analysis of multiple studies, rather than rely on a single exploratory one). As noted even with such heavily studied areas as adolescent smoking prevention, few interventions may be rigorously evaluated in terms of their behavioral effects, much less their long-term health effects. Considering the increased pressure for information disclosure in other domains, especially for pharmaceutical and financial products, there is likely to be increasing research on how to convey the quality of data needed for decision making.

Over the past half century decision science has developed a large body of theory, methods, and results in diverse application areas. There have, however, been few applications to disease prevention in nonclinical settings, especially for chronic health conditions such as diabetes. Extending decision science to diabetes prevention and treatment could both improve health and advance basic science by having it confront the novel theoretical issues in ways that promote collaboration of behavioral and decision scientists. That combination of promise and challenge could encourage basic researchers to work on diabetes prevention and treatment, building on basic and applied research on related problems.

■ References

Beyth-Marom R et al. (1993). Perceived consequences of risky behaviors. *Developmental Psychology* **29**, 549–63.

Bostrom A, Fischhoff B, Morgan MG (1992). Characterizing mental models of hazardous processes: a methodology and an application. *Journal of Social Issues* **48**, 85–100.

Brewer NT et al. (2007). Meta-analysis of the relationship between risk perception and health behavior: the example of vaccination. *Health Psychology*, **26**, 136–45.

Brownson RC, Haire-Joshu D, Luke, DA (2006). Shaping the context of health: a review of environmental and policy approaches in the prevention of chronic diseases, *Annual Review of Public Health* **27**, 341–70.

Bruine de Bruin W, Parker AM, Fischhoff B (2007). Can teens predict significant life events? *Journal of Adolescent Health* **41**, 208–10.

Caban A, Walker EA (2006). A systematic review of research on culturally relevant issues for Hispanics with diabetes. *The Diabetes Educator* **32**, 584–95.

Casalino L et al. (2003). External incentives, information technology, and organized processes to improve health care quality for patients with chronic diseases, *JAMA* **289**, 434–41.

Centers for Disease Control and Prevention (CDC) (2007). Summary Health Statistics for U.S. Adults: National Health Interview Survey, 2006. *Vital and Health Statistics* **10**, 1–153.

Chodosh J et al. (2005). Meta-analysis: chronic disease self-management programs for older adults. *Annals of Internal Medicine* **143**, 427–38.

Christakis NA, Fowler JH (2007). The spread of obesity in a large social network over 32 years. *New England Journal of Medicine* **357**, 370–9.

Crandall JP et al. (2008). The prevention of type 2 diabetes. *Nature Clinical Practice Endocrinology & Metabolism* **4**, 382–93.

Dawes RM, Corrigan B (1974). Linear models in decision making. *Psychological Bulletin* **81**, 95–106.

Diabetes Control and Complications Trial (DCCT) Research Group (1993). The effect of intensive treatment of diabetes on the development of long-term complications in insulin dependent diabetes mellitus. *New England Journal of Medicine* **329**, 977–86.

Downs JS et al. (2004). Interactive video behavioral intervention to reduce adolescent females' STD risk: a randomized controlled trial. *Social Science & Medicine* **59**, 1561–72.

Engelgau MM, Narayan KM, Herman WH (2000). Screening for type 2 diabetes. *Diabetes Care* **23**, 1563–80.

Fischhoff B (1994). What forecasts (seem to) mean. *International Journal of Forecasting* **10**, 387–403.

Fischhoff B (1996). The real world: what good is it? *Organizational Behavior and Human Decision Processes* **65**, 232–48.

Fischhoff B (1999). Why (cancer) risk communication can be hard. *Journal of the National Cancer Institute Monographs* **25**, 7–13.

Fischhoff B (2005). Decision research strategies. *Health Psychology* **21**, S9–16.

Fischhoff B (2009). Risk perception and communication. In: Detels R et al., eds. *Oxford Textbook of Public Health,* 5th ed., pp 940–52. Oxford: Oxford University Press.

Fisher EB et al. (2002). Behavioral science research in prevention of diabetes: status and opportunities. *Diabetes Care* **25**, 599–606.

Gardner GT, Stern PC (2008). The short list: the most effective actions U.S. households can take to curb climate change. *Environment* **50**, 12–25.

Garg AX et al. (2005). Effects of Computerized Clinical Decision Support Systems on Practitioner Performance and Patient Outcomes: A Systematic Review, *JAMA* **293**, 1223–38.

Herman WH et al. (2005). The cost-effectiveness of lifestyle modification or metformin in preventing type 2 diabetes in adults with impaired glucose tolerance. *Annals of Internal Medicine* **142**, 323–32.

Hill JO, Peters JC, Wyatt HR (2007). The role of public policy in treating the epidemic of global obesity. *Clinical Pharmacology and Therapeutics* **81**, 772–5.

Jia H, Santana A, Lubetkin EI (2004). Measuring risk perception among low-income minority primary care patients. *Journal of Ambulatory Care Management* **27**, 314–27.

Jones H et al (2003) Changes in diabetes self-care behaviors make a difference in glycemic control: the Diabetes Stages of Change (DiSC) study. *Diabetes Care* **26**, 732–7.

Knowler WC et al. (2002). Reduction in the incidence of type 2 diabetes with lifestyle intervention or metformin. *New England Journal of Medicine* **346**, 393–403.

Langer E (1975). The illusion of control. *Journal of Personality and Social Psychology* **32**, 311–28.

Lerner JS, Keltner D (2000). Beyond valence: toward a model of emotion-specific influences on judgement and choice. *Cognition & Emotion* **14**, 473–93.

Lewis MA, Neighbors C (2006). Social norms approaches using descriptive drinking norms education: a review of the research of personalized normative feedback. *Journal of American College Health* **54**, 213–8.

Loewenstein G (1996). Out of control: visceral influences on behavior. *Organizational Behavior and Human Decision Processes* **65**, 272–92.

Morgan MG et al. (2001). *Risk Communication: The Mental Models Approach.* New York: Cambridge University Press.

Munro S et al. (2007). A review of health behaviour theories: how useful are these for developing interventions to promote long-term medication adherence for TB and HIV/AIDS? *BMC Public Health* **7**, 104.

O'Connor AM et al. (1999). Decision aids for patients facing health treatment or screening decisions: systematic review. *British Medical Journal* **319**, 731–4.

Say R, Murtagh M, Thomson R (2006). Patients' preference for involvement in medical decision making: a narrative review. *Patient Education and Counseling* **60**, 102–14

Seymour JD et al. (2004). Impact of nutrition environmental interventions on point-of-purchase behavior in adults: a review. *Preventive Medicine* **39**, 108–36.

Simon HA (1956). Rational choice and the structure of the environment. *Psychological Review* **63**, 129–38.

Slovic P, ed. (2001). *Perception of risk.* New York: Cambridge Univeresity Press.

Slovic P et al. (2007). The affect heuristic. *European Journal of Operational Research* **177**, 1333–52.

Sunstein CR, Thaler RH (2003). Behavioral economics, public policy, and paternalism: libertarian paternalism. *American Economic Review* **93**, 175–9.

Thaler RH, Sunstein CR. (2008). *Nudge.* New Haven: Yale University Press.

Thom T et al. (2006). Heart disease and stroke statistics—2006 update: a report from the American Heart Association Statistics Committee and Stroke Statistics Subcommittee. *Circulation* **113**, e85–151.

Tversky A, Kahneman D (1974). Judgment under uncertainty: heuristics and biases. *Science* **185**, 1124–31.

Tversky A, Kahneman D (1981). The framing of decisions and the psychology of choice. *Science* **211**, 453–8.

UK Prospective Diabetes Study (UKPDS) Group (1998). Intensive blood-glucose control with sulphonylureas or insulin compared with conventional treatment and risk of complications in patients with type 2 diabetes. *Lancet* **352**, 837–53.

Walker EA et al. (2003). Risk perception for developing diabetes. *Diabetes Care* **26**, 2543–8.

Walter FM et al. (2004). Lay understanding of familial risk of common chronic diseases: a systematic review and synthesis of qualitative research. *Annals of Family Medicine* **2**, 583–94.

Webb TL, Sheeran P (2006). Does changing behavioral intentions engender behavior change? A meta-analysis of the experimental evidence. *Psychological Bulletin* **132**, 249–68.

Weinstein N (1987). Unrealistic optimism about susceptibility to health problems: conclusions from a community-wide sample. *Journal of Behavioral Medicine* **10**, 481–500.

Weinstein N (1993). Testing four competing theories of health-protective behavior. *Health Psychology* **12**, 324–33.

Weinstein N (2007). Misleading tests of health behavior theories. *Annals of Behavioral Medicine* **33**, 1–10.

32. PUBLIC HEALTH POLICY DECISIONS AND DIABETES

Considerations and Case Studies

Frank Vinicor

■ Main Public Health Messages

- The interactions of patients with their physicians are influenced by many factors that go far beyond the physicians' training, education, and accumulated knowledge—these factors can be called *policies*.
- A large number of policies currently influence the prevention and management of diabetes mellitus in the United States.
- Simple changes in policy, even as small as having patients' shoes and socks removed before they are seen in the examining room, can have major effects on the practice of preventive medicine by clinicians.
- The Chronic Care Model is useful for structuring the outpatient care of patients with diabetes.
- A diabetes registry that keeps track of glycosylated hemoglobin (A1C) values is one example of linking diabetes problems, politics, and policies in today's world.
- In the United States, coverage of diabetes services by Medicare has improved.
- The World Health Organization now recognizes diabetes as a "threat to the world," the first time this organization has described a chronic disease in this way.

■ Introduction

In the minds of most a visit to the medical office eventually will involve a one-to-one interaction with an individual health professional. Should that interaction involve a physician, the imagery is one of a discussion of the nature of the patient's concerns, a physical examination of some variety, and perhaps blood tests, x-rays, and other diagnostic testing. Ultimately, recommendations are made by the doctor in cooperation with the patient, with the latter assuming that the physician's advice reflects a synthesis of formal training and education as well as additional experience-based accumulation of knowledge.

The physician-patient interaction is very personal and private, with the physician relating to the patient in what appears to be a closed one-to-one system. Presumably, most patients assume that their physician is neither encumbered nor limited by any outside factor, nor influenced by the ideas and thoughts of people with whom the doctor, let alone the patient, does not have a known and personal relationship. Two people—the patient and the doctor—are talking directly to one another to understand and resolve a specific health problem.

Surrounding this important and personal interaction, however, are often more general and impersonal factors in the form of rules, regulations, traditions, guides, guidelines, and other influences on the physician's behavior. These "quiet" and perhaps even "hidden" factors fall under the general rubric of "policies." Formally, a policy is a "plan or course of action, as of a government, political party or business, intended to influence and determine decisions, actions and other matters." (*American Heritage Dictionary of the English Language* 1981). Within the medical world, policies have certain interesting characteristics: (1) they generally are established to improve perceived deficiencies in some aspect of medical care; (2) they are most often established by *groups* of people and/or organizations that do not have a direct or personal relationship with the great majority of the patients affected; (3) they affect many people and groups other than patients, including physicians and insurers; and (4) considerable time is involved in their establishment, implementation, and, in the end, regular use.

At present, the number of policies that affect some aspect of medicine is remarkably large (Oliver, 2006). Whereas many affect the field of health care generally, e.g., the quality of care, requirements for medical records, some are specific to a particular disease, medical procedure, or laboratory test or have some other particular focus (Oliver 2006). Reimbursement plans, the use of specific medications for patients with an acute myocardial infarction on their admission to an intensive care unit (ICU), e.g., ASA (acetylsalicylic acid), β-blockers, and acceptable laboratory procedures and standards for lipid or hemoglobin A1C (glycosylated hemoglobin) assays are but a few examples of policies based on efficacious science that affect the actions of individual physicians each day.

Within this large and growing list of policies there are many that specifically target important challenges in the prevention and management of diabetes. Indeed, diabetes is frequently viewed as a model chronic disease for the development of clinical and public health guidelines because of the high cost and burden it imposes on the United States and because successful reduction of diabetes-related morbidity is thought to depend on actions made by the patient, provider, health system, and broader community. Rather than review all of these policies, this chapter demonstrates the breadth and "power" of selected diabetes policies, moving from ones that are relatively simple and could be directly implemented within a clinic without great difficulty to policies of such potential impact that they could ultimately influence *all* people with diabetes in a large metropolitan area, in a country such as the United States, or even throughout the world. Policies of such potential impact are, not surprisingly, both challenging and controversial.

■ Preventing Lower-Extremity Amputations among Persons with Diabetes Mellitus

Policy Change in the Clinic

Diabetes mellitus is the most common cause of nontraumatic lower-extremity amputations in the United States, if not the world (Gregg et al. 2004). During the past few decades important scientific investigations have identified the contributions of impaired vascular and neuropathic systems to the genesis of foot and leg disorders associated with diabetes (Pecorino, Reiter, and Burgess 1990).

With the proper use of relatively simple clinical tests, patients with diabetes who have "high-risk feet" and are therefore prone to lower-extremity diseases and subsequent amputations can now be identified (Lento et al. 1996). Most important, there is good evidence that among those individuals with high-risk feet, relatively simple efforts can reduce the incidence of foot ulcers and possibly subsequent amputations (Lento et al. 1996).

To identify a high-risk foot, however, the lower extremity must be examined. In extremely busy clinics and other medical facilities, when many *other* aspects of diabetes demand attention, the feet are often not examined (Reiber, Boyce, and Smith 1995). Certainly, the use of traditional "educational maneuvers" such as lectures, handouts, demonstrations, and reminders can be helpful, but the time and effectiveness of these approaches must be questioned.

More than two decades ago, Cohen demonstrated the "power of policy" by having office staff remove the shoes and socks of patients after they had seated them in the examination room (Cohen 1983). Even in the absence of any additional and "traditional" educational efforts, physicians were more than three times as likely to perform foot examinations when patients were presented barefoot than when they were still wearing shoes and socks. Even for busy clinicians, simply seeing naked feet increased the use of foot exams to approximately 60%. Although evidence that this policy resulted in reduced rates of foot lesions or amputation was not available, the point remains that a relatively simple policy change in the diabetes clinic's routine appeared to have a major impact on the practice of preventive medicine in this busy setting.

■ Policies at the Clinical and Health System Levels

In the example above, a single and relatively simple policy change in one clinic resulted in an important improvement in preventive care for persons with diabetes.

But most hospital facilities are far more complex than outpatient clinics, with needs for a broad range of laboratory testing, the timely availability of records, modern communications systems, and so forth. In general policies need to be in place that would result in careful, accurate, and timely integration of all the parts of this "total clinic" to ensure a "productive interaction" between an individual patient and the health care provider.

The "Chronic Care Model" (CCM) and its associated policies is an example of a template for restructuring the interactions of the several components of a busy and full medicine clinic, including those facilities that care primarily for persons with diabetes (Robert Wood Johnson Foundation 2007). The CCM has six essential components: support for self-management, the design of a delivery system, decision support, a clinical information system, a structured health care organization, and community interactions. When policies are in place to establish each of these components, and when they are functioning seamlessly and appropriately, diabetes management and care improve (Bodenheimer, Wagner, and Grumbach 2002; Wagner 2004). Although describing the CCM in detail is beyond the scope of this chapter, applying the policies that underlie this model has been tested in three very different clinical settings, with evidence of improved diabetes care in each as well as greater satisfaction among the health professionals working in this environment (Heisler and Wagner 2004; Landon et al. 2007; McCulloch et al. 2004; Piatt et al. 2006). For example, within an underserved community in Pennsylvania, CCM was associated with improvements in A1C (–0.6 percentage points), lipid components, and scores on both knowledge and empowerment (Piatt et al. 2006). In essence, in each of these facilities, the necessary ingredients of an effective and efficient clinic were identified, and policies were established that would allow the six critical components to function as a total single unit. Although associated with periodic difficulties, the CCM nevertheless represents on a larger scale how thoughtful policies can result in successful models of care, especially for chronic conditions such as diabetes.

■ The Use of a Diabetes Registry as a Policy Tool

In the United States, states are a major loci for delivering public health programs (Wagner, Austin, and Von Orff 1996). Although some activities also take place at the national or local level, the states assume major responsibility for most types of public health efforts (Gostin 2000). Within the past century, however, some U.S. cities have become very active in public health policy and action. An effort being tested in New York City reflects the juxtaposition of (1) a disturbing increase in its rates of diabetes and associated complications and (2) the practical advantage of having most A1C measurements performed in public health laboratories (Steinbrook 2006). Because of these two factors, New York City's Board of Health and Public Health Department created an "A1C Registry" that can serve as a marker of the quality of care for diabetes (Steinbrook 2006). The concept is that if A1C values exceed a certain value, say 8%, both the patients and their health care providers will be contacted, with the expectation that those patients will be given additional help in trying to improve glycemic control (and ultimately decrease the likelihood of diabetes complications and thus expenses for the city).

Not unexpectedly, this program, now in its early pilot stages, has created much attention and controversy. Issues of privacy, the challenges of data collection and analyses (>1 million A1C tests are performed each year in New York City), and the effectiveness of the planned interventions are but some of the challenges that must be resolved. Regardless, within the context of this chapter the key point is that a policy created for diabetes patients by health professionals who *do not* have a one-to-one relationship with these patients is attempting to draw on existing city resources and facilities (the public clinical laboratory) to improve care. This creative policy, clearly not without its problems, would at least identify those persons whose glycemic control is in a "dangerous zone," and it includes a reminder system that could ultimately help to improve diabetes management.

How well and widely this policy will evolve remains to be seen, but it is a good example of the potential linkages of problems, policies, and politics as municipalities intervene in the clinical world of diabetes.

■ Reimbursement Policies and Diabetes Mellitus

Perhaps no diabetes policies have been as controversial as those pertaining to reimbursement for diabetes care, medications, supplies, and, especially, patient education. It is interesting to examine reimbursement policies for diabetes before and after 2003, the year of the Medicare Modernization Act (CMS Legislative Summary 2003). Even in the early years of Medicare, several aspects of diabetes care outside the hospital, including training in self-management, were covered by Medicare (Ashkenazy and Abrahamson 2006). However, the reimbursement was limited in terms of both the amount of reimbursement and the items covered (Leichter 1999). Further, any additional services needed to be certified/requested by a physician only, and initially they had to be delivered within the hospital. As major diabetes organizations such as the American Diabetes Association (ADA) and the American Association of Diabetes Educators, as well as individual diabetes practitioners (especially certified diabetes educators), began to work closely and strongly with the Health Care Financing Administration to improve the coverage of all diabetes services (Ashkenazy and Abrahamson 2006), the situation improved. Especially important in the demands for diabetes patient education outside the hospital were political activities that resulted in policies contained within in the Balanced Budget Act of 1997 that solidified Medicare coverage for diabetes supplies and added language to expand the availability of diabetes education and reimbursement for that activity (Ashkenazy and Abrahamson 2006; Leichter 1999).

The 1997 Balanced Budget Act notwithstanding, the path for expanding services in diabetes education has been a rocky and difficult one. Developing clear definitions of "diabetes education" and establishing the validity and importance of training in diabetes self-management for preventing complications and other undesirable outcomes have been major challenges for the entire diabetes community, even within the hospital setting (Leichter 1999). Fortunately the Medicare Modernization Act of 2003 expanded many policies on coverage for persons with diabetes, including reimbursement for medications and a variety of screening tests for diabetes complications and associated conditions, e.g., cardiovascular disease, and finally, outpatient diabetes education—but only if that education met the strict criteria of such organizations as the ADA or the Indian Health Service (CMS Legislative Summary 2003). However, even with the Medicare Modernization Act's greater attention to diabetes in several areas, plus its stipulation of reimbursement for the screening of patients for previously unrecognized diabetes, the components of this act remain complex, and interpretations of their meaning continue to change (Nettles 2005). Resolution and clarification of these various uncertainties by the Centers for Medicare & Medicaid Services remain critical for two major reasons: (1) most people hospitalized for diabetes are over the age of 65 and are thus probably covered by Medicare (Rice 2007), and (2) policy decisions made by the Centers for Medicare & Medicaid Services often serve as the model for private insurance programs.

In essence then, in terms of policies that address reimbursement for various dimensions of diabetes, progress has occurred over the past several years, and especially since 2003. Still the element that most health professionals would consider a core part of diabetes management—education—remains both not fully resolved and, for many practitioners, a frustrating issue (Leichter 1999). Perhaps the lesson learned with this series of policies is that although they appear to be simple (and they do need to be set forth in a formal manner), sometimes these are the very policies that are most complex in design and the slowest to be implemented (CMS Legislative Summary 2003)—in part because of the mix of policies with politics (Kingdon 1984) and the core issue of "reimbursement."

■ Diabetes Policies and "The World"

As described above a policy can affect an individual person, a procedural component of a clinic, an entire outpatient clinical structure, a whole city, or, in the United States, all patients with confirmed or suspected diabetes who are covered by Medicare. Why not create policies for the world? Globally, it is estimated that more than 200 million persons are living with diabetes today. Even more disconcerting, that number is expected to exceed 400 million within the next half century (King, Aubert, and Herman 1999), in part because there will be a striking aging of the world's population (King, Aubert, and Herman 1999). The United Nations, through its major health entity, the World Health Organization (WHO), and its regional offices, such as the Pan American Health Organization, which benefit from WHO's policies and prestige, has traditionally addressed acute and especially infectious diseases such as HIV/AIDS, malaria, and tuberculosis. But as data accumulate regarding noninfectious or chronic conditions such as diabetes, it has become apparent to many that major international health organizations must begin to recognize the devastating impact of chronic diseases already wreaking havoc all over the world—devastation that will likely worsen (Adeyl, Smith, and Robles 2007).

Through the efforts of many countries, especially those labeled as developing countries, through the International Diabetes Federation, and through persistent action on the part of thousands of individuals throughout the world, the General Assembly of the United Nations passed a landmark resolution on December 20, 2006, describing diabetes as a "threat to the world" (United Nations Resolution on Diabetes 2006). This "international policy"—the first to specifically address a chronic disease—identifies diabetes as a health priority in individual nations, establishes recognition of the human, social, and economic burden of this noninfectious disease, and reinforces the notions that (1) *all* with diabetes must receive appropriate care, especially access to insulin, and that (2) much of type 2 diabetes can be prevented by changes in lifestyle (United Nations Resolution on Diabetes 2006). The specific consequences of this very broad and encouraging policy must now be converted to *action*. As reflected in a recent news release by WHO (World Health Organization 2007), the creation of such a diabetes policy provides both framework and ethic to actively and respectfully engage in the "political arena" (Kingdon 1984; Oliver 2006) with WHO, WHO Regions, and especially with nations that are members of the WHO General Assembly and have signed the diabetes proclamation. Very difficult decisions will need to be made by these nations, which are facing many health challenges, but chronic diseases like diabetes mellitus must now be on the list of society-threatening conditions.

■ Summary

Improving preventive and management services for diabetes requires two inter-related elements: (1) committed and capable *individuals,* health care professionals and patients alike, and (2) an *environment or context* in which these individuals can apply their skills and knowledge. For those of us who still have responsibilities for individual patients, it is easy not to think about all the policies that influence our individual clinical care activities. But they are present, and they can be quite powerful and influential. In this chapter, five examples of policies directed toward diabetes—each with a different purpose, target, breadth of impact, and level of complexity—have been briefly described. There are many others, and more will be proposed and established in the future. The creation and implementation of these policies are two essential responsibilities of public health (Oliver 2006). When done wisely in cooperation with experienced health care professionals, when they are based on solid science, and when they are closely evaluated after implementation, these policies can result in a reverse in the extent and future threat of diabetes in the United States.

■ References

Adeyl O, Smith O, Robles S (2007). *Public policy and the challenge of chronic noncommunicable diseases*. Washington, DC: The World Bank.

Ashkenazy R, Abrahamson M (2006). Medicare coverage for patients with diabetes: a national plan with individual consequences. *Journal of General Internal Medicine* **21**, 386–92.

Bodenheimer T, Wagner EH, Grumbach K (2002). Improving primary care for patients with chronic illness. *JAMA* **288**, 1775–9.

CMS Legislative Summary (2003). Summary of H.R.1 Medicare prescription drug, improvement, and modernization act of 2003, Public Law 108-173. Available at http://www.cms.hhs.gov/MMAUpdate/downloads/PL108-173summary.pdf. Accessed February 5, 2009.

Cohen SJ (1983). Potential barriers to diabetes care. *Diabetes Care* **6**, 499–500.

Gostin L (2000). Public health law in a new century: part 1: law as a tool to advance the community's health. *JAMA* **283**, 2837–41.

Gregg EW et al. (2004). Prevalence of lower-extremity disease in the U.S. adult population =/> 40 years of age with and without diabetes: 1999 National Health and Nutrition Examination Survey. *Diabetes Care* **27**, 1591–7.

Heisler M, Wagner E (2004). Improving diabetes treatment quality in managed care organizations: some progress, many challenges. *American Journal of Managed Care* **10**, 115–7.

King H, Aubert R, Herman W (1999). Global burden of diabetes, 1995–2025: prevalence, numerical estimates and projections. *Diabetes Care* **22**, 1414–31.

Kingdon JW (1984). *Agendas, Alternatives, and Public Policies*. Boston: Little, Brown.

Landon B et al. (2007). Improving the management of chronic disease at community health centers. *New England Journal of Medicine* **356**, 921–34.

Leichter S (1999). The business of diabetes education before and after new Medicare regulations. *Clinical Diabetes* **17**, 127–32.

Lento S et al. (1996). Risk factors predicting lower extremity amputations in patients with NIDDM. *Diabetes Care* **19**, 607–12.

McCulloch D et al. (2004). Constructing a bridge across the quality chasm: a practical way to get healthier, happier patients, providers and health care delivery systems. *Diabetes Spectrum* **17**, 92–6.

Nettles A (2005). Patient education in the hospital. *Diabetes Spectrum* **18**, 44–8.

Oliver T (2006). The politics of public health policy. *Annual Review of Public Health* **27**, 195–233.

Pecorino R, Reiter G, Burgess E (1990). Pathways to diabetic limb amputation: basis for prevention. *Diabetes Care* **13**, 513–21.

Piatt GA et al. (2006). Translating the chronic care model into the community: results from a randomized control trial of a multifaceted diabetes care intervention. *Diabetes Care* **29**, 811–7.

Reiber G, Boyce E, Smith D (1995). Lower extremity foot ulcers and amputations in diabetes. In: Harris M et al., eds. Diabetes in America, 2nd ed., pp. 47–67. Bethesda, MD: National Institutes of Health. DHHS publication no. 95-1468.

Rice D (2007). A little more talk, a lot more action: defining the future of diabetes education. *Diabetes Educator* **33**, 353–4.

Robert Wood Johnson Foundation (2007). The chronic care model. Princeton, NJ: Robert Wood Johnson Foundation.

Steinbrook R (2006). Facing the diabetes epidemic—mandatory reporting of glycosylated hemoglobin values in New York City. *New England Journal of Medicine* **354**, 545–8.

The American Heritage Dictionary of the English Language (1981). Boston: Houghton Mifflin Co.

United Nations Resolution on Diabetes (2006). New York: United Nations.

Wagner E (2004). Chronic disease care. *British Medical Journal* **328**, 177–8.

Wagner E, Austin B, Von Orff M (1996). Organizing care for patients with chronic diseases. *Milbank Quarterly* **74**, 511–44.

World Health Organization (2007). Press release. World Health Assembly. Geneva: WHO.

33. DIABETES PUBLIC HEALTH INFORMATION RESOURCES

Joanne M. Gallivan and Matt Petersen

■ Main Public Health Messages

- A wide range of materials on diabetes can be obtained from organizations in the federal government, voluntary and professional organizations, and the private sector.
- Numerous entities within the federal government or the private sector underwrite research in diabetes.

■ Introduction

This chapter summarizes the major Web-based information, education, and research resources on diabetes prevention and control that are available to public health researchers and practitioners from organizations in the federal government, voluntary and professional organizations, and the private sector. Informational and educational resources are described for public health researchers and practitioners and for public and patient audiences.

Resources Available from Organizations in the Federal Government

Public health researchers and practitioners can access a wide range of useful tools and resources on the Internet to advance their work in diabetes prevention and control. All of the resources from organizations in the federal government are available copyright-free and may be downloaded and reproduced at no charge. Resources described in the following section include clinical guidelines, resources to produce systems change, clinical practice tools, offerings in continuing education, and research articles and statistics. See Table 33.1 for a list of governmental diabetes resources for public health researchers and practitioners.

The authors wish to thank Rachel Greenberg and James Ott for their help in preparing this manuscript.

TABLE 33.1 *Resources for Public Health Researchers and Practitioners*

Organization	Practice Guidelines	System Change Resources	Clinical Practice Tools	CME Offerings	Research and Statistics	Printer-Friendly Patient Materials
Federal Government Organizations						
Agency for Healthcare Research and Quality www.ahrq.gov	•	•			•	
CDC, Division of Diabetes Translation www.cdc.gov/diabetes					•	•
Indian Health Service, Division of Diabetes Treatment and Prevention www.ihs.gov/medicalprograms/diabetes/	•	•	•			
National Diabetes Education Program www.ndep.nih.gov	•	•	•	•	•	•
National Diabetes Education Program www.betterdiabetescare.nih.gov			•		•	•
National Diabetes Education Program www.diabetesatwork.org			•			•
National Diabetes Information Clearinghouse www.diabetes.niddk.nih.gov	•		•		•	•
National Guideline Clearinghouse ™ www.guideline.gov	•		•		•	
National Heart, Lung and Blood Institute www.nhlbi.nih.gov	•	•	•	•	•	•
National Kidney Disease Education Program www.nkdep.nih.gov	•	•	•		•	•

Resource						
National Library of Medicine www.nlm.nih.gov			•		•	
Veterans Affairs Diabetes Program http://www1.va.gov/diabetes/	•		•		•	
Voluntary and Professional Organizations						
American Association of Clinical Endocrinologists www.aace.com		•	•	•	•	
American Association of Diabetes Educators www.aadenet.org		•	•	•	•	
American Diabetes Association www.diabetes.org	•	•	•	•	•	•
American Dietetic Association www.eatright.org	•		•			
American Heart Association www.americanheart.org	•	•	•	•	•	
Barbara Davis Center for Childhood Diabetes www.uchsc.edu/misc/diabetes/index.html			•		•	•
Diabetes Research Institute www.diabetesresearch.org	•		•		•	
Joslin Diabetes Center www.joslin.org	•		•	•	•	•
Juvenile Diabetes Research Foundation www.jdrf.org			•		•	•
International Organizations						
World Health Organization www.who.int/en			•		•	•
International Diabetes Federation www.idf.org	•				•	•

To help public health researchers and practitioners stem the growing epidemic of diabetes, governmental organizations have developed a wealth of resources to inform and educate people with diabetes and those at risk for the disease. Resources are available that focus on diabetes prevention and control; key lifestyle behaviors such as weight control, healthy eating, and physical activity; insurance benefits; and materials for high-risk and special-needs audiences as well as public education materials and Web links. See Table 33.2 for a list of governmental diabetes resources for patient and public audiences.

Agency for Healthcare Research and Quality (AHRQ)

Web site: www.ahrq.gov/.
Mission: To improve the quality, safety, efficiency, and effectiveness of health care for all Americans.

The AHRQ Web site provides current and archived clinical practice guidelines from governmental, health professional, and medical specialty organizations; evidence based practice information such as scientific reviews and evidence reports; research on outcomes and effectiveness; comparative data on the clinical effectiveness of pharmaceuticals, devices, and health care services; technology assessments; and U.S. Preventive Services Task Force guidelines. AHRQ funds the National Guideline Clearinghouse™ (see below).

Centers for Disease Control and Prevention (CDC), Division of Diabetes Translation

Web site: www.cdc.gov/diabetes
Mission: To eliminate the preventable burden of diabetes through leadership, research, programs, and policies that translate science into practice.

The CDC Division of Diabetes Translation Web site includes fact sheets, statistics, publications, and information about state Diabetes Prevention and Control Programs that develop and maintain state and local programs in diabetes. CDC distributes several publications, including a guide for people with diabetes (available in English and Spanish) and the eight-page *National Diabetes Fact Sheet: National Estimates and General Information on Diabetes in the United States*. Other CDC divisions that provide information and resources relevant to diabetes prevention and control include the Division of Adolescent and School Health [www.cdc.gov/nccdphp/dash] and the Division of Nutrition and Physical Activity [www.cdc.gov/nccdphp/dnpa].

Centers for Medicare & Medicaid Services (CMS)

Web site: www.medicare.gov/health/diabetes.asp
Mission: To provide information on which diabetes services, screening, and supplies are covered by Medicare.

TABLE 33.2 Resources for Patient and Public Audiences

Organization	Diabetes Prevention	Diabetes Control	Weight Control	Healthy Eating and Physical Activity	Insurance Benefits	Easy-to-Read Materials	Multilingual Multicultural	Special Needs	Awareness Campaigns
Federal Government Organizations									
CDC Division of Diabetes Translation www.cdc.gov/diabetes	•	•	•	•		•	•		•
CDC Division of Adolescent and School Health www.cdc.gov/nccdphp/dash			C¹	C		C	C		
CDC Division of Nutrition, Physical Activity, and Obesity www.cdc.gov/nccdphp/dnpa			•	•			•		•
Centers for Medicare and Medicaid Services www.medicare.gov/health/diabetes.asp	OA	OA	OA	OA	OA		OA		
Food and Drug Administration, Diabetes Information Section www.fda.gov/diabetes/		•	•	•			•		•

(continued)

TABLE 33.2 (*continued*)

Organization	Diabetes Prevention	Diabetes Control	Weight Control	Healthy Eating and Physical Activity	Insurance Benefits	Easy-to-Read Materials	Multilingual Multicultural	Special Needs	Awareness Campaigns
National Diabetes Education Program www.ndep.nih.gov	•	•	•	•		•	•	•	•
National Diabetes Information Clearinghouse www.diabetes.niddk.nih.gov	•	•	•	•		•	•	•	
National Eye Health Education Program www.nei.nih.gov		•					•	B	•
National Heart, Lung, and Blood Institute www.nhlbi.nih.gov		•	•	•		•	•		•
National Kidney Disease Education Program www.nkdep.nih.gov		•				•	•		•
National Library of MedicineMedline Plus www.ncbi.nlm.nih.gov	•	•	•	•			•		

Office of Minority Health Resource Center www.omhrc.gov	•	•	•	•	•	•	•	
U.S. Department of Agriculture www.usda.gov/wps/portal/usdahome	•	•	•	•	•	•	•	
Weight-control Information Network www.niddk.nih.gov/health/nutrit/win.htm		•	•	•		•	B	
Voluntary and Professional Organizations								
American Association of Clinical Endocrinologists www.aace.com		•	•	•		•		•
American Diabetes Association www.diabetes.org	•	•	•	•	•	•	•	
American Dietetic Association (ADA) www.eatright.org		•	•					
American Heart Association www.americanheart.org		•	•					•

(continued)

TABLE 33.2 *(continued)*

Organization	Diabetes Prevention	Diabetes Control	Weight Control	Healthy Eating and Physical Activity	Insurance Benefits	Easy-to-Read Materials	Multilingual Multicultural	Special Needs	Awareness Campaigns
Barbara Davis Center for Childhood Diabetes www.uchsc.edu/misc/diabetes/index.html	•	•		•					
Friends With Diabetes www.friendswithdiabetes.org		•		•			•		
Joslin Diabetes Center www.joslin.org		C				C	•		
Juvenile Diabetes Research Foundation www.jdrf.org		C	C	C		C			
Kids Health www.kidshealth.org		C	C	C		C	•		

The Naomi Berrie Diabetes
Center www.nbdiabetes.org

International Organizations

World Health Organization
www.who.int/en

International Diabetes
Federation www.idf.org

[1]Key: C = children, OA = older adults, B = blind, H = handicapped, etc.

The CMS Web site provides information on Medicare's coverage for diabetes services, supplies, and screening. The Web site also includes a comprehensive list of links to other diabetes sites.

Food and Drug Administration (FDA), Diabetes Information

Web site: www.fda.gov/diabetes/
Mission: To assure that diabetes medicines, insulin, and medical products for diabetes care are safe and that they work as well as claimed.

The FDA's diabetes Web site contains detailed information and news for consumers on glucose meters and other diabetes management devices, insulin, diabetes pills, lancing devices, food and meal planning, complications of diabetes, and questions and answers about diabetes and the role of the FDA in regulating devices and medications. Also included is information on the regulation and labeling of food and dietary supplements and links to other governmental and nongovernmental diabetes resources.

Indian Health Service (IHS), Division of Diabetes Treatment and Prevention

Web site: www.ihs.gov/medicalprograms/diabetes/
Mission: To develop, document, and sustain clinical and public health efforts to treat and prevent diabetes in American Indian and Alaska Native communities.

The IHS Division of Diabetes Treatment and Prevention (DDTP) Web site contains consensus-based guidelines on care of patients with type 2 diabetes and for adults with prediabetes and metabolic syndrome, with special emphasis on addressing the unique aspects of care for American Indians and Alaska Natives. DDTP also has developed a comprehensive set of consensus-based Diabetes Best Practices to improve diabetes care in clinical and community settings.

National Diabetes Education Program (NDEP)

Web site: www.ndep.nih.gov
Mission: To reduce the morbidity and mortality associated with diabetes and its complications and to prevent onset of the disease.

The NDEP is the federal government's leading public education program promoting diabetes prevention and control. The main NDEP Web site, www.ndep.nih.gov, contains numerous clinical practice tools, patient education materials for lower-literacy audiences in English, Spanish, and 15 Asian or Pacific Islander languages, public awareness campaigns, and statistical fact sheets on diabetes prevention and control. NDEP materials may be downloaded or ordered online from the Web site.

The NDEP's www.betterdiabetescare.nih.gov Web site provides health care professionals with steps, models, guidelines, resources, and tools for making and evaluating effective systems changes. Tools featured on the site include recommendations for clinical practice, risk assessments, algorithms, and support for patient education. Primary care providers, diabetes educators, specialists, office managers, and managed care organization staff who use www.betterdiabetescare.nih.gov may receive continuing education (CE) or continuing medical education (CME) credit from Indiana University.

The NDEP's www.diabetesatwork.org Web site is a comprehensive Web-based resource designed to help public health organizations, businesses, and managed care systems assess the impact of diabetes in the workplace. The site also provides information to help employees manage their diabetes and take steps toward reducing risks for related complications, such as heart disease.

National Eye Health Education Program (NEHEP)

Web site: http://www.nei.nih.gov/nehep/
Mission: To protect and prolong the vision of the American people.

The NEHEP Web site provides professional and patient education materials related to diabetic eye disease (retinopathy) and its treatment, including literature for patients, guides for health professionals, education kits for community health workers and pharmacists, and a clinical studies database.

National Guideline Clearinghouse (NGC)™

Web site: www.guideline.gov
Mission: To provide a comprehensive, searchable, Web-based database of evidence-based clinical practice guidelines and related documents.

The NGC provides health professionals, health plans, health care purchasers, and others a mechanism for obtaining objective, detailed information on clinical practice guidelines. Key components of the NGC Web site include structured abstracts of the guidelines, links to full-text guidelines, Palm-based PDA Downloads of guidelines, a Guideline Comparison utility for generating comparisons of two or more guidelines, and an Annotated Bibliography database where users can search for citations for publications and resources about guidelines.

National Heart, Lung, and Blood Institute (NHLBI)

Web site: www.nhlbi.nih.gov
Mission: To provide leadership for a national program in diseases of the heart, blood vessels, lung, and blood; blood resources; and sleep disorders.

The NHLBI Web site provides comprehensive education and information resources for professional and public audiences on preventing and managing cardiovascular disease and associated risk factors. Health professional resources include clinical practice guidelines, clinical resource tools, and continuing medical education programs. Resources for consumers include tools for assessing health risk, educational tutorials, recipes for healthy eating, and other publications to promote healthy lifestyles.

National Institute of Diabetes and Digestive and Kidney Diseases (NIDDK)

www.niddk.nih.gov
Mission: To conduct and support research on many of the most serious diseases affecting public health.

The NIDDK of the National Institutes of Health provides information services on diabetes prevention and control to health care professionals and consumers through its National Diabetes Information Clearinghouse (NDIC). The NDIC Web site includes information on treatments for diabetes and its complications, statistics on diabetes, clinical trials, and practice guidelines. Resources for consumers include patient education materials for lower-literacy audiences in English and Spanish. Health professionals can access the online NIDDK Image Library. NDIC materials may be downloaded or ordered online from the Web site.

National Kidney Disease Education Program (NKDEP)

Web site: www.nkdep.nih.gov/
Mission: To reduce the morbidity and mortality caused by kidney disease and its complications.

The NKDEP raises awareness of the seriousness of kidney disease, the importance of testing those at high risk (those with diabetes, high blood pressure, or a family history of kidney failure), and the availability of treatment to prevent or to slow kidney failure. The NKDEP Web site includes current information and statistics about chronic kidney disease (CKD), clinical practice and patient education tools on diabetes and kidney disease, and links to guidelines on managing CKD and related risk factors.

National Library of Medicine (NLM)

Web site: www.nlm.nih.gov
Mission: To collect biomedical and genetics articles and materials and provide information and research services in all areas of biomedicine and health care.

PubMed is a service of the NLM that includes over 19 million citations from MEDLINE and other life science journals for biomedical articles dating back to the 1950s. PubMed includes links to full-text articles and other related resources. The result of a MEDLINE/PubMed search is a list of citations (including authors, title, source, and often an abstract) to journal articles and an indication of free electronic full-text availability. Searching is free of charge and does not require registration. NLM's MedlinePlus provides consumers with links to extensive information from the National Institutes of Health and other trusted sources on over 700 diseases and conditions, including diabetes.

Office of Minority Health Resources Center (OMHRC)

Web site: www.omhrc.gov
Mission: To improve and protect the health of racial and ethnic minority populations through the development of health policies and programs that will eliminate health disparities.

The OMHRC Web site contains information on a variety of health topics, including diabetes, that is geared for minority audiences. The diabetes section provides numerous links to publications on diabetes prevention and control, in English and Spanish. Contents include diabetes statistics and fact sheets on diabetes management, healthy eating, lifestyle changes, and diabetes complications.

U.S. Department of Agriculture (USDA)

Web site: www.usda.gov
Mission: To provide leadership on food, agriculture, natural resources, and related issues based on sound public policy, the best available science, and efficient management.

The USDA Web site provides extensive information and educational resources on food and nutrition, including links to many diabetes resources. The Web site features the "My Pyramid: Steps to a Healthier You" plan that helps people choose the right foods in the right amounts. The "My Pyramid Tracker" helps people assess their food intake and physical activity level. In addition, the USDA site contains a "What's in the food you eat" search tool that has nutrient profiles for 13,000 foods commonly eaten in the United States (in familiar portion sizes).

U.S. Department of Veterans Affairs (VA) Diabetes Program

Web site: www1.va.gov/diabetes/
Mission: To provide excellence in patient care, veterans' benefits, and customer satisfaction.

The VA Web site includes links to numerous diabetes resources as well as a downloadable version of the VA's Guidelines on Management of Diabetes Mellitus. The guideline draws heavily from the American Diabetes Association, the National Cholesterol Education Program, and National Kidney Foundation guidelines for people with diabetes.

Weight-control Information Network (WIN)

Web site: http://win.niddk.nih.gov
Mission: To provide the general public, health professionals, the media, and Congress with up-to-date, science-based information on obesity, weight control, physical activity, and related nutritional issues.

WIN is an information service of the NIDDK of the National Institutes of Health. WIN provides up-to-date, science-based information on obesity, weight control, physical activity, and related nutritional issues.

Voluntary/Nonprofit Resources

Many nonprofit organizations provide a range of patient and professional education materials on the Internet. The following section highlights the most prominent sources of diabetes information and some noteworthy sources of information on specific topics or for specific patient populations.

American Association of Clinical Endocrinologists (AACE)

Web site: www.aace.com
Mission Statement: AACE is a medical professional community of clinical endocrinologists committed to enhancing its members' ability to provide the highest quality of care.
Mission Statement: To transform the lives of patients by enabling one another to practice leading-edge, proactive, ethical and cost-effective medicine.
The AACE Web site has clinical practice guidelines and a range of professional education pieces, including "clinical conversation" Webcasts. The site also has practice management forms for members.

American Association of Diabetes Educators (AADE)

Web site: www.diabeteseducator.org
Mission: To drive professional practice to promote healthy living through self-management of diabetes and related conditions.
AADE offers a range of CE-accredited online professional education opportunities for nurses, dietitians, and pharmacists for a small fee. For patient education the site features educational materials available for purchase, including a comprehensive set of educational videos.

American Diabetes Association (ADA)

Web site: www.diabetes.org
Mission: To prevent and cure diabetes and to improve the lives of all people affected by diabetes.
The ADA Web site has a broad range of professional and patient education materials. Patient education materials on all aspects of diabetes management are provided in both HTML text and PDF format. There are a handful of tools available, including a food guide and menu planner, a simple diabetes risk test, an advanced health risk calculator (Diabetes PHD), and an interactive tool for tracking physical activity. Materials range from basic introductory material for the newly diagnosed

to more advanced self-management information. Many materials are available in Spanish as well as English. The site also features moderated forums and discussion groups.

For professional education, the new "Diabetes Pro" section of the ADA site provides access to all ADA professional journals, meeting abstracts, Webcasts, clinical trial data, and CE-accredited educational activities. Access to all these materials, including CE activities, is free with the exception of journal articles or Webcasts that are less than 6 months from release.

American Dietetic Association (ADA)

Web site: www.eatright.org
Mission: To improve the nation's health and advance the profession of dietetics through research, education, and advocacy.

The ADA Web site has patient and professional information materials in HTML and PDF formats on healthy eating and medical nutrition therapy. There is a limited amount of material devoted to nutrition that is specific to diabetes.

American Heart Association (AHA)

Web site: www.americanheart.org
Mission: To build healthier lives free of cardiovascular diseases and stroke.

The AHA has a range of materials on diabetes, especially as it relates to cardiovascular disease and stroke. There are basic information pieces in English and Spanish on managing diabetes for both patients and professionals with links to AHA scientific guidelines and statements.

The most robust materials on the AHA Web site are available in its "The Heart of Diabetes" program, access to which requires a free registration. For patients "The Heart of Diabetes" includes informational pieces on diabetes, a 12-week course on improving physical activity, and a monthly newsletter with tips and information on achieving a healthy lifestyle. For professionals there is a limited range of patient education materials, including slides and PDF handouts.

Barbara Davis Center for Childhood Diabetes (BDC)

www.uchsc.edu/misc/diabetes/index.html
Mission: To provide care for children and adults with type 1 diabetes, to provide a unique environment to foster clinical and basic biomedical research, and to support the development and application of research for the prevention, cure, and understanding of the disease process that leads to type 1 diabetes.

The BDC has two comprehensive, free, online books available on its Web site. *Understanding Diabetes* is written for parents or for children who can read at the 8th-grade level. The book reviews the entire spectrum of issues related to managing diabetes from an overview of the etiology to blood glucose management, handling sick days, nutrition, exercise, and insulin administration. *Type 1 Diabetes: Cellular, Molecular & Clinical Immunology* covers a wide array of issues in the science and medicine of type 1 diabetes, including etiology and pathophysiology, genetics, epidemiology, and islet transplantation. Most chapters are accompanied by PowerPoint slide sets.

Diabetes Research Institute (DRI)

Web site: www.diabetesresearch.org
Mission: To develop and rapidly apply the most promising research to treat and cure those now living with diabetes.

The primary focus of the DRI Web site is on DRI research activities with explanations of the DRI research program and information about ongoing clinical trials. The site has a number of professional education materials, including a monograph on initiating basal/bolus insulin therapy and a range of Webcasts on topics such as initiating insulin therapy, treating hypoglycemia, and understanding the etiology and prevention of complications.

Friends with Diabetes (FWD)

Web site: http://www.friendswithdiabetes.org/
Mission: To offer quality education about controlling diabetes and incorporating it into the Jewish tradition and lifestyle.

The FWD Web site has information materials in English, Yiddish, and Hebrew on topics relevant to observant Jews with diabetes, including guidance on diabetes management issues as they relate to fasting and to observing the Sabbath. (The unrelated Jewish Diabetes Association Web site, www.jewishdiabetes.org, has similar information in English only.)

Joslin Diabetes Center

http://www.joslin.org
Mission: To improve the lives of people with diabetes and its complications through innovative care, education, and research that will lead to prevention and cure of the disease.

Joslin is an ACCME (Accreditation Council for Continuing Medical Education)-accredited education provider. The Joslin Web site features a changing array of CE-credited symposia, satellite broadcasts, videotapes, CDs, DVDs, and monographs. In general the educational materials are provided through the support of industry sponsorship and are free to the user. For health care providers the site includes clinical practice guidelines on specific topics such as diabetes in pregnancy and managing weight in type 2 diabetes. For consumers the site includes patient education materials in English and Spanish in both HTML and printer-friendly formats, and there is a dedicated site for children and teens, http://www.joslin.org/KidsTeens_Index_2610.asp, with youth-targeted information and discussion groups.

Juvenile Diabetes Research Foundation International (JDRF)

Web site: www.jdrf.org
Mission: To find a cure for diabetes and its complications through the support of research.

The JDRF Web site offers materials containing practical advice for patients in HTML and PDF formats. There are a number of pieces devoted to school issues for both parents and school staff. The site also has a variety of educational materials on self-management of type 1 diabetes. There are no professional education materials.

Kids Health

Web site: www.kidshealth.org
Mission: To improve the health and spirit of children.

Kids Health is a Web site from the Nemours Foundation, established in 1936 by philanthropist Alfred I. duPont. The Kids Health site provides information on a wide range of childhood health topics, including diabetes. The site's diabetes section has information for parents on type 1 and type 2 diabetes, with basic diabetes information, recipes, advice on medications, and blood glucose testing. There are some simple tools for tracking diet and blood glucose levels.

The Naomi Berrie Diabetes Center (NBDC)

Web site: www.nbdiabetes.org/index.html
The NBDC Web site has a small number of information items for parents of children with type 1 diabetes on topics such as nutrition and carbohydrate counting. The site also has PDF forms for tracking diet and blood glucose meter readings.

International Resources

The Web sites of the World Health Organization (WHO) and the International Diabetes Federation (IDF) are the two primary online international sources of information about diabetes. There are many international sites maintained by nongovernmental organizations and other agencies around the world that contain diabetes information, primarily for patients, in a wide range of languages. The IDF site has an extensive list of Web sites for these organizations.

World Health Organization (WHO)

Web site: www.who.int/en
Mission: The attainment by all peoples of the highest level of health.

The portion of the WHO Web site that is devoted to diabetes focuses primarily on the disease's epidemiology with some basic material for patient education. Substantial portions of WHO's site can be navigated in six different languages: Arabic, Chinese, English, French, Russian, and Spanish. Some, but not all, of the information on the site about diabetes is also in those six languages; one booklet that provides broad, basic information about diabetes, "Diabetes Action Now," is available in English, French, and Spanish.

The Pan American Health Organization (PAHO) is a regional division of WHO with its own Web site. The site contains a limited amount of professional education materials in English and Spanish, primarily epidemiologic information about the prevalence of diabetes in the Americas.

International Diabetes Federation

Web site: www.idf.org
Mission: To promote diabetes care, prevention, and a cure worldwide.

IDF has a substantial amount of information on its Web site for both patients and professionals, both as online resources and in the form of printer-friendly downloads. The site includes epidemiologic data, practice guidelines, and position statements. IDF's 80-page practice guideline is available in English, Spanish, Russian, Indonesian, and Turkish.

There are several patient brochures on understanding diabetes and its complications. Most of the IDF materials are available in English, French, and Spanish. One limitation of the materials for the United States is that all values are expressed in European units (e.g., mmol/L) instead of mg/dL, and the U.S. equivalents are not always provided. One of the key features of the IDF site is an extensive list of Web sites and contact information for all of the IDF member organizations. These member organization Web sites sometimes offer diabetes information to patients in their native language, although they usually lack an English translation, and thus only a native speaker could verify the suitability and accuracy of the information presented.

Private Industry Resources

The major pharmaceutical companies and manufacturers of diabetes-related equipment and supplies have Web sites containing information for patients and health care professionals. People with diabetes can find extensive information and resources for managing their diabetes; health care professionals can find downloadable patient education materials and links to the latest practice guidelines, drug information, and continuing education programs. Virtually all device and drug manufacturers provide their FDA-approved information for their products (e.g., package inserts) as PDFs on their sites.

Some pharmaceutical company Web sites provide information on their programs to help patients cover the cost of diabetes medicines. In addition, pharmaceutical companies and device manufacturers have formed coalitions to work together with the leading diabetes voluntary organizations to improve diabetes treatment and outcomes.

Research Funding Organizations

Numerous federal government and voluntary/nonprofit organizations listed in Tables 33.1 and 33.2 provide funding opportunities for research—from basic to behavioral research on type 1 and type 2 diabetes. The Web sites of these organizations contain details about the goals of their research programs and application procedures.

The Diabetes Center Program of the National Institute of Diabetes and Digestive and Kidney Diseases (NIDDK)

Web site: http://www2.niddk.nih.gov/Research

Mission: The NIDDK funds Diabetes Endocrinology Research Centers (DERCs) and Diabetes Research and Training Centers (DRTCs) across the United States. Both types of centers are designed to support and enhance the national research effort in diabetes and related endocrine and metabolic diseases.

DERCs support three primary research-related activities: biomedical research cores, a Pilot and Feasibility (P&F) program, and an Enrichment program. DRTCs possess all elements of a DERC, with additional dedicated core services and P&F awards to support research in diabetes prevention and control. All activities pursued by diabetes centers are designed to enhance the efficiency, productivity, effectiveness, and multidisciplinary nature of research in Diabetes Center topic areas. Following are the funded Diabetes Centers as of 2010.

Diabetes and Endocrinology Research Centers (DERCs)

University of California/Los Angeles and San Diego
University of Colorado Health Science Center
Yale University
Boston Area Consortium
Joslin Diabetes Center
University of Massachusetts
Columbia University
University of Pennsylvania
Baylor College of Medicine
University of Washington

Diabetes Research and Training Centers (DRTCs)

University of Alabama at Birmingham

University of Chicago
University of Michigan
Washington University
Johns Hopkins University/University of Maryland
Albert Einstein College of Medicine
Vanderbilt University

INDEX

Note: Page references followed by "*f*" and "*t*" denote figures and tables, respectively.